PROSTATE CANCER – DIAGNOSTIC AND THERAPEUTIC ADVANCES

Edited by **Philippe E. Spiess**

Prostate Cancer – Diagnostic and Therapeutic Advances
Edited by Philippe E. Spiess

Published by InTech
Janeza Trdine 9, 51000 Rijeka, Croatia

Publishing Process Manager Marija Radja

Technical Editor Teodora Smiljanic

Cover Designer InTech Design Team

Additional hard copies can be obtained from orders@intechopen.com

Prostate Cancer – Diagnostic and Therapeutic Advances, Edited by Philippe E. Spiess
p. cm.
ISBN 978-953-307-319-4

For EU product safety concerns:
IN TECH d.o.o., Prolaz Marije Krucifikse Kozulić 3, 51000 Rijeka, Croatia,
info@intechopen.com or visit our website at intechopen.com.

Meet the editor

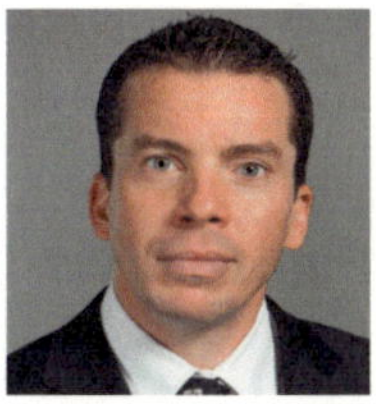

Dr Philippe E. Spiess is an assistant professor with dual appointment in the department of Genitourinary Oncology at the Moffitt Cancer Center and the department of Urology at the University of South Florida in Tampa, Florida. Dr Spiess was born and raised in Montreal, Canada where he completed his urological training at McGill University. He subsequently completed his urologic oncologic training at the M. D. Anderson Cancer Center in Houston, Texas. Dr Spiess has published over 80 peer reviewed scientific papers in urologic oncology in addition to being a nationally and internationally recognized expert in the management of genitourinary malignancies. He has dedicated much of his research efforts to optimizing the surgical management of locally advanced and locally recurrent prostate cancer. He currently sits on the NCCN Panel for bladder and penile cancer in addition to being the video section editor of the International Brazilian Journal of Urology.

Contents

Preface

In this book titled "Prostate Cancer - Diagnostic and Therapeutic Advances", we highlight many of the significant advances made in our treatment armamentarium of prostate cancer. This book is a tribute to our pioneering urologists and allied healthcare professionals who have continually pushed forward our traditional therapeutic envelope. The present book is subdivided into four sections termed: 1) novel diagnostic approaches, 2) surgical treatments options, 3) radiation therapy and its potential sequelae, and 4) medical management and its treatment complications. After reading the present book , readers will be very familiar with the major clinical advances made in our multifaceted treatment approach to prostate cancer over the past decade.

As editor-in-chief of this book, I would like to acknowledge the significant efforts made by all of the contributing authors and entire editorial team in the publishing of this work. Their dedication to the publication of the most contemporary and comprehensive scientific data has resulted in this truly excellent work. I would like to dedicate this book to my clinical mentors at both McGill University and the University of Texas M.D.Anderson Cancer Center. You have taught me not only to manage genitourinary malignancies using the highest quality surgical and medical care but as well have instilled in me a sense of responsibility to our scientific community to contribute in a meaningful way and to continually improve myself as a person and clinician. I practice medicine today following the principle your engrained with me which is to treat each individual patient as if this was my own close family member.

Philippe E. Spiess, Editor-In-Chief
Assistant Professor, Dept of Genitourinary Oncology
H. Lee Moffitt Cancer Center, Tampa, Florida
USA

Scott Eggener, M.D.
Assistant Professor, Department of Urology
University of Chicago, Chicago
USA

Vladimir Mourariev, M.D., Ph.D.
Department of Urology, University of Cincinnati, Ohio
USA

Matthew Biagioli, M.D.
Assistant Professor, Department of Radiation Oncology
Moffitt Cancer Center, Tampa
USA

Kevin Zorn, M.D.
Assistant Professor, Department of Urology
Universite de Montreal, Montreal
Canada

Shahrokh Shariat, M.D., Ph.D.
Associate Professor, Department of Urology
Weill Cornell Medical Center, New York
USA

Dr Alejandro Rodriguez
Assistant Professor, Department of Urology
University of South Florida, Tampa
USA

Part 1

Novel Diagnostic Approaches

1

Biomarkers of Aggressiveness in Prostate Cancer

Cuvillier Olivier and Malavaud Bernard
CNRS, Institut de Pharmacologie et de Biologie Structurale, Toulouse
Université de Toulouse, UPS, IPBS, Toulouse
Hôpital Rangueil, Service d'Urologie et de Transplantation Rénale, Toulouse
France

1. Introduction

Although significant progress in the investigation of prostate cancer biomarkers, some men are overdiagnosed with indolent prostate cancer while others die from aggressive disease diagnosed too late. The introduction of PSA (Prostate Specific Antigen) in clinical practice has resulted in early detection and reduced mortality from prostate cancer (Schroder et al., 2009). Despite its great utility for prostate cancer detection and prognostication, PSA as a single test has several limitations. Prostate cancer screening remains thus controversial, because of the risk of overdiagnosis reduced mortality and overtreatment and the inability to detect a significant proportion of aggressive tumors. To extend the limited information provided by PSA testing, other biomarkers that could discriminate between indolent from aggressive cancers are therefore an absolute must. Despite numerous studies of biomarker candidates have been presented the last decade, the identification of the most aggressive subsets of this disease is still not possible. This review will cover last years development in this area and highlight the most promising biomarkers in prostate cancer, which have been divided into three groups; protein-based, DNA-based and RNA-based markers.

2. Protein biomarkers

2.1 Prostate Stem Cell Antigen (PSCA)

PSCA (Prostate Stem Cell Antigen) is a membrane glycoprotein with 30% homology to stem cell antigen type 2 (SCA-2), an immature lymphocyte cell surface marker. Like SCA-2, PSCA is attached to the membrane by a GPI anchor which can be cleaved by a phospholipase. Because of its homology with SCA-2, PSCA was named inaccurately since it is not a marker for stem cells nor is it uniquely expressed in the prostate (Saeki et al., 2010). Initially, PSCA was identified as a tumor antigen overexpressed in the prostate (Reiter et al., 1998), and subsequent studies have revealed that it is also up-regulated in other cancers including bladder and pancreas. PSCA has been proposed as a promising tumor marker of diagnostic and prognosis, as well as a potential therapeutic target for patients with metastatic prostate cancer. PSCA expression indeed increases with high gleason score, advanced stage and bone metastasis (Gu et al., 2000; Han et al., 2004; Lam et al., 2005; Zhigang & Wenlv, 2004). The levels of PSCA are also amplified in the prostate intraepithelial neoplasia (PIN) lesions that subsequently progressed to cancer compared to those that did not progress (Zhigang & Wenlu, 2007). PSCA might also represent a useful marker for metastasis detection as almost 95% of lymph nodes and bone samples with metastasis have been found positive for PSCA expression (Ananias et al., 2009). It was originally observed that PSCA mRNA bearing cells circulating in peripheral blood were identified at higher rates in prostate cancer patients with extraprostatic disease (Hara et al., 2002). The presence of *PSCA* transcripts in the peripheral blood has found to be a significant predictor of biochemical recurrence after prostatectomy in high-risk prostate cancer (Joung et al., 2010). Of note, PSCA has also been investigated as a potential target for tumor-targeted immunotherapy and for suppression by anti-PSCA antibody in animals. Further evaluation of PSCA as a clinical prostate cancer marker of aggressiveness needs to be validated.

2.2 Prostate Secretory Protein 94 (PSP94)

The ELISA dosage of β-microseminoprotein (MSP) ou PSP94 (Prostate Secretory Protein of 94 amino acids) - one of three predominant proteins secreted by the human prostate gland (Lilja & Abrahamsson, 1988) - could be potentially interesting. In a case-control study of 1,212 men with no previous history of prostate cancer, Nam et al. found that patients with low PSP94 levels had a high probability for having prostate cancer diagnosed at biopsy (Nam et al., 2006). The authors also suggested that those cancers that maintain PSP94 expression tend to be well differentiated and less aggressive, as reported in previous immunohistochemistry studies (Abrahamsson et al., 1988). In serum, PSP94 can be complexed with PSPBP (PSP-binding protein), a glycoprotein of 50 kDa sharing significant identity with the CRISP (cystein-rich seccretory protein) family of proteins (Reeves et al., 2005). In a study comprising 185 patients, it was showed that PSPBP is negatively associated with recurrence after radical prostatectomy (Reeves et al., 2006). On the contrary, PSP94 immunohistochemistry performed on 59 radical prostatectomy specimens was associated with worsened survival outcomes (Girvan et al., 2005). Another immunohistochemistry study conducted on 945 patients found a high expression of PSP94 in tumor cells patients to be associated with a longer time to postprostatectomy biochemical recurrence (Bjartell et al., 2007) in agreement with serum studies. Further studies will be needed to determine whether PSP94 and its binding protein represent novel prognostic factors in the clinic.

However, it is interesting to note that genome-wide association studies identified several SNPs in a region on chromosome 10 that harbors the *PSP94* gene (Eeles et al., 2008; Thomas et al., 2008). Its location and the strength of the association raises the possibility that this SNP may be causally related to disease risk, but resequencing and further analyses will be needed clarify the functional basis of this association.

2.3 Early Prostate Cancer Antigens ECPA and ECPA-2

ECPA and ECPA-2 (Early Prostate Cancer Antigens) are nuclear matrix proteins those alterations are commonly associated with prostate cancer (Getzenberg et al., 1991; Lakshmanan et al., 1998). Initially, immunohistochemical studies on men with negative biopsies who were ultimately found to have prostate cancer could identify individuals as much as 5 years earlier than the current diagnostic (Dhir et al., 2004). ECPA positivity was hypothesized to be an early event in disease progression, as there was no correlation between ECPA staining and Gleason grade or pT stage (Uetsuki et al., 2005). In 2005, an ECPA-based ELISA showed 92% sensitivity and 94% specificity in prostate cancer detection in patients undergoing radical prostatectomy, however only 46 blood samples were examined (Paul et al., 2005). ELISA used for initial serum EPCA measurement in 112 men with isolated high-grade prostatic intraepithelial neoplasia (HGPIN), showed a significantly higher serum ECPA level in isolated HGPIN patients with subsequent cancer than those without cancer (Zhao & Zeng, 2010). Pretreatment serum EPCA levels were also determined with an ELISA in 77 patients with clinically localized prostate cancer who underwent radical prostatectomy and 51 patients with locally advanced or metastatic disease who received primary androgen deprivation therapy, and were correlated with clinicopathological variables and disease progression. Patients with locally advanced and metastatic prostate cancer had significantly higher serum EPCA level than those with clinically localized disease. These data suggest that EPCA level correlates significantly with the poor prognosis, showing prediction potential for prostate cancer progression (Zhao et al., 2011). Unrelated to the original ECPA, the nuclear protein ECPA-2 was recently described (Leman et al., 2007). Carried out on 385 blood samples, the ECPA-2 ELISA was able to differentiate between men with and without prostate cancer with 92% specificity and 94% sensitivity, whereas the specificity of PSA was only 65% in the same population (Leman et al., 2007). More importantly, in contrast to PSA, ECPA-2 is able to discriminate men with non-organ-confined prostate cancer from those with organ-confined diseases. Although additional validation studies are needed to show the performance of ECPA-2 in a more representative population, these results lend support to the development of a more accurate blood-based assay to identify aggressive prostate cancer.

2.4 uPA/uPAR

A wealth of reports suggest a key role for the urokinase-type plasminogen activator and its receptor (uPA/uPAR) in invasion and metastatic dissemination (Duffy, 2004). uPA is is a member of the serine protease family synthetized and secreted as a pro-enzyme, whose activation is markedly accelerated upon binding with high affinity to specific membrane-bound or soluble cell surface uPAR. Once activated, the uPA/uPAR system efficiently converts plasminogen into plasmin, a protease which then modulates extracellular matrix degradation, tumor cell invasion and growth factor activation (Duffy, 2004). In prostate cancer, overexpression of uPA and uPAR (transcripts and proteins) have been reported in tumor tissues suggesting that both proteins could be associated with tumor progression. Immunohistochemical studies have shown an incremental increase in uPA/uPAR expression from benign epithelium to primary organ-confined prostate cancer, to disease extending beyond the prostate capsule, and to bone metastases (Cozzi et al., 2006; Gavrilov et al., 2001; Pulukuri et al., 2007; Usher et al., 2005). In addition, overexpression of uPA and its inhibitor PAI-1 are associated with aggressive prostate cancer recurrence in men treated with radical prostatectomy (Gupta et al., 2009). Elevated circulating levels of uPA and/or uPAR have been associated with advanced prostate cancer and bone metastases (Hienert et al., 1988a; Hienert et al., 1988b; Miyake et al., 1999). Shariat et al. have recently reported that plasma levels of uPA and uPAR are not only higher in men with prostate cancer than in healthy controls, but decrease significantly after prostatectomy (suggesting that direct local production by malignant cells significantly contributes to increased uPA and uPAR circulating levels of these markers in patients), then increase with disease progression (Shariat et al., 2007). Of note, higher preoperative uPA and uPAR were both significantly associated with shorter progression PSA doubling times, failure to respond to salvage local radiation therapy, and /or development of distant metastases (Shariat et al., 2007). Larger studies are needed to validate the promising role of uPA and uPAR as biomarkers of aggressive prostate cancer.

3. DNA biomarkers

3.1 Epigenetic markers

Epigenetic alterations, i.e., alterations in gene expression without changes in the DNA sequence, include global genomic hypomethylation, promoter hypermethylation of CpG islands and loss of imprinting. The most common somatic genome alteration during prostate cancer development appears to be the hypermethylation in the regulatory region of certain genes, most commonly in the promoter of the π-class glutathione-*S*-transferase (*GSTP1*) gene (Lee et al., 1994). GSTP1 is a member of a large family of glutathione transferases that protect DNA from free radicals (Hayes & Strange, 1995). Men with a positive preoperative serum analysis for *GSTP1* CpG island hypermethylation were at significant risk to experience PSA recurrence within the first several years following radical prostatectomy (Bastian et al., 2005). A high frequency of *GSTP1* methylation in the urine of men with high-stage cancer was also recently reported (Woodson et al., 2008). Other candidate genes have been examined for hypermethylation along with *GSTP1*. A recent study suggested that men with advanced prostate cancer and biochemical recurrence experience a significant increase in promoter hypermethylation between initial diagnosis (first blood analysis) and time to progression (second blood analysis) in the four genes with the highest methylation frequencies (*GSTP1, APC, RARβ2* and *RASSF1α*) in prostate cancer patients compared to age-matched controls (Roupret et al., 2008). This study suggests that multiple gene methylation analysis in circulating cell DNA could be a good biomarker for early detection of prostate cancer recurrence.

3.2 Gene fusion proteins

Based on a bioinformatics strategy Tomlins et al. described for the first time in prostate cancer a series of genetic rearrangements between the 5′-untranslated region of TMPRSS2 (21q22) and some members of the ETS family of transcription factors, such as ERG (21q22), ETV1 (7p21) and ETV4 (17q21), which have important roles in several oncogenic pathways (Tomlins et al., 2005). Approximatively 50% of prostate cancers from serum PSA-screened cohorts harbor recurrent gene fusions (Kumar-Sinha et al., 2008), which can be detected by fluorescent *in situ* hybridisation (FISH). Conflicting results have been reported regarding the prognosis value of prostate cancer harboring TMPRESS2:ERG gene fusions. Earlier studies reported associations with high stage, metastasis, and prostate cancer-specific death (Attard et al., 2008; Demichelis et al., 2007; Nam et al., 2007), but more recent reports found no association with outcome (Gopalan et al., 2009; Leinonen et al., 2010; Mehra et al., 2007), an association with favorable outcome (Saramaki et al., 2008), or a similar percentage of TMPRSS2:ERG gene fusion in minute and nonminute adenocarcinomas (Albadine et al., 2009), all suggesting its lack of value as a marker of aggressive prostate cancer. The analysis of the relationship between TMPRSS2:ERG fusion and morphological features of prostate cancer has produced diverging results. Most studies have found no statistically significant association between TMPRSS2:ERG rearrangement and Gleason score, while some have demonstrated an association with either higher (Attard et al., 2008; Demichelis et al., 2007) or lower Gleason scores (Fine et al., 2010; Gopalan et al., 2009). Taken together, it seems like the TMPRSS2:ERG fusion gene is an early event related to development of prostate cancer rather than a marker for progressive disease. Of note, the TMPRSSE:ERG fusion has potential for noninvasive prognosis of prostate cancer. Although RNA-based urinary tests demonstrate in general a high specificity and sensitivity to detect prostate cancer, no significant relationship was found between the presence of fusion transcripts and Gleason score or clinical stage (Hessels et al., 2007; Rice et al., 2010).

3.3 Loss of heterozygosity

The loss of heterozygosity (LOH) is a frequent genetic alteration in prostate cancer, in particular on chromosome arms 7q, 8p, 10q, 12p, 13q, 16q, 17q and 18q (Dong, 2006). Studies on chromosomal deletions of 8p22 by fluorescence in situ hybridization technique revealed 8p22 deletion to be the strongest parameter to predict disease progression in patients undergoing surgery (Matsuyama et al., 2001). If some LOH have been shown to be associated with early stages of prostate cancer (Lu & Hano, 2008), others seem to indicate the presence of tumor suppressor genes whose inactivation is correlated with aggressive and metastatic tumors (Dong et al., 2000; Kibel et al., 2000; Matsuyama et al., 2007). A recent study reported the development of a noninvasive method to detect early stages of prostate cancer using LOH analysis of 7q31, 8p22, 12p13, 13q14, 16q23.2 and 18q21. Indeed LOH could be found in cells from urine obtained by prostatic massage (Thuret et al., 2005). In patients who underwent radical prostatectomy, LOH was confirmed from the prostatic tissue with a concordance of 86%. This noninvasive approach warrants further investigation to bring pronostic information on prostate cancer aggressiveness.

4. RNA biomarkers

4.1 PCA3

PCA3 (formerly known as DD3) is a non-coding RNA very prostate specific (Bussemakers et al., 1999; de Kok et al., 2002). PCA3 mRNA levels can be measured in the urine specimens and several studies have shown that the PCA3 score is superior to serum PSA for predicting biopsy outcome (Groskopf et al., 2006; Haese et al., 2008; van Gils et al., 2007). The relationship between PCA3 score and parameters of cancer aggressiveness has also been studied and differ. Some studies report a positive relationship between PCA3 scores and parameters of more serious disease (Nakanishi et al., 2008; Whitman et al., 2008), while other studies could not find such a relationship (Hessels et al., 2010). Further studies are requested to evaluate the potential of PCA3 testing as prognostic test for prostate cancer.

4.2 AMACR

α-methylacyl-CoA racemase (AMACR) is a catalyst in the peroximal beta-oxidation of branched chain fatty acids found in dietary sources (Wanders et al., 2001), such as red meat and dairy products, the consumption of which has been associated with increased prostate cancer risks (Hsing & Chokkalingam, 2006). AMACR has been identified as a potential biomarker based on its overexpression in localized prostate cancer as compared to benign prostate epithelium (Luo et al., 2002; Rhodes et al., 2002; Rubin et al., 2002). In fact, immunostaining for AMACR is commonly performed in prostate biopsies to help distinguish benign from malignant tissue. Of note, AMACR expression was found consistently lower both at the transcriptional (cDNA expression arrays and RT-PCR) and at the protein level (immunohistochemistry and western-blot) in metastatic prostate cancer compared to localized prostate cancer (Kuefer et al., 2002; Rubin et al., 2004). An association between low AMACR protein expression at diagnosis and an increased risk of biochemical recurrence and fatal prostate cancer was reported in patients diagnosed with a localized prostate cancer who underwent radical prostatectomy or not (Rubin et al., 2005). Recent findings from the same group confirmed that down-regulation of AMACR expression is associated with poorer outcomes in a cohort of 920 men diagnosed with prostate cancer. However the lack of statistical significance suggests that tumor AMACR expression at diagnosis is not a useful prognostic biomarker for lethal disease after treatment (Barry et al., 2011). Although AMACR protein can been detected in urine by western-blot, its concentration is low in serum, making the development of a serum test difficult (Rogers et al., 2004). Circulating concentrations of AMACR mRNA in urine or serum quantified by RT-PCR have been found elevated in patients but these pilot studies are limited to small series (Zehentner et al., 2006; Zielie et al., 2004).

4.3 MicroRNAs

MicroRNAs are small RNAs found to regulate mRNA function by modulating both mRNA stability and the translation of mRNA into protein. Their expression is commonly altered in solid tumors and multiple microRNAs have been shown to have oncogenic properties or act like tumor suppressor genes. Besides their therapeutic potential, microRNAs hold unique characteristics that herald them as ideal tumor markers including their stability and ease of detection (Heneghan et al., 2010). Despite the large body of work that has been published to date, only limited information is available regarding the expression levels of specific microRNAs in relation to the aggressiveness of prostate cancer. Taking advantage of the stability of tumor-derived microRNAs in circulating blood, Mitchell and co-workers found a remarkably higher level of miR-141 (46-fold increase) in a patients with metastatic prostate cancer compared to healthy control men (Mitchell et al., 2008). The first evidence of a possible prognostic relevance of microRNAs in prostate cancer was obtained from a study examining the tissue expression of 40 patients undergoing prostatectomy. The increased expression of miR-135b and miR-194 was associated with biochemical recurrence within 2 years of surgery (Tong et al., 2009). Another study, conducted on matched tumor and adjacent normal tissues obtained from 76 patients, found that high expression of miR-96 was associated with cancer recurrence after radical prostatectomy, and that prognostic information was confirmed by an independent tumor sample set from 79 pateints (Schaefer et al., 2010). The miR-221 expression is also progressively reduced in aggressive prostate cancer and metastasis and predicts clinical recurrence in patients (n=92) undergoing radical prostatectomy (Spahn et al., 2010). More recently, miR-143 and miR-145 were identified as being associated with bone metastasis of prostate cancer and involved in the regulation of epithelial-mesenchymal transition (Peng et al., 2011). Interestingly, the loss of miR-101 expression during cancer progression in human tumors has been associated with overexpression of histone methytransferase EZH2 (enhancer of zeste homolog 2) (Varambally et al., 2008). Amounts of both EZH2 mRNA and EZH2 protein are increased in metastatic prostate cancer; in addition, clinically localized prostate cancers that express higher concentrations of EZH2 show a poorer prognosis (Varambally et al., 2002). In cancer cell lines, the expression and function of EZH2 are inhibited by miR-101 (Varambally et al., 2008).

Thus, dysregulated expression of EZH2 may be involved in the progression of prostate cancer, and miR101 might represent a marker that distinguishes indolent prostate cancer from those at risk of lethal progression

5. Other potential biomarkers

5.1 Metabolomics

Metabolite profiling or metabolomics, the analysis of endogenous metabolites in a biological system was recently suggested to be a promising approach to identify novel metabolites or their changes (Fredolini et al., 2010). In practice, however, analysis of the metabolome is complex because of the large range of detectable metabolites. By screening 110 samples from men's urine and blood and 42 tissue samples, Chinnaiyan and collaborators recently identified 1,126 metabolites. They identified 87 that distinguish normal prostate from prostate cancer, then narrowed down the list to 6 whose levels were higher in samples linked to localized prostate cancer and higher still in metastatic disease (Sreekumar et al., 2009). Sarcosine, an *N*-methyl derivative of the amino acid glycine, was identified as a differential metabolite that was highly increased during prostate cancer progression to metastasis. Surprisingly, the authors also provided evidence using cell cultures for a functional role of sarcosine in promoting invasive properties in these cells, whereas lowering the level of the enzyme producing sarcosine reduces invasiveness (Sreekumar et al., 2009). The potential role of urinary was reevaluated in another study, which showed that sarcosine in urine after digital rectal examination fails as a marker in prostate cancer detection and identification of aggressive tumors (Jentzmik et al., 2010). In addition to this work, the same group showed no correlation with sarcosine level in tissues and tumor stage, tumor grade or biochemical recurrence in 92 samples obtained after radical prostatectomy (Jentzmik et al., 2011). Although the lack of metastatic tissue samples was a limitation, this study establishes that sarcosine measurement in prostate tissue is not suitable to predict cancer aggressiveness or biochemical progress.

5.2 Disseminated tumor cells

The shedding of tumor cells into the circulation is a necessary condition for metastasis dissemination and the clinical relevance of the detection of disseminated tumors cells (DTCs) in bone marrow (the most prominent metastatic site in prostate and breast cancer) or in peripheral blood of patients free of apparent metastasis in under investigation. So far, only large breast cancer studies have confirmed the independent prognostic value of the bone marrow status (Berg et al., 2007). Recent studies have demonstrated an association between DTCs in bone marrow at diagnosis of nonmetastastic prostate cancer (Berg et al., 2007; Kollermann et al., 2008). Although a DTC-positive bone marrow status was associated with grading and increased risk of metastasis, the study by Berg et al. on 266 patients did not find a correlation of DTC detection and survival (Berg et al., 2007). In contrast, Köllermann et al. demonstrated the prognostic relevance of DTCs in bone marrow patients with clinically localized prostate cancer submitted to neo-adjuvant hormonal therapy followed by radical prostatectomy and a median follow-up of 44 months (Kollermann et al., 2008). This study is the first one on a large series of patients with sufficient long follow-up to clearly demonstrate an adverse prognostic effect of the presence of DTCs at the time of initial diagnostic.

Markers	Strategy of Detection	Comments
PSCA	RT-PCR (blood), Protein expression (tissue)	Potential therapeutic target
PSP94	ELISA (blood), Protein expression (tissue)	One of the major secretory proteins of the prostate gland
ECPA/ECPA-2	ELISA (blood), Protein expression (tissue)	
uPA/uPAR	ELISA (blood), Protein expression (tissue)	uPAR expression in DTCs (bone marrow, peripheral blood), Potential therapeutic target
Epigenetic markers (eg. GSTP1)	Methylation specific PCR (blood, urine)	Potential Multiplex test with other urine biomarkers
Gene fusion proteins (eg. TMPRSS2 :ERG)	RT-PCR (urine) FISH (tissue)	Potential Multiplex test with other urine biomarkers
Loss of heterozygoty	PCR (blood, urine)	
PCA3	Transcription-mediated amplification assay (urine)	Potential Multiplex test with other urine biomarkers
AMACR	RT-PCR (blood, urine) Protein expression (tissue)	Potential Multiplex test with other urine biomarkers, Potential therapeutic target
MicroRNAs	RT-PCR (blood, urine, tissue)	Potential therapeutic targets
Metabolomics	Profiling (urine, blood)	
Disseminated Tumor Cells	Enumeration (blood, bone marrow)	

Table 1. Potential biomarkers and their strategy of detection

Despite bone marrow analysis provides important information, peripheral blood studies are more acceptable in the clinical management than invasive BM aspirations. However, identification of circulating tumor cells (DTCs) require extremely sensitive analytical methods that are usually combined with enrichment procedures. Although promising results from patients with advanced stages demonstrate the value of CTCs technology (currently evaluated and validated in clinical trials as a predictor and surrogate endpoint of treatment response), studies on patients at earlier stages are hampered by the low CTC counts. A recent study from Haber and collaborators shows that tumor cells obtained from the blood of cancer patients were monitored before and after surgery, most circulating cells rapidly declined shortly after surgery while others persisted months thereafter, suggesting that postoperative CTCs might derive from preestablished non prostatic sites of disease that continue to shed CTCs into the circulation (Stott et al., 2010). If confirmed, these observations support the potential application of CTC monitoring as a marker of invasive localized disease before the establishment of viable metastatic lesions.

6. Conclusion

We have here attempted to give some examples of potential DNA-based, RNA-based and protein-based markers of aggressiveness in prostate cancer. Comparisons between studies are often difficult because of some inconsistencies between study cohorts, collection methods and handling of samples. It is unlikely that a single biomarker (evaluated on conventional approach looking at a single molecular predictor significantly up- or down-regulated) will provide the information requested to tell how aggressive a diagnosed prostate cancer is. New research methods (proteomics, metabolomics…) are also emerging, and high-throughput technologies will facilitate biomarker discovery. Therefore, future advances in this field will probably have to integrate proteomics, transcriptomics and multiplex approaches and identify combinations of multiple biomarkers in order to improve the characterization of aggressive prostate cancers.

7. Acknowledgments

The authors are supported by the Association Française d'Urologie, the Association pour la Recherche sur les Tumeurs de Prostate, the Institut National du Cancer, the Ligue Nationale contre le Cancer (Equipe labellisée), the Université Paul Sabatier de Toulouse, the Hôpitaux de Toulouse.

8. References

Abrahamsson, P.A.; Lilja, H.; Falkmer, S.& Wadstrom, L.B. (1988). Immunohistochemical distribution of the three predominant secretory proteins in the parenchyma of hyperplastic and neoplastic prostate glands. Prostate, Vol.12, No.1, pp.39-46, ISSN 0270-4137

Albadine, R.; Latour, M.; Toubaji, A.; Haffner, M.; Isaacs, W.B.; E, A.P.; Meeker, A.K.; Demarzo, A.M.; Epstein, J.I.& Netto, G.J. (2009). TMPRSS2-ERG gene fusion status in minute (minimal) prostatic adenocarcinoma. Mod Pathol, Vol.22, No.11, (Nov), pp.1415-1422, ISSN 1530-0285

Ananias, H.J.; van den Heuvel, M.C.; Helfrich, W.& de Jong, I.J. (2009). Expression of the gastrin-releasing peptide receptor, the prostate stem cell antigen and the prostate-specific membrane antigen in lymph node and bone metastases of prostate cancer. Prostate, Vol.69, No.10, (Jul 1), pp.1101-1108, ISSN 1097-0045

Attard, G.; Clark, J.; Ambroisine, L.; Fisher, G.; Kovacs, G.; Flohr, P.; Berney, D.; Foster, C.S.; Fletcher, A.; Gerald, W.L.; Moller, H.; Reuter, V.; De Bono, J.S.; Scardino, P.; Cuzick, J.& Cooper, C.S. (2008). Duplication of the fusion of TMPRSS2 to ERG sequences identifies fatal human prostate cancer. Oncogene, Vol.27, No.3, (Jan 10), pp.253-263, ISSN 1476-5594

Barry, M.; Dhillon, P.K.; Stampfer, M.J.; Perner, S.; Ma, J.; Giovannucci, E.; Kurth, T.; Mucci, L.A.& Rubin, M.A. (2011). alpha-Methylacyl-CoA racemase expression and lethal prostate cancer in the Physicians' Health Study and Health Professionals Follow-up Study. Prostate, (Jun 28), ISSN 1097-0045

Bastian, P.J.; Palapattu, G.S.; Lin, X.; Yegnasubramanian, S.; Mangold, L.A.; Trock, B.; Eisenberger, M.A.; Partin, A.W.& Nelson, W.G. (2005). Preoperative serum DNA GSTP1 CpG island hypermethylation and the risk of early prostate-specific antigen recurrence following radical prostatectomy. Clin Cancer Res, Vol.11, No.11, (Jun 1), pp.4037-4043, ISSN 1078-0432

Berg, A.; Berner, A.; Lilleby, W.; Bruland, O.S.; Fossa, S.D.; Nesland, J.M.& Kvalheim, G. (2007). Impact of disseminated tumor cells in bone marrow at diagnosis in patients with nonmetastatic prostate cancer treated by definitive radiotherapy. Int J Cancer, Vol.120, No.8, (Apr 15), pp.1603-1609, ISSN 0020-7136

Bjartell, A.S.; Al-Ahmadie, H.; Serio, A.M.; Eastham, J.A.; Eggener, S.E.; Fine, S.W.; Udby, L.; Gerald, W.L.; Vickers, A.J.; Lilja, H.; Reuter, V.E.& Scardino, P.T. (2007). Association of cysteine-rich secretory protein 3 and beta-microseminoprotein with outcome after radical prostatectomy. Clin Cancer Res, Vol.13, No.14, (Jul 15), pp.4130-4138, ISSN 1078-0432

Bussemakers, M.J.; van Bokhoven, A.; Verhaegh, G.W.; Smit, F.P.; Karthaus, H.F.; Schalken, J.A.; Debruyne, F.M.; Ru, N.& Isaacs, W.B. (1999). DD3: a new prostate-specific gene, highly overexpressed in prostate cancer. Cancer Res, Vol.59, No.23, (Dec 1), pp.5975-5979, ISSN 0008-5472

Cozzi, P.J.; Wang, J.; Delprado, W.; Madigan, M.C.; Fairy, S.; Russell, P.J.& Li, Y. (2006). Evaluation of urokinase plasminogen activator and its receptor in different grades of human prostate cancer. Hum Pathol, Vol.37, No.11, (Nov), pp.1442-1451, ISSN 0046-8177

de Kok, J.B.; Verhaegh, G.W.; Roelofs, R.W.; Hessels, D.; Kiemeney, L.A.; Aalders, T.W.; Swinkels, D.W.& Schalken, J.A. (2002). DD3(PCA3), a very sensitive and specific marker to detect prostate tumors. Cancer Res, Vol.62, No.9, (May 1), pp.2695-2698, ISSN 0008-5472

Demichelis, F.; Fall, K.; Perner, S.; Andren, O.; Schmidt, F.; Setlur, S.R.; Hoshida, Y.; Mosquera, J.M.; Pawitan, Y.; Lee, C.; Adami, H.O.; Mucci, L.A.; Kantoff, P.W.; Andersson, S.O.; Chinnaiyan, A.M.; Johansson, J.E.& Rubin, M.A. (2007). TMPRSS2:ERG gene fusion associated with lethal prostate cancer in a watchful waiting cohort. Oncogene, Vol.26, No.31, (Jul 5), pp.4596-4599, ISSN 0950-9232

Dhir, R.; Vietmeier, B.; Arlotti, J.; Acquafondata, M.; Landsittel, D.; Masterson, R.& Getzenberg, R.H. (2004). Early identification of individuals with prostate cancer in negative biopsies. J Urol, Vol.171, No.4, (Apr), pp.1419-1423, ISSN 0022-5347

Dong, J.T. (2006). Prevalent mutations in prostate cancer. J Cell Biochem, Vol.97, No.3, (Feb 15), pp.433-447, ISSN 0730-2312

Dong, J.T.; Chen, C.; Stultz, B.G.; Isaacs, J.T.& Frierson, H.F., Jr. (2000). Deletion at 13q21 is associated with aggressive prostate cancers. Cancer Res, Vol.60, No.14, (Jul 15), pp.3880-3883, ISSN 0008-5472

Duffy, M.J. (2004). The urokinase plasminogen activator system: role in malignancy. Curr Pharm Des, Vol.10, No.1, pp.39-49, ISSN 1381-6128

Eeles, R.A.; Kote-Jarai, Z.; Giles, G.G.; Olama, A.A.; Guy, M.; Jugurnauth, S.K.; Mulholland, S.; Leongamornlert, D.A.; Edwards, S.M.; Morrison, J.; Field, H.I.; Southey, M.C.; Severi, G.; Donovan, J.L.; Hamdy, F.C.; Dearnaley, D.P.; Muir, K.R.; Smith, C.; Bagnato, M.; Ardern-Jones, A.T.; Hall, A.L.; O'Brien, L.T.; Gehr-Swain, B.N.; Wilkinson, R.A.; Cox, A.; Lewis, S.; Brown, P.M.; Jhavar, S.G.; Tymrakiewicz, M.; Lophatananon, A.; Bryant, S.L.; Horwich, A.; Huddart, R.A.; Khoo, V.S.; Parker, C.C.; Woodhouse, C.J.; Thompson, A.; Christmas, T.; Ogden, C.; Fisher, C.; Jamieson, C.; Cooper, C.S.; English, D.R.; Hopper, J.L.; Neal, D.E.& Easton, D.F. (2008). Multiple newly identified loci associated with prostate cancer susceptibility. Nat Genet, Vol.40, No.3, (Mar), pp.316-321, ISSN 1546-1718

Fine, S.W.; Gopalan, A.; Leversha, M.A.; Al-Ahmadie, H.A.; Tickoo, S.K.; Zhou, Q.; Satagopan, J.M.; Scardino, P.T.; Gerald, W.L.& Reuter, V.E. (2010). TMPRSS2-ERG gene fusion is associated with low Gleason scores and not with high-grade morphological features. *Mod Pathol*, Vol.23, No.10, (Oct), pp.1325-1333, ISSN 1530-0285

Fredolini, C.; Liotta, L.A.& Petricoin, E.F. (2010). Application of proteomic technologies for prostate cancer detection, prognosis, and tailored therapy. *Crit Rev Clin Lab Sci*, Vol.47, No.3, (May-Jun), pp.125-138, ISSN 1040-8363

Gavrilov, D.; Kenzior, O.; Evans, M.; Calaluce, R.& Folk, W.R. (2001). Expression of urokinase plasminogen activator and receptor in conjunction with the ets family and AP-1 complex transcription factors in high grade prostate cancers. *Eur J Cancer*, Vol.37, No.8, (May), pp.1033-1040, ISSN 0959-8049

Getzenberg, R.H.; Pienta, K.J.; Huang, E.Y.& Coffey, D.S. (1991). Identification of nuclear matrix proteins in the cancer and normal rat prostate. *Cancer Res*, Vol.51, No.24, (Dec 15), pp.6514-6520, ISSN 0008-5472

Girvan, A.R.; Chang, P.; van Huizen, I.; Moussa, M.; Xuan, J.W.; Stitt, L.; Chin, J.L.; Yamasaki, Y.& Izawa, J.I. (2005). Increased intratumoral expression of prostate secretory protein of 94 amino acids predicts for worse disease recurrence and progression after radical prostatectomy in patients with prostate cancer. *Urology*, Vol.65, No.4, (Apr), pp.719-723, ISSN 1527-9995

Gopalan, A.; Leversha, M.A.; Satagopan, J.M.; Zhou, Q.; Al-Ahmadie, H.A.; Fine, S.W.; Eastham, J.A.; Scardino, P.T.; Scher, H.I.; Tickoo, S.K.; Reuter, V.E.& Gerald, W.L. (2009). TMPRSS2-ERG gene fusion is not associated with outcome in patients treated by prostatectomy. *Cancer Res*, Vol.69, No.4, (Feb 15), pp.1400-1406, ISSN 1538-7445

Groskopf, J.; Aubin, S.M.; Deras, I.L.; Blase, A.; Bodrug, S.; Clark, C.; Brentano, S.; Mathis, J.; Pham, J.; Meyer, T.; Cass, M.; Hodge, P.; Macairan, M.L.; Marks, L.S.& Rittenhouse, H. (2006). APTIMA PCA3 molecular urine test: development of a method to aid in the diagnosis of prostate cancer. *Clin Chem*, Vol.52, No.6, (Jun), pp.1089-1095, ISSN 0009-9147

Gu, Z.; Thomas, G.; Yamashiro, J.; Shintaku, I.P.; Dorey, F.; Raitano, A.; Witte, O.N.; Said, J.W.; Loda, M.& Reiter, R.E. (2000). Prostate stem cell antigen (PSCA) expression increases with high gleason score, advanced stage and bone metastasis in prostate cancer. *Oncogene*, Vol.19, No.10, (Mar 2), pp.1288-1296, ISSN 0950-9232

Gupta, A.; Lotan, Y.; Ashfaq, R.; Roehrborn, C.G.; Raj, G.V.; Aragaki, C.C.; Montorsi, F.& Shariat, S.F. (2009). Predictive value of the differential expression of the urokinase plasminogen activation axis in radical prostatectomy patients. *Eur Urol*, Vol.55, No.5, (May), pp.1124-1133, ISSN 1873-7560

Haese, A.; de la Taille, A.; van Poppel, H.; Marberger, M.; Stenzl, A.; Mulders, P.F.; Huland, H.; Abbou, C.C.; Remzi, M.; Tinzl, M.; Feyerabend, S.; Stillebroer, A.B.; van Gils, M.P.& Schalken, J.A. (2008). Clinical utility of the PCA3 urine assay in European men scheduled for repeat biopsy. *Eur Urol*, Vol.54, No.5, (Nov), pp.1081-1088, ISSN 0302-2838

Han, K.R.; Seligson, D.B.; Liu, X.; Horvath, S.; Shintaku, P.I.; Thomas, G.V.; Said, J.W.& Reiter, R.E. (2004). Prostate stem cell antigen expression is associated with gleason score, seminal vesicle invasion and capsular invasion in prostate cancer. *J Urol*, Vol.171, No.3, (Mar), pp.1117-1121, ISSN 0022-5347

Hara, N.; Kasahara, T.; Kawasaki, T.; Bilim, V.; Obara, K.; Takahashi, K.& Tomita, Y. (2002). Reverse transcription-polymerase chain reaction detection of prostate-specific antigen, prostate-specific membrane antigen, and prostate stem cell antigen in one milliliter of peripheral blood: value for the staging of prostate cancer. *Clin Cancer Res*, Vol.8, No.6, (Jun), pp.1794-1799, ISSN 1078-0432

Hayes, J.D.& Strange, R.C. (1995). Potential contribution of the glutathione S-transferase supergene family to resistance to oxidative stress. *Free Radic Res*, Vol.22, No.3, (Mar), pp.193-207, ISSN 1071-5762

Heneghan, H.M.; Miller, N.& Kerin, M.J. (2010). MiRNAs as biomarkers and therapeutic targets in cancer. *Curr Opin Pharmacol*, Vol.10, No.5, (Oct), pp.543-550, ISSN 1471-4973

Hessels, D.; Smit, F.P.; Verhaegh, G.W.; Witjes, J.A.; Cornel, E.B.& Schalken, J.A. (2007). Detection of TMPRSS2-ERG fusion transcripts and prostate cancer antigen 3 in urinary sediments may improve diagnosis of prostate cancer. *Clin Cancer Res*, Vol.13, No.17, (Sep 1), pp.5103-5108, ISSN 1078-0432

Hessels, D.; van Gils, M.P.; van Hooij, O.; Jannink, S.A.; Witjes, J.A.; Verhaegh, G.W.& Schalken, J.A. (2010). Predictive value of PCA3 in urinary sediments in determining clinico-pathological characteristics of prostate cancer. *Prostate*, Vol.70, No.1, (Jan 1), pp.10-16, ISSN 1097-0045

Hienert, G.; Kirchheimer, J.C.; Christ, G.; Pfluger, H.& Binder, B.R. (1988a). Plasma urokinase-type plasminogen activator correlates to bone scintigraphy in prostatic carcinoma. *Eur Urol*, Vol.15, No.3-4, pp.256-258, ISSN 0302-2838

Hienert, G.; Kirchheimer, J.C.; Pfluger, H.& Binder, B.R. (1988b). Urokinase-type plasminogen activator as a marker for the formation of distant metastases in prostatic carcinomas. *J Urol*, Vol.140, No.6, (Dec), pp.1466-1469, ISSN 0022-5347

Hsing, A.W.& Chokkalingam, A.P. (2006). Prostate cancer epidemiology. *Front Biosci*, Vol.11, pp.1388-1413, ISSN 1093-4715

Jentzmik, F.; Stephan, C.; Lein, M.; Miller, K.; Kamlage, B.; Bethan, B.; Kristiansen, G.& Jung, K. (2011). Sarcosine in prostate cancer tissue is not a differential metabolite for prostate cancer aggressiveness and biochemical progression. *J Urol*, Vol.185, No.2, (Feb), pp.706-711, ISSN 1527-3792

Jentzmik, F.; Stephan, C.; Miller, K.; Schrader, M.; Erbersdobler, A.; Kristiansen, G.; Lein, M.& Jung, K. (2010). Sarcosine in urine after digital rectal examination fails as a marker in prostate cancer detection and identification of aggressive tumours. *Eur Urol*, Vol.58, No.1, (Jul), pp.12-18; discussion 20-11, ISSN 1873-7560

Joung, J.Y.; Cho, K.S.; Kim, J.E.; Seo, H.K.; Chung, J.; Park, W.S.; Choi, M.K.& Lee, K.H. (2010). Prostate stem cell antigen mRNA in peripheral blood as a potential predictor of biochemical recurrence in high-risk prostate cancer. *J Surg Oncol*, Vol.101, No.2, (Feb 1), pp.145-148, ISSN 1096-9098

Kibel, A.S.; Faith, D.A.; Bova, G.S.& Isaacs, W.B. (2000). Loss of heterozygosity at 12P12-13 in primary and metastatic prostate adenocarcinoma. *J Urol*, Vol.164, No.1, (Jul), pp.192-196, ISSN 0022-5347

Kollermann, J.; Weikert, S.; Schostak, M.; Kempkensteffen, C.; Kleinschmidt, K.; Rau, T.& Pantel, K. (2008). Prognostic significance of disseminated tumor cells in the bone marrow of prostate cancer patients treated with neoadjuvant hormone treatment. *J Clin Oncol*, Vol.26, No.30, (Oct 20), pp.4928-4933, ISSN 1527-7755

Kuefer, R.; Varambally, S.; Zhou, M.; Lucas, P.C.; Loeffler, M.; Wolter, H.; Mattfeldt, T.; Hautmann, R.E.; Gschwend, J.E.; Barrette, T.R.; Dunn, R.L.; Chinnaiyan, A.M.& Rubin, M.A. (2002). alpha-Methylacyl-CoA racemase: expression levels of this novel cancer biomarker depend on tumor differentiation. *Am J Pathol*, Vol.161, No.3, (Sep), pp.841-848, ISSN 0002-9440

Kumar-Sinha, C.; Tomlins, S.A.& Chinnaiyan, A.M. (2008). Recurrent gene fusions in prostate cancer. *Nat Rev Cancer*, Vol.8, No.7, (Jul), pp.497-511, ISSN 1474-1768

Lakshmanan, Y.; Subong, E.N.& Partin, A.W. (1998). Differential nuclear matrix protein expression in prostate cancers: correlation with pathologic stage. J Urol, Vol.159, No.4, (Apr), pp.1354-1358, 0022-5347 (Print)

Lam, J.S.; Yamashiro, J.; Shintaku, I.P.; Vessella, R.L.; Jenkins, R.B.; Horvath, S.; Said, J.W.& Reiter, R.E. (2005). Prostate stem cell antigen is overexpressed in prostate cancer metastases. Clin Cancer Res, Vol.11, No.7, (Apr 1), pp.2591-2596, 1078-0432 (Print)

Lee, W.H.; Morton, R.A.; Epstein, J.I.; Brooks, J.D.; Campbell, P.A.; Bova, G.S.; Hsieh, W.S.; Isaacs, W.B.& Nelson, W.G. (1994). Cytidine methylation of regulatory sequences near the pi-class glutathione S-transferase gene accompanies human prostatic carcinogenesis. *Proc Natl Acad Sci U S A*, Vol.91, No.24, (Nov 22), pp.11733-11737, ISSN 0027-8424

Leinonen, K.A.; Tolonen, T.T.; Bracken, H.; Stenman, U.H.; Tammela, T.L.; Saramaki, O.R.& Visakorpi, T. (2010). Association of SPINK1 expression and TMPRSS2:ERG fusion with prognosis in endocrine-treated prostate cancer. *Clin Cancer Res*, Vol.16, No.10, (May 15), pp.2845-2851, ISSN 1078-0432

Leman, E.S.; Cannon, G.W.; Trock, B.J.; Sokoll, L.J.; Chan, D.W.; Mangold, L.; Partin, A.W.& Getzenberg, R.H. (2007). EPCA-2: a highly specific serum marker for prostate cancer. *Urology*, Vol.69, No.4, (Apr), pp.714-720, ISSN 1527-9995

Lilja, H.& Abrahamsson, P.A. (1988). Three predominant proteins secreted by the human prostate gland. *Prostate*, Vol.12, No.1, pp.29-38, ISSN 0270-4137

Lu, T.& Hano, H. (2008). Deletion at chromosome arms 6q16-22 and 10q22.3-23.1 associated with initiation of prostate cancer. *Prostate Cancer Prostatic Dis*, Vol.11, No.4, pp.357-361, ISSN 1476-5608

Luo, J.; Zha, S.; Gage, W.R.; Dunn, T.A.; Hicks, J.L.; Bennett, C.J.; Ewing, C.M.; Platz, E.A.; Ferdinandusse, S.; Wanders, R.J.; Trent, J.M.; Isaacs, W.B.& De Marzo, A.M. (2002).

Alpha-methylacyl-CoA racemase: a new molecular marker for prostate cancer. *Cancer Res*, Vol.62, No.8, (Apr 15), pp.2220-2226, ISSN 0008-5472

Matsuyama, H.; Oba, K.; Matsuda, K.; Yoshihiro, S.; Tsukamoto, M.; Kinjo, M.; Sagiyama, K.; Takei, M.; Yamaguchi, A.; Sasaki, K.& Naito, K. (2007). Haploinsufficiency of 8p22 may influence cancer-specific survival in prostate cancer. *Cancer Genet Cytogenet*, Vol.174, No.1, (Apr 1), pp.24-34, ISSN 0165-4608

Matsuyama, H.; Pan, Y.; Oba, K.; Yoshihiro, S.; Matsuda, K.; Hagarth, L.; Kudren, D.; Naito, K.; Bergerheim, U.S.& Ekman, P. (2001). Deletions on chromosome 8p22 may predict disease progression as well as pathological staging in prostate cancer. *Clin Cancer Res*, Vol.7, No.10, (Oct), pp.3139-3143, ISSN 1078-0432

Mehra, R.; Tomlins, S.A.; Shen, R.; Nadeem, O.; Wang, L.; Wei, J.T.; Pienta, K.J.; Ghosh, D.; Rubin, M.A.; Chinnaiyan, A.M.& Shah, R.B. (2007). Comprehensive assessment of TMPRSS2 and ETS family gene aberrations in clinically localized prostate cancer. *Mod Pathol*, Vol.20, No.5, (May), pp.538-544, ISSN 0893-3952

Mitchell, P.S.; Parkin, R.K.; Kroh, E.M.; Fritz, B.R.; Wyman, S.K.; Pogosova-Agadjanyan, E.L.; Peterson, A.; Noteboom, J.; O'Briant, K.C.; Allen, A.; Lin, D.W.; Urban, N.; Drescher, C.W.; Knudsen, B.S.; Stirewalt, D.L.; Gentleman, R.; Vessella, R.L.; Nelson, P.S.; Martin, D.B.& Tewari, M. (2008). Circulating microRNAs as stable blood-based markers for cancer detection. *Proc Natl Acad Sci U S A*, Vol.105, No.30, (Jul 29), pp.10513-10518, ISSN 1091-6490

Miyake, H.; Hara, I.; Yamanaka, K.; Gohji, K.; Arakawa, S.& Kamidono, S. (1999). Elevation of serum levels of urokinase-type plasminogen activator and its receptor is associated with disease progression and prognosis in patients with prostate cancer. *Prostate*, Vol.39, No.2, (May), pp.123-129, ISSN 0270-4137

Nakanishi, H.; Groskopf, J.; Fritsche, H.A.; Bhadkamkar, V.; Blase, A.; Kumar, S.V.; Davis, J.W.; Troncoso, P.; Rittenhouse, H.& Babaian, R.J. (2008). PCA3 molecular urine assay correlates with prostate cancer tumor volume: implication in selecting candidates for active surveillance. *J Urol*, Vol.179, No.5, (May), pp.1804-1809; discussion 1809-1810, ISSN 1527-3792

Nam, R.K.; Reeves, J.R.; Toi, A.; Dulude, H.; Trachtenberg, J.; Emami, M.; Daigneault, L.; Panchal, C.; Sugar, L.; Jewett, M.A.& Narod, S.A. (2006). A novel serum marker, total prostate secretory protein of 94 amino acids, improves prostate cancer detection and helps identify high grade cancers at diagnosis. *J Urol*, Vol.175, No.4, (Apr), pp.1291-1297, ISSN 0022-5347

Nam, R.K.; Sugar, L.; Yang, W.; Srivastava, S.; Klotz, L.H.; Yang, L.Y.; Stanimirovic, A.; Encioiu, E.; Neill, M.; Loblaw, D.A.; Trachtenberg, J.; Narod, S.A.& Seth, A. (2007). Expression of the TMPRSS2:ERG fusion gene predicts cancer recurrence after surgery for localised prostate cancer. *Br J Cancer*, Vol.97, No.12, (Dec 17), pp.1690-1695, ISSN 0007-0920

Paul, B.; Dhir, R.; Landsittel, D.; Hitchens, M.R.& Getzenberg, R.H. (2005). Detection of prostate cancer with a blood-based assay for early prostate cancer antigen. *Cancer Res*, Vol.65, No.10, (May 15), pp.4097-4100, ISSN 0008-5472

Peng, X.; Guo, W.; Liu, T.; Wang, X.; Tu, X.; Xiong, D.; Chen, S.; Lai, Y.; Du, H.; Chen, G.; Liu, G.; Tang, Y.; Huang, S.& Zou, X. (2011). Identification of miRs-143 and -145 that Is Associated with Bone Metastasis of Prostate Cancer and Involved in the Regulation of EMT. *PLoS One*, Vol.6, No.5, pp.e20341, ISSN 1932-6203

Pulukuri, S.M.; Estes, N.; Patel, J.& Rao, J.S. (2007). Demethylation-linked activation of urokinase plasminogen activator is involved in progression of prostate cancer. *Cancer Res*, Vol.67, No.3, (Feb 1), pp.930-939, ISSN 0008-5472

Reeves, J.R.; Dulude, H.; Panchal, C.; Daigneault, L.& Ramnani, D.M. (2006). Prognostic value of prostate secretory protein of 94 amino acids and its binding protein after radical prostatectomy. *Clin Cancer Res*, Vol.12, No.20 Pt 1, (Oct 15), pp.6018-6022, ISSN 1078-0432

Reeves, J.R.; Xuan, J.W.; Arfanis, K.; Morin, C.; Garde, S.V.; Ruiz, M.T.; Wisniewski, J.; Panchal, C.& Tanner, J.E. (2005). Identification, purification and characterization of a novel human blood protein with binding affinity for prostate secretory protein of 94 amino acids. *Biochem J*, Vol.385, No.Pt 1, (Jan 1), pp.105-114, ISSN 1470-8728

Reiter, R.E.; Gu, Z.; Watabe, T.; Thomas, G.; Szigeti, K.; Davis, E.; Wahl, M.; Nisitani, S.; Yamashiro, J.; Le Beau, M.M.; Loda, M.& Witte, O.N. (1998). Prostate stem cell antigen: a cell surface marker overexpressed in prostate cancer. *Proc Natl Acad Sci U S A*, Vol.95, No.4, (Feb 17), pp.1735-1740, ISSN 0027-8424

Rhodes, D.R.; Barrette, T.R.; Rubin, M.A.; Ghosh, D.& Chinnaiyan, A.M. (2002). Meta-analysis of microarrays: interstudy validation of gene expression profiles reveals pathway dysregulation in prostate cancer. *Cancer Res*, Vol.62, No.15, (Aug 1), pp.4427-4433, ISSN 0008-5472

Rice, K.R.; Chen, Y.; Ali, A.; Whitman, E.J.; Blase, A.; Ibrahim, M.; Elsamanoudi, S.; Brassell, S.; Furusato, B.; Stingle, N.; Sesterhenn, I.A.; Petrovics, G.; Miick, S.; Rittenhouse, H.; Groskopf, J.; McLeod, D.G.& Srivastava, S. (2010). Evaluation of the ETS-related gene mRNA in urine for the detection of prostate cancer. *Clin Cancer Res*, Vol.16, No.5, (Mar 1), pp.1572-1576, ISSN 1078-0432

Rogers, C.G.; Yan, G.; Zha, S.; Gonzalgo, M.L.; Isaacs, W.B.; Luo, J.; De Marzo, A.M.; Nelson, W.G.& Pavlovich, C.P. (2004). Prostate cancer detection on urinalysis for alpha methylacyl coenzyme a racemase protein. *J Urol*, Vol.172, No.4 Pt 1, (Oct), pp.1501-1503, ISSN 0022-5347

Roupret, M.; Hupertan, V.; Catto, J.W.; Yates, D.R.; Rehman, I.; Proctor, L.M.; Phillips, J.; Meuth, M.; Cussenot, O.& Hamdy, F.C. (2008). Promoter hypermethylation in circulating blood cells identifies prostate cancer progression. *Int J Cancer*, Vol.122, No.4, (Feb 15), pp.952-956, ISSN 1097-0215

Rubin, M.A.; Bismar, T.A.; Andren, O.; Mucci, L.; Kim, R.; Shen, R.; Ghosh, D.; Wei, J.T.; Chinnaiyan, A.M.; Adami, H.O.; Kantoff, P.W.& Johansson, J.E. (2005). Decreased alpha-methylacyl CoA racemase expression in localized prostate cancer is associated with an increased rate of biochemical recurrence and cancer-specific death. *Cancer Epidemiol Biomarkers Prev*, Vol.14, No.6, (Jun), pp.1424-1432, ISSN 1055-9965

Rubin, M.A.; Zerkowski, M.P.; Camp, R.L.; Kuefer, R.; Hofer, M.D.; Chinnaiyan, A.M.& Rimm, D.L. (2004). Quantitative determination of expression of the prostate cancer protein alpha-methylacyl-CoA racemase using automated quantitative analysis (AQUA): a novel paradigm for automated and continuous biomarker measurements. *Am J Pathol*, Vol.164, No.3, (Mar), pp.831-840, ISSN 0002-9440

Rubin, M.A.; Zhou, M.; Dhanasekaran, S.M.; Varambally, S.; Barrette, T.R.; Sanda, M.G.; Pienta, K.J.; Ghosh, D.& Chinnaiyan, A.M. (2002). alpha-Methylacyl coenzyme A racemase as a tissue biomarker for prostate cancer. *JAMA*, Vol.287, No.13, (Apr 3), pp.1662-1670, ISSN 0098-7484

Saeki, N.; Gu, J.; Yoshida, T.& Wu, X. (2010). Prostate stem cell antigen: a Jekyll and Hyde molecule? *Clin Cancer Res*, Vol.16, No.14, (Jul 15), pp.3533-3538, ISSN 1078-0432

Saramaki, O.R.; Harjula, A.E.; Martikainen, P.M.; Vessella, R.L.; Tammela, T.L.& Visakorpi, T. (2008). TMPRSS2:ERG fusion identifies a subgroup of prostate cancers with a favorable prognosis. *Clin Cancer Res*, Vol.14, No.11, (Jun 1), pp.3395-3400, ISSN 1078-0432

Schaefer, A.; Jung, M.; Mollenkopf, H.J.; Wagner, I.; Stephan, C.; Jentzmik, F.; Miller, K.; Lein, M.; Kristiansen, G.& Jung, K. (2010). Diagnostic and prognostic implications of microRNA profiling in prostate carcinoma. *Int J Cancer*, Vol.126, No.5, (Mar 1), pp.1166-1176, ISSN 1097-0215

Schroder, F.H.; Hugosson, J.; Roobol, M.J.; Tammela, T.L.; Ciatto, S.; Nelen, V.; Kwiatkowski, M.; Lujan, M.; Lilja, H.; Zappa, M.; Denis, L.J.; Recker, F.; Berenguer, A.; Maattanen, L.; Bangma, C.H.; Aus, G.; Villers, A.; Rebillard, X.; van der Kwast, T.; Blijenberg, B.G.; Moss, S.M.; de Koning, H.J.& Auvinen, A. (2009). Screening and prostate-cancer mortality in a randomized European study. *N Engl J Med*, Vol.360, No.13, (Mar 26), pp.1320-1328, ISSN 1533-4406

Shariat, S.F.; Roehrborn, C.G.; McConnell, J.D.; Park, S.; Alam, N.; Wheeler, T.M.& Slawin, K.M. (2007). Association of the circulating levels of the urokinase system of plasminogen activation with the presence of prostate cancer and invasion, progression, and metastasis. *J Clin Oncol*, Vol.25, No.4, (Feb 1), pp.349-355, ISSN 1527-7755

Spahn, M.; Kneitz, S.; Scholz, C.J.; Stenger, N.; Rudiger, T.; Strobel, P.; Riedmiller, H.& Kneitz, B. (2010). Expression of microRNA-221 is progressively reduced in aggressive prostate cancer and metastasis and predicts clinical recurrence. *Int J Cancer*, Vol.127, No.2, (Jul 15), pp.394-403, ISSN 1097-0215

Sreekumar, A.; Poisson, L.M.; Rajendiran, T.M.; Khan, A.P.; Cao, Q.; Yu, J.; Laxman, B.; Mehra, R.; Lonigro, R.J.; Li, Y.; Nyati, M.K.; Ahsan, A.; Kalyana-Sundaram, S.; Han, B.; Cao, X.; Byun, J.; Omenn, G.S.; Ghosh, D.; Pennathur, S.; Alexander, D.C.; Berger, A.; Shuster, J.R.; Wei, J.T.; Varambally, S.; Beecher, C.& Chinnaiyan, A.M. (2009). Metabolomic profiles delineate potential role for sarcosine in prostate cancer progression. *Nature*, Vol.457, No.7231, (Feb 12), pp.910-914, ISSN 1476-4687

Stott, S.L.; Lee, R.J.; Nagrath, S.; Yu, M.; Miyamoto, D.T.; Ulkus, L.; Inserra, E.J.; Ulman, M.; Springer, S.; Nakamura, Z.; Moore, A.L.; Tsukrov, D.I.; Kempner, M.E.; Dahl, D.M.; Wu, C.L.; Iafrate, A.J.; Smith, M.R.; Tompkins, R.G.; Sequist, L.V.; Toner, M.; Haber, D.A.& Maheswaran, S. (2010). Isolation and characterization of circulating tumor cells from patients with localized and metastatic prostate cancer. *Sci Transl Med*, Vol.2, No.25, (Mar 31), pp.25ra23, ISSN 1946-6242

Thomas, G.; Jacobs, K.B.; Yeager, M.; Kraft, P.; Wacholder, S.; Orr, N.; Yu, K.; Chatterjee, N.; Welch, R.; Hutchinson, A.; Crenshaw, A.; Cancel-Tassin, G.; Staats, B.J.; Wang, Z.; Gonzalez-Bosquet, J.; Fang, J.; Deng, X.; Berndt, S.I.; Calle, E.E.; Feigelson, H.S.; Thun, M.J.; Rodriguez, C.; Albanes, D.; Virtamo, J.; Weinstein, S.; Schumacher, F.R.; Giovannucci, E.; Willett, W.C.; Cussenot, O.; Valeri, A.; Andriole, G.L.; Crawford, E.D.; Tucker, M.; Gerhard, D.S.; Fraumeni, J.F., Jr.; Hoover, R.; Hayes, R.B.; Hunter,

D.J.& Chanock, S.J. (2008). Multiple loci identified in a genome-wide association study of prostate cancer. *Nat Genet*, Vol.40, No.3, (Mar), pp.310-315, ISSN 1546-1718

Thuret, R.; Chantrel-Groussard, K.; Azzouzi, A.R.; Villette, J.M.; Guimard, S.; Teillac, P.; Berthon, P.; Houlgatte, A.; Latil, A.& Cussenot, O. (2005). Clinical relevance of genetic instability in prostatic cells obtained by prostatic massage in early prostate cancer. *Br J Cancer*, Vol.92, No.2, (Jan 31), pp.236-240, ISSN 0007-0920

Tomlins, S.A.; Rhodes, D.R.; Perner, S.; Dhanasekaran, S.M.; Mehra, R.; Sun, X.W.; Varambally, S.; Cao, X.; Tchinda, J.; Kuefer, R.; Lee, C.; Montie, J.E.; Shah, R.B.; Pienta, K.J.; Rubin, M.A.& Chinnaiyan, A.M. (2005). Recurrent fusion of TMPRSS2 and ETS transcription factor genes in prostate cancer. *Science*, Vol.310, No.5748, (Oct 28), pp.644-648, ISSN 1095-9203

Tong, A.W.; Fulgham, P.; Jay, C.; Chen, P.; Khalil, I.; Liu, S.; Senzer, N.; Eklund, A.C.; Han, J.& Nemunaitis, J. (2009). MicroRNA profile analysis of human prostate cancers. *Cancer Gene Ther*, Vol.16, No.3, (Mar), pp.206-216, ISSN 1476-5500

Uetsuki, H.; Tsunemori, H.; Taoka, R.; Haba, R.; Ishikawa, M.& Kakehi, Y. (2005). Expression of a novel biomarker, EPCA, in adenocarcinomas and precancerous lesions in the prostate. *J Urol*, Vol.174, No.2, (Aug), pp.514-518, ISSN 0022-5347

Usher, P.A.; Thomsen, O.F.; Iversen, P.; Johnsen, M.; Brunner, N.; Hoyer-Hansen, G.; Andreasen, P.; Dano, K.& Nielsen, B.S. (2005). Expression of urokinase plasminogen activator, its receptor and type-1 inhibitor in malignant and benign prostate tissue. *Int J Cancer*, Vol.113, No.6, (Mar 1), pp.870-880, ISSN 0020-7136

van Gils, M.P.; Hessels, D.; van Hooij, O.; Jannink, S.A.; Peelen, W.P.; Hanssen, S.L.; Witjes, J.A.; Cornel, E.B.; Karthaus, H.F.; Smits, G.A.; Dijkman, G.A.; Mulders, P.F.& Schalken, J.A. (2007). The time-resolved fluorescence-based PCA3 test on urinary sediments after digital rectal examination; a Dutch multicenter validation of the diagnostic performance. *Clin Cancer Res*, Vol.13, No.3, (Feb 1), pp.939-943, ISSN 1078-0432

Varambally, S.; Cao, Q.; Mani, R.S.; Shankar, S.; Wang, X.; Ateeq, B.; Laxman, B.; Cao, X.; Jing, X.; Ramnarayanan, K.; Brenner, J.C.; Yu, J.; Kim, J.H.; Han, B.; Tan, P.; Kumar-Sinha, C.; Lonigro, R.J.; Palanisamy, N.; Maher, C.A.& Chinnaiyan, A.M. (2008). Genomic loss of microRNA-101 leads to overexpression of histone methyltransferase EZH2 in cancer. *Science*, Vol.322, No.5908, (Dec 12), pp.1695-1699, ISSN 1095-9203

Varambally, S.; Dhanasekaran, S.M.; Zhou, M.; Barrette, T.R.; Kumar-Sinha, C.; Sanda, M.G.; Ghosh, D.; Pienta, K.J.; Sewalt, R.G.; Otte, A.P.; Rubin, M.A.& Chinnaiyan, A.M. (2002). The polycomb group protein EZH2 is involved in progression of prostate cancer. *Nature*, Vol.419, No.6907, (Oct 10), pp.624-629, ISSN 0028-0836

Wanders, R.J.; Vreken, P.; Ferdinandusse, S.; Jansen, G.A.; Waterham, H.R.; van Roermund, C.W.& Van Grunsven, E.G. (2001). Peroxisomal fatty acid alpha- and beta-oxidation in humans: enzymology, peroxisomal metabolite transporters and peroxisomal diseases. *Biochem Soc Trans*, Vol.29, No.Pt 2, (May), pp.250-267, ISSN 0300-5127

Whitman, E.J.; Groskopf, J.; Ali, A.; Chen, Y.; Blase, A.; Furusato, B.; Petrovics, G.; Ibrahim, M.; Elsamanoudi, S.; Cullen, J.; Sesterhenn, I.A.; Brassell, S.; Rittenhouse, H.; Srivastava, S.& McLeod, D.G. (2008). PCA3 score before radical prostatectomy predicts extracapsular extension and tumor volume. *J Urol*, Vol.180, No.5, (Nov), pp.1975-1978; discussion 1978-1979, ISSN 1527-3792

Woodson, K.; O'Reilly, K.J.; Hanson, J.C.; Nelson, D.; Walk, E.L.& Tangrea, J.A. (2008). The usefulness of the detection of GSTP1 methylation in urine as a biomarker in the diagnosis of prostate cancer. *J Urol*, Vol.179, No.2, (Feb), pp.508-511; discussion 511-502, ISSN 1527-3792

Zehentner, B.K.; Secrist, H.; Zhang, X.; Hayes, D.C.; Ostenson, R.; Goodman, G.; Xu, J.; Kiviat, M.; Kiviat, N.; Persing, D.H.& Houghton, R.L. (2006). Detection of alpha-methylacyl-coenzyme-A racemase transcripts in blood and urine samples of prostate cancer patients. *Mol Diagn Ther*, Vol.10, No.6, pp.397-403, ISSN 1177-1062

Zhao, Z.; Ma, W.; Zeng, G.; Qi, D.; Ou, L.& Liang, Y. (2011). Serum Early Prostate Cancer Antigen (EPCA) Level and Its Association with Disease Progression in Prostate Cancer in a Chinese Population. *PLoS One*, Vol.6, No.5, pp.e19284, ISSN 1932-6203

Zhao, Z.& Zeng, G. (2010). Increased serum level of early prostate cancer antigen is associated with subsequent cancer risk in men with high-grade prostatic intraepithelial neoplasia. *Endocr Relat Cancer*, Vol.17, No.2, (Jun), pp.505-512, ISSN 1479-6821

Zhigang, Z.& Wenlu, S. (2007). Prostate stem cell antigen (PSCA) mRNA expression in prostatic intraepithelial neoplasia: implications for the development of prostate cancer. *Prostate*, Vol.67, No.11, (Aug 1), pp.1143-1151, ISSN 0270-4137

Zhigang, Z.& Wenlv, S. (2004). Prostate stem cell antigen (PSCA) expression in human prostate cancer tissues and its potential role in prostate carcinogenesis and progression of prostate cancer. *World J Surg Oncol*, Vol.2, pp.13, ISSN 1477-7819

Zielie, P.J.; Mobley, J.A.; Ebb, R.G.; Jiang, Z.; Blute, R.D.& Ho, S.M. (2004). A novel diagnostic test for prostate cancer emerges from the determination of alpha-methylacyl-coenzyme a racemase in prostatic secretions. *J Urol*, Vol.172, No.3, (Sep), pp.1130-1133, ISSN 0022-5347

2

The Influence of Obesity on Prostate Cancer Diagnosis and Treatment

Piotr Bryniarski, Andrzej Paradysz and Mieczysław Fryczkowski
Medical University of Silesia in Katowice, Department of Urology in Zabrze
Poland

1. Introduction

To date there were only a few risk factors for developing prostate cancer (Pca) like advanced age, skin color and family history (Crawford, 2003). For the long time obesity was considered a negative feature which may contribute to chronic diseases like hypertension or diabetes, but its relationship with cancers was unknown. Last years revealed the obvious truth that such relationship exists and may be very strong. The problem seems to be very important given that obesity is very common, especially in western countries.

Over the past 25 years, the number of obese men has increased from 15% to 30% in USA. In 2000 66% of adults in U.S were classified as overweight or obese (Flegal et al., 2002) Nowadays no one denies that overweight and obesity is an independent risk factor for developing colon cancer or post-menopausal breast cancer.

Relationship with other cancers is still discussed especially in case of Pca. While the connection between obesity and chronic internal diseases is simple to explain, its relation to cancers is not so unequivocal. Most theories indicate the permanent chronic inflammation in obese which may contribute to oncogenesis.

Dishormonose observed in obese consists of high levels of insulin, insulin growth factor - 1 (IGF-1) (Chan et al., 1998, 2002), leptin, estrogens, and low levels of androgens. Insulin and IGF -1 are strong mitosis activators which may explain such "oncopotential". On the other hand low levels of testosterone and high of estrogen should protect men from developing Pca. It is only a simple example why the relation between obesity and prostate cancer may be very complex.

2. Nutrition

Several products are thought to be associated with increased risk for developing prostate cancer, others are known to act protectively. To the first group we may include saturated fats, red meat and dairy products (Kondo et al., 1994; Shirai, et al., 1997; Torniainen et al., 2007). In the second group we will find vitamin A, D and E, selenium, lycopene, fitoestrogens and isoflavones (Clark et al., 1998; Heinonen et al., 1998; Imaida et al., 2001; Kato et al., 2000; Schwartz et al., 1990). Vitamin A, D, E, selenium, lycopene and fitoestrogens are the compounds of fruits, vegetables, soya and tea. Vitamin A is known to improve cell apoptosis (Pienta et al., 1993; Young et al., 1994). Vitamin D facilitates cell differentiation (Hedlund et al., 1997). It was hypothesized that it may increase PSA doubling time (PSA DT) (Beer et al., 2003). Selenium is a known antioxidant (Clark et al., 1996). In Asia, where soya and tea consumption (fitoestrogens) is higher in comparison to western countries, the prevalence of prostate cancer is lower (Adlercreutz et al., 1993; Fotsis et al., 1993). Several studies tried to prove the favorable impact of vitamin E in Pca prevention (Knekt et al., 1990; The Alpha-Tocopherol, Beta-Carotene Cancer Prevention Study Group, 1994).

However, it has to be stressed that such influences are still rather hypothesis than evidence based facts. SELECT (Selenium and Vitamin E Comparison Trial) trial failed to demonstrate the favorable impact of selenium and vitamin E on Pca morbidity (Ledesma et al., 2011).

3. Obesity

It is of paramount significance to distinguish between high-risk and low-risk patients depending on extent of obesity. There are many ways to determine the range of overweight and obesity. The most prevalent is body mass index developed by World Health Organization. However, it does not differentiate fat mass from muscle mass. That is why waist - hip ratio (WHR) is more commonly applied while assessing the central adiposity, and correlates much stronger with hormonal alterations (the importance of that finding is emphasized later in the text) than BMI.

There are various theories concerning the influence of obesity on the natural development, diagnostics or progression after radical treatment of Pca. The Health Professional Follow-Up Study was based on 47757 men who were observed for 14 years and showed that relative risk for developing prostate cancer was 0,52 in obese compared to non-obese men (Giovannucci et al., 2003).

The 5 times increased percentage of biochemical recurrence after radical prostatectomy observed in Afro-Americans, compared to Euro-Americans, is sometimes explained by 3 times more frequent presence of overweight or obesity among the former. It also may result from the polymorphism of the androgen receptor which causes higher PSA concentration in Afro-Americans. On the other hand two large studies failed to demonstrate disastrous impact of obesity on prostate cancer morbidity (Andersson et al., 1997; Rapp et al., 2005).

Not only the absolute value of BMI seems to be important when assessing the patient's risk. It was shown that also gaining weight at the greatest rate of ≥ 1.5 kg/year between 25 years of age and time of Pca diagnosis will result in more rapid biochemical failure after radical treatment (Strom et al., 2005).

The influence of obesity on Pca is definitely negative, including the following:

1. dishormonose – abnormal hormone concentrations, which induces the intensification of diagnostics and at the same time postpones proper treatment
2. comorbidities, which pushes the prostate diagnostics into the background and consequently patients suffer from more advanced forms of prostate cancer
3. difficulties in per rectum examination in obese patients,
4. difficulties during transrectal ultrasound (TRUS) of the prostate and prostate biopsy (due to larger prostates in obese patients) (Freedland et al., 2006).
5. difficulties during radical prostatectomy and radical radiotherapy due to:
    a. technical problems (larger hooks, smaller operational field)
    b. larger prostates observed in obese patients (much problem while conducting nerve-sparing technique)

6. Unfavorable postoperative features especially higher rate of:
   a. high grade disease
   b. positive surgical margins
   c. extraprostatic extension (pT3a)
   d. lymph node metastases (N+)
   e. biochemical recurrence
   f. fatal disease
7. hemodilution (explained later)

Lastly it was proved that the unfavorable impact of obesity on Pca may be explained by genetic examinations. It was hypothesized that the AA genotype of rs9939609, which is associated with an increase in BMI, would protect against non-aggressive prostate tumors whilst increasing the risk of aggressive prostate tumors (Lewis et al., 2010). The abovementioned study gave us only weak proof of such correlation.

4. Prostate cancer cells and adipocytes

Skeletal metastases are most common in advanced Pca. Metastases are known to be osteoblastic ones. Prostate cancer cells are absorbing lipids directly to develop and progress, that is why bone marrow is so common place of metastases.

It was also experimentally shown that bone marrow without adypocytes is less attractive for prostate cancer cells to residue (Brown et al., 2006). It was even suggested that lowering lipid levels with statins will impact the progression of prostate cancer, but this assumption turned out not to be true (Platz et al., 2006).

5. Sex hormones

As stated in the introduction in obese levels of sex hormones are different from that observed in normal weight people. Prostate is hormone-sensitive gland and therefore androgens are needed for its development.

Also prostate cancer is hormone-sensitive and testosterone is known to accelerate its progression to advanced and metastatic form while estrogens inhibit such progress. This finding led us to application of castration (surgical or pharmacological) in the treatment of advanced or metastatic prostate cancer.

However, the relation between dishormonese and prostate cancer is not so unequivocal. Testosterone also influences the differentiation of prostate cells (but not prostate cancer cells) to mature forms, while estrogens have contrary impact and therefore may lead to poorly differentiated Pca (Massengill et al. 2003; Schatzl et al., 2001).

6. Aggressive prostate cancer

It is also assumed that PCa in overweight people is more aggressive. Usually it was stated that Pca with Gleason score > 7 was significantly more frequent in obese patients. Not all authors agree with that hypothesis (Chyou et al., 1994; Major et al., 2011; Nilsen et al., 1999; Rodriguez et al., 2007; Schuurman et al., 2000; Snowdon et al., 1984).

Authors emphasize that central obesity as the outcome of excessive fat accumulation results in glucose intolerance, high blood pressure, atherosclerosis, cardiovascular disease, insulin resistance, altered metabolic profile, metabolic syndrome, and obesity-related lipid disorders (Hsing et al., 2007). Especially insulin resistance, higher IGF-1 and leptin levels are recognized responsible for such aggressiveness (Hedlund et al., 1994; Prabhat et al., 2010). IGF-1 is involved in angiogenesis, responsible for bone metastases and developing androgen-independent progression of Pca. Leptin is responsible for cell migration and growth factor expression in hormone-resistant cells of Pca.

It is not proven that worse treatment outcomes in obese patients are due to unfavorable features of prostate cancer itself. In one of the studies it was reported that obesity was positively correlated with clinical progression independently of prostate cancer grade, stage and primary treatment (Gong et al., 2007).

Higher rate of cancer progression is also due to unfavorable features of obese men after radical prostatectomy. It was proven that increased BMI is associated with high grade disease, positive surgical margins, extraprostatic extension of the disease and lymph node metastases. Biochemical recurrence after radical prostatectomy is also more frequent in obese patients compared to non-obese men (Freedland et al., 2005).

7. Androgen deprivation therapy (ADT)

Pharmacological castration with GnRH agonists is the standard treatment for patients with locally advanced or metastatic Pca. However, it is burdened with several adverse effects like osteoporosis, loss of libido, erectile dysfunction and finally metabolic syndrome. Increased levels of total cholesterol, LDL and decreased HDL, diabetes and hypertension contribute to higher risk of acute coronary syndrome (ACS).

Obese patients receiving ADT are at highest risk for developing ACS as ADT therapy and obesity shares the cardiovascular risk through the metabolic syndrome. They should be constantly monitored and treated accordingly (Cleffi et al., 2011). Osteoporosis in Pca is not only the result of cancer itself. Osteoblastic metastases of prostate cancer contribute to pathologic spine fractures which may be fatal eventually. Immediate spine decompression in orthopedics department is indicated in such condition.

The situation may be worse when patient is given ADT. I was proven that hypogonadism leads to osteopenia and finally to osteoporosis. As obese patients have lower levels of testosterone, abovementioned unfavorable factors may contribute to pathologic fractures.

To prevent such mournful course patients are advised to take bisphospfonates (alendronic, zolendronic, clodronic acid, etc.) or denosumab (RANK ligand inhibitor) which inhibit osteoclasts and slow down progression of the disease.

8. Hemodilution

Undoubtedly, a negative feature of PSA concentration is the fact that it is subject to hemodilution. Some authors claim that in overweight and obese patients PSA concentration is lower, which is, in the first place, caused by the aforementioned phenomenon. This phenomenon is supposed to consist in the dissolution of PSA mass in a large amount of plasma, finally resulting in lower PSA concentration. PSA is a protease which physiological function consists in liquefying semen.

Every man is characterized by a quite invariable amount (mass) of this secreted into the blood protein, depending on age, the size of prostate, the presence of cancer or other prostate diseases. However, standard PSA determination means that PSA mass is dissolved in plasma volume which is mainly dependant on the obesity extent. This led some authors to explore new markers independent of hemodilution (Bryniarski et al., 2011). PSA mass meets these criteria, but further studies are needed to demonstrate its superiority over standard PSA concentration.

9. Author's contribution

Hereby we present our work on hemodilution (Bryniarski et al., 2011). The aim of our study was to prove the superiority of PSA mass over standard PSA concentration in predicting biochemical recurrence after radical prostatectomy.

9.1 Material and methods

From 1994 until the end of 2007 206 radical retropubic prostatectomies in Caucasian men suffering from prostate cancer were carried out in the Department of Urology in Zabrze, Medical University of Silesia in Katowice. The patients who underwent preoperative anti-androgen therapy, chemotherapy or radiotherapy were excluded from the research (29 patients).

177 patients were qualified for the research. In our group two types of data were subject to analysis. Preoperative data, such as: age, height, weight, BMI, PSA concentration (immunoenzymatic Elecsys test; Cobas 6000 Hitachi) and postoperative data: the extent of histopathologic differentiation of prostate tissue in Gleason score, extracapsular extension (pT3), the presence of lymph nodes metastases and the presence of positive surgical margins.

Patients are under constant control in the Hospital Outpatient Clinic, thanks to which data concerning progression (biochemical recurrence, local recurrence, death) were also collected and the cancer-specific survival time was determined. The total volume of plasma and the PSA mass were calculated on the basis of the formulas (Table 1) (Boer, 1984; Du Bois & Du Bois, 1916).

Estimated Body Surface (EBS)	Plasma volume [liters] (PV)	PSA mass [μg]
$(weight)^{0,425}$ x $(height)^{0,72}$ x 0,007184	EBS x 1,670	PV x PSA concentration

Table 1. The formulas to estimate plasma volume and PSA mass.

The group of 177 patients was divided according to:

1. BMI – into 3 groups: I – 45 patients with normal weight (BMI < 25), II – 95 overweight patients (BMI – 25 – 29,9), III – 37 obese patients (BMI ≥ 30).
2. Preoperative PSA concentration – into 3 groups: I – 79 patients with PSA < 10 ng/ml, II – 66 patients with PSA 10 – 19,9 ng/ml, III – 32 patients with PSA ≥ 20 ng/ml.
3. Preoperative PSA mass – into 3 groups: I – 71 patients with PSA < 40 μg, II – 78 patients with PSA 40 – 69,9 μg and III – 28 patients with PSA ≥ 70 μg.

The characteristics of each group is shown in tables 2 and 3.

		BMI (kg/m²)			PSA (ng/ml)			PSA mass (μg)		
		I	II	III	I	II	III	I	II	III
Age (years)	mean	62,8	62,2	62,1	63	61,4	62,6	62,8	61,8	62,7
	SD	6,7	5,9	6	5,7	6,9	5,5	5,8	6,5	6
	range	50-76	48-74	49-71	49-74	48-76	52-72	49-74	48-76	52-72
BMI (kg/m²)	mean	23,4	27,4	32,6	27,1	28	27,4	26,9	27,8	28,2
	SD	1,4	1,3	2,3	2,9	4	3,3	2,9	3,6	4
	range	17,9-24,9	25-29,9	30,1-40,3	20-37,5	17,9-40,3	22,1-35	20-37,5	17,9-40,3	22,1-38
Plasma volume (liters)	mean	3,1	3,2	3,45	3,2	3,3	3,2	3,2	3,2	3,2
	SD	0,13	0,2	0,2	0,2	0,2	0,2	0,2	0,2	0,2
	range	2,9-3,4	2,8-3,9	2,9-4,1	2,7-3,7	2,8-4,1	2,9-3,7	2,7-3,7	2,8-4,1	2,9-3,9
PSA concentration (ng/ml)	mean	12,8	14,1	14,2	6,4	14,2	31,3	6,1	14,1	32,6
	SD	8,9	11,9	7,7	1,9	2,8	11,6	1,7	3,5	11,9
	range	2,8-51,8	1,8-61,7	4,2-43,4	1,8-9,8	10-19,8	20,4-61,7	1,8-9,6	9-21,8	18-61,7
Gleason score	median	5	6	6	5	6	6	5	6	6
PSA mass (μg)	mean	56,6	46,2	48,9	20,8	47	101,1	19,7	46,2	106,7
	SD	27,4	39	25,1	6,37	10,3	37,1	5,6	11,3	36,5
	range	31,9-156,6	6,5-196,6	13,7-129,5	6,5-32,7	30,3-71	64,2-196,6	6,5-29,8	30,3-69,6	70,7-196,6

Table 2. Characteristics of patients in groups of BMI, PSA concentration and PSA mass.

All constant variables distributions were analyzed with regard to normality by means of Kolmogorov-Smirnov and Lilliefors tests. By means of descriptive statistics the following characteristics have been determined: mean or median, standard deviation as well as maximal and minimal value.

In order to determine differences between the groups, where variables are of categorical character, Chi-square test has been used. In order to determine differences between a number of independent groups, where continuous variables have distribution other than normal, Kruskal-Wallis test has been used.

In order to eliminate the influence of factors disrupting the correlation between BMI and PSA concentration, such as: age, the extent of prostate cancer differentiation in Gleason score, extracapsular extension (pT3) or positive surgical margins, multiple regression has been used to create a model which would describe the aforesaid relationship. The aforementioned disrupting factors have been incorporated into the model.

		BMI (kg/m²)			PSA concentration (ng/ml)			PSA mass (µg)		
		I	II	III	I	II	III	I	II	III
pT3	Yes	12 (18,1%)	33 (50%)	21 (31,9%)	14 (21,2%)	32 (48,5%)	20 (30,3%)	13 (19,6%)	34 (51,5%)	19 (28,7%)
	No	33 (29,7%)	62 (55,8%)	16 (14,5%)	65 (58,5%)	34 (30,6%)	12 (10,9%)	58 (52,2%)	44 (39,6%)	9 (8,1%)
Positive lymph nodes	Yes	2 (20%)	4 (40%)	4 (40%)	1 (10%)	5 (50%)	4 (40%)	1 (10%)	3 (30%)	6 (60%)
	No	43 (25,7%)	91 (54,5%)	33 (19,8%)	78 (46,7%)	61 (36,5%)	28 (16,7%)	70 (41,9%)	75 (44,9%)	22 (13,1%)
Positive surgical margin	Yes	13 (26%)	28 (56%)	9 (18%)	9 (18%)	27 (54%)	14 (28%)	7 (14%)	29 (58%)	14 (28%)
	No	32 (25,1%)	67 (52,7%)	28 (22%)	70 (55,1%)	39 (30,7%)	18 (14,1%)	64 (50,3%)	49 (38,5%)	14 (11%)
Biochemical recurrence	Yes	13 (20%)	34 (52,3%)	18 (27,6%)	15 (23%)	30 (46,1%)	20 (30,7%)	14 (21,5%)	33 (50,7%)	18 (27,6%)
	No	32 (28,5%)	61 (54,4%)	19 (16,9%)	64 (57,1%)	36 (32,1%)	12 (10,7%)	57 (50,8%)	45 (41,1%)	10 (8,9%)
Local recurrence	Yes	4 (20%)	10 (50%)	6 (30%)	5 (25%)	9 (45%)	6 (30%)	5 (25%)	7 (35%)	8 (40%)
	No	41 (26,1%)	85 (54,1%)	31 (19,7%)	74 (47,1%)	57 (36,3%)	26 (16,5%)	66 (42%)	71 (45,2%)	20 (12,7%)
Death	Yes	1 (6,6%)	6 (40%)	8 (53,3%)	1 (6,6%)	10 (66,6%)	4 (26,6%)	0 (0%)	9 (60%)	6 (40%)
	No	44 (27,1%)	89 (54,9%)	29 (17,9%)	78 (48,1%)	56 (34,5%)	28 (17,2%)	71 (43,8%)	69 (42,5%)	22 (13,5%)

Table 3. Characteristics of patients in groups of BMI, PSA concentration and PSA mass.

In order to evaluate and compare the odds ratio of biochemical recurrence together with the elevated concentration and mass of the PSA, the model of logistic regression has been used. The model has been adjusted to Gleason score (<8 and ≥ 8) in postoperative specimen. As both the concentration and the PSA mass did not show normal distribution, the logarithmic (decimal) transformation of data has been performed. 10 patients who have been diagnosed with metastases in the surrounding lymph nodes have been removed from the model because the presence of metastases would distort the results of the observation.

Cancer-specific survival of patients has been evaluated by means of Kaplan-Meier analysis, while the significance of differences between them has been evaluated by means of Gehan's Wilcoxon test.

Receiver operating characteristic (ROC) curves compared predictive variables.

For all statistical tests the critical level of significance has been adopted at $p<0,05$. The statistical analysis has been calculated by means of StatSoft Statistica 8.0.

9.2 Results

The values PSA mass in the research has a statistically significant influence on extracapsular extension ($p<0,001$), the presence of metastases in the surrounding lymph nodes ($p<0,001$), the frequency of positive surgical margins ($p<0,001$), the presence of biochemical ($p<0001$) and local recurrence ($p<0,001$) and the rate of death ($p<0,001$).

The research has shown that BMI does not influence preoperative PSA concentration and PSA mass (Fig.1 and 2). Differences in preoperative PSA concentration between the 3 groups of patients are statistically insignificant ($p = 0,28$). The total plasma volume is higher in obese patients ($p<0,001$).

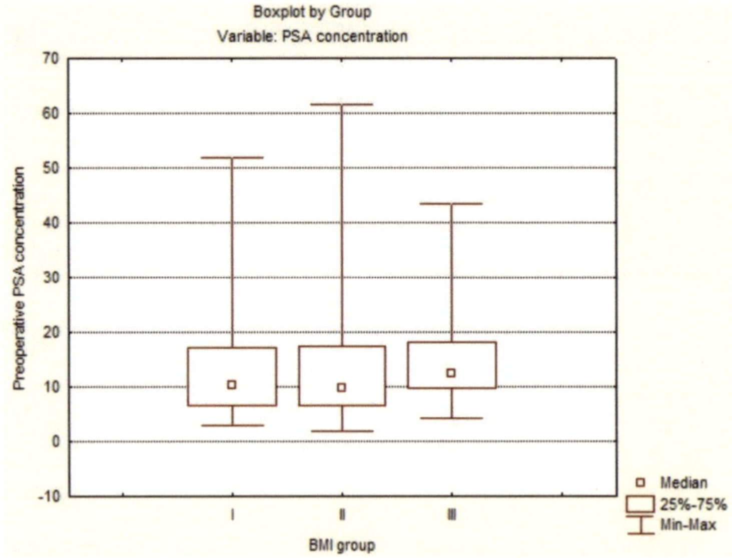

Fig. 1. Comparison of preoperative PSA concentration (ng/ml) in BMI groups.

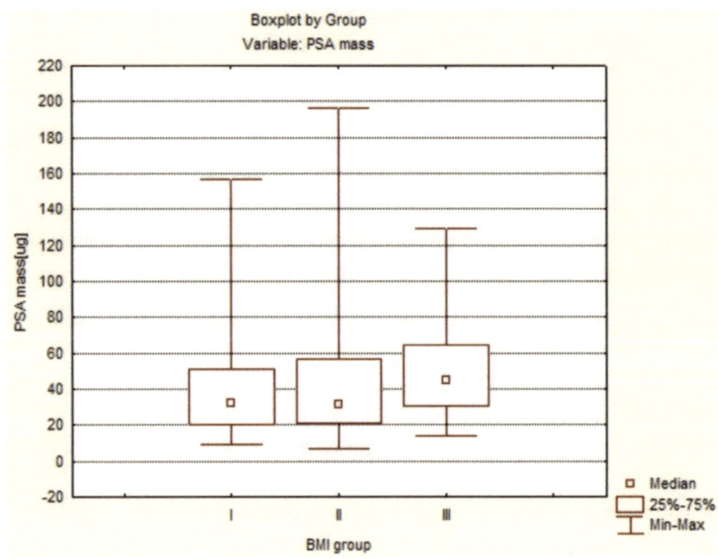

Fig. 2. Comparison of preoperative PSA mass in BMI groups.

The model of multiple regression has proved the lack of statistically significant correlation between preoperative PSA concentration and BMI (p = 0,99). The research has proved that the elevated preoperative value of PSA mass (p = 0,02) is the factor which influences the cancer-specific survival of patients with prostate cancer after RP (Fig.3).

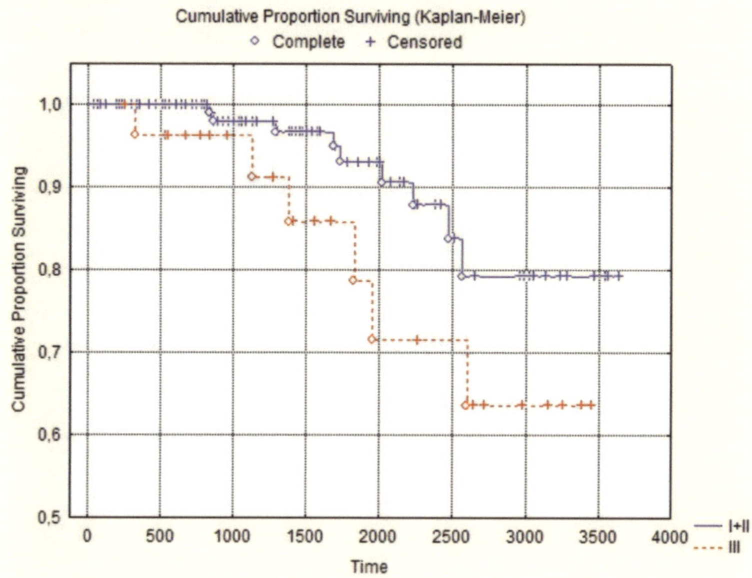

Fig. 3. Comparison of overall survival time (days) in patients with prostate cancer depending on the PSA mass.

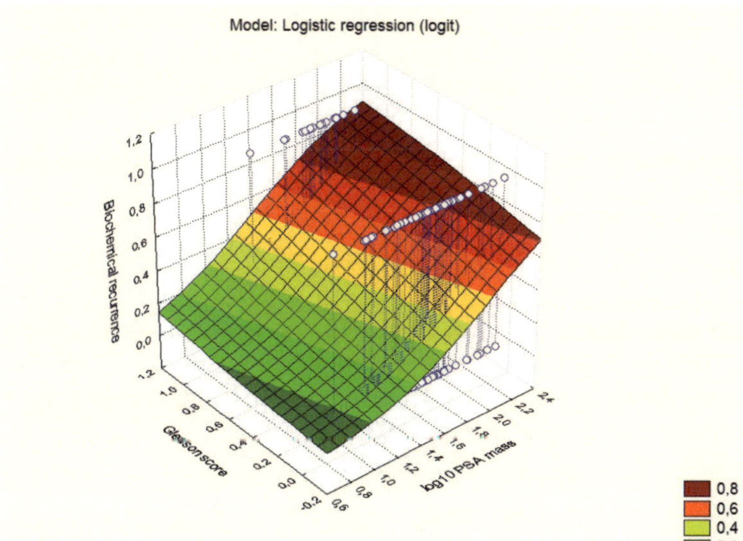

Fig. 4. Three-dimensional model of logistic regression with two independent variables (Gleason score and decimal logarithm from the value of PSA mass) and dependent dychotomic variable (biochemical recurrence).

The odds ratio of biochemical recurrence, with the PSA mass increased 10 times, is equal to 8,64 (95% CI: 2,54 - 29,3; p<0,001) (Fig. 4). The odds ratio of biochemical recurrence, with the PSA concentration increased 10 times, is equal to 7,66 (95% CI: 2,25 - 26; p<0,001).
ROC curves for preoperative PSA mass and PSA concentration showed an area under curve (AUC) of 0,72 and 0,65 respectively for biochemical recurrence after RP (Fig. 5). The difference between these two predictors (AUC) was statistically significant (p=0,04).

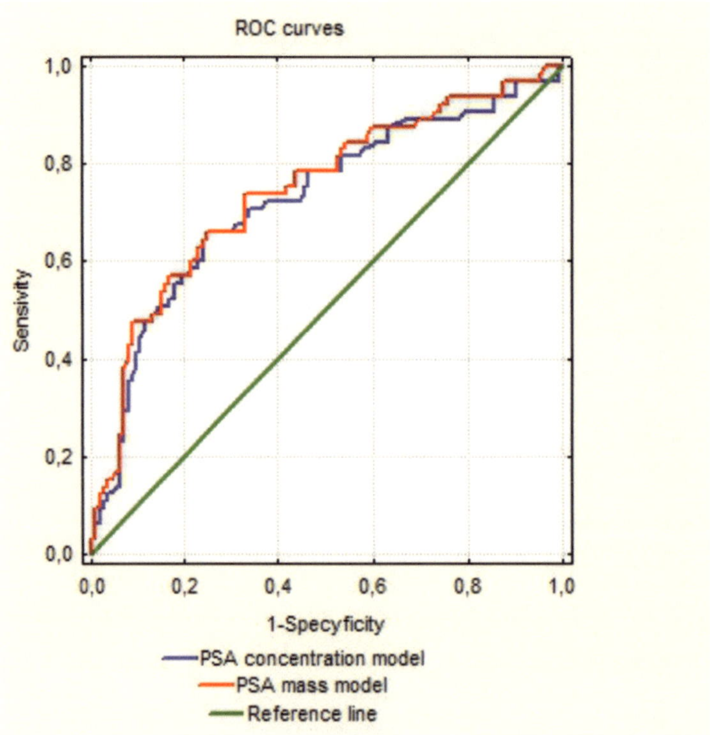

Fig. 5. ROC curves for PSA mass as a preoperative predictor of biochemical recurrence after RP (Area Under Curve - 0,72).

9.3 Discussion

There are various theories concerning the influence of obesity on the natural development, diagnostics or progression after radical treatment of prostate cancer. The 5 times increased percentage of biochemical recurrence observed in Afro-Americans, compared to Euro-Americans, is sometimes explained by 3 times more frequent presence of overweight or obesity among the former (Spangler et al., 2007).
Its influence is definitely negative, including the following:

1. difficulties in per rectum examination in obese patients (Bray, 2006),
2. dishormonose (Hsing et al., 2002; Kaaks et al., 2000) - abnormal hormone concentrations, which induces the intensification of diagnostics and at the same time postpones proper treatment,
3. comorbidities, which pushes the prostate diagnostics into the background and consequently patients suffer from more advanced forms of prostate cancer

Some authors suggest another factor, namely, lower PSA concentration in obese patients (Baillargeon et al., 2005). The consequence of the aforesaid correlation may impact on prostate cancer diagnosis and evaluation of progression after its radical treatment. Other authors disclaim the abovementioned connection (Freedland et al., 2006).

The authors who prove that obese patients are characterized by lower PSA concentration, refer to the phenomenon of hemodilution. The supporters of that theory claim that obesity is characterized by a larger amount of circulating blood, so theoretically the constant PSA mass circulating in the organism would be dissolved in a large amount of plasma, resulting in a lower PSA concentration.

However, our research has not proved that the elevated BMI has a significant influence on the preoperative PSA concentration. In order to explain the inconsistency we will call upon racial differences between the analyzed groups. The following research has been done on a group of patients of Caucasian race, while the aforesaid research has been frequently based on ethnically heterogeneous groups. The cause of differences between the outcomes can result from the polymorphism of the androgen receptor which causes higher PSA concentration in Afro-Americans, as well as statistically significant bigger obesity of this group (Xu et al., 2002). The influence of ethnical differences can, of course, be dismissed by appropriate statistical manipulations, nevertheless, it seems that research done on homogenous groups is characterized by greater statistical power.

In order to exclude the potential influence of hemodilution on the PSA concentration, the PSA mass in each patient has been calculated. Thanks to mathematical formulas used to estimate the total amount of circulating blood, its amount can be quite precisely determined. It has to be underlined that the phenomenon of hemodilution in obese patients had no statistically significant influence on PSA concentration. Also, having excluded other factors influencing PSA concentration, such as: cancer differentiation in Gleason score, the extracapsular extension (pT3), positive surgical margins or the patient's age, no significant correlation between BMI and the preoperative PSA concentration has been found.

However, comparing both parameters (PSA concentration and the PSA mass) it has to be stressed that the probability of biochemical recurrence after RP is better predicted by PSA mass, which surely results from the fact that the PSA mass includes the element eliminating the phenomenon of hemodilution. Despite the fact that both preoperative parameters "equally well" evaluate the progression after RP, the PSA mass seems to be a little more sensitive parameter (which is indicated by the difference in the odds ratio and AUC).

9.4 Conclusions

1. Increased preoperative value of the PSA mass is connected with:
    a. more frequent cancer diagnosis of pT3 prostate cancer,
    b. more frequent diagnosis of metastases in the surrounding lymph nodes,
    c. more frequent recognition of the positive surgical margin,
    d. shorter cancer-specific survival time,
    e. higher percentage of progression.
2. The preoperative PSA mass is a better predictor of biochemical recurrence after RP than PSA concentration.
3. The total plasma volume is higher in obese patients, however, it does not influence the preoperative PSA concentration significantly.

10. References

Crawford, ED. (2003). Epidemiology of prostate cancer. *Urology*. Vol. 62, No. 6, (December 2003), Supplement 1, pp. 3–12, ISSN 0090-4295

Flegal, KM., Carroll, MD., Ogden, CL. & Johnson, CL. (2002). Prevalence and trends in obesity among US adults, 1999-2000. *JAMA*. Vol. 288, No. 14, (October 2002), pp. 1723-7, ISSN 0098-7484

Chan, JM., Stampfer, MJ., Giovannucci, E., Gann, PH., Ma, J., Wilkinson, P., Hennekens, CH. & Pollak, M. (1998). Plasma insulin like growth factor-I and prostate cancer risk: a prospective study. *Science*. Vol. 279, No. 5350, (January 1998), pp. 563-6, ISSN 0036-8075

Chan, JM., Stampfer, MJ., Ma, J., Gann, P., Gaziano, JM., Pollak, M. & Giovannucci, E. (2002). Insulin-like growth factor-I (IGF-I) and IGF binding protein-3 as predictors of advanced-stage prostate cancer. *J Natl Cancer Inst*. Vol. 94, No. 14, (July 2002), pp. 1099-106, ISSN 0027-8874

Kondo, Y., Homma, Y., Aso, Y. & Kakizoe, T. (1994). Promotional effect of two-generation exposure to a high-fat diet on prostate carcinogenesis in ACI/Seg rats. *Cancer Res*. Vol. 54, No. 23, (December 1994), pp. 6129-32, ISSN 0008-5472

Shirai, T., Sano, M., Tamano, S., Takahashi, S., Hirose, M., Futakuchi, M., Hasegawa, R., Imaida, K., Matsumoto, K., Wakabayashi, K., Sugimura, T. & Ito, N. (1997). The prostate: a target for carcinogenicity of 2-amino-1-methyl-6-phenylimidazo[4,5-b]pyridine (PhIP) derived from cooked foods. *Cancer Res*. Vol. 57, No. 2, (January 1997) pp. 195-8, ISSN 0008-5472

Torniainen, S., Hedelin, M., Autio, V., Rasinperä, H., Bälter, KA., Klint, A., Bellocco, R., Wiklund, F., Stattin, P., Ikonen, T., Tammela, TL., Schleutker, J., Grönberg, H. & Järvelä, I. (2007). Lactase persistence, dietary intake of milk, and the risk for prostate cancer in Sweden and Finland. *Cancer Epidemiol Biomarkers Prev. Vol.* 5, No. 5, (May 2007), pp. 956-61, ISSN 1055-9965

Kato, K., Takahashi, S., Cui, L., Toda, T., Suzuki, S., Futakuchi, M., Sugiura, S. & Shirai, T. (2000). Suppressive effects of dietary genistin and daidzin on rat prostate carcinogenesis. *Jpn J Cancer Res*. Vol. 91, No. 8, (August 2000), pp. 786-91, ISSN 0910-5050

Imaida, K., Tamano, S., Kato, K., Ikeda, Y., Asamoto, M., Takahashi, S., Nir, Z., Murakoshi, M., Nishino, H. & Shirai, T. (2001). Lack of chemopreventive effects of lycopene and curcumin on experimental rat prostate carcinogenesis. *Carcinogenesis*. Vol. 22, No. 3, (March 2001), pp. 467-72, ISSN 0143-3334

Clark, LC., Dalkin, B., Krongrad, A., Combs, GFJr., Turnbull, BW., Slate, EH., Witherington, R., Herlong, JH., Janosko, E., Carpenter, D., Borosso, C., Falk, S. & Rounder, J. (1998). Decreased incidence of prostate cancer with selenium supplementation: results of a double-blind cancer prevention trial. *Br J Urol*. Vol. 81, No. 5, (May 1998), pp. 730-4, ISSN 0007-1331

Heinonen, O., Albanes, D. & Virtamo, J. (1998). Prostate cancer and supplementation with alpha-tocopherol and beta-carotene: incidence and mortality in a controlled trial. *J Natl Cancer Inst*. Vol. 90, No. 6, (March 1998), pp. 440-6, ISSN 0027-8874

Schwartz, GG. & Hulka, BS. (1990). Is vitamin D deficiency a risk factor of prostate cancer? (Hypothesis). *Anticancer Res*. Vol. 10, No. 5A, (September 1990), pp. 1307-11, ISSN 0250-7005

Pienta, KJ., Nguyen, NM. & Lehr JE. (1993). Treatment of prostate cancer in the rat with the synthetic retinoid fenretinide. *Cancer Res*. Vol. 53, No. 2, (January 1993), pp. 224-6, ISSN 0008-5472

Young, CY., Murtha, PE., Andrews, PE., Lindzey, JK. & Tindall DJ. (1994). Antagonism of androgen action in prostate tumor cell by retinoic acid. *Prostate*. Vol. 25, No. 1, (July 1994), pp. 39-45, ISSN 0270-4137

Hedlund, TE., Moffatt, KA., Uskokovic, MR. & Miller, GJ. (1997). Three synthetic vitamin D analogues induce prostate-specific acid phosphatase and prostate-specific antigen while inhibiting the growth of human prostate cancer cell in a vitamin D receptor-dependent fashion. *Clin Cancer Res*. Vol. 3, No. 8, (August 1997), pp. 1331-8, ISSN 1078-0432

Beer, TM., Lemmon, D., Lowe, BA., & Henner, WD. (2003). High-dose weekly oral calcitriol in patients with a rising PSA after prostatectomy or radiation for prostate carcinoma. *Cancer*. Vol. 97, No. 5, (March 2003), pp. 1217-24 ISSN 1097-0142

Clark, LC., Combs, GF Jr., Turnbull, BW., Slate, EH., Chalker, DK., Chow, J., Davis, LS., Glover, RA., Graham, GF., Gross, EG., Krongrad, A., Lesher, JL Jr., Park, HK., Sanders, BB Jr., Smith, CL. & Taylor JR. (1996). Effects of selenium supplementation for cancer prevention in patients with carcinoma of the skin. *JAMA* Vol. 276, No. 24, (December 1996), pp. 1957-63, ISSN 0098-7484

Fotsis, T., Pepper, M., Adlercreutz, H., Fleischmann, G., Hase, T., Montesano, R. & Schweigerer, L. (1993). Genistein, a dietary-derived inhibitor of in vitro angiogenesis. *Proc Natl Acad Sci USA*. Vol. 90, No. 7, (April 1993), pp. 2690-4, ISSN 0027-8424

Adlercreutz, H., Markkanen, H. & Watanabe, S. (1993). Plasma concentrations of phytooestrogens in Japanese men. *Lancet*. Vol. 342, No. 8881, (November 1993), pp. 1209-10, ISSN 0140-6736

Knekt, P., Aromaa, A., Maatela, J., Alfthan, G., Aaran, RK., Hakama, M., Hakulinen, T., Peto, R. & Teppo L. (1990). Serum selenium and subsequent risk of cancer among Finnish men and women. *J Natl Cancer Inst*. Vol. 82, No. 10, (May 1990), pp. 864-8, ISSN 0027-8874

The Alpha-Tocopherol, Beta-Carotene Cancer Prevention Study Group. (1994). The effect of vitamin E and 3-carotene on the incidence of lung cancer and other cancers in male smokers. *N Engl J Med*. Vol. 330, No. 15, (April 1994), pp. 1029-35, ISSN 0028-4793

Ledesma, MC., Jung-Hynes, B., Schmit, TL., Kumar, R., Mukhtar, H. & Ahmad, N. (2011). Selenium and vitamin E for prostate cancer: post-SELECT (Selenium and Vitamin E Cancer Prevention Trial) status. *Mol Med*. Vol.17, No. 1-2, (January-February 2011), pp. 134-43, ISSN 1076-1551

Giovannucci, E., Rimm, EB., Liu, Y., Leitzmann, M., Wu, K., Stampfer, MJ. & Willett WC. (2003). Body mass index and risk of prostate cancer in U.S. health professionals. *J Natl Cancer Inst*. Vol. 95, No. 16, (August 2003), pp. 1240-4, ISSN 0027-8874

Rapp, K., Schroeder, J., Klenk, J., Stoehr, S., Ulmer, H., Concin, H., Diem, G., Oberaigner, W., & Weiland SK. (2005). Obesity and incidence of cancer: a large cohort study of over 145,000 adults in Austria. *Br J Cancer*. Vol. 93, No. 9, (October 2005), pp. 1062-7 ISSN 0007-0920

Andersson, SO., Wolk, A., Bergström, R., Adami, HO., Engholm, G., Englund, A. & Nyrén O. (1997). Body size and prostate cancer: a 20-year follow-up study among 135006 Swedish construction workers. *J Natl Cancer Inst*. Vol. 89, No. 5, (March 1997), pp. 385-9 ISSN 0027-8874

Strom, SS., Wang, X., Pettaway, CA., Logothetis, CJ., Yamamura, Y., Do, KA., Babaian, RJ. & Troncoso P. (2005). Obesity, weight gain, and risk of biochemical failure among prostate cancer patients following prostatectomy. *Clin Cancer Res*. Vol. 11, No. 19, (October 2005), pp. 6889-94 ISSN 1078-0432

Freedland, SJ., Giovannucci, E. & Platz, EA. (2006) Are Findings from Studies of Obesity and Prostate Cancer Really in Conflict? *Cancer Causes Control*. Vol. 17, No. 1, (February 2006) pp. 5–9, ISSN 0957-5243

Lewis, SJ., Murad, A., Chen, L., Davey Smith, G., Donovan, J., Palmer, T., Hamdy, F., Neal, D., Lane, JA., Davis, M., Cox, A. & Martin RM. (2010) Associations between an obesity related genetic variant (FTO rs9939609) and prostate cancer risk. *PLoS One*. Vol. 19, No. 10, (October 2010), pp. e13485 ISSN 1932-6203

Brown, MD., Hart, CA., Gazi, E., Bagley, S. & Clarke, NW. (2006). Promotion of prostatic metastatic migration towards human bone marrow stoma by Omega 6 and its inhibition by Omega 3 PUFAs. *Br J Cancer*. Vol. 94, No. 6, (March 2006), pp. 842–53, ISSN 0007-0920

Platz, EA., Leitzmann, MF., Visvanathan, K., Rimm, EB., Stampfer, MJ., Willett, WC. & Giovannucci E. (2006). Statin drugs and risk of advanced prostate cancer. *J Natl Cancer Inst*. Vol. 98, No. 24, (December 2006), pp. 1819–25, ISSN 0027-8874

Massengill, JC., Sun, L., Moul, JW., Wu, H., McLeod, DG., Amling, C., Lance, R., Foley, J., Sexton, W., Kusuda, L., Chung, A., Soderdahl, D. & Donahue T. (2003). Pretreatment total testosterone level predicts pathological stage in patients with localized prostate cancer treated with radical prostatectomy. *J Urol*. Vol. 169, No. 5, (May 2003), pp. 1670–5, ISSN 0022-5347

Schatzl, G., Madersbacher, S., Thurridl, T., Waldmüller, J., Kramer, G., Haitel, A. & Marberger, M. (2001). High-grade prostate cancer is associated with low serum testosterone levels. *Prostate*. Vol. 47, No. 1, (April 2001), pp. 52–8, ISSN 0270-4137

Snowdon, DA., Phillips, RL. & Choi, W. (1984). Diet, obesity, and risk of fatal prostate cancer. *Am J Epidemiol*. Vol. 120, No. 2, (August 1984), pp. 244-50, ISSN 0002-9262

Chyou, PH., Nomura, AM. & Stemmermann GN. (1994). A prospective study of weight, body mass index and other anthropometric measurements in relation to site-specific cancers. *Int J Cancer*. Vol. 57, No. 3, (May 1994), pp. 313-7, ISSN 1097-0215

Rodriguez, C., Freedland, SJ., Deka, A., Jacobs, EJ., McCullough, ML., Patel, AV., Thun, MJ. & Calle, EE. (2007). Body mass index, weight change, and risk of prostate cancer in the Cancer Prevention Study II Nutrition Cohort. *Cancer Epidemiol Biomarkers Prev*. Vol. 16, No. 1, (January 2007), pp. 63-9, ISSN 1055-9965

Schuurman, AG., Goldbohm, RA., Dorant, E. & van den Brandt, PA. (2000). Anthropometry in relation to prostate cancer risk in the Netherlands Cohort Study. *Am J Epidemiol*. Vol. 151, No. 6, (March 2000), pp. 541-9, ISSN 0002-9262

Nilsen, TI. & Vatten, LJ. (1999). Anthropometry and prostate cancer risk: a prospective study of 22,248 Norwegian men. *Cancer Causes Control*. Vol. 10, No. 4, (August 1999), pp. 269-75 ISSN 0957-5243

Major, JM., Klonoff-Cohen, HS., Pierce, JP., Slymen, DJ., Saltzstein, SL., Macera, CA., Mercola, D. & Kattan MW. (2011). Prostate cancer postoperative nomogram scores and obesity. *PLoS One*. Vol. 6, No. 2, (February 2011), pp. e17382 ISSN 1932-6203

Hsing, AW., Sakoda, LC. & Chua, S Jr. (2007). Obesity, metabolic syndrome, and prostate cancer. *Am J Clin Nutr*. Vol. 86, No. 3, (September 2007), pp. 843–57, ISSN 0002-9165

Prabhat, P., Tewari, R., Natu, SM., Dalela, D., Goel, A., Tandon, P., Goel, MM. & Singh, K. Is central obesity, hyperinsulinemia and dyslipidemia associated with high-grade prostate cancer? A descriptive cross-sectional study. *Indian J Urol*. Vol. 26, No. 4, (October 2010), pp. 502-6 ISSN 0970-1591

Hedlund, TE. & Miller, GJ. (1994). A serum-free defined medium capable of supporting growth of four established human prostatic carcinoma cell lines. *Prostate*. Vol. 24, No. 5, (May 1994), pp. 221–8, ISSN 0270-4137

Gong, Z., Agalliu, I., Lin, DW., Stanford, JL. & Kristal, AR. (2007) Obesity is associated with increased risks of prostate cancer metastasis and death after initial cancer diagnosis in middle-aged men. *Cancer*. Vol. 109, No. 6, (March 2007), pp. 1192–202, ISSN ISSN 1097-0142

Freedland, SJ., Grubb, KA., Yiu, SK., Humphreys, EB., Nielsen, ME., Mangold, LA., Isaacs, WB. & Partin, AW. (2005). Obesity and risk of biochemical progression following radical prostatectomy at a tertiary care referral center. *J Urol*. Vol. 174, No. 3, (September 2005), pp. 919-22, ISSN 0022-5347

Cleffi, S., Neto, AS., Reis, LO., Maia, P., Fonseca, F., Wroclawski, ML., Neves, M., Pompeo, AC., Del Giglio, A., Faria, EF. & Tobias-Machado, M. (2011) Androgen Deprivation Therapy And Morbid Obesity: Do They Share Cardiovascular Risk Through Metabolic Syndrome? *Actas Urol Esp*. Vol. 35, No. 5, (May 2011), pp. 259-265, ISSN 0210-4806

Bryniarski, P., Paradysz, A. & Fryczkowski, M. PSA mass as a marker of prostate cancer progression after radical prostatectomy. (2011). *Med Sci Monit*. Vol. 17, No. 2, (February 2011), pp. 104-9, ISSN 1234-1010

Boer, P. (1984). Estimated lean body mass as an index for normalization of body fluid volumes in humans. *Am J Physiol*. Vol. 247, No. 4 Pt 2, (October 1984), pp. 632-6, ISSN 0363-6135

Du Bois, D. & Du Bois, EF. (1916) A formula to estimate the approximate surface area if height and weight be known. *Arch Intern Med*. Vol. 17, No. 5, (October 1916), pp. 863-871, ISSN 0899-9007

Spangler, E., Zeigler-Johnson, CM., Coomes, M., Malkowicz, SB., Wein, A. & Rebbeck, TR. (2007). Association of obesity with tumor characteristics and treatment failure of prostate cancer in African-American and European American men. *J Urol*. Vol. 178, No. 5, (November 2007), pp. 1939-44, ISSN 0022-5347

Bray, GA. (2006). Obesity: the disease. *J Med Chem*. Vol. 49, No. 14, (July 2006), pp. 4001-7, ISSN 0022-2623

Hsing, AW., Reichardt, JK. & Stanczyk, FZ. (2002). Hormones and prostate cancer: current perspectives and future directions. *Prostate*. Vol. 52, No. 3, (August 2002), pp. 213-35, ISSN 0270-4137

Kaaks, R., Lukanova, A. & Sommersberg, B. (2000). Plasma androgens, IGF-1, body size, and prostate cancer risk: a synthetic review. *Prostate Cancer Prostatic Dis.* Vol. 3, No. 3, (November 2000), pp. 157-72, ISSN 1365-7852

Baillargeon, J., Pollock, BH., Kristal, AR., Bradshaw, P., Hernandez, J., Basler, J., Higgins, B., Lynch, S., Rozanski, T., Troyer, D. & Thompson, I. (2005). The association of body mass index and prostate-specific antigen in a population-based study. *Cancer.* Vol. 103, No. 5, (March 2005), pp. 1092-5, ISSN 1097-0142

Freedland, SJ., Platz, EA., Presti, JC Jr., Aronson, WJ., Amling, CL., Kane, CJ. & Terris, MK. (2006). Obesity, serum prostate specific antigen and prostate size: implications for prostate cancer detection. *J Urol.* Vol. 175, No. 2, (February 2006), pp. 500-4, ISSN 0022-5347

Xu, J., Meyers, DA., Sterling, DA., Zheng, SL., Catalona, WJ., Cramer, SD., Bleecker, ER. & Ohar, J. (2002). Association studies of serum prostate-specific antigen levels and the genetic polymorphisms at the androgen receptor and prostate-specific antigen genes. *Cancer Epidemiol Biomarkers Prev.* Vol. 11, No. 7, (July 2002), pp. 664-9, ISSN 1055-9965

3

Renewing Perspectives on Men's Prostate Cancer Literacy and Engagement Along the Disease Continuum

Margareth Santos Zanchetta[1], Margot Kaszap[2], Marko Monteiro[3], Franklin Gorospe IV[4] and Roger Pilon[5]
[1]*Ryerson University, Faculty of Community Services*
Daphne Cockwell School of Nursing, Toronto, ON
[2]*University Laval, Faculty of Education, Quebec, QC*
[3]*State University of Campinas, Dept. of Science and Technology Policy, Campinas, SP*
[4]*Humber Institute of Technology and Advanced Learning, School of Health Sciences*
Nursing Program & University Health Network - Toronto General Hospital, Toronto, ON
[5]*Laurentian University, School of Nursing, Sudbury, ON*
[1,2,4,5]*Canada*
[3]*Brazil*

1. Introduction

In this chapter, we intend to familiarize readers with the complex scope of the experience of being a man with prostate cancer in current societies and dealing with scientific and popular health knowledge related to prostate cancer. We discuss issues of taking care of one's male body, being an older learner learning while facing a chronic degenerative disease, as well as the questions that social and health care professionals may encounter from men in providing meaningful health care. The provision of health care to men seems controversial, due to the lack of national policies on men's health in most countries as well as scarcity of men's health promotion programs in multicultural societies.

This chapter presents a brief overview of the state of knowledge about masculinities and gender, health literacy, and age - all major social determinants of health for men. The authors of each section present scientific knowledge produced in their qualitative research to contextualize other scholars' ideas and arguments. At the end of each section are clinical vignettes and reflection questions related to the contents of each section.

2. Men, masculinities, health and prostate cancer: Complex technology, body control, and decision making

In this section we address the issue of control that may coexist with other needs facing men, from prostate cancer detection through rehabilitation. Being in control relates to both the social enactments of masculinities and to how men understand current trends in health and technology. Control has been discussed as an important signifier of virility in different cultural contexts (Almeida, 1996; Bourdieu, 2001) and as a factor in men's perception of their bodies and assessment of the emotional and physiological care they receive. For men, losing control is seen as a negative experience, which may lead to negative experiences of preventative methods or care (Courtenay, 2000). Control is also a powerful metaphor for how current medicine, through increasingly technological interventions in the body, is being shaped by technoscience (Clarke et al., 2003; Steinberg, 1997). This "virile" [our emphasis] biomedical agenda should be tempered by attention to what some call "subjective variables," which we call "social or cultural factors". These factors include how men experience different types of masculinities and how these experiences and values inform men's attitudes toward health (Zanchetta et al., 2010). Social/cultural factors are relevant to every aspect of health and disease, and taking them into account will open professionals' perception to the complexity and richness of gender-related experiences of health practices.

2.1 Control in men's studies

The issue of control in the context of men's health is rooted in the upsurge of so-called men's studies in international academic literature, an upsurge that followed debates about gender in what is now known as the second wave of feminism (Butler, 1990; Scott, 1989). Men's studies tried to consider seriously the feminist claim that gender was not only about women, but should involve a close analysis of the relationships between genders. In addition, power relations emerged as a concomitant issue in debates about control. Such relations were not only analyzed in terms of how men relate to women, but also how men relate among themselves, and any claims that biology determined gender practices and power relations were to be vigorously denied. Gender was to be seen as socially constructed, not necessarily derivative of one's biological make-up. Men's studies scholars believed gender relationships are pervasive in our understanding of the world and that, therefore, our practices are deeply influenced by gendered understandings (Courtenay, 2000; Monteiro, 2000, 2001).

Studies of masculinities or men's studies became an important, separate subfield in the early 1980s and 1990s, especially in North America, Western Europe, and Australia (Carrigan et al., 1985; Cornwall & Lindisfarne, 1994; Gilmore, 1990; Kimmel, 1987). Masculinity was then increasingly incorporated into critical discourse on gender and power, instead of being an unquestioned universal category within discourse, culture, and politics (Monteiro, 2000). Authors began to discuss the unequal distribution of power between men and women, and among men themselves. The idea of hegemonic masculinities (Connell, 1995) became central to studies of masculinities, for example, because it enabled both deconstruction of masculinity as a uniform category that could be applied to all men and a discussion of power inequalities that affected men. Without construing men as merely victims of social expectations, these discussions opened up talk about plural masculinities in the study of men.

2.2 Masculinity, health, and prostate cancer

When discussing diversity among men, it then became important to address the challenges involved in becoming a man. Different masculinities are not purely biological or self-evident; they emerge in a process that is at the same time social, cultural, historical, etc. With the process of becoming a man seen as a process of men incorporating certain expectations, social roles, and practices (Bourdieu, 1997, 2001), masculinities can then be seen as also problematic, complex, and sometimes burdensome to men and their health. When men are viewed as a diverse group, with some men having better access to social prestige and power than other men and women, dynamics of gender and gender inequality become clearer and richer. Also, viewing men as diverse enables exploration of links between gender dynamics and health, a research agenda in progress.

Researchers pursuing this agenda has begun to explore the close relationships between masculinities and health (Courtenay, 2000), in the sense that gender perceptions and gender-related differences aid in explaining differences in health risks, and how health practices play a role in gender differences. Taking care of oneself, for example, might be considered effeminate in some contexts, leading to higher incidence of easily preventable diseases. When men embody masculinities that promote risky behavior as proof of virility, sexual conquests or failure to use condoms may put men (and their sexual partners) at higher risk for sexually transmitted diseases. In the case of prostate cancer, both the fear of bodily fragility (before and after treatment) and a masculinity that discourages care may be relevant to understanding how men experience their bodies and diseases (Mahalik et al., 2007).

Lohan (2007) suggests that, rather than focusing on men's studies and concepts such as hegemonic masculinities, researchers should embrace critical studies on men, a research area more attuned to feminist critiques of gender and power relations in society, in order to assess which factors explain how gender and health connect. Critical studies on men not only incorporate culture and behavior, but contextualize discussions of men's health in a wider explanatory framework including psychological, biological, and other factors. This context can be relevant to increasingly technological health interventions that regard differences (such as race and gender) in different terms than traditional health interventions. As biological difference becomes understood in genetic terms, for example, and as health research incorporates these advances in genetics, researchers of men's health will need to rethink how health, biology, and bodily differences are being lived in real life by men.

Men's experiences with health and prostate cancer should not be understood in a merely cultural register, however. Although cultural factors, such as the idea of "men don't cry" [our emphasis], are very important in understanding how men experience prostate cancer and care (Chapple & Ziebland, 2002), embodied factors, such as side effects of surgical and other interventions, reduce men's sense of their own virility (Chapple & Ziebland, 2002). Understanding embodied factors demands an understanding of masculinities that goes beyond social construction and embraces the complex interaction of many factors. Masculinities contradict each other, vary locally and nationally, and comprise complex hierarchies, for example (Connell & Messerschmidt, 2005; Wall & Kristjanson, 2005). They are also deeply infused with technology in varied contexts (Mellstrom, 2004).

2.3 Control in men's health-related experiences

Men's need and search for control, and attempts to be in control, suggest avenues to understanding the context for possible associations of cultural, embodied, and technological factors in men's experiences with prostate cancer. Such complex associations, because they help to constitute men's emotional and embodied experiences with disease and gender, may be crucial to understanding how men experience disease and recovery differently and thus how successful prevention and treatment can be. Control is multifaceted for men: Control over one's body and its diseases; control over other men, over women, over one's feelings, and over the public sphere, are some examples. As part of performing masculinities successfully, men generally avoid situations where they may lose control. Such situations may include preventive care and other actions that may improve health or prospects for survival (Kimmel, 1995; Lohan, 2007). Control is also at stake in current medical interventions, where advances in genetics, nanotechnology and other fields potentially enable control over every bodily process (Channel, 1991; Hogle, 2005). Proponents of this "virile" [our emphasis] approach to health and disease, we argue, need to pay attention to the complexity of men's lived experiences and gender differences in order to enhance the approach's effectiveness.

2.4 Control and the delivery of health care

Control is a general trend in how health and disease are being tackled by modern, techno-scientific medicine. The trend, called "bio-medicalization" (Clarke et al., 2003) describes how techno-science is becoming the dominant framework through which the concepts of health and the body are understood, as well as how health interventions are researched and used (Hogle, 2005; Lenoir, 2002a; Lenoir, 2002b). Bio-medicalization frames many health-related actions, from how we perceive the body visually, to the increasing use of technologies that make body interiors available for display and intervention (Taylor, 2005; Van Dijck, 2005), to ways of designing bodily interventions that are increasingly mediated by technology (Lenoir, 2004). This trend toward the incorporation of technology in health is increasingly evident as genetics becomes a dominant language to describe and understand diseases, including diabetes (Hedgecoe, 2002), cancer (Chung et al., 2002; Fujimura, 1996; Monteiro, 2009), and many others (Fullwiley, 2007). Not only has prostate cancer begun to be reinterpreted as a genetic disease, along with cancer in general, but the search is ongoing for genes to classify prostate cancer, diagnose it early, and refine surgical interventions (Shen & Abate-Shen, 2010). As prostate cancer becomes "molecularized" (Monteiro, 2009), its amenability to intervention is also transforming (Monteiro, 2011).

With a new, biomedical and techno-scientific approach to health and disease, control over bodily processes has been sought in ways unimaginable in the past. From increasingly precise interventions in the body, to the search for genes that would enable early diagnosis and even modeling of future behavior (Monteiro & Keating, 2009), control is at the center of how health is understood and practiced today. This effort to control bodily processes through increasingly sophisticated technology may, however, ignore the particularities of gender and masculinities, as discussed above. Nonetheless, an approach to prostate cancer that relies increasingly on techno-science to classify, diagnose, and surgically intervene can offer exciting new ways to approach the disease. Improving outcomes and enabling new methods for treatment and diagnosis will hopefully help circumvent some of the barriers towards self-care present in traditional masculinities, which usually see self-care as contrary to an ideal of the male body as impenetrable. New genetic tests could replace existing methods for examining the prostate, which many men find invasive. Establishing molecular bio-markers for prostate cancer that could reliably establish risk for the disease, for example, may enable early diagnosis, early treatment, and higher survival rates. Bio-markers would avoid, for example, uncomfortable examinations and unreliable prostate-specific-antigen (PSA) tests. However, an assumption of technological progress overlooks the many pitfalls such technology-based treatments could face. For instance, given discussion on the centrality of socio-cultural factors in explaining how men relate to their bodies and to health, it is not certain whether men will accept the idea of knowing in advance their risks for cancer. They may fear of loss of control over their health or fear becoming cancer "patients in waiting" at an early age before any cancer symptoms appear (Rajan, 2006). Mere knowledge that one carries genes that make one susceptible to cancer does not necessarily lead men to adopt preventive behavior. Indeed, it is clear that men avoid such behavior due to social expectations (Mahalik et al., 2007). Also, risks inherent in currently available prostate-cancer treatments are problematic for many men, in spite of any other considerations relating to their knowledge about preventing and monitoring cancer (Chapple & Ziebland, 2002).

When powerful trends to reinterpret health and disease in terms of new technologies (genetic or otherwise) dominate, researchers run the risk of ignoring the rich debate over socio-cultural factors that affect gender and health/disease. Although new technologies offer wonderful prospects for diagnosis and treatment, social factors such as gender, behavior, and culture should not be underestimated in terms of their contributions to understanding health and risk behaviors. Control, an attribute of hegemonic masculinity, is often associated with science and technology (two very male-dominated fields in some respects). This traditionally Western logic should be enriched with an understanding of how culture, society, and history explain health, disease, and treatment.

This debate about control, genetics, and technology is meaningful to social and health professionals who care for and advise men and their significant others throughout the prostate-cancer trajectory. Professionals should reflect on their beliefs about masculinity and prostate cancer, and their professional practice. Knowing that control is central to many men's experiences of masculinity, professionals should take a cautionary approach when presenting decision aids and discussing options about which they ask men to make immediate decisions. Caution is recommended mainly when men make decisions without professional guidance, because men may postpone reflection in favor of taking immediate action, thereby trying to demonstrate autonomy and willingness to decide. Men have been highly influenced by medicalization of erectile dysfunction in advertising for sexual-performance-enhancing drugs, advertising that focuses on the social importance of erections to virility. Therefore, professionals need to expand their understanding of the values and meaning that men attribute to diseases that threaten their sense of masculinity, and therefore their sexual and emotional health.

2.5 Informing professional practice

Knowledge of multiple aspects of culture, society, and history is important to help social and health professionals decode behavior expected of men as engaged partners in their own treatment and rehabilitation. Societies are becoming more and more multicultural, giving men opportunities to learn new meanings of being a man, and new attitudes to men's health, men's self-care, men's sexuality, and facts and myths related to prostate cancer (Zanchetta et al., 2010). For professionals, it is difficult to gather scientific evidence on men's behaviors, due to men's resistance to participating in clinical and behavioral studies (Deslauriers & Deslauriers, 2010). Again, gender-related discourse and perceived lack of control over data-collection encounters may affect men's participation in studies. To counteract resistance, researchers recommend allowing men to feel in control of their disclosure of personal information, such as feelings, fears, disagreeable symptoms, threatening thoughts, and awareness of uncertainties (Deslauriers & Deslauriers, 2010). Such research fieldwork strategies may also be helpful for assessment and follow-up interviews in clinical contexts, where professionals can use a conversational style with men, instead of a professional authoritative style of asking direct and probing questions. Despite a culturally and socially constructed trend of men being attracted to technology (Lerman et al., 2003;

Mellstrom, 2004) and technological advances in prostate-cancer-risk identification, early detection, treatment, and rehabilitation, men still perceive that technological interventions reduce their capacity to control the responses of their bodies and emotions to such interventions (Chapple & Ziebland, 2002).

Widespread public access to prostate cancer information in popular and scientific media has uncovered current discourse surrounding uncertainty about prostate cancer among researchers and health care professionals. Certainly, men are less likely to trust the health care system's assurance that current technologies are helpful and to rely on information from health care professionals in their decision making. Regardless of men's personal level of education and health literacy, they should be supported in enhancing their ability to perceive and differentiate levels of risk when making informed decisions about treatments. Gender-related experiences are, again, important to consider in the clinical context, because men's health experiences tend not to be solitary. Men's experiences are, instead, influenced by the roles of women (mothers, wives, partners, daughters, nieces, aunts, etc.) and other caring figures (fathers, same-sex partners, coaches, etc.) in their lives. Together, caring figures influence men's decisions to seek medical help, adhere to treatments, and most important, transcend the limitations and changes imposed by prostate cancer. Such a collective view of men's health experiences challenges current organizational policies requiring that personal information remain private and neglects the social and cultural fact that men are human beings, who (in less publicly demonstrative ways than women) are influenced by intimate others in seeking health and well being (Zanchetta et al., 2010).

2.6 Reflecting on control in men's experiences with prostate cancer screening

Below are some true stories with fictitious names as clinical vignettes and reflection questions to help readers identify control as a key concept in men's experience of prostate cancer and reflect on how control plays out in clinical practice. No answers are provided, because we want to stimulate readers' recall of their own experience so that they can construct appropriate answers to the reflection questions.

2.6.1 Clinical vignettes

- John, a 56-year-old accountant, was urged by his wife to get screened for prostate cancer. After months of postponing his decision, he agrees to make an appointment for an annual physical. During the history taking, he tells the doctor that he feels fine and does not understand why he should have a physical. John says, "If it isn't broken, why fix it?"
- Charles, a 50-year-old engineer, comes to the clinic for his annual physical and discusses prostate screening with his family doctor. They discuss the merits of DRE versus PSA testing. His doctor explains both screening tests. Charles is reluctant to have a DRE test, given the invasive nature of the procedure. In spite of the information his doctor provides about the limited sensitivity and specificity of the PSA test, Charles decided to have the PSA test done, because he believes that it will be less invasive than the DRE test.
- Silvio, a 50-year-old computer designer, is a newcomer to Canada who speaks and understands English at an intermediate level. After arriving, he looked for a family doctor to monitor a recurrent inflammation in his prostate as well as have his annual PSA test. Due to pain and urinary troubles, the doctor ordered an abdominal

ultrasound. Silvio remembers that he barely understood his doctor`s explanations about the ultrasound. He had it in a hospital without any problems but is worried about the presence of blood in his urine for the last 5 days, which he does not understand. He believes that the doctor "saw something" during the ultrasound. He feels lost, with no clues about his situation and really wants to do something about that. Unfortunately, he must wait three to four weeks for a follow-up medical consultation.

2.6.2 Questions

- Why is control important when it comes to men's health?
- What strategies could health care professionals consider that might promote men's empowerment as active participants in planning preventative health actions for prostate cancer and its treatment?
- What barriers might contribute to men feeling a loss of control over early detection of prostate cancer?

3. A contemporary view of educating elders for health: Insights for educational practice in clinical and community settings

This section focuses on the relationship between older people and health education, as it relates to men with prostate cancer. Men's knowledge and understanding of learning about health, both in a biomedical and socio-cultural sense, is essential during the prostate cancer trajectory. Davis et al. (2008) discuss the importance for health care professionals of recognizing factors that contribute to elder's low health literacy, which may be increasing. Health literacy is a central to successful communication between health care professionals and elderly patients. It is not only essential for elderly patients to be equipped with appropriate knowledge of the disease process so as to be actively involved in their care, but health education must support patients to become more autonomous. Education for empowerment, as pioneered by Paulo Freire, requires a health education process centered in dialog between educators and learners (Wallerstein & Bernstein, 1988). Educating today's older people about cancer requires new educational strategies, particularly new education technologies that simplify complex cancer information and facilitate learning. Older people are active users of computers and the internet; misconceptions to the contrary must not shape health care professionals' beliefs about older people's ability to learn about their health (Alpay et al., 2004).

3.1 Older patients' acquisition of formative learning

A discussion involving knowledge and learning implies talking about "alphabetization" and literacy, or even about various literacy levels and literacy backgrounds. Traditionally, literacy was defined in general terms but, currently, we tend to differentiate among a range of literacy concepts. The new term "alphabetization" belongs to the old literacy paradigm in which we assessed individuals in terms of their ability to read, write, and use numbers. The goal was to rank individuals according to their literacy level, what we now call the "degree of alphabetization." Today, some literacy researchers work within a new literacy paradigm: as a social practice reflecting the literacy background of the person (Barton et al., 1998, 2000). Kaszap and Clerc (2008) clarify both alphabetization and literacy concepts and suggest how to use them.

The degree of *health alphabetization* may indicate - at a specific time in one's life - competence in searching for, identifying, collecting, understanding, critiquing, and interpreting health information. This information is used to create and communicate messages about one's health status, to make choices in preventing disease, to recover or preserve health, to solve problems related to one's health using language (written, oral, visual, audible, tactile, etc.) in a variety of contexts in day-to-day life (at the world, community, school, and individual levels). Health alphabetization can frequently be measured by tests, and other reporting and self-appraisal methods. On the other hand, the concept of *health literacy* comprises several assets (translation of Kaszap & Clerc, 2008, as cited in Kaszap & Zanchetta, 2009). First, it sums all health information acquired from family, school, social, cultural, and professional sources (formal and informal) during a continuous, gradual learning process. Second, it sums all the values, beliefs, fears, habits, attitudes, and behaviors that each person holds in all the aspects of life related to health. Third, health literacy comprises one's specific background: (a) health culture and health knowledge, (b) the type of health education to which one was exposed, individual's attitudes, behaviours, and feelings, values and beliefs; (c) practices in searching for health information, reading and decoding it, and communicating it (in oral or written form), and (d) using numerical information and health information to solve health problems in everyday life.

Seen from the above-described point of view, measurement of health literacy is neither feasible nor possible. However, it is a state, or even a set of personal practices, that can be described more or less accurately. Seen this way, health literacy can be more or less broad, more or less adequate - or inadequate- for a situation or a context. Zanchetta (2002) describes the origin of men's prostate cancer literacy as follows:

All men reported that during childhood, school and family constituted the sources of available health information during the formation of their informational background on health matters. Health information in childhood was synonymous with consuming healthy food, having good hygiene, and receiving vaccinations at school. (p. 191)

Men's learning experiences with prostate cancer build on lifelong learning about health and its incorporation into daily life. Zanchetta (2002) proposes a definition of health literacy about prostate cancer based on survivors' experiences:

Older men live and deal with health information through the handling of the imprints of their beliefs, and representations, as well as life, learning, and illness experience. For this, a supportive environment is primordial to enable them to regain the sense of illness, the decision-making power upon one's body and destiny, as well as to redefine the social roles by reconstructing partnerships with the social and informational network. (p. 294)

The definition above shows that the construction of health literacy is multidimensional and involves social factors, such as life stories, cumulative experience, social learning, autonomy, and social interactions. Seminal studies have demonstrated a strong relationship between low literacy and poor health (Brown et al., 1993; Davis et al., 1991; Francis, 1991; Mayeaux et al., 1996; Weiss et al., 1992, 1994; Weiss & Coyne, 1997) and proposed health literacy as a new social determinant of health (Rootman et al., 2007; Zanchetta et al., 2011). Therefore, we suggest that inadequate health literacy may impede other social determinants of health, which in turn may worsen one's ability to use health information in making decisions.

Considering the above-mentioned factors, we propose a conceptual framework (Figure 1) that shows alphabetization as an integral part of health literacy, within the social determinants of health. Together with a supportive environment, health literacy may influence individuals' response to particular health situations and contexts as well as their awareness of existing resources and ways to accessing them. Perlow (2010) reports that low health literacy has major impacts on health disparities and adverse health outcomes throughout the lifespan, including hospitalization, chronic disease, and higher health care costs.

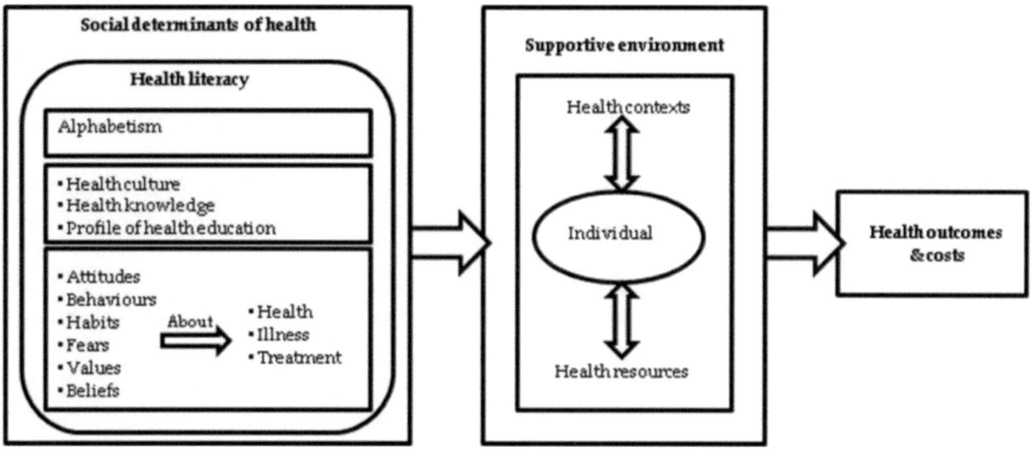

Fig. 1. The health literacy conceptual framework

With the growing elderly population in developed and developing countries, health costs (financial, human, material, physical, emotional, etc.) are anticipated to grow. The emerging worldwide movement of supporting patients to be autonomous, aware partners in health care is also leading education and health professionals to rethink the role of health educators. To promote health literacy, health educators are facing demands to renew and expand their toolboxes of educational aids and to adopt teaching innovations to sustain the mobilization of learning potential among older patients. The next section presents some considerations for health educators to think about.

3.2 Strategies in health education

Over time, health education has been done mostly in a traditional way by health professionals, according to health curricula. In this approach, information is given on disease, and treatments are explained in a "you have to" way. This approach is basically one-way knowledge transmission, from professionals to patients and not vice versa. Using this traditional approach, professionals scarcely have time to learn what health literacy patients already have. Patients do not have time to discuss their fears, values, and conceptions. The traditional approach to health education has brought with it serious problems. For example, recent research tells us that inadequate literacy often reveals misconceptions about different aspects of health, such as patient's erroneous understanding of how a body change in enduring diseases, long term effects of drugs or other treatments (Buston & Wood, 2000; Kaszap et al., 2000, 2006), and false beliefs about popular treatments (e.g., magical peas or liniments) with supposedly spectacular effects on blood pressure (Kaszap et al., 2000). With older men, health educators should take such health-related misconceptions and false beliefs into account and propose new strategies for health education.

Health education should not merely be transmission of information, because recipients of transmitted information may filter it through faulty premises; for example, misconceptions about bodies, health, and treatments and false beliefs about natural products that supposedly have miraculous effects on various diseases. Before delivering health information, health professionals should seek to understand the literacy backgrounds of older men: what they know, their beliefs, fears, habits, conceptions, and behaviors concerning their health, illness, medications, and treatments. Torres et al. (2008) reveal the importance of such exploration to understand and address the deeply rooted web of ideology, norms, and practices that influence health decision making and behavioral responses. Kruger et al. (2007) argue that professionals must ask elders questions about their functional and emotional health status. Health professionals should understand older men's "supportive environments" (Zanchetta, 2002, p. 294), comprising their families and their social and information networks. Without this baseline information about older men, health professionals will not be able to teach them appropriately, to enhance their understanding of diseases and treatment, to persuade them to follow medication and treatment regimes, or to prepare them to choose among treatment options (Kaszap & Drolet, 2009).

Transmitting information does not imply that its recipients agree with it and will immediately act upon it. New knowledge needs to be constructed. Knowledge construction means, therefore that, when new knowledge is offered, it needs to be discussed, even challenged, before it can be accepted and integrated in an individual's own existing knowledge system. Construction of health-related knowledge requires time, but taking this time will save time and money in the long run: time lost in repeated explanations, time and money lost in preventable hospitalization and preventable health deterioration. Moon (2011) explains that elder experience transformative learning with success but as a process which takes time and need support. Knowledge construction happens within relationships between older individuals and health professionals when professionals explore with elders their health backgrounds - their values, beliefs, fears, habits, attitudes, conceptions, and behaviors; and when professionals respect each patient's learning style: their individual ways of listening, asking questions and answering them. Knowledge construction also happens when explanations are meaningful (neither too technical nor childish) and use appropriate terminology, examples, or visual aids, such as photos and drawings. Concomitantly, lack of trust in relationships between health professionals and older individuals may jeopardize their engagement in teaching-learning initiatives, due their fear of disclosing personal information about their health problems (Kaszap & Drolet, 2009). Professionals need to find out about older men's misconceptions and false beliefs by asking questions about their health, illness, and treatment. By 'misconceptions', we mean erroneous explanations from erroneous understandings. By 'false beliefs', we mean beliefs based on superstitions and popular knowledge, not on scientific proof. All together, they are erroneous premises. These erroneous premises should be challenged and deconstructed prior to proposing new knowledge. Deconstructing knowledge means that professionals need to ask questions about an older man's conceptions or beliefs to be able to understand why the older man thinks the way he does. Where did he get that explanation? Then professionals need to start a dialog about both sides of the argument and give examples and explanations based on scientific knowledge. Professionals need to drive the discussion in a way that older men will adopt the scientific position because, when older people do not properly understand their disease and the needed treatments, when they are not adhering with their treatments or medication, they become severely ill and need to be hospitalized.

3.3 Evolution from existing to new educational technologies

Despite well documented challenges in educational initiatives with older learners, some researchers interested in promoting older learners' health literacy are incorporating new technological tools into health teaching to enhance learning. Most older individuals are willing to learn about new technology, even to use and master it, especially if they are under 80 years old and in good mental health (Kaszap et al., 2002; Gil-Gómez et al., 2011; Jensen et al., 2010; Mackert et al., 2009; Saposnik et al., 2010; Wallington, 2008). It seems to be just a matter of having help in learning how to use new technology and having enough time to understand and practice it. Kaszap et al. (2000), in a study exploring the experiences of rural and urban older individuals with various technologies, documented elders' preference for information-gathering contexts (see Figure 2). They preferred private contexts (such as a visit to a professional's office) for gathering information on personal matters and group

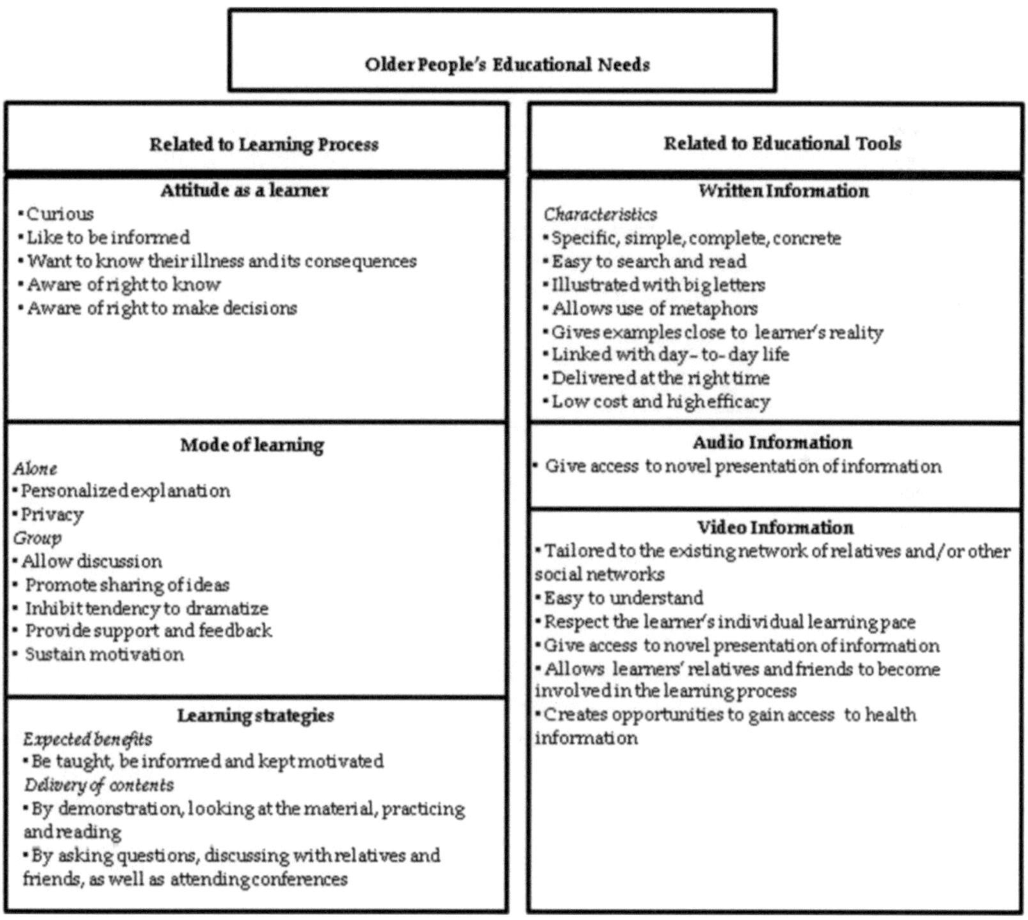

Fig. 2. Older individuals' views on different aspects of health learning

contexts (among relatives and friends, even strangers) for gathering general information about health, illness, and treatment, because belonging to a group allows discussion, idea sharing, support, and maintains motivation for continuous learning. Golding (2011) reports that older men in community settings learn when education is social, local, practical, situated, and in groups, particularly isolated men. Prins et al. (2009) argue that social interactions are needed to support elders, and Bergsma (2004) adds that personal and social change are possible through empowerment education.

In libraries nowadays, it is common to see elders looking for information on the Web, writing emails, or chatting on Skype. Community initiatives to develop computer literacy among older learners are undoubtedly opening new avenues for learning about health, for both already and newly computer-literate elders. Twenty-first century elders are becoming more familiar with technologies such as cell phones, videos, and computers. Even interactive video games (Nintendo Wii and Wii balance board) have been introduced to older patients for curative and rehabilitation purposes (Gil-Gómez et al., 2011; Saposnik et al., 2010). Elders are open to, and like, new experiences in the context of playing and exercising in rehabilitation and homecare settings. In the news, we see older people bowling via Wii to improve their balance after surgery and using Wii-based yoga and light exercise to regain vitality after hospitalization. Technological possibilities now exist that encourage elders to access information and take care of themselves in a variety of contexts. Health educators should support them through teaching older people to make use of these new opportunities for learning about health, illness, and treatments. Along with face-to-face discussion, virtual chatting can enhance older people's lives, despite any health conditions.

3.4 Rethinking prostate cancer and prostate health education

To prevent prostate cancer and deal with the disease throughout its trajectory, both prostate cancer information and prostate cancer literacy are important. The complexity of scientific knowledge make prostate cancer education with men of all ages and education levels a real challenge, in particular with older men having low degrees of alphabetization, whose social and information networks are crucial supports for decision making (Zanchetta, 2002). According to Kaszap and Drolet (2009), health literacy appraisal should explore a person's ability to acknowledge his/her own prior knowledge, current fears, beliefs, values, misconceptions, attitudes, habits, and behaviours - all of which build the foundation for constructing new knowledge. Innovations in clinical practice will certainly be needed to reveal the dynamic relationships between health knowledge, health literacy, the internet as a source of health information along with professional guidance (Jensen et al., 2010), especially for older people who are hard to reach (Macker et al., 2009), and the advantages of other technology used in rehabilitation and prostate cancer education. Levasseur and Carrier (2010) stress that rehabilitation and health literacy share goals: both see as important individuals' overall capacities for self-care, enhancing functioning, facilitating individuals' participation in their own health care, client-centered care, and equity in access to services, for example. Inspired by Zanchetta (2002) and knowledge construction theories (Jonnaert, 2009), education about prostate health can be expanded to include all men, regardless of their conceptual and experiential knowledge.

Older individuals may actively participate in transformative learning initiatives if time and supportive social interactions to foster learning are available to them (Moon, 2011; Prins et al., 2009). Support can include helping older individuals understand how to find information on the internet and how to mobilize a supportive network of groups or individuals in the community (Wallington, 2008). Health educators should use age-specific tools and elder-client-centered instructions to promote older people's health literacy (Morrow et al., 2007). Educational materials should be prepared for specific purposes and complex information delivered in forms other than writing (Roberts & Partridge, 2011), such as story telling (Wilkin & Ball-Rokeach, 2006). Discussions should using common terminology and repeat contents taught through learner-teach-back techniques. Professionals should apply medical information to topics familiar to elders (Prasauskas & Spoo, 2006), for which professionals need to understand older patients' literacy backgrounds. No more than four essential points should be provided at a time, with any written information reflecting learners' colloquial language, framed by learners' own health culture, and stating expected health behaviors (Prasauskas & Spoo, 2006).

It may take time for health professionals to learn about each elder's fears, beliefs, habits, behaviours, and conceptions of health before it is possible to discuss disease and their treatment (Orel et al., 2005). However, learning older men's communication styles and literacy backgrounds will help professionals to begin talking about prostate cancer treatment and to gain clients' trust, without inspiring too much fear. Health professionals should let older men absorb the fact that they have prostate cancer before discussing solutions - absorbing such information also takes time. The educational process should occur in several steps; otherwise it will be perceived as challenging older men's sense of masculinity. Such caution in communication is particularly relevant for physicians, who are advised to inquire, in all consultations, about older men's functional and emotional health status (Kruger et al., 2007). Finally, it is important that older men themselves examine their assumptions (about, for example, masculinity) before constructing new knowledge and accept the need to make changes in their lives; for example, they may need to change their food choices to supplement medical treatment of their prostate cancer (Mróz et al., 2011).

3.5 Reflecting on men's accounts of prostate cancer health education

In the clinical vignettes presented below we present the experiences of some older men in learning about prostate cancer, including why they sought information and how engagement in learning helped them move toward better prostate health.

3.5.1 Clinical vignettes

- Claudio, a 59-year-old flooring installer, receives a diagnosis of prostate cancer. He tells his urologist that he has no symptoms and feels just fine. Because he feels well, he is not concerned about the diagnosis and decides that he will not let this diagnosis affect him in any way. He is not interested in discussing treatment options and decides to leave the physician's office.
- When Constantin, a 67-year-old newspaper columnist, receives the diagnosis of prostate cancer, he tells his oncologist that his father had prostate cancer and experienced serious side effects from the treatment. Constantin does not want to go through what his father experienced and decides refuse any and all prostate cancer treatment offered to him. In fact, he is so concerned about possible side effects that he does not even want to discuss treatment options with the oncologist.
- When Bernardo, a 69-year-old retired parole officer, receives a diagnosis of prostate cancer, he is initially surprised. However, within a few days he tells his wife that he has gained the distinction of joining the brotherhood of prostate cancer. Bernardo is, has lived a full life and refuses to let the prostate cancer diagnosis define who he is. Bernardo has a great sense of humor and subscribes to the adage that laughter is the best medicine.

3.5.2 Questions

- What are some principles of adult learning that can guide health professionals in teaching older men about prostate cancer?
- Identify strategies that could foster learning among older men about their health and their bodies.
- What teaching strategies should health professionals consider when promoting literacy about health and prostate cancer among older men?

4. Information strategies and health behaviors related to levels of prostate-cancer literacy

In Section 3, we contextualized health literacy within the perspective of men's experiences with prostate cancer. In this section, we present the results of a qualitative study with 14 Francophone Canadian men. The study documented men's strategies for dealing with prostate cancer information and their self-rated levels of health literacy (Zanchetta, 2002). The study demonstrated that levels of health literacy were not influenced by older men's self-reported general literacy (Zanchetta et al., 2007) and that, despite differences in their levels of health literacy, older men reported similar strategies for dealing with prostate cancer information: comparison, deduction, and hypothesis formation (Zanchetta et al., 2007). These information strategies revealed the importance of communication through social, intimate, and interpersonal interactions in enhancing older men's health literacy.

4.1 Older men's construction of health literacy

Older men's health literacy is influenced by several factors, such as seeking health-related information to promote and maintain health, leading to personal empowerment (World Health Organization, 1998), reading and numeracy skills, comprehension, and decision making (Oldfield & Dreher, 2010); opportunities to obtain health-related information; concepts of masculinity (Peerson & Saunders, 2010; Zanchetta et al., 2010); and congruency between health-related information and personal views of masculinity (Zanchetta, 2002).

To guide decision making in collaboration with physicians, men with prostate cancer face great challenges in learning about and understanding their disease (Barry, 2010). Two of these uncertainties relate to prostate cancer's trajectory and the complex information patients receive about their prognosis and treatment options (Nanton et al., 2009). These uncertainties influence men's ability to participate in decision making about their care. In Zanchetta et al.'s (2007) study, men's various information strategies allowed them to participate in making decisions about their complex care. Low health literacy rates are another prominent challenge. Low health literacy rates limit men's understanding of prostate cancer information (Easton et al., 2010). Another challenge to the health literacy of men with prostate cancer is the lack of consensus among health care professionals about the most effective decision aids and the safest methods for screening and monitoring (Gwede & McDermott, 2006). Nor does consensus exist among health professionals on whether prostate cancer screening improves health outcomes (Krist et al., 2007) or what harmful consequences prostate cancer treatment has for men's physical and sexual functioning (Barry, 2010).

All of the above challenges, added to contradictions in information from health care professionals, contribute to men's confusion in trying to understand scientific discourse about prostate cancer and the impact of treatment on men's sexual function. Men's goal for learning about prostate cancer becomes clear: They seek information they can use to survive the disease, not scientific understanding of the disease process (Zanchetta et al., 2007). Erectile dysfunction, one potential consequence of prostate cancer treatment, represents failed masculinity (Knight & Latini, 2009) for men who adopt traditional masculinities. This representation undermines their motivation to learn about prostate cancer and its treatment.

4.2 A new understanding of older men's construction of prostate cancer literacy

Through a discourse analysis technique called "abduction in communication" (Boudon, 1998, 1999, 2000), reasons why men with disparate levels of education (from three years of home schooling to doctorate) used similar information strategies were identified. Three analytical assumptions guided the analysis that revealed the similarity of these cognitive processes: (a) men's attempts to connect general health information with prostate cancer information would disclose the *modus operandi* of becoming prostate cancer literate, (b) men's key motivations for learning would determine the strategies they used to construct information strategies, and (c) external factors initially considered negative, non-collaborative, and obstructive would motivate men to construct more information strategies. The results of the analysis are (presented in the rest of Section 4.2 and in Figure 3 to 6) portray how older men's use of prostate cancer information and their discourse about prostate cancer was framed by ideas of space, distance, and possibility. Men's use of information responded to their need to deal with notions of truth, lies, and the possibility of errors; plausible and non-plausible uses of information; possible and impossible decisions; fact and illusion, and so on. In addition, men dealt with how long they might live; whether they would remain in their own homes as they grew older or move to retirement homes or seniors' apartments; and where they might ultimately die.

4.2.1 Core information strategies men use to become prostate-cancer literate

Despite differences in men's self-reported levels of schooling and self-rated health literacy, with survival as an ultimate goal for learning, men looked for new informational support among peers, other individuals, relatives, media, and health professionals. Men mainly used hypothetical reasoning to decode the prostate cancer information they acquired from health professionals and informal sources (newspapers, television, internet, books, pamphlets, etc.). Men's struggles to become prostate cancer literate included reflecting on life and death as well as using the cognitive processes of hypothesizing, deducting, and comparing. To do that, they combined prostate cancer information they gathered from medical journals and their physicians with information from their own illness experiences. Figure 3 presents the general analytical categories and shows how the interpretative poles oscillate between the positive and negative impacts of decoded information related to the dimensions of health, diagnosis of prostate cancer and illness, men's socio-cultural identity, the external world, and the imprints of life and prostate cancer-related information. One of the key strategies men used to decode information was to compare information from different sources about the accuracy of medical prognoses, changes in lifestyle due to cancer, recovery expectations, and expected difficulties in end-of-life situations. As men felt more certain about the predictability of medical prognoses, some men's attitudes changed. Although some remained socially isolated, others enrolled in prostate cancer support groups, became more committed to their own health, or to men's collective health. Certainty also brought to older men a greater will to live and a peaceful acceptance of possible death from prostate cancer.

In the figures 3 to 6, the arrow going from bottom left to top right of each figure means the paradigm of understanding from a negative to a positive pole.

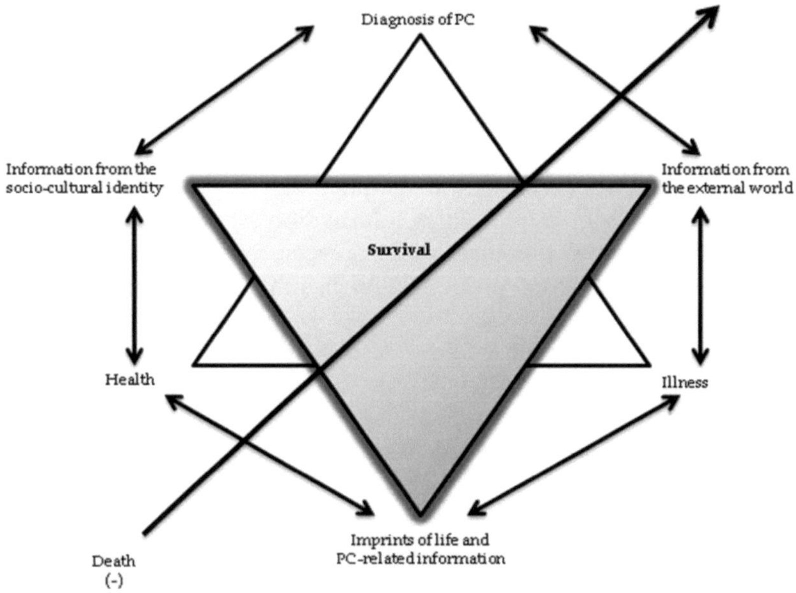

Fig. 3. General analytical categories related to core information strategies

4.2.2 Strategies for dealing with prostate cancer-related information within the paradigm of health literacy

Older men also used their new prostate-cancer health literacy to create multiple possibilities for living with prostate cancer. They used their accumulated knowledge to transform previous representations about life after prostate cancer and the disease itself. From their contacts with other individuals in their social networks, men learned how to survive better and longer with prostate cancer. Particularly relevant in this transformation were information exchanges with other prostate cancer survivors, sharing information with undiagnosed men, and new information provided by significant others.

Analysis of men's accounts of exchanges of information also revealed controversies about whether information gathered through the process mentioned above actually contributed to men's prostate cancer literacy. First, older men seemed to be more interested in communicating information and personal experiences with prostate cancer than in the process of learning itself. Second, partial, imprecise, or superficial information about prostate cancer could either stagnate or propel older men's learning about prostate cancer. Third, the hypotheses (deductive and inductive) those men generated after contact with prostate cancer information impelled them to either confirm or refute the hypotheses. In doing so, older men built the core of their interpretative logic and thereby created meaning out of their experiences with prostate cancer. The information strategies thus fueled men's determination to transform all future contact they had with prostate cancer information. Figure 4 presents how men compared their situations with those of other individuals living with cancer and, whether they had low or high levels of health literacy, formed hypotheses, made comparisons, and decisions.

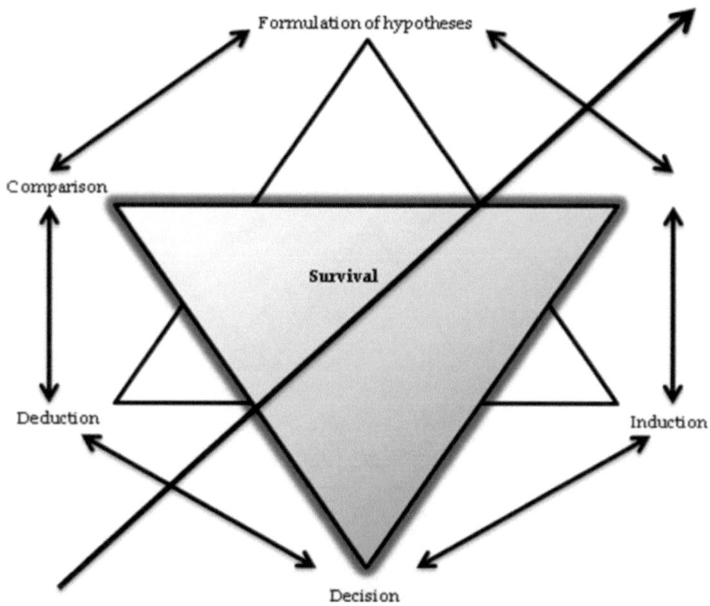

Fig. 4. Strategies for dealing with prostate cancer-related information

4.2.3 Strategies men use to make sense of prostate cancer information

Men's use of hypothesizing and of deductive and inductive reasoning varied in intensity and frequency, depending on older men's self-rated level of health literacy and the uncertainty they faced about their medical conditions. Men's use of these analytical techniques was congruent with their tendency to assess information logically by seeking to understand events and facts and by decoding large amounts of (sometimes contradictory) prostate cancer information. The intensity and frequency of men's hypothesizing, deduction, and induction seemed to be associated with the importance they attributed to the process of decision making, regardless of its domain. The cognitive processes of hypothesizing and deducting also influenced men's acceptance or refusal of prostate cancer information, because men selected information based on their values. Selecting, valuing, and incorporating prostate cancer information, and other information indirectly related to prostate cancer, can be explained by men's increasing interest in information seeking. Men's main focus was learning what to do to ensure their survival and how to do it. This focus led men to value what could help them understand clinical facts. Men sought to find, in each piece of prostate cancer information, anything that could contribute to a pragmatic plan for surviving cancer. Men valued information that was personally relevant to them and could contribute to decision-making. In this information-selection process, men's participation in information networks and the information support that they received from significant others were important.

Men's constant hypothesizing seemed to be an attempt to understand and compare information from multiple sources, information that created doubts in their minds. With these doubts, men constantly struggled to reduce abstraction and uncertainty in the information they gathered. The difficulty with abstraction related most often to descriptions of cellular processes and cell-level responses to treatment, as expressed by levels of PSA, prostate cancer recurrence, and metastasis. Without being able to understand this complex information, men could not evaluate its pertinence and quality.

Men needed to evaluate this information to construct meaning by comparing it to their own health experiences, as well as with health and prostate cancer information they had already gathered. Figure 5 displays the key factors that influenced the way older men lived with prostate cancer information.

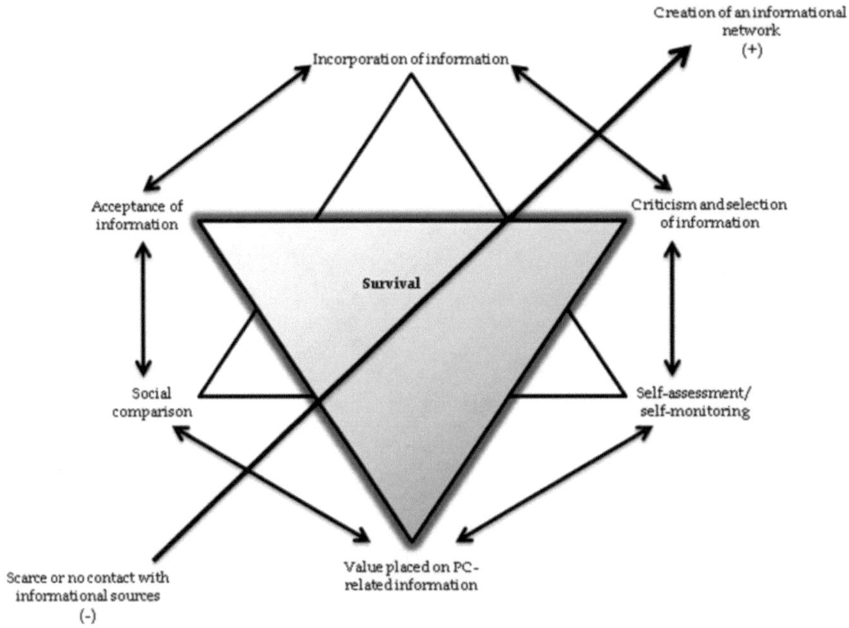

Fig. 5. Key factors influencing the way men live with prostate cancer-related information

4.2.4 Key factors underlying older men's information strategies

For older men, the utility of all information men found relevant was its contribution to solving problems, filling knowledge gaps, and helping men learn how to live with prostate cancer. The relevance individual men attributed to information revealed differences among older men in their critical attitudes to the information they gathered. Men either focused on analyzing the information's technical content or applied the information to political and collective aspects of men's experiences with prostate cancer.

These critical attitudes revealed how men came in contact with and joined information networks to explore their social environments. Men who had little or no contact with sources of health information other than their urologists lived in cognitive isolation. On the other hand, men who gradually constructed networks comprising health professionals (other than urologists) and lay people slowly incorporated new knowledge into their lives through collective learning and exchanging experiences, knowledge that supplemented and complemented information from their urologists.

Incorporation of information into men's lives was a goal shared by men with prostate cancer and other individuals who were directly or indirectly involved with their new lives after medical recovery. Before being able to decode prostate cancer information, some men confronted the reality that other men and women live with cancer that was more or less severe than theirs. This confrontation raised men's awareness of the potential impact of prostate cancer on their own lives. Comparing their lives to the lives of others allowed men to ascertain the relevance of prostate cancer information and incorporate it into their daily lives, specifically into self-assessment and self-monitoring. Men valued information that responded to their pragmatic needs, rather than theoretical information that was difficult to decode. Once they found enough information to answer their questions, men stopped searching.

The quality of prostate cancer information was another factor men used to evaluate the credibility of information sources and whether or not to accept information from them. When men perceived new information to be high quality, even if it contradicted information that they deemed valuable, they were open to comparing it to contradictory information. The issues of quality, criticism, and acceptance explained men's unwavering acceptance of medical diagnoses of prostate cancer, their strong tendency not to seek second medical opinions, and their unconditional acceptance of medical therapies recommended by their physicians. Moreover, other issues were at play in this process: men's lack of knowledge about the disease and its medical treatment, trust in the technical competence and scientific knowledge of their physicians, and what value men placed on prostate cancer information.

Figure 6 displays the dynamics of how men lived their daily lives (outside of hospitals and clinics) with the prostate cancer information they gathered through information networks. Men's prostate cancer literacy depended on the effects of experiences with prostate cancer within or outside such networks. Men would create and be part of information networks to build their individualized knowledge about prostate cancer. Being part of information networks helped them understand and make meaning out of their own illness experiences. Men's understanding of the disease was a shared construction of experiences of others in their immediate social environment. This shared construction filled men's knowledge gaps and resolved misunderstandings, allowing men to construct new social roles inspired by their awareness of the need to share knowledge and gain empirical skills to manage prostate cancer. Therefore, men tended to transmit information about the prevention and early detection of prostate cancer, as well as how men already touched by the disease had improved the quality of their lives.

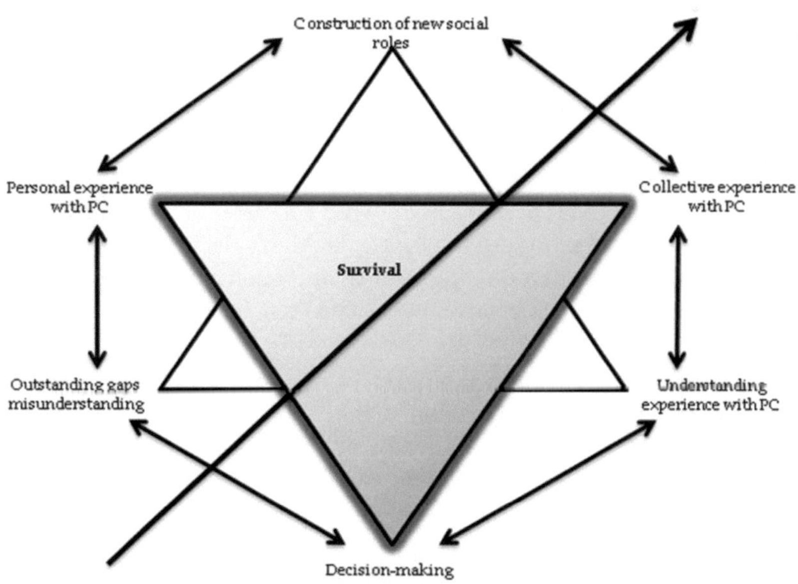

Fig. 6. Dynamics of living with prostate cancer-related information

4.3 Ultimate goals in constructing information strategies for becoming prostate-cancer literate

As described above, the process of becoming prostate-cancer literate unfolded along the life-death continuum; levels of health literacy (from low to high); levels of contact with information networks (from no contact to creation of one's own information network); and illness experiences within or outside information networks. Men's information strategies came out of the desire to preserve their moral integrity, self-image, and to maintain their social roles (as husbands, fathers, grandfathers, friends, and peer counsellors). Awareness of loss, regret, deception, and hope encouraged older men to remain in their social roles, while sharing their wisdom about how to live well[1] with prostate cancer (Zanchetta, 2004). Living well with prostate cancer included creating a new body free of embarrassing conditions (e.g., urinary incontinence), a new masculinity, and a new perception of control. Living well also included redefining one's sense of successful adaptation and, most important, adopting new familial and other social roles while being aware of one's own vulnerability (Kelly, 2009). Men's experience with uncertainty throughout their prostate cancer trajectory was affected by their knowledge about the disease, the disease's stage, and the availability of informal support networks (Nanton et al., 2009). These factors may, in turn, have affected men's desire to survive prostate cancer.

One of older men's primary goals was to understand their illness experiences, an understanding which would enable them to tackle their other primary goal: to regain decisional power over their own bodies and destiny. Guided by hope of surviving prostate cancer, older men decided either to make their journey solitary or collective - experiences shared with family, friends, peers, and strangers. It was between these two extremes of experience with prostate cancer that construction of new social roles, even new social identities, occurred. These new roles and identities preserved the integrity of men's masculine self-images, despite suffering related to loss of sexual functioning.

Men reborn out of collective prostate-cancer journeys distinguished between sharing their own experiences and transmitting information about prostate cancer. They also discerned with which strangers to talk about their experiences of prostate cancer and with which strangers to share its private issues. In contrast, men emerging out of solitary prostate-cancer journeys felt unprotected from the dehumanizing health care system and its professionals. They felt restrained in their freedom to share their cancer experiences with others and believed that silence among men about prostate cancer was natural. Despite these differences in men's preferences for living with prostate cancer, we can identify in the participants' accounts the same underlying rationale. Men's decisions about disclosing their experience with prostate cancer were explained by the intensity of their wishes, as fathers and husbands as well as friends, to protect their loved ones from worry.

4.4 Contributions of this research to the practice of social and health professionals

The research findings described in Section 4 may challenge clinicians' perception that academic education level is the only indicator of patients' ability to understand health information and that less educated patients will be unable to do so. For example,

---

[1] Because none of the research participants was free of prostate cancer, it is beyond the scope of this section to discuss men's perspectives on being free of the disease, feeling safe, or having the disease under control.

sometimes physicians' communication style (e.g., rapid transmission of brief information, underestimating men's capacity to capably make decisions) can push men to adopt a critical, reflective attitude toward the information physicians transmit. In the research described above, this paradox supported older men's determination to educate themselves about prostate cancer and general health. Therefore, social and health professionals should view men's process of becoming prostate cancer literate as a collective, affective, and social process involving other men, women, and other significant others. Medical information about treatment options and their impacts on sexual health is less important to men with prostate cancer than prostate cancer's impacts on men's social identity.

4.5 Reflecting on men's accounts of constructing prostate cancer literacy

In Section 4, we discussed how men construct their prostate cancer literacy throughout the disease process. Below are some accounts to guide readers' reflection about the multiple dimensions of literacy that underpin the process of becoming prostate cancer literate. There are no correct answers to the reflection questions. We hope that reflecting on your own experience as health care professionals will help you answer the questions.

4.5.1 Clinical vignettes

- Michael, a 56-year-old underground miner, was recently diagnosed with prostate cancer. He arrives at an appointment with his oncologist to discuss treatment options. Michael is presented with two options: hormone therapy and orchiectomy. The oncologist discusses the potential outcomes of each of these options. Michael is quite concerned about hormones' possible side effects, such as hot flashes, growth of the mammary glands, and reduction in sexual stamina. Neither option is particularly appealing to Michael. He decides that he needs time to consider the treatment options and discuss them with his wife of 30 years.
- Frank, a 67-year-old retired postal worker, shares with his doctor his experience of participating in a support group for men undergoing prostate cancer treatment. At first he thought this group might be a good source of support as he navigated the often complex world of prostate cancer treatment. After attending a few meetings, however, he discovered that all the men in the support group do is complain. He was also surprised that their complaints were not about discomfort or side effects that they had experienced as a result of their treatments but, instead, about their difficulties getting information and answers to their questions.
- Raymond, a 51-year-old registered nurse, was diagnosed with prostate cancer six months ago. He began hormone therapy two months ago. As a health care professional, his is well acquainted with medication side effects. During a routine follow-up visit with his urologist, Raymond reports that he has been experiencing numerous side effects which he believes are related to the hormone therapy. In addition, and perhaps more concerning, is the fact that his sex drive has severely diminished and he is now experiencing erectile dysfunction. His symptoms are so intense that he finds himself unable to work. He reports that he has been doing some reading on alternative and more natural methods of treatment and wants to discuss discontinuing his hormone therapy. He tells the urologist that his quality of life is so affected by the hormone therapy that he is not willing to continue living like this.

Questions

- What new facilitators for learning can professionals give men, to help them decode prostate cancer information?
- How should professionals incorporate discussion about issues of masculinity when teaching men about modalities of screening, monitoring, treatment, and rehabilitation?
- What are the advantages, for professionals, of learning about how men construct personally relevant meaning from prostate cancer information?
- What innovations should be introduced into prostate-cancer-teaching practices to move from a treatment-focused teaching toward a gender- focused approach?
- Which simple strategies could you create to assess the health literacy of men with prostate cancer in your clinical practice?

5. Health literacy: Impact on survival of the prostate cancer patient, significant others, and clinicians

Health professionals demonstrate growing interest in the functional aspect of health literacy (Oldfield, & Dreher, 2010), despite their concomitant concern about how to assess and deal with it in daily professional practice. According to Peerson and Saunders (2009), "Because health literacy involves knowledge, motivation and activation, it is a complex thing to measure and to influence" (p. 285). Professionals' interest in health literacy focuses on individuals' understanding of health messages, which can enable them to participate more actively in their treatment and be successful in self-management of their illnesses. For years, research on the multiple factors related to health literacy has been guided by several conceptual and theoretical models: information seeking (Bagley-Burnett, 1992; Lenz, 1984), information needs (Derdiarian, 1987), uncertainty in illness (Mishel, 1990), and unaided decisions in health care (Pierce, 1996). Relevant psychological features of information-seeking behavior were explored in some seminal studies. These features are anxiety, resulting in the tendency to attribute responsibility for decision making to others; avoidance or receptivity to learning about one's disease; motivation to seek disease-specific information; and attributing the cause of cancer to fate or personal fault (Lavery & Clarke, 1999; Siegel & Raveis, 1997; Walker et al., 1996). Furthermore, studies have shown that representations of a disease tend to shape individuals' preferences for the type, amount, nature, and use of health information (Fieler et al., 1996; Gollop, 1997a, 1997b; Griffiths & Leek, 1995; Ko et al., 1997; Meischke & Johnson, 1995). Other studies opened new avenues for understanding individuals' preferences for the content of health information: the *how, when, why, who,* and *where* of prognosis, treatments, management, and control of illness (Chalmers et al., 1996; Davison & Degner, 1997; Fieler et al., 1996; Hack et al., 1994; Shaw et al., 1994).

5.1 Health literacy as a survival tool for the patient

If patients' ultimate goal in obtaining health information is to survive, health literacy plays a key role in individuals' sense of self-determination (Zanchetta, & Moura, 2006) and in their ability to deal with illness uncertainty (Zanchetta, 2005). Despite the impressive number of studies related to learning about health issues, few researchers have explored the influences of health learning on individuals' illness experiences within the context of their community life. This learning experience, framed by community features, seems to be particularly critical to older individuals living with cancer, because they report decreased social and community involvement as well as shrinking social networks (Houldin & Wasserbauer, 1996). Cutilli and Bennett (2009) demonstrated that men perform worse than women on health-literacy-assessment tests, due to factors such as education, language, income, information-seeking behavior, and type of health insurance. For older men, such predictors of low performance on health literacy assessments are particularly relevant, because marital status, education, and perceived health status predict health-information seeking (Elder et al., 2010). Low literate individuals tend to have difficulty understanding health information and using the health care system. The reasons for this difficulty include (a) limited comprehension of written and verbal health information, (b) not trusting written health information and preferring to gather health information through personal communication, (c) inability to understand health terms and concepts, (d) insufficient information about the health system, and (e) feelings of shame and embarrassment in revealing their limitations (Health Canada, 1999). The paramount issue, low health literacy, seems to be related to cultural, cognitive, and social aspects of having access to, understanding, and using health information (Oldfield & Dreher, 2010). In particular, low literate individuals who have low levels of numeracy and general knowledge may have difficulty dealing with treatment-related information containing ratios, probabilities, or percentages. Such information, about cures, treatment complications, and/or side effects, is usually given to patients in the contexts of decision making or informed consent. Certainly, one's ability to understand complex health information can either undermine or enhance one's interest in gathering health information.

Studies have also demonstrated that older men consider information on self-management of their diseases too superficial (Walker et al., 1998), especially because of aging-related problems such as cognitive impairment and decrease in vitality. The search for, processing of, incorporation of, and meaning attached to health information seems to be directly affected by older men's level of disease awareness (Morasso et al., 1997), which may decline with cognitive impairment. The nature of prostate cancer treatment demands that health professionals provide clinical education that responds to older men's knowledge deficits and addresses the physical and psychological problems men experience after treatment (Miaskowski, 1999). For example, men who undergo cryosurgical ablation of the prostate may face complications, such as urethrorectal fistulae, bladder-outlet-obstruction incontinence, impotence, and urinary tract infections. Radical prostatectomy may lead to anxiety, bladder spasms, pain, high risk of hemorrhage, and pulmonary embolisms. The complications surrounding external beam radiation include fatigue, diarrhea, and cystitis. Finally, hormone therapy leads to impotence, hot flashes, gynecomastia, and high risk of pathologic fractures (Giddens, 2004). The impact of such complications can affect men's self-image, and dealing with complex medical information can become challenging for older men. To become health literate, they must make sense of health information, find congruency between their past and new knowledge (Craig, 1987), and incorporate health information into their daily lives in a meaningful way.

Interestingly, incorporation of new knowledge about prostate cancer and other medical issues differs according to men's self-reported level of health literacy and unfolds within the multiple, interconnected dimensions of their lives. Zanchetta (2002) showed that health information is incorporated into daily life only if it is congruent with the following factors: men's individual identities; their social trajectories within a specific masculine identity, health-education experience, and life stories; representations of aging, body, cancer/prostate cancer, and health/illness. Table 1 summarizes key definitions of health literacy applicable to learning about prostate cancer in a clinical context.

As consumers of prostate cancer information, men with prostate cancer reveal common strategies for using information (Zanchetta, 2004). Older men tend to perceive prostate cancer as an innocuous disease and react nonchalantly to prostate cancer diagnosis. They usually receive partial information and lack comprehension of clinical conditions and/or the evolutionary stages of prostate cancer. Nonetheless, they enjoy reading, which leads to an interest in reading books about other men's experiences with prostate cancer, the prostate gland, prostate-cancer survival, prognosis, and treatments. They also enjoy learning about principles of chemotherapy, preparation for undergoing chemotherapy and its effects, and modes of adaptation to prostate cancer. They do not believe information displayed in medical pamphlets, due their lack of identification of the pamphlet's authors. Frequently, older men assess their own clinical conditions and the effectiveness of their treatments by tracking changes in their PSA test results. They tend not to seek second opinions from urologists other than their own to either confirm the need for therapy or the quality of scientific evidence in health information. However, men correlate the health information they have with new information they find. Finally, because older men value their physicians' professional competence and trust them, men do not gather health information from other (formal or informal) sources (Zanchetta, 2002).

Conceptual definitions of health literacy – ability to:
Access, read, or listen to; process; and appraise textual, graphic, and numeric health information. Build new meanings from health information. Understand health messages and communicate them in users' social environments. Navigate the health care system. Use textual, numeric, and graphic health information to inform decision making, reduce health risks, and enhance quality of life. Use health information to access health care in a medical culture that requires self-defense and health vigilance. Evaluate and communicate health information to improve one's own and one's family's life. Solve health problems by using multiple forms of language (written, oral, visual, tactile, etc.), at multiple levels (individual, family, community, world) and in multiple contexts (home, work, school). Use all family, school, social, cultural, and professional assets gathered through continual learning (formal or informal), through regular contact with information, knowledge, attitudes, and health behaviors in all aspects of life.

Source: Kaszap & Zanchetta (2009)

Table 1. Conceptual definitions of health literacy

Zanchetta (2002) observed, during a community information session with a total of 50 participants (women, and men with and without prostate cancer) about the epidemiological, treatment, and rehabilitation aspects of prostate cancer, that most men's questions were about technical procedures. These questions indicated lack of comprehension, difficulty with basic interpretation of the medical content of health information, and knowledge gaps, and thereby revealed the participants' world of living with prostate cancer. Table 2 gives the questions men asked, in their original form and grouped into themes. In the same study, men's learning needs were raised by two chairmen of a prostate cancer support group, who had compiled the accounts of several other men. The chairmen said that becoming literate about prostate cancer is not a linear, one-dimensional process. According to them, men become aware of their lack of knowledge about prostate cancer and motivated to seek information about it for the following reasons: (a) acknowledgment that, for men, ageing is usually accompanied by prostate problems, (b) symptoms of excessive prostate enlargement launch information seeking about early signs/symptoms of prostate cancer, (c) men's new awareness of their vulnerability to disease after receiving a prostate cancer diagnosis, (d) receiving information about treatment side effects and their impacts on men's lives, (e) men's perception and experience of treatment and its side-effects, (f) recurrence of prostate problems after treatment, and (g) psychological and social impacts of treatment of prostate cancer.

Theme	Questions
Epidemiology	Why do the rates of prostate cancer increase? What are the environmental risk factors? Are the risk factors presented in the slides in conformity with their degree of importance? Is there something that one can do about the family risks factors? What is the most dangerous type of cancer? Rectal, bladder, or prostate?
Screening procedures	When must one begin PSA testing? What do you recommend as preventive action? After what age must one have an examination? After the age of 50, what is the suggested interval between examinations?
Causes	Is there any link with stress? Does drinking alcoholic beverage cause prostate cancer? Does bleeding during the biopsy transmit cancer? Is it true that sitting for long periods may cause prostate cancer? Could a vasectomy cause prostate cancer? Could hormone therapy cause prostate cancer?
Knowledge issues	What is serum testosterone? Is there another type of testosterone? What is its source of production? What does a gland full of granulomatosis mean? What are the meanings of the letters and degrees used to classify cancer?

Theme	Questions
Diagnostic procedures	Can a prostate cancer diagnosis be made using a blood test? If the cancer is in its beginning stage, can a biopsy indicate its presence?
Self-assessment	Does prostate irritation mean prostate cancer? Does the presence of blood in the sperm indicate prostate cancer?
Technical procedures	What does a rectal examination indicate? What justifies the removal of the testes? Does an examination exist that allows us to see the whole prostate? During a rectal examination, does the physician feel just a part of the prostate? Can a physician identify prostate cancer simply by looking at the prostate? How can one see the prostate with an echography? How is the result of an echography analyzed with the PSA? What can one do after having lymph nodes removed? Is radiation therapy applied through the rectum? Is chemotherapy as efficient as surgery? What is the likelihood of bleeding after radiation therapy?
Interpretation of PSA titration levels	What are the normal limits of the PSA test? Does the PSA have another type of utility? Could it indicate another type of disease?

Table 2. Scope of men's questions about prostate cancer

Men may also learn about prostate cancer through the collective experience offered in prostate cancer support groups. In these support groups, men learn from each other as well as from invited speakers; exchange information and experience; offer and obtain mutual help, advice, and support; and advocate for their rights as health consumers and citizens. Despite these multiple opportunities, some men still believe that other men come together in prostate cancer support groups to complain and cry "like a woman" (F. S. and W. K., personal communication, Kingston, Canada, March 2004). Such a misconception may explain why men from ethnic minorities tend not to enrol in prostate cancer support groups and why some men only attend them after treatment, despite their physicians' recommendations or referrals. In other cases, doctors referred men to prostate cancer support groups after treatment, which may imply that these men decided on treatments with only partial knowledge of their consequences and later regretted their decisions (D. G., personal communication, Montreal, Canada, June 2001).

Other ethno-cultural influences also influenced study participants' behavior related to prostate cancer. First, most of the Caucasian men (who self-identified as being of European descent) were socially expected to keep silent about disease and any suffering. Second, their mothers taught them to promote their own health and take preventive action against diseases, mainly through nutrition (Zanchetta et al., 2004). Given such expectations of stoic silence, men need professional mentoring and assistance to acknowledge that time is required to deal effectively with the diagnosis of prostate cancer, adequately comprehend medical information, consider available alternatives, and reflect on the potential outcomes of their decisions. Such an investment of time will ultimately generate a greater sense of control over men's life choices and a greater degree of normalcy in their lives.

5.2 Impact of men's prostate cancer literacy on their significant others

The impact of a prostate cancer diagnosis on couple and family dynamics is frequently reported in the scientific literature. However, other than shared stress, other experiences of men's significant others with prostate cancer information remain poorly explored. Men themselves report feeling embarrassed in revealing to their wives that prostate-biopsy results confirm their urologists' suspicion of prostate cancer (Zanchetta, 2004). Another gap in the literature concerns partners' unidentified or unmet information needs (Sinfield et al., 2008). For partners, becoming prostate-cancer literate would facilitate their participation in decision making as well as collaboration in all stages of treatment - as information gatherers, care providers, promoters of adherence with treatments, and even advocates for health and social services. As most of partners of men with prostate cancer are women, likely also elderly and living with their own diseases, we can expect that men's partners are knowledgeable consumers of health services who are able to sustain their partners' struggles to learn about prostate cancer. Because close interpersonal relationships influence illness experiences and transform the solitary cancer journey into a joint experience (Illingworth et al., 2010), partners can discover, learn about, and transcend limitations to redefining the meaning of prostate cancer.

Another impact of prostate cancer literacy is men's decision to share their illness experiences with their sons. This decision relates to genetic predisposition to cancer, early detection, and screening procedures (Zanchetta, 2002, 2004). However, a "code of silence between men" can prevent disclosure of diagnosis. In Zanchetta's (2002) study, decision to inform sons and sons was explained from two opposite perspectives. Fathers who shared their illness experiences with their sons did so because of feelings of fatherhood and its perceived inherent responsibilities, and a concomitant desire to protect their sons. These fathers were concerned about the possibility of another case of prostate cancer in the family, felt confident in talking about prostate cancer, valued talking about illness experience to improve their own well-being, and perceived themselves as being open minded. Fathers who did not share their illness experiences with their sons felt unable to discuss parental subjects with their children, did not want to upset their sons with the daily problems caused by prostate cancer, felt that their sons were not concerned about prostate cancer, and had difficulty revealing personal experiences that provoked feelings of frustration and regret.

5.3 Surviving multiple professional challenges to sustain men's prostate cancer literacy

Health professionals utilize evidence-based practice to bridge the theory–practice gap and to guide patient care with the best available evidence (Paley et al., 2007). The goal of health and social professionals in the prostate cancer care continuum (screening, detection/diagnosis, treatment, rehabilitation) is to provide instrumental care and information that combines effective medical and social science with optimal technology, allied to a humanistic approach. However, to provide services that respond to the specific needs of men, according to the World Health Organization (2002), professionals need to acknowledge gender-specific roles and biological distinctions as well as differences among men in needs, power, access to resources, obstacles, and opportunities. Gender equity is needed in the delivery of health services to overcome the structural oppression that grants women access to a humanist approach in health care relationships, but denies men access to the same humanist approach. Zanchetta et al. (2010), in discussing the role of health and social professionals in supporting men's preventative prostate health behaviors, warn that "men today also define their relationships according to trustworthiness. For this reason, professionals should learn how to build trusting relationships with men, to facilitate a new men's culture of seeking preventive care for diseases that threaten men's self-identity" (p. 266). Although Kelly (2009) found that health professionals acknowledge the need to establish trusting relationships with men and aim to overcome communication barriers with them, men in the same study reported that not being taught to deal with physical changes after undergoing prostate cancer treatment led them to feel betrayed by the health care system.

Prostate cancer can significantly impact every aspect of a man's life. Jonsson et al. (2009) conclude that men with prostate cancer "are placed in a new life situation, against their will" (p. 273). These patients move through their illness experience with feelings of fear and uncertainty. Although scientific advances continue to enhance preventative, screening, diagnosis and treatment options, patients continue to experience the prostate cancer journey as separate silos of care. Patient-centered care is one approach that could reconnect these silos into a care continuum. Patient-centered care, which has gained momentum in the last two decades, is an approach to providing health care in which the patient is the focal point. According to the Picker Institute (2011), the eight guiding principles of professional practice in organizations committed to patient-centered care are (a) respect for patients' values, preferences, and expressed needs, (b) coordination and integration of care, (c) information, communication, and education, (d) physical comfort, (e) emotional support and alleviation of fear and anxiety, (f) involvement of family and friends, (g) continuity and transition, and (h) access to care.

The application of these principles coexists with challenges that professionals may face to satisfactorily implementing patient-centered care to ultimately sustain men's prostate cancer literacy. The first challenge is the unresponsiveness of professional practice to the needs of male patients. Despite the patient centered-care movement, patients are continually *cared for* not *cared with*; for instance, professionals present patients with complex treatment options, seeking yes or no decisions about life-changing, high-risk treatments but allowing little time for men to reflect, learn about, and discuss options. Professionals who provide direct care, such as nurses, are faced with the difficult choice of dividing their time among a complex array of institutional demands. These other priorities ultimately result in less time for teaching their patients about health. Professionals are driven by their technical expertise, leading to the transfer of knowledge from 'expert health care professional' to 'patient'. Is this prevalent practice effective? Does men's motivation to seek care rest on the attainment of 'patient knowledge'? Or does their need to survive underpin all the other tasks that men living with prostate cancer must undergo? Ethnic-minority men are less likely than Caucasians to share health information with care providers that they obtained elsewhere. Those whose first languages are not

English tend to complain about disrespect and racial discrimination and are thus less likely than Caucasians to advocate for tests and treatments (Elder et al., 2010). Older men with co-morbidities do not extensively seek information on prostate cancer and its treatment, relying more on the technical expertise of health professionals (Nanton et al., 2009). How do health professionals deal with all these simultaneous and synergistic factors?

The second challenge is twofold: first, it concerns the complexity of the health teaching needed for men to become partners in their care; second, it concerns the similarly complex health teaching needed for men to become decision-making partners. A prostate cancer diagnosis may give a man the opportunity to revisit his life priorities and to learn more about health and how to face health threats (Mishel et al., 2002). For this reason, promotion of health literacy goes beyond simple provision of information; instead, men's lived experience must be taken into account to facilitate their discovery of health information within their unique masculine contexts of living, learning, and applying knowledge. Throughout the prostate cancer trajectory, health education will offer men reassurance, knowledge, and understanding about how to balance the changes they are expected to face.

For prostate cancer screening, Gaster et al. (2010) suggest an "Ask-Tell-Ask" approach that fosters open, interactive dialog between health professionals and men. *Ask* initiates discussion that enables the health professional to explore a man's need for information; *Tell* provides a patient-focused response by the health professional, tailoring information to the patient's needs; and *Ask* allows for reflection and summation of the dialog. This approach facilitates therapeutic interaction between health professional and patient, actively focusing on the patient's own perspective and situation. It enables the patient to move beyond receiving the information toward understanding, internalizing, reflecting, and ultimately, discovering prostate-cancer-care information as it intertwines with sense of himself as a person. No matter what the presentation tool (simple paper or Web-based decision-making aid), the Ask-Tell-Ask approach engages men in learning about prostate cancer screening and making decisions about it (Krist et al., 2007).

Application of patient-centered care to prostate cancer promotes reciprocation and interactivity, allowing patients to be active partners with health professionals in the delivery of care. The one-way, linear communication in traditional prostate cancer care is less effective in engaging men with their own care (Gaster et al., 2010). Individualized teaching may better satisfy men's knowledge needs. Feldman-Stewart et al. (2009) found that men most often asked questions about treatment: first, because of their need to understand and, second, because of their desire to make decisions and plan. Even if men living with prostate cancer did want a lot of information, the amount of and details of information they asked for varied enormously, due to personal reasons. For example, with recent technological advances in the treatment of prostate cancer, men have the opportunity to consider various treatment options. Open prostatectomy procedures can now be performed by surgeons with success rates similar to those with laparascopic or robot-assisted prostatectomy (Lallas & Trabulsi, 2010). Despite these options, patients' feelings of vulnerability when facing complex information about treatment options can be overpowering. Health professionals ask men with prostate cancer to make life-altering decisions about complex, high-risk treatments they know little about. Men are expected to reduce their experience of prostate cancer to a simple *yes* or *no* consent to treatments. When health professionals focus only on outcomes of the procedures, they leave behind the process by which the outcomes are achieved. In contrast, men not only focus on the outcomes of care, but more important to them, the process of care (Jayadevappa et al., 2010). The way that health professionals deliver prostate cancer care can significantly influence men's active engagement in their care (Martinez et al., 2009). Knowledge of disease progression and response to treatments is key for men living with advanced or recurrent prostate cancer, because they need instrumental knowledge to deal with uncertainty about how long their bodies will be able to respond to therapies (Nanton et al., 2009).

Being a partner in care means being a decision maker. Stacey et al. (2010) report that men want more opportunity to decide than they are allowed. Their vehemence remains unchanged if they are not offered decision aids or the opportunity to discuss the details of treatment with health professionals. This vehemence applies equally to the informed consent process, which usually requires more in-depth information and clearer explanations to support men's understanding. Moreover, men want more information on potential harms of therapies, since health professionals tend to present more often the benefits. As discussed in Section 5.2, men's partners should be considered in the process of decision-making. To include men's partners, Illingworth et al. (2010) propose that health professionals talk to men about their significant others and all spheres of their lives. These authors emphasize the central role of men's interpersonal relationships in their experiences with prostate cancer.

Finally, the last challenge for professionals relates to collaboration within their own professions and with other health and social professions. It is known that limited professional links between family physicians and urologists erect structural barriers for health care delivery to older men (Greene & Adelman, 2003). It is beyond the scope of this section to suggest that other members of multidisciplinary cancer-care teams change their practice, due to ethical principles. However, we would like to highlight that Zanchetta (2004), at the time an oncology nurse interested in health literacy, made some recommendations to nurses to counteract misconceptions about older men's health literacy. These recommendations may inspire other professionals. Aiming to awake and enhance nurses' awareness of their opportunity, and responsibility, to expand professional knowledge about men's health literacy, Zanchetta (2004) recommended that nurses (a) be aware that functional health literacy is a result of a broad, socially constructed process, rather than a set of abilities comprising reading, counting, and recognition of words, (b) be particularly attentive to the nature and extension of individual men's social networks, (c) encourage men to collaborate with nurses in creating educational materials, (d) invite physicians to co-create educational materials that respond to knowledge gaps and misunderstandings about prostate cancer, (e) redesign, with men, innovative strategies to communicate others' experiences with cancer, and (f) record their clinical observations of the differences among men's information behaviors.

Enhancing the quality of prostate cancer care involves more than advances in science and technology. It requires engaging patients in treatment-related decisions and fostering a health care environment that facilitates health literacy among patients. The patient-centered care approach enables health care professionals to focus on patients as well as their significant others, as they journey through the prostate cancer trajectory. Engaging patients through patient-centered care allows their collaboration with health care professionals to fulfil the goal of *caring with the patient*.

5.4 Reflecting on the complexity of patient-centred care and survival in prostate cancer

Our aim in the following exercise is to present some insights into the complexity of patient centred care and men's experience of prostate cancer literacy as a survival tool. While reading each clinical vignette, we suggest that readers consider how difficult it is for men to decode medical information in order to make decisions, as well as how challenging it is for professionals to promote men's health and prostate-cancer literacy.

5.4.1 Clinical vignettes

- Juan, a 49-year-old elementary school teacher, comes into the clinic for a follow-up appointment with his urologist/oncologist after undergoing a prostatectomy and radiation therapy. He has been having his PSA level monitored regularly since he was diagnosed and underwent surgery and treatment. Juan's doctor tells him that his PSA level remains unchanged following radiation therapy and that they will continue to monitor it over time. Juan is not satisfied with this report and wants the doctor to tell him conclusively whether his cancer is cured. The doctor responds that time will tell.
- Hassan, a 55-year-old car salesman, is diagnosed with prostate cancer. His urologist discusses possible treatment options, including surgery and radiation. Hassan was recently remarried, to a much younger woman, and explains that their sex life is quite active. They have been discussing the possibility of having a baby. Hassan is concerned that prostate-cancer treatment could lead to erectile dysfunction, which could end his happy, active sex life. He is unwilling to take a chance that his sex life will be affected and that he could jeopardize his chance of having a baby with his new wife.
- Roberto, a 45 year-old Crown attorney, receives a diagnosis of prostate cancer. He is devastated. His father died of advanced prostate cancer at the age of 55. Roberto reports that he has a strong faith in God and that he plans on praying for a miracle. He refuses any and all treatment that is offered to him, because he believes that, through prayer, he will be healed. Roberto's physician attempts to convince him that, if he refuses treatment, he risks the same outcome as his father. The physician tells Roberto that, because he is a young man and the cancer was detected early, the outcome could be favorable if he considers treatment.

5.4.2 Reflection questions

- What factors contribute to men's difficulty in understanding prostate cancer information and utilizing the health care system?
- What impact can men's experience of prostate cancer have on significant others, and how can that impact be attenuated by new professional attitudes and practices?
- What changes in professional practice relating to prostate cancer literary will acknowledge the importance of different perceptions of masculinity?
- How could education, social, and health professionals collaborate to develop age- and gender-appropriate, sensitive educational tools?
- How do you foresee education about prostate cancer focusing on aspects of men's lives other than sexuality?

6. Conclusion

In this chapter, we presented a multidisciplinary view of men's health literacy in prostate cancer, drawing from the disciplines of medical anthropology, education, and nursing. We intended to expand readers' vision of health literacy beyond measurable personal skills toward a view of health literacy as a personal asset that individuals build throughout social interactions within the multiples spheres of their lives. We also intended to portray men's experience of prostate cancer as an experience that goes beyond failures and improvement in sexual performance to a much broader and more significant masculine experience. Health literacy for older men with prostate cancer can preserve their moral integrity, social identity, and self-perception of masculinity. Health education for men with prostate cancer should expand their awareness of health challenges, guide them in correctly interpreting prostate cancer information, and create new ways of enjoying life after prostate cancer. Uncertainties, challenges, and doubts are shared with significant others, who may also have difficulty talking openly about the impacts of prostate cancer, present and future, on the men they love and care for. For this reason, significant others should also be educated about prostate cancer. To create collaboration among men, health educators, social and health professionals, and significant others to improve men's prostate cancer literacy, it will be necessary to redesign current communication approaches. Communication needs to be innovative, creative, and sensitive to men's social networks, age, cultures, general literacy, and, of course, gender. Men differ in the way they understand and live their own masculinity. Not all men are equally health literate; health literacy depends on the collective project of health education. The kind of prostate cancer literacy that we envision is one that will liberate men from any sense of powerlessness and hopelessness, enabling men to transcend any limitations imposed by prostate cancer.

7. Acknowledgements

We acknowledge Yasmin Taher and Mohamed Mohamed for their support as research assistants and Ms Margaret Oldfield for editing the manuscript's text.
Funding: Faculty of Community Services Publications Grant, Ryerson University and Faculté des sciences d'éducation, Université Laval.

8. References

Alpay, L. L.; Toussaint, P. J.; Ezendam, N. P. M.; Rovekamp, T. J. M.; Graafmans, W. C. & Westendorp, R. G. J. (2004). Easing Internet Access of Health Information for Elderly Users. *Health Informatics Journal.* Vol.10, No.3, (September), pp. 185-194, ISSN 1741-2811

Almeida, M. V. de (1996). *The Hegemonic Male: Masculinity in a Portuguese Town,* Berghahn Books, ISBN 157181891X, London, United Kingdom

Bagley-Burnett, C. (1992). Measuring Information-seeking Behaviors. In: *Instrumental for Clinical Nursing Research,* M. Frank-Stromborg (Ed.), 151-169, Jones & Bartlett, ISBN 0867203404, Norwalk, Connecticut. United States

Barry, M. J. (2010). Shared Decision Making Supported by Patient Decision Aids for Prostate Cancer Screening and Treatment. *Psicooncología,* vol.7, No 2-3, pp. 257-267, ISSN 16967240

Barton, D.; Hamilton, M. & Ivanic, R. (2000). *Situated Literacies: Reading and Writing in Context*, Routledge, ISBN 0-415-20670-7, London, United Kingdom

Barton, D. & Hamilton, M. (1998). *Local Literacies: Reading and Writing in One Community*. Routledge, ISBN 0-415-17150-4, London, United Kingdom

Bergsma, L. J. (2004). Empowerment education: The Link Between Media Literacy and Health Promotion. *American Behavioral Scientist*, Vol.48, No.2, (October), pp. 152-164, ISSN 1552-3381

Boudon, P. (2000). Entre Rhétorique et Dialectique: La Constitution des Figures d'argumentation [Between Rhetoric and Dialetic: The Constitution of the Figures of Argumentation]. *Langages*, Vol. 34, No.137, pp. 63-86, ISSN 0458-726X

Boudon, P. (1999). *Le Réseau du Sens: Une Approche Monadologique pour la Compréhension du Discours* [The Network of Meaning: An Approach to Understanding the Monadological Discourse] Allemagne: Éditions scientifiques européennes, Peter Lang, ISBN 3906761959, Bern, Switzerland

Boudon, P. (1998). L'abduction et le Champ Sémiotique. Le Tiers Communicationnel, 255-284, Harmattan, Montréal, Canada

Bourdieu, P. (1977). *Outline of a Theory of Practice*, Cambridge University Press, ISBN 0 521 29164, Cambridge, United Kingdom

Bourdieu, P. (2001). *Masculine Domination*, Stanford University Press, ISBN 0-8047-3818-1, Stanford, United States

Brown, P.; Ames, N.; Mettger, W.; Smith, T. J.; Gramarossa, G. L.; Friedell, G. H.; & McDonald, S. S. (1993). Closing the Comprehension Gap: Low Literacy and the Cancer Information Service. *Journal of the National Cancer Institute*. Monographs. Vol. 14, (November), pp. 157-163, ISSN 1052-6773

Buston, K. M. & Wood, S. F. (2000). Non-Compliance amongst Adolescents with Asthma: Listening to What They Tell Us about Self-Management, *Family Practice*, Vol.17, No.2, (April), pp. 134-138, ISSN 0263-2136

Butler, J. (1990) *Gender Trouble: Feminism and the Subversion of Identity*, Routledge, ISBN 0415900425, New York, United States

Barry, M. J. (2010). Shared Decision Making Supported by Patient Decision Aids for Prostate Cancer Screening and Treatment. *Psicooncología*, vol.7, No 2-3, pp. 257-267, ISSN 16967240

Barton, D.; Hamilton, M. & Ivanic, R. (2000). *Situated Literacies: Reading and Writing in Context*, Routledge, ISBN 0-415-20670-7, London, United Kingdom

Barton, D. & Hamilton, M. (1998). *Local Literacies: Reading and Writing in One Community*. Routledge, ISBN 0-415-17150-4, London, United Kingdom

Bergsma, L. J. (2004). Empowerment education: The Link Between Media Literacy and Health Promotion. *American Behavioral Scientist*, Vol.48, No.2, (October), pp. 152-164, ISSN 1552-3381

Boudon, P. (2000). Entre Rhétorique et Dialectique: La Constitution des Figures d'argumentation [Between Rhetoric and Dialetic: The Constitution of the Figures of Argumentation]. *Langages*, Vol. 34, No.137, pp. 63-86, ISSN 0458-726X

Boudon, P. (1999). *Le Réseau du Sens: Une Approche Monadologique pour la Compréhension du Discours* [The Network of Meaning: An Approach to Understanding the

Monadological Discourse] Allemagne: Éditions scientifiques européennes, Peter Lang, ISBN 3906761959, Bern, Switzerland

Boudon, P. (1998). L'abduction et le Champ Sémiotique. Le Tiers Communicationnel, 255-284, Harmattan, Montréal, Canada

Bourdieu, P. (1977). *Outline of a Theory of Practice,* Cambridge University Press, ISBN 0 521 29164, Cambridge, United Kingdom

Bourdieu, P. (2001). *Masculine Domination,* Stanford University Press, ISBN 0-8047-3818-1, Stanford, United States

Brown, P.; Ames, N.; Mettger, W.; Smith, T. J.; Gramarossa, G. L.; Friedell, G. H.; & McDonald, S. S. (1993). Closing the Comprehension Gap: Low Literacy and the Cancer Information Service. *Journal of the National Cancer Institute.* Monographs. Vol. 14, (November), pp. 157-163, ISSN 1052-6773

Buston, K. M. & Wood, S. F. (2000). Non-Compliance amongst Adolescents with Asthma: Listening to What They Tell Us about Self-Management, *Family Practice,* Vol.17, No.2, (April), pp. 134-138, ISSN 0263-2136

Butler, J. (1990) *Gender Trouble: Feminism and the Subversion of Identity,* Routledge, ISBN 0415900425, New York, United States

Carrigan, T.; Connel, R. & Lee, J. (1985). Towards a New Sociology of Masculinity. *Theory and Society,*Vol.14, No.5, (November), pp. 551-604, ISSN 0304-2421

Chalmers, K.; Thomson, K. & Degner, L. F. (1996). Information, Support, and Communication Needs of Women with a Family History of Cancer. *Cancer Nursing,* Vol.19, No.3, (June), pp. 204-213, ISSN 0162-220X

Channel, D. F. (1991) *The Vital Machine: A Study of Technology and Organic Life,* Oxford University Press, ISBN 0195060407, New York, United States

Chapple, A. & Ziebland, S. (2002). Prostate Cancer: Embodied Experience and Perceptions of Masculinity. *Sociology of Health and Illness,* Vol.24, No.6, (October), pp. 820-841, ISSN 0141-9889

Chung, C. H.; Bernard, P. S. & Perou, C.M. (2002). Molecular Portraits and the Family Tree of Cancer. *Nature Genetics,* Vol.32, (December), Supp:533-540, ISSN 1061-4036

Clarke, A. E.; Shim, J. K.; Mamo, L.; Forsket, J. R. & Fishman, J. R. (2003). Biomedicalization: Technoscientific Transformations of Health, Illness and U.S. Biomedicine. *American Sociological Review,* Vol.68, No.2, (April), pp. 161-194, ISSN 0003-1224

Cutilli, C. C. & Bennett, I. M. (2009). Understanding the Health Literacy of America: Results of the National Assessment of Adult Literacy. *Orthopaedic Nursing,* Vol.28, No.1, (January-February), pp. 27-32, ISSN 0744-6020

Connell, R. (1995). *Masculinities,* University of California Press, ISBN 0520089995, Berkeley, United States

Connel, R. W. & Messerschmidt, J. W. (2005) Hegemonic Masculinity: Rethinking the Concept. *Gender and Society,* Vol.19, No.6, (December), pp. 829-859, ISSN 1552-3977

Connor, A.; Layne, L. & Thomisee, K. (2010). Providing Care for Migrant Farm Worker Families in Their Unique Sociocultural Context and Environment. *Journal of Transcultural Nursing,* Vol.21, No.2, (April), pp. 159-166, ISSN 1552-7832

Cornwall, A. & Lindisfarne, N. (1994) (Eds.). *Dislocating Masculinity: Gender, Power and Anthropology,* Routledge, ISBN 0-203-39343-0, London, United Kingdom

Courtenay, W. (2000). Constructions of Masculinity and Their Infuence on Men's Well-Being: A Theory of Gender and Health. *Social Science and Medicine,* Vol.50, No.10, (May), pp. 1385-1401, ISSN 0277-9536

Craig, L. L. (1987). *Characteristics of Older Men and Their Ability to Comprehend Printed Health Education Materials.* Unpublished doctoral dissertation. University of Alabama at Birmingham, Birmingham

Davis, T. C.; Crouch, M. A.; Long, S. W.; Jackson, R. H.; Bates, P.; George, R. B. & Bairnsfather, L. E. (1991). Rapid Assessment of Literacy Levels of Adult Primary Care Patients. *Family Medicine.* Vol. 23, No.6, (August), pp. 433-435, ISSN 0742-3225

Davis, T. C.; Williams, M. V.; Marin, E.; Parker, R. M. & Glass, J. (2008). Health Literacy and Cancer Communication. *Cancer Journal for Clinicians,* Vol.52, No.3, (May-June), pp. 134-149, ISSN 0007-9235

Davison, J. & Degner, L. F. (1997). Empowerment of Men Newly Diagnosed with Prostate Cancer. *Cancer Nursing,* Vol.20, No.3, (June), pp. 187-196, ISSN 0162-220X

Derdiarian, A. (1987). Informational Needs of Recently Diagnosed Cancer Patients: A Theoretical Framework. Part I. *Cancer Nursing,* Vol.10, No.2, (April), pp. 107-115, ISSN 0162-220X.

Deslauriers, J.-P. & Deslauriers, J.-M. (2010). La Recherche Auprès des Hommes: Défis et Enjeux. [Research with Men: Challenges and Issues] In: *Regards Sur les Hommes et les Masculinités: Comprendre et Intervenir,* [Vision about Men and Masculinities: Understanding and Intervention], J.-M. Deslauriers, G. Tremblay, S. G. Dufault, D. Blanchette & J.-Y Desgagnés, 153-172, Les Presses de l'Université Laval, ISBN 978-2-7637-8954-5, Québec, Canada

Easton, P.; Entwistle, V. A. & Williams, B. (2010). Health in the 'Hidden Population' of People with Low Literacy: A Systematic Review of the Literature. *BMC Public Health,* Vol.10, (August), pp. 459-468, ISSN 1471-2458

Elder, K. T.; Wilshier, J. C.; McRoy, L.; Campbell, D.; Gary, L. C. & Safford, M. (2010). Men and Differences by Racial/Ethnic Group in Self Advocacy during the Medical Encounter. *Journal of Men's Health,* Vol.7, No.2, (June), pp. 135-144, ISSN 1875-6867

Feldman-Stewart, D.; Brennenstuhl, S.; Brundage, M. D. & Siemens, D. R. (2009). Overall Information Needs of Early-Stage Prostate Cancer Patients over a Decade: Highly Variable and Remarkably Stable. *Support Care Cancer,* Vol.17, No.4, (April), pp. 429-435, ISSN 1433-7339

Fieler, V. K.; Wlasowicz, G. S.; Mitchell, M. L.; Jones, L. S. & Johnson, J. E. (1996). Information Preferences of Patients Undergoing Radiation Therapy. *Oncology Nursing Forum,* Vol. 23, No.10, pp.1603-1608, ISSN 0190-535X

Francis, C. K. (1991). Hypertension, Cardiac Disease, and Compliance in Minority Patients. *The American Journal of Medecine.* Vol. 91, No.1A, (July), pp. 29S-36S, ISSN 0002-9343

Fujimura, J. (1996) *Crafting Science: A Sociohistory of the Quest for the Genetics of Cancer* Harvard University Press, ISBN 0 674 15553 0, Cambridge, United Kingdom

Fullwiley, D. (2007). The Molecularization of Race: Institutionalizing Human Difference in Pharmacogenetics Practice. *Science as Culture,* Vol.16, No.1, (March), pp. 1-30, ISSN 0950-5431

Gaster, B.; Edwards, K.; Trinidad, S. B.; Gallagher, T. H. & Braddock, C. H. (2010). Patient-Centred Discussions about Prostate Cancer Screening: A Real World Approach. *Annals of Internal Medicine,* Vol.123, No.10, (November), pp. 661-667, ISSN 1539-3704

Giddens, J. F. (2004). Nursing Management-Male Reproductive Problems. In: *Medical-Surgical Nursing: Assessment and Management of Clinical Problems,* S. M. Lewis, M. M. Heitkemper, & S. R. Dirksen, (6th Ed.), 1435-1462, Mosby, ISBN 9780323036900, St. Louis, Missouri, United States

Gil-Gómez, J. A.; Lloréns, R.; Alcañiz, M. & Colomer, C. (2011). Effectiveness of a Wii Balance Board-Based System (eBaViR) for Balance Rehabilitation: A Pilot Randomized Clinical Trial in Patients with Acquired Brain Injury. *Journal of Neuroengineering and Rehabilitation,* Vol.8, No.1, (May), pp. 30. Available from http://www.jneuroengrehab.com/content/8/1/30SSN 1743-0003

Gilmore, D. (1990). *Manhood in the Making: Cultural Concepts of Masculinity,* Yale University Press, ISBN 9780300050769, New Haven, United States

Golding, B. G. (2011). Social, Local, and Situated: Recent Findings about the Effectiveness of Older Men's Informal Learning in Community Contexts. *Adult Education Quarterly,* Vol.20, No.10, (May), pp. 1–18, ISSN 1552-3047

Gollop, C. J. (1997a). Health Information-Seeking Behavior and Older African American Women. *Bulletin of the Medical Library Association,* Vol.85, No.2, (April), pp. 141-146, ISSN 0025-7338

Gollop, C. J. (1997b). Where Have All the Nice Old Ladies Gone? Researching the Health Information-Seeking Behavior of Older African American Women. In: *Oral Narrative Research with Black Women,* K. M. Vaz (Ed.), 143-155, Sage, ISBN 9780803974296, Thousand Oaks, California, United States

Greene, M. G. & Adelman, R. D. (2003). Physician-Older Patient Communication about Cancer. *Patient Education Counselling,* Vol.50, No.1, (May), pp. 55-60, ISSN 0738-3991 Griffiths, M. & Leek, C. (1995). Patient Education Needs: Opinions of Oncology Nurses and Their Patients. *Oncology Nursing Forum,* Vol.22, No.1, (January-February), pp. 139-144, ISSN 0190-535X

Gwede, C. K. & McDermott, R. J. (2006). Prostate Cancer Screening Decision Making Under Controversy: Implications for Health Promotion Practice. *Health Promotion Practice,* Vol.7, No.1, (January), pp. 134-146, ISSN 1524-8399

Hack, T. F.; Degner, L. F. & Dyck, D. G. (1994). Relationship Between Preferences for Decisional Control and Illness Information among Women with Breast Cancer: A Quantitative and Qualitative Analysis. *Social Science & Medicine,* Vol.39, No.2, (July), pp. 279-289, ISSN 0277-9536

Health Canada (March 24, 1999). Literacy French- Profile. Available: http: //www.hc-sc.gv.ca/hppb/developpement-promotion/pubf/literacy-health/literacyfr2.htm

Hedgecoe, A. (2002). Reinventing diabetes: Classification, Division and the Geneticization of Disease. *New Genetics and Society*, Vol.21, No. (August), pp. 7-27, ISSN 1469-9915

Hogle, L. F. (2005). Enhancement Technologies and the Body. *Annual Review of Anthropology*, Vol.34, (October), pp. 695-716, ISSN 0084-6570

Houldin, A. D. & Wasserbauer, N. (1996). Psychosocial Needs of Older Cancer Patients: A Pilot Study. *MEDSURG Nursing*, Vol.5, No. 4, (August), pp. 253-256, ISSN 1092-0811

Illingworth, N.; Forbat, L.; Hubbard, G. & Kearney, N. (2010). The Importance of Relationships in the Experience of Cancer: A Re-working of the Policy Ideal of the Whole-Systems Approach. *European Journal of Oncology Nursing*, Vol.14, No.1, (February), pp. 23-28, ISSN 1532-2122

Jayadevappa, R.; Schwartz, S.; Chatre, S.; Wein, A. J. & Malkowicz, S. B. (2010). Satisfaction with Care: A Measure of Quality of Care in Prostate Cancer Patients. *Medical Decision Making*, Vol.30, No.2, (March-April), pp. 234-245, ISSN 1552-681X

Jensen, J. D.; King, A. J.; Davis, L. A. & Guntzviller, L. M. (2010). Utilization of Internet Technology by Low-Income Adults: The Role of Health Literacy, Health Numeracy, and Computer Assistance. *Journal of Aging and Health*, Vol.22, No.6, (September), pp. 804-826, ISSN 1552-6887

Jonsson, A.; Aus, G. & Bertero, C. (2009). Men's Experience of Their Life Situation when Diagnosed with Advanced Prostate Cancer. *European Journal of Oncology Nursing*, Vol.13, No.4, (September), pp. 268-273, ISSN 1532-2122

Jonnaert, P. (2009) *Créer des Conditions D'apprentissage: Un Cadre de Rréférence Socio-constructiviste pour une Formation Didactique des Enseignants*. [Create Conditions for Learning: A Socio-constructivist Framework for a Pedagogical Education of Teachers], De Boeck, ISBN 2804131548, Bruxelles, Belgium

Kaszap, M.; Viens, C.; Fortin, J. Ajar, D.; Ollivier, É. & Vandal, S. (2000). Rapport de Recherche. *Besoins D'éducation à la Santé Chez une Clientèle Âgée Peu Alphabétisée Atteinte de Maladies Cardio-vasculaires: Une Étude Exploratoire*. [Research Report. Health Education Needs of Low Literate Seniors Living with Cardiovascular Diseases: An Exploratory Study], Groupe de recherche Alpha-santé Éditeur, ISBN 2-98069 19-0-9, Québec, Canada

Kaszap, M.; Viens, C.; Ajar, D.; Ollivier, É.; Leclerc, L.-P. & Bah, Y. M. (2002). Rapport de Recherche. *Évaluation de L'applicabilité des Nouvelles Technologies de L'information et de la Communication dans le Domaine de L'éducation à la Santé des Adultes Peu Alphabétisés Atteints de Maladies Cardio-vasculaires*. [Research Report. Evaluation of the Applicability of New Information and Communication Technology for Health Education of Low Literate Seniors Living with Cardiovascular Diseases], Groupe de recherche Alpha-santé Éditeur, ISBN 2-9806919-1-7, Québec, Canada

Kaszap, M. (2006). Understanding Low Literate Elderly's Health Decisions by Recording Their Misconceptions and Metaphors. *Proceedings of the 12th Qualitative Health Conference*, p. 75, Edmonton, Alberta, Canada, April 2-5, 2006

Kaszap, M.; Drolet, M. & Gagné, I. (2008). Formation des Professionnels de la Santé et des Intervenants Communautaires à L'épistémologie de la Littératie en Santé des Personnes Âgées; Une Approche Socioconstructiviste Basée sur la Chronologie

Iconographique Thématique. [Education of Health Professionals and Community Workers According to the Epistemology of Seniors' Health Literacy: A Socioconstructivist Approach based on a Chronological, Iconography Theme], *Proceedings, 15th International Conference on Globalization and Education Towards A Knowledgeable Society*, Vol.1, pp. 447-448, Marrakech, Morocco, June 2-6, 2008

Kaszap, M. ; &Clerc, I. (2008). Réflections autour des concepts d'alphabétisme et de littératie. [Reflection on the concepts of alphabetization and literacy]. Rapport: Suites à donner au 2e Forum national de recherche en santé des communautes francophones en situation minoritaire, Unpublished manuscript. Ottawa, Canada, Novembre 22-24, 2007

Kaszap, M. & Drolet M. (December 2009) Rapport de Recherche. *L'animation Télévisuelle en Santé.* [The Tele-visual Animation in Health]. Available: http://www.ccl-cca.ca/CCL/Research/FundedResearch/201007Kaszap-FoodTV-2.html

Kaszap, M. & Zanchetta, M. S. (2009). La Littératie en Santé, Vécue dans la Simplicité mais Comprise à Travers la Complexité: Regard sur les Communautés Culturelles (Francophones, Minoritaires et Multiethniques) [Health Literacy, Lived in Simplicity but Understood Through Complexity: Issues of Cultural Communities (Francophone, Minority and Multiethnicity], In: *Les littératies multiples: lire au 21e siècle* [Multiple literacies: Reading in the 21st century], D. Masny (Ed.), 287-325, Les Presses de l'Université d'Ottawa, ISBN 978-2-7603-0702-5, Ottawa, Ontario, Canada

Kelly, D. (2009). Changed men: The Embodied Impact of Prostate Cancer. *Qualitative Health Research,* Vol.19, No.2, (February), pp. 151-163, ISSN 1049-7323

Kimmel, M. (1987). Rethinking Masculinity: New Directions in Research, In: *Changing men: new directions in research on men and masculinities,* M. Kimmel (Ed.), 9-24, Sage, ISBN 0803929978, Thousand Oaks, California, United States

Kimmel M. (1995). *Manhood in America: A Cultural History,* Free Press, ISBN 978-0-02-874067-6, New York, United States

Ko, N. Y.; Shiau, C. & Sheu, S. L. (1997). Informational Needs and Information-seeking Behaviors of Recently Diagnosed HIV Seropositive Gay Men. *Hu Li Za Zhi* (The Journal of Nursing), Vol.44, No.3, (June), pp. 32-40, ISSN 0047-262X.

Krist, A. H.; Woolf, S. H.; Johnson, R. E. & Kerns, J. W. (2007). Patient Education on Prostate Cancer Screening and Involvement in Decision Making. *Annals of Family Medicine,* Vol.5, No.2, (March-April), pp. 112-119, ISSN 1544-1717

Knight, S. J. & Latini, D. M. (2009). Sexual Side Effects and Prostate Cancer Treatment Decisions: Patient Information Needs and Preferences. *Cancer Journal,* Vol.15, No.1, (January-February), pp. 41-44, ISSN 1528-9117

Kruger, J.; Prohaska, T. R. & Furner, S. E. (2007). Preferences for Health Inquiry among Adults Aged 50 and Over. *Research on Aging,* Vol.29, No.4 (July), pp. 283-296, ISSN 1552-7573

Lallas, C. D. & Trabulsi, C. J. (2010). Laparascopic and Robotic Radical Prostatectomy. In: *Glenn's Urologic Surgery* (7th Ed.), S.D. Graham & T.E. Keane (Ed.), 867-880, Lippincott Williams & Wilkins, ISBN 0781791413, Philadelphia, Pennsylvania, United States

Lavery, J. F. & Clarke, V. A. (1999). Prostate Cancer: Patients' and Spouses' Coping and Marital Adjustment. *Psychology, Health & Medicine,* Vol.4, No.3 (August), pp. 289-302, ISSN 1354-8506

Lenoir, T. (2002a). Makeover: Writing the Body into the Posthuman Technoscape Part Two: Corporeal Axiomatics. *Configurations,* Vol.10, No.3 (September), pp. 373-385, ISSN 1063-1801

Lenoir, T. (2002b). Makeover: Writing the Body into the Posthuman Technoscape Part One: Embracing the Posthuman. *Configurations,* Vol.10, No.2 (April), pp. 203-220, ISSN 1063-1801

Lenoir, T. (2004). The Virtual Surgeon: New Practices for an Age of Medialization, In: *Data Made Flesh: Embodying Information,* R. Mitchell and P. Thurtle (Eds.), 137-153, Routledge, ISBN 9780415969055, New York, United States

Lenz, E. R. (1984). Information-seeking: A Component of Client Decisions and Health Behavior. *Advances in Nursing Science,* Vol.6, No.3, (April), pp. 59-72, ISSN 0161-9268

Lerman, N.; Oldenziel, R.; Mohun, A. (2003) (Eds.). *Gender and Technology: A Reader,* Johns Hopkins University Press, ISBN 0-8018-7259-6, Baltimore, Maryland, United States

Levasseur, M. & Carrier, A. (2010). Do Rehabilitation Professionals Need to Consider Their Clients' Health Literacy for Effective Practice? *Clinical Rehabilitation,* Vol.24, No.8, (August), pp. 756-765, ISSN 1477-0873

Lohan, M. (2007). How Might We Understand Men's Health Better? Integrating Explanations from Critical Studies on Men and Inequalities in Health. *Social Science and Medicine,* Vol.65, No.3 (August), pp. 493-504, ISSN 0277-9536

Mackert, M.; Love, B. & Whitten, P. (2009). Patient Education on Mobile Devices: An E-health Intervention for Low Health Literate Audiences. *Journal of Information Science,* Vol.35, No.1, (October), pp. 82–93, ISSN 1741-6485

Mahalik, J.; Burns S. & Syzdek, M. (2007). Masculinity and Perceived Normative Health Behaviors as Predictors of Men's Health Behaviors. *Social Science and Medicine,* Vol.64, No.11, (June), pp. 2201-2209, ISSN 0277-9536

Martinez, L. S.; Schwartz, J. S.; Freres, D.; Fraze, T. & Hornik, R. C. (2009). Patient-clinician Information Engagement Increases Treatment Decision Satisfaction among Cancer Patients Through Feeling of Being Informed. *Patient Education and Counseling,* Vol.77, No.3, (December), pp. 384-390, ISSN 1873-5134

Mayeaux, E. J.; Murphy, P. W.; Arnold, C.; Davis, T. C.; Jackson, R. H. & Sentell, T. (1996). Improving Patient Education for Patients with Low Literacy Skills. *American Family Physician.* Vol.53, No.1, (January), pp. 205-211, ISSN 0002-838X

Meischke, H. & Johnson, D. (1995). Women's Selection of Sources for Information on Breast Cancer Detection. *Health Values,* Vol.19, No.5 (December), pp. 30-38, ISSN 0147-0353

Mellstrom, U. (2004). Machines and Masculine Subjectivity: Technology as an Integral Part of Men's Life Experiences. *Men and Masculinities,* Vol.6, No.4 (April), pp. 368-382, ISSN 1097-184X

Miaskowski, C. (1999). Prostate Cancer. In: *Oncology Nursing: Assessment and Clinical Care,* C. Miaskowski & P. Buchsel (Eds.), 1471-1501, Mosby, ISBN 978-081-5169-90-1, St. Louis, Missouri, United States

Mishel, M. H. (1990). Reconceptualization of the Uncertainty in Illness Theory. *Image: Journal of Nursing Scholarship,* Vol.22, No.4, (December), pp. 256–262, ISSN 0743-5150

Mishel, M. H.; Belyea, M.; Germino, B.; Stewart, J. L.; Bailey, D. E. & Robertson, C. (2002). Helping Patients with Localized Prostate Carcinoma Manage Uncertainty and Treatment Side Effects: Nurse Delivered Psychoeducational Intervention Over the Telephone. *Cancer,* Vol.94, No.6, (March), pp. 1854–1866, ISSN 0008-543X

Monteiro, M. (2000). *"Tenham Piedade dos Homens!": Masculinidades em Mudança* ["Have Pity on Men!": ChangingMasculinities], FEME, ISBN 85-86913-06-5, Juiz de Fora, Brazil

Monteiro, M. (2001). Corpo e Masculinidade na Revista VIP Exame [Body and Masculinity in VIP Exame Magazine], *Cadernos Pagu,* No.16 (December), pp. 235-266, ISSN 0104-8333

Monteiro, M. (2011). *Dilemas do Humano: Reinventando o Corpo Numa Era (Bio)tecnologica* [Dilemmas of the Human: Reinventing the Body in a (Bio)technological Era]. Social Sciences, São Paulo: Annablume. (in press)

Monteiro, M. (2009). Molecular representations: Reflections on microarrays and prostate cancer. *Leonardo Electronic Almanac,* Vol.16, (May), pp. 1-12

Monteiro, M. & Keating, E. (2009). Managing Misunderstandings: The Role of Language in Interdisciplinary Scientific Collaboration. *Science Communication* Vol.31, No.1, (February), pp. 6-28, ISSN 1552-8545

Moon, P. J. (2011). Bereaved Elders: Transformative Learning in Late Life. *Adult Education Quarterly,* Vol.61, No.1 (February), pp. 22-39, ISSN 1552 3047

Morasso, G.; Alberisio, A.; Capelli, M.; Rossi, C.; Baracco, G. & Costantini, M. (1997). Illness Awareness in Cancer Patients: A Conceptual Framework and a Preliminary Classification Hypothesis. *Psycho-Oncology,* Vol.6, No. 3, (September), pp. 212-217, ISSN 1057 9249

Morrow, D. G.; Weiner, M.; Steinley, D.; Young, J. & Murray, M. D. (2007). Patients' Health Literacy and Experience with Instructions : Influence Preferences for Heart Failure Medication Instructions. *Journal of Aging & Health,* Vol.19, No.4 (August), pp. 575-593, ISSN 0898-2643

Mróz, L. W.; Chapman, G. E.; Oliffe, J. L. & Bottorff J. L. (2011). Men, Food, and Prostate Cancer: Gender Influences on Men's Diets. *American Journal of Men's Health,* Vol.5, No.2, (March), pp. 177-187, ISSN 1557-9891

Nanton, V.; Docherty, A.; Meystre, C. & Dale, J. (2009). Finding a Pathway: Information and Uncertainty along the Prostate Cancer Patient Journey. *British Journal of Health Psychology,* Vol.14, No.3 (September), pp. 437-458, ISSN 1359-107X

Oldfield, S. R. &Dreher, H. M. (2010). The Concept of Health Literacy within the Older Adult Population. *Holistic Nursing Practice,* Vol.24, No.4, (July-August), pp. 204–212, ISSN 1550-5138

Orel, N. O.; Spence, M. & Steele, J. (2005). Getting the Message Out to Older Adults: Effective HIV Health Education Risk Reduction Publications. *Journal of Applied Gerontology,* Vol.24, No.5, (November), pp. 490-508, ISSN 1552-4523

Paley, J.; Cheyne, H.; Dalgleish, L.; Duncan, E. A. S. & Niven, C. A. (2007). Nursing's Ways of Knowing and Dual Process of Theories of Cognition. *Journal of Advanced Nursing,* Vol.60, No.6, (December), pp. 692-701, ISSN 0309-2402

Peerson, A. & Saunders, M. (2009). Health Literacy Revisited: What Do We Mean and Why Does it Matter? *Health Promotion International,* Vol.24, No.3, (September), pp. 285-296. ISSN 1460-2245

Perlow, E. (2010). Accessibility: Global Gateway to Health Literacy. *Health Promotion Practice,* Vol.11, No.1, (January), pp. 123–131, ISSN 1524 8399

Picker Institute. *About.* Retrieved May 30, 2011, from http://pickerinstitute.org/about

Pierce, P. F. (1996). When the Patient Chooses: Describing Unaided decisions in Health Care. *Human Factors,* Vol.38, No.2 (June), pp. 278-287, ISSN 0018-7208

Prasauskas, R. & Spoo, L. (2006). Literally Improving Patient Outcomes. *Home Health Care Management Practice,* Vol.18, No.4, (June), pp. 270-271, ISSN 1552-6739

Prins, E.; Willson, B.; Kai, T. & Schafft, A. (2009). Social Interaction and Support among Women in Adult Education and Family Literacy. *Adult Education Quarterly,* Vol.59, No.4, (August), pp. 335-352, ISSN 0741-7136

Prout, A.; Hayes, L. & Gelder, L. (1999). Medicines and the Maintenance of Ordinariness in the Household Management of Childhood Asthma. *Sociology of Health & Illness* Vol. 21, No.2, (December), pp. 137–162, ISSN 0141–9889

Rajan, K. S. (2006). *Biocapital: The Constitution of Postgenomic Life,* Duke University Press, ISBN 0-8223-3720-7, Durham, North Carolina, United States

Roberts, N. J. & Partridge, M. R. (2011). Evaluation of a Paper and Electronic Pictorial COPD Action Plan. *Chronic Respiratory Disease,* Vol.8, No.1, (February), pp. 31–40, ISSN 1479-9731

Rootman, I.; Frankish, J. & Kaszap, M. (2007). Health Literacy in Canada, In: *Health Promotion in Canada,* M. O'Neill, A. Pederson, S. Dupere & I. Rootman (Eds.), 61-74, Canadian Scholars' Press, ISBN 1551303256, Toronto, Ontario, Canada

Saposnik, G.; Teasell, R.; Mamdani, M.; Hall, J.; Mcllroy, W.; Cheung, D.; Thorpe, K. E.; Cohen, L. G. & Bayley M. (2010). Effectiveness of Virtual Reality Using Wii Gaming Technology in Stroke Rehabilitation: A Pilot Randomized Clinical Trial and Proof of Principle. *Stroke,* Vol.41, No.7, (July), pp. 1477-1484, ISSN 1524-4628

Scott, J. (1989). *Gender and the Politics of History,* Columbia University Press, ISBN 0-231-11857-0, New York, United States

Shaw, C. R.; Wilson, S. A. & O'Brien, M. E. (1994). Information Needs Prior to Breast Biopsy. *Clinical Nursing Research,* Vol.3, No.2 (May), pp. 119-131, ISSN 1054-7738

Shen, M. & Abate-Shen, C. (2010). Molecular Genetics of Prostate Cancer: New Prospects for Old Challenges. *Genes and Development,* Vol.24, No.18, (September), pp. 1967-2000, ISSN 1549-5477

Siegel, K. & Raveis, V. (1997). Perceptions of Access to HIV-related Information, Care, and Services among Infected Minority Men. *Qualitative Health Research,* Vol.7, No.1, (February), pp. 9-31, ISSN 1552-7557

Sinfield, P.; Baker, R.; Agarwal, S. & Tarrant, C. (2008). Patient-Centred Care: What Are the Experiences of Prostate Cancer Patients and Their Partners? *Patient Education and Counseling* Vol.73, No.1, (October), pp. 91–96, ISSN 0738-3991

Stacey, D.; Paquet, L. & Samant, R. (2010). Exploring Cancer Treatment Decision-making by Patients: A Descriptive Study. *Current Oncology,* Vol.17, No.4, (August), pp. 85-93, ISSN 1198-0052

Steinberg, D. L. (1997). *Bodies in Glass: Genetics, Eugenics, Embryoethics,* Manchester University Press, ISBN 978-0719046681, Manchester, Greater Manchester, United Kingdom

Taylor, J. S. (2005). Surfacing the Body Interior. *Annual Review of Anthropology,* Vol.34, No. (June), pp. 741-56, ISSN 0084-6570

Torres, M. I.; Marquez, D. X.; Carbone, E. T.; Stacciarini, J-M. R. & Foster, J. W. (2008). Culturally Responsive Health Promotion in Puerto Rican Communities: A Structuralist Approach. *Health Promotion Practice,* Vol.9, No.2 (April), pp. 149-158, ISSN 1524-8399.

Van Dijck, J. V. (2005). *The Transparent Body: A Cultural Analysis of Medical Imaging,* University of Washington Press, ISBN 0-295-98490-2, Seattle, Washington, United States

Walker, B. L.; Nail, L. M.; Larsen, L.; Magill, J. & Schwartz, A. (1996). Concerns, Affect, and Cognitive Disruption Following Completion of Radiation Treatment for Localized Breast or Prostate Cancer. *Oncology Nursing Forum,* Vol.23, No.8, (September), pp. 1181-1187, ISSN 0190-535X

Walker, L. G.; Köhler, C. R. D.; Heys, S. D. & Eremin, O. (1998). Psychosocial Aspect of Cancer in the Elderly. *European Journal of Surgical Oncology,Vol.*24, No.5, (October), pp. 375-378, ISSN 0748 7983

Wall, D. & Kristjanson L. (2005). Men, Culture and Hegemonic Masculinity: Understanding the Experience of Prostate Cancer. *Nursing Inquiry,* Vol.12, No.2 (June), pp. 87-97, ISSN 1320-7881

Wallerstein, N. & Bernstein, E. (1988). Empowerment Education: Freire's Ideas Adapted to Health Education. *Health Education & Behavior,* Vol.15, No.4, (December), pp. 379-394, ISSN 1552-6127

Wallington, S. F. (2008). The Internet as an Emerging Patient Education Tool Among African American Men With Prostate Cancer: An Exploratory Study. *American Journal of Men's Health,* Vol. 2, No.2 (June), pp. 106-121, ISSN 1557 9891

Weiss, B. D.; Hart, G.; McGee, D. L. & D'Estelle, S. (1992). Health Status of Illiterate Adults: Relation Between Literacy and Health Status Among Persons with Low Literacy Skills. *Journal of American Board Family Practice,* Vol. 5, No.3, (May-June), pp.257-264, ISSN 0893-8652

Weiss, B. D.; Blanchard, J. S.; McGee, D. L.; Hart, G.; Warren, B.; Burgoon, M. & Smith, K. J. (1994). Illiteracy Among Medicaid Recipients and its Relationship to Health Care Costs. *Journal of Health Care for the Poor and Underserved,* Vol. 5, No.2, (August), pp. 99-111, ISSN 1049-2089

Weiss, B. D. & Coyne, C. (1997). Communication with Patients Who Cannot Read. *The New England Journal of Medecine,* Vol. 337, No.4, (July), pp. 272-273, ISSN 1049-2089

Wilkin, H. A. & Ball-Rokeach, S. J. (2006). Reaching at Risk Groups: The Importance of Health Storytelling in Los Angeles Latino Media. *Journalism,* Vol.7, No.3 (August), pp. 299-320, ISSN 1741-3001

World Health Organization (2002). *Mainstreaming Gender Equity in Health: The Need to Move Forward- Madrid Statement.* Gender Mainstreaming Programme, WHO Regional Office for Europe. Copenhagen, Denmark World Health Organization. Available from http://www.euro.who.int/__data/assets/pdf_file/0008/76508/A75328.pdf

World Health Organization (January 1998). Division of Health Promotion, Education and Communications Health Education and Health Promotion Unit. *Health Promotion Glossary.* Geneva, Switzerland: World Health Organization. Available from http://www.who.int/hpr/NPH/docs/hp_glossary_en.pdf

Zanchetta, M.; Kaszap, M.; Mohamed, M.; Racine, L.; Maheu, C.; Masny, D.; Cèsar, I.; Maltais, C.; Sangwa-Lugoma, G.; Lussier, N. & Kinslikh, D. (2011). Lessons Learned from Francophone Families' Health Literacy: Linguistic Minority Status As a New Social Determinant of Health. Unpublished manuscript

Zanchetta, M.; Monteiro, M. S.; GorospeIV.; F. F.; Pilon, R. S. & Peña, A. (2010). Ideas of Masculinities in Latin America Countries and Their Influences on Immigrant Men's Attitudes toward Health, Prostate Cancer Prevention: An Analysis of Literature. *International Men's Health and People,* Vol.7, No.3, (October), pp. 259-269, ISSN 1875-6867.

Zanchetta, M. S.; Perreault, M.; Kaszap, M. & Viens, C. (2007). Patterns in Information Strategies Used by Older Men to Understand and Deal with Prostate-cancer-related Information: An Application of the Modélisation Qualitative Research Design. *International Journal of Nursing Studies,* Vol.44, No.6 (August), pp. 961-972, ISSN 0020-7489

Zanchetta, M. S.; Cognet, M.; Xenocostas, S.; Aoki, D. & Talbot, Y. (2007). Prostate Cancer among Canadian Men: A Transcultural Representation. *International Journal of Men's Health,* Vol.6, No.3, (September), pp. 224-258, ISSN 1532-6306

Zanchetta, M. S. & Moura, S. (2006). Self-determination and Information-seeking in End Stage of Cancer. *Clinical Journal of Oncology Nursing,* Vol.10, No.6, (December), pp. 803-807, ISSN 1092-1095

Zanchetta, M. S. (2005). Uncertainty and Health Information-seeking Behavior. *Online Brazilian Journal of Nursing,* Vol.4, No.2. Available from: www. uff.br/neape/obj402zanchetta.htm, ISSN 1676-4285

Zanchetta, M.; Cognet, M.; Xenocostas, S.; Talbot, Y.; Upshur, E. G. R.; Aoki, D. & Wildfong, D. (2004). *Family Values and Ethno-cultural Background Underlie Attitudes and Beliefs about Prostate Cancer: Time + Urgency+ Effectiveness…a Challenging Equation.* "Hospitals in a culturally diverse Europe" International conference on quality-assured health care and health promotion for migrants and ethnic minorities. December 9-11, Amsterdam, Netherlands. (Abstracts book, pp. 89-90). Available from: http: //www.mfh-eu.net/conf/results/poster2

Zanchetta, M. S. (2004). Understanding Functional Health Literacy in Experiences with Prostate Cancer: Older Men as Consumers of Health Information. *Online Brazilian Journal of Nursing*, Vol.3, No.2, (July), ISSN 1676-4285. Available from http://www.uff.br/nepae/siteantigo/objn302zanchetta.htm

Zanchetta, M. S. (2002). *Older Men's Self-reported Levels of Functional Health Literacy and the Process of Constructing Strategies to Live and Deal with Prostate Cancer-related Information within Their Natural Environments: A Qualitative Model*. Unpublished PhD. Thesis, Université de Montréal. Publication number NQ75925

4

Prostate Specific Membrane Antigen as Biomarker and Therapeutic Target for Prostate Cancer

Philipp Wolf
Department of Urology, University Medical Centre Freiburg
Germany

1. Introduction

The Prostate Specific Membrane Antigen (PSMA) is considered to be the most well established target antigen in prostate cancer, since it is highly and specifically expressed at all tumor stages on the surface of prostate tumor cells. This chapter outlines the structure, function, and expression of PSMA, its relevance as prognostic and diagnostic biomarker, and different therapeutic approaches targeting this antigen.

2. The Prostate Specific Membrane Antigen (PSMA)

2.1 Structure, function and expression

PSMA, also known as Glutamate Carboxypeptidase II (GCPII, EC 3.4.17.21), N-acetyl-α-linked acidic dipeptidase I (NAALADase) or folate hydrolase, is a type II transmembrane protein, which is anchored in the cell membrane of prostate epithelial cells (Carter et al., 1996; Pinto et al., 1996). In 1998, the gene encoding PSMA was mapped to chromosome 11p11-p12, where it encompasses 19 exons spanning about 60 kb of genomic DNA (O'Keefe et al., 1998). The cDNA of PSMA codes for a glycoprotein of 750 amino acids (aa) with a molecular mass of about 100 kDa. The protein is partitioned into a small intracellular domain of 19 aa, a transmembrane domain of 21 amino acids, and a large extracellular domain of 707 aa. Crystallization data revealed that the extracellular domain of PSMA folds into three distinct structural and functional domains: a protease domain (aa 56-116), an apical domain (aa 117-351), and a C-terminal domain (aa 592-750). Furthermore, it was shown that PSMA is expressed as a compact homodimer, which is highly glycosylated with oligosaccharides accounting up to 25% of the molecular weight (Davis et al., 2005; Mesters et al., 2006).

PSMA contains a binuclear zinc site and can act as glutamate carboxypeptidase or folate hydrolase, catalyzing the hydrolytic cleavage of glutamate from poly-γ-glutamated folates (Ghosh & Heston, 2003). Therefore, PSMA is thought to play a role in the folate metabolism of the prostate. This hypothesis is supported by recent studies, where PSMA expression correlated with proliferation and folate uptake of PSMA transfected cells (Yao & Bacich, 2006; Yao et al., 2009).

In contrast to other prostate-related antigens, like prostate specific antigen (PSA), prostate acidic phosphatase (PAP) or prostate secretory protein (PSP), PSMA is not secreted into circulation. Instead of that, PSMA undergoes constitutive internalization, which is about threefold enhanced after antibody binding (Liu et al., 1998). It is therefore suggested that PSMA has transport function and that anti-PSMA antibodies might act as surrogates for a yet unknown ligand. The endocytic pathways of PSMA after antibody binding were specified in a recent study and comprise clathrin-mediated endocytosis, macropinocytosis, and clathrin-, calveolae-independent endocytosis (Liu et al., 2009b).

To examine the PSMA expression in the prostate, immunohistochemical analyses were performed. In a study with prostate tissue specimen from 184 patients with prostate cancer, the percentage of PSMA positive stained cells averaged about 69.5% (range 20%-90%) in the benign epithelium, 77.9% (range 30-100%) in high grade prostatic intraepithelial neoplasia (PIN) and was highest in adenocarcinomas with a mean of 80.2% (range 30-100%). In contrast, tumor stroma, urothelium, normal vasculature and, with rare exceptions, basal cells were PSMA negative (Bostwick et al., 1998). Other immunohistochemical studies demonstrated a heterogeneous, weak to moderate staining of normal prostate epithelial cells, and a homogeneous, extensive staining of prostate adenocarcinomas and metastases (Silver et al., 1997; Wolf et al., 2010a).

PSMA expression is highly organ specific. An extraprostatic expression was only detected in secretory cells of the salivary glands (Israeli et al., 1994; Troyer et al., 1995; Wolf et al., 2010a), in cryptic cells of the duodenal brush border (Chang et al., 1999; Wolf et al., 2010a), and in a subset of proximal renal tubules (Liu et al., 1997; Silver et al., 1997; Chang et al., 1999). In some studies, an additional expression was found in the brain and in the colon, but these results are controversially discussed (Troyer et al., 1995; Silver et al., 1997; Chang et al., 1999; Sacha et al., 2007). Nonetheless, potential side effects of anti-PSMA therapeutics against PSMA expressing normal organs were not described until today.

Interestingly, PSMA is also discussed as an unique anti-angiogenetic target, since it is expressed in the neovascularization of numerous solid tumors (bladder, kidney, breast, pancreas, lung, melanoma), but not in normal blood vessels (Liu et al., 1997; Chang et al., 1999; Chang et al., 2001; Baccala et al., 2007). In this respect, it was found that PSMA regulates cell invasion and tumor angiogenesis by modulating integrin signal transduction in endothelial cells (Conway et al., 2006).

2.2 PSMA as prognostic and diagnostic biomarker

Generally, prostate carcinoma tissues show a higher PSMA expression and an increased enzymatic activity of PSMA compared with normal prostate and benign prostate hyperplasia (BPH) tissues (Lapidus et al., 2000; Burger et al., 2002). Therefore, the question was raised, if PSMA might serve as a valuable biomarker for the management of prostate cancer.

Indeed, in different studies a direct correlation between PSMA expression and the Gleason score, which is used for the staging of prostate cancer, was determined for adenocarcinomas (Su et al., 1995; Kawakami & Nakayama, 1997; Burger et al., 2002). Moreover, an upregulation of PSMA was shown in tumor cells of patients with hormone-refractory prostate cancer (Wright et al., 1996; Kawakami & Nakayama, 1997). In a study with tissue specimen from 136 patients it was demonstrated that PSMA can serve as a prognostic biomarker, because it significantly correlates with adverse prognostic factors, like tumor grade, pathological stage, aneuploidy, and biochemical recurrence, and therefore independently predicts disease outcome (Ross et al., 2003).

Recently, a new splice variant (PSM-E) was described, which is specifically overexpressed in prostate carcinomas and which correlates with the Gleason score (Cao et al., 2007). PSM-E, which is expressed in the cytoplasm, could account for the lack of correlation between histological positive staining of anti-PSMA antibodies with clinical grade (stage) (Mannweiler et al., 2009).

Despite of such controversies, it is apparent that the enhanced expression and enzymatic activity of PSMA in aggressive prostate tumors is indicative of a selective advantage on the part of cells expressing it and that it contributes to prostate carcinogenesis.

PSMA was found to associate with the anaphase-promoting complex and to induce chromosomal instability (Rajasekaran et al., 2008). Moreover, PSMA favoured prostate cancer development in a permissive folate environment (Yao & Bacich, 2006; Yao et al., 2009). One mechanism by which PSMA contributes to prostate tumor growth is its ability to activate IL-6 and CCL5 synthesis. These cytokines acted synergistically to enhance the growth of LNCaP cells by activating the MAPK pathway (Colombatti et al., 2009).

Taken together, assessment of PSMA levels, either alone or in combination with PSA status, might prove useful in future for the diagnosis of metastatic prostate cancer, risk assessment, and the prognosis of disease outcome.

2.3 PSMA as therapeutic target

Specific characteristics of PSMA concerning its structure, function and expression make it an ideal candidate as a target antigen for the treatment of advanced prostate cancer. (1) Its high and specific expression on the prostate cancer cell surface and the fact that it is not shed into the circulation allows an effective systemic delivery of PSMA targeting therapeutics. (2) Its high organ specificity leads to a minimal binding of anti-PSMA drugs to normal organs and therefore to a maximal reduction of potential side effects. (3) Its expression at all tumor stages enables a therapeutic intervention at any time of the disease. (4) Its internalization after ligand binding can be used for the targeted delivery of intracellular acting drugs. (5) Its enzymatic activity allows the cleavage of prodrugs to active molecules on the surface of prostate cancer cells.

Many preclinical and clinical studies were performed in the last years, which used PSMA as target antigen. They include radioimmunotherapy, the use of immunotoxins, targeted virotherapy, retargeting of immune cells, PSMA vaccination, prodrug activation, photodynamic therapy, and PSMA targeting nanoparticles.

2.3.1 Anti-PSMA radioimmunotherapy

Radioimmunoconjugates generally consist of an antibody moiety as target domain coupled to a therapeutic radionuclide (alpha- or beta-particle) with the biologic effect of high linear energy transfer (LET) radiation. Compared to conventional radiotherapy, radioimmunoconjugates allow the targeted delivery of reduced radiation doses to the tumor, which ideally leads to a reduction of side effects. Moreover, the radiation of a radioimmunoconjugate is not restricted to cells presenting the target antigen. It also affects neighboring cells with a heterogeneous antigen expression or insufficient vascularization, which is so called "bystander effect" (Rzeszowska-Wolny et al., 2009).

An initial immunoscintigraphic approach targeting PSMA was done with the ^{111}Indium (^{111}In) labeled anti-PSMA monoclonal antibody 7E11 (Capromab Pendetide (Prosta Scint®), Cytogen, Philadelphia, PA) (Kahn et al., 1994; Sodee et al., 1996; Kahn et al., 1998). With this radioimmunoconjugate a higher sensitivity was reached in the imaging of prostate cancer soft tissue metastases compared to Computed Tomography (CT) or Magnetic Resonance Tomography (MRT) (Murphy et al., 1998). Therefore, Prosta Scint® received approval from the U.S. Food and Drug Administration (FDA) for the detection and imaging of prostate cancer soft tissue metastases (Rosenthal et al., 2001). The reason, why Prosta Scint® is only suitable for the detection of soft tissue metastases, is based on the fact that the 7E11 antibody recognizes an intracellular epitope of PSMA. Therefore, it can not bind to viable tumor cells, but only to PSMA molecules in damaged, dead or dying cells. Lymph node or bone metastatic lesions tend to be relatively small and do not characteristically own a high percentage of apoptotic or necrotic cells. Indeed, in a radioimmunotherapeutic trail with the ^{90}Yttrium-(^{90}Y) labeled 7E11, no objective or biochemical remissions could be measured (Deb et al., 1996; Kahn et al., 1999).

Therefore, monoclonal antibodies, which bind to the extracellular domain of PSMA, were used for the construction of radioimmunoconjugates in subsequent studies. Three anti-PSMA antibodies, called 3/A12, 3/E7, and 3/F11, which recognize different extracellular epitopes, were labeled with ^{64}Copper (^{64}Cu) and used for Positron Emission Tomography (PET) imaging of human prostatic tumors in the SCID mouse xenograft model. Whereas excellent tumor uptakes of all antibodies between 31.6 and 35.1%ID/g were measured in tumors of the PSMA expressing androgen-independent LNCaP subline C4-2, only activities at background levels were detected in PSMA negative DU 145 control xenografts (Elsasser-Beile et al., 2009; Alt et al., 2010). In a first preclinical experiment, the antibody 3/F11 was labeled with the beta particle emitter ^{177}Lutetium (^{177}Lu) and was used for the radioimmunotherapy of mice bearing C4-2 tumors xenografts. Biodistribution studies revealed a tumor to muscle ratio of more than 70 and a tumor to blood ratio of more than 4.5 after 72 h. Treatment of mice with the conjugate resulted in tumor growth inhibition and in a more than 2-fold enhanced survival after application of a single dose of 1 MBq. However, in this study the therapeutic window was small, because mice treated with a dose of 2 MBq apparently died of myelotoxicity (Behe et al., 2011).

Another panel of antibodies binding to extracellular PSMA (J415, J533, and J591) was tested in preclinical and clinical trials for radioimmunotherapy. J591 was labeled with the alpha particle emitter ^{213}Bismuth (^{213}Bi), which is well suited for the radiation of single cell neoplasms and micrometastases in a range between 0.07 and 0.1 mm. [^{213}Bi]J591 caused a high cytotoxicity against LNCaP cells *in vitro. In vivo*, a significant improvement of tumor free survival in nude bearing LNCaP tumors was reached, which was accompanied by a significant reduction of PSA serum levels (McDevitt et al., 2000). In another study, the biodistribution of the ^{131}Iod (^{131}I) labeled antibodies J591, J415, and 7E11 was examined. High tumor uptakes were measured with all antibodies in LNCaP tumor xenografts, which were up to 20-fold higher than in PSMA negative DU 145 or PC-3 tumors. Autoradiographic studies showed that the extracellular binding antibodies J415 and J591 preferentially recognized areas of viable tumor cells, whereas the intracellular binding antibody 7E11 mainly detected necrotic tumor areas (Smith-Jones et al., 2003).

The antibody J591 was chosen for further radioimmunotherapeutic experiments. To reduce a possible immunogenicity of the mouse antibody in prostate cancer patients, J591 was humanized by site directed mutagenesis of putative B- and T-cell epitopes of the variable domains and by exchanging the mouse constant domains into human ones. The humanized antibody J591 (huJ591) was then labeled with ^{131}I and ^{90}Y. Doses of 3.7 to 11.1 MBq ^{131}I-hu591 and of 3.7 to 4.7 MBq ^{90}Y-hu591 led to a reduction of mean tumor volumes between 15 and 90% in nude mice bearing LNCaP tumors. Additionally, both radioimmunoconjugates effected an 2 to 3-fold increase of median survival relative to untreated controls (Vallabhajosula et al., 2004).

In a first phase I clinical trail, prostate cancer patients initially received the ^{111}In-labeled huJ591 for immunoscintigraphy followed by application of ^{90}Y-huJ591 for therapy. With ^{111}In-huJ591 total body images demonstrated a significant metabolism of the radioimmunoconjugate in the liver and to a lesser extend in the kidneys and spleen. Additionally, bone and soft tissue metastases were efficiently targeted. One week later, ^{90}Y-huJ591 was applicated and a maximal tolerated dose (MTD) of 17.5 mCi/m^2 could be determined. PSA stabilisation was noted in 6/29 patients and 2 patients showed a PSA decline of 70 and 85% lasting 8 and 8.6 months, respectively (Milowsky et al., 2004). Another cohort of 35 patients received ^{177}Lu-labeled huJ591 at doses between 10 and 75 mCi/m^2. Blood and urinary pharmacokinetics were similar to those of ^{90}Y-huJ591. But the MTD of 70 mCi/m^2 was about 4-fold higher. Patients treated with 75 mCi/m^2 ^{177}Lu-huJ591 developed grade 3 and 4 thrombocytopenia and grade 4 neutropenia, but retreatment with 30 mCi/m^2 was well tolerated. In 4 patients a PSA decline of more than 50% and in 16 patients a PSA stabilisation was noted (Milowsky et al., 2004). In both clinical trials with radiolabeled huJ591 myelosuppression was dose-limiting. Whereas no clear correlation between myelotoxicity and therapeutic dose was determined for ^{90}Y-huJ591, myelotoxicity and especially thrombocytopenia correlated well with the applicated doses and the bone marrow doses for ^{177}Lu-huJ591 (Vallabhajosula et al., 2005).

To verify PSMA as a target for an anti-angiogenesis therapy, ^{111}In-huJ591 was used for the imaging of known metastases in patients with different solid tumors. Indeed, this radioimmunoconjugate showed a high uptake in metastases of 7/10 kidney cancer patients, 4/4 colon carcinoma patients, 3/3 lung cancer patients, 3/3 pancreatic cancer patients, 1/3 bladder cancer patients, 2/3 breast cancer patients, and 1/1 melanoma patient (Milowsky et al., 2007).

2.3.2 Anti-PSMA immunotoxins

PSMA was also used as a target for the generation of immunotoxins against prostate cancer. Immunotoxins are constructs, where a PSMA binding domain (antibody, antibody fragment, RNA aptamer, peptide) is coupled to a toxin domain. The toxin domain is targeted by the PSMA binding domain to the prostate cancer cell and is cytotoxic after internalization.

Ricin from *Ricinus communis* acts as a very common toxin for the construction of immunotoxins. It consists of the ricin A chain and the ricin B chain held together by a disulfide bond. The ricin A chain is the enzymatically active subunit, which inactivates the protein biosynthesis machinery by irreversible hydrolysis of the N-glycosidic bond of an adenine (A4324) within the 28S rRNA. The ricin B chain binds ubiquitous to cell surface structures and facilitates membrane translocation and intracellular trafficking of the ricin A chain (Sandvig et al., 2002).

The first generation of anti-PSMA immunotoxins was made by chemically coupling of anti-PSMA antibodies to ricin A. An immunotoxin consisting of J591 and ricin A elicited a 50% reduction in cell viability (IC_{50}) of LNCaP cells at a concentration of about 265 pM and showed a more than 5000-fold potentation of cytotoxicity compared to the unconjugated ricin A chain (Fracasso et al., 2002). For another ricin A-based immunotoxin with the rat monoclonal antibody E6 an IC_{50} value of 60 pM was measured. Additionally, a significant inhibition of LNCaP tumor growth in the mouse xenograft model was reached with this molecule (Huang et al., 2004).

In a recent study, the humanized antibody huJ591 was linked to the plant toxin saporin. Saporin is produced is seeds and leaves of the plant *Saponaria officinalis* and belongs to class I ribosome inactivating proteins. With the saporin-based immunotoxin, a percentage of 60.3% apoptotic cells and an IC_{50} value of 140 pM was determined on LNCaP cells after 72 h incubation. Furthermore, a significant inhibition of tumor growth was measured in the LNCaP tumor xenograft model. However, due to its high molecular weight of about 280 kDa, the immunotoxin is thought to have a high immunogenicity and a limited diffusion into tumor tissues. Therefore, further development is focused on saporin-based constructs of smaller size less inherent immunogenicity (Kuroda et al., 2010).

The anti-PSMA antibody J591 was also used for the construction of an immunotoxin containing the melittin-like peptide 101 from honey bee (*Apis mellifera*) venom. This construct successfully inhibited the growth of LNCaP-LN3 tumors and led to a slight improvement of the median survival of treated mice. However, the high affinity of peptide 101 to lipid bilayer membranes also led to a high non-specific cytotoxicity (Russell et al., 2004).

A further immunotoxin was generated by coupling huJ591 to the chemotherapeutic drug maytansinoid 1 (DM1) (Henry et al., 2004), which is a microtubule-depolymerizing analogue of maytansine (Chari et al., 1992). Maytansine is a naturally occurring ansa macrolide and was evaluated as a chemotherapeutic agent in the 1970s and 1980s. Unfortunately, maytansine caused severe, dose-limiting gastrointestinal and central neurological toxicities and was therefore not developed further (Blum et al., 1978). With the DM1-based anti-PSMA immunotoxin, called MLN2704, a growth delay of CWR22Rv1 tumor xenografts of more than 100 days was achieved at an optimized dosage schedule of 60 mg/kg every 14 days (Henry et al., 2004). MLN2704 was also tested in a clinical phase I trial in 9 patients with prostate cancer. Two of these patients, treated with 264 or 343 mg/m^2 immunotoxin respectively, had a more than 50% decrease in their PSA serum level. Additionally, the patient treated with 264 mg/m^2 showed a measurable tumor regression (Galsky et al., 2008).

In another approach, a fully human anti-PSMA antibody was generated in transgenic mice and was conjugated to monomethylauristatin E (MMAE), which is a potent inhibitor of tubulin polymerization. With this construct IC_{50} values of 83 pM on LNCaP cells and of 65 pM on C4-2 cells could be determined. Furthermore, a significant improvement of the median survival of tumor bearing mice 9-fold relative to the controls was reached without any signs of toxicity. Interestingly, 2/5 animals treated with a maximal dose of 6 mg/kg immunotoxin had no detectable tumor or measurable PSA at day 500 and could therefore considered as cure (Ma et al., 2006).

Obstacles of chemically conjugated immunotoxins to be optimal therapeutic agents comprise a high immunogenicity, a possible influence of chemical modifications on antigen binding, and inhomogeneous preparations. This can, at least in part, be overcome by second generation, recombinant immunotoxins.

For the construction of the first recombinant immunotoxin against PSMA, an anti-PSMA single chain antibody fragment (scFv), consisting of one variable domain of the heavy chain (V_H) and one variable domain of the light chain (V_L) connected by a flexible linker, was generated from the monoclonal antibody 3/A12 by phage display. This scFv was called A5.

As toxin domain, the truncated form of *Pseudomonas* exotoxin A (PE40), consisting of the transmembrane domain and the enzymatically active domain of the toxin, was used. The virulence factor *Pseudomonas* Exotoxin A from the human pathogenic bacterium *Pseudomonas aeruginosa* is able to ADP-ribosylate the eukaryotic elongation factor 2 (eEF-2) of a target cell, which leads to the inhibition of protein biosynthesis and finally to apoptosis (Wolf & Elsasser-Beile, 2009). The bacterially expressed anti-PSMA immunotoxin, called A5-PE40, specifically bound to prostate cancer cells with IC_{50} values in the low pM range. Moreover, it induced a significant growth inhibition of C4-2 tumors in the SCID mouse xenograft model (Wolf et al., 2006; Wolf et al., 2008).

A similar immunotoxin was recently generated by using the scFv D7 from the anti-PSMA antibody 3/F11. This immunotoxin, termed D7-PE40, also showed a high binding to C4-2 cells and led to a significant growth inhibition of subcutaneously implanted tumors. In toxicity studies, D7-PE40 was well tolerated in mice at single, but at higher doses the immunotoxin was lethal. Blood analyses indicated that the death of the animals was based on a severe hepatotoxicity, which was marked by increased aspartate transaminase (AST) and alanine transaminase (ALT) serum levels. Histopathological examinations revealed a marked damage of the hepatic parenchyma with disappearance of sinusoidal structures based on apoptosis and vacuolar degeneration of hepatocytes (Wolf et al., 2010b). Hepatotoxicity is a very common side effect of *Pseudomonas* Exotoxin A based immunotoxins and is presumably attributed to a TNF-alpha release of Kupffer cells (Onda et al., 1999). Different strategies are therefore under investigation to reduce the hepatotoxicity, e.g. by PEGylation or lowering of the isoelectric points of the immunotoxins (Onda et al., 2001). Another main research comprises the reduction of the immunogenicity by elimination of immunodominant B-cell epitopes (Onda et al., 2006).

Alternatively to antibodies or antibody fragments, RNA aptamers can be used for the construction of immunotoxins, which are considered to be advantageous with respect to a higher stability, ease of synthesis and lower production costs. One immunotoxin was constructed by coupling of an anti-PSMA RNA aptamer to the plant toxin gelonin from *Gelonium multiflorum*, which has high N-glycosidase activity on the 28S RNA unit of eukaryotic ribosomes. This molecule was found to be toxic against prostate cancer cells with an IC_{50} value of 27 nM (Onda et al., 2006).

Recently, a chemical ligand, termed 2-[3-(1,3-dicarboxypropyl)ureido] pentanedioic acid (DUPA), was synthesized that selectively binds to PSMA (Kularatne et al., 2010). After coupling to different chemotherapeutic drugs, this molecule was capable to mediate the targeted killing of LNCaP cells (Kularatne et al., 2010).

2.3.3 Targeted virotherapy

In a recent study, measles viruses of a live attenuated strain were used for a targeted anti-PSMA virotherapy (Liu et al., 2009a). Measles viruses are very effective against a variety of tumor types, including prostate cancer (Blechacz & Russell, 2008; Msaouel et al., 2009). Generally, measles viruses infect host cells via one of two measles receptors, CD64 or SLAM. CD64 is ubiquitously present on the surface of human cells, whereas SLAM is expressed on immune cells. The viruses take their oncolytic effect by induction of an extensive intracellular fusion between infected cells and neighboring cells to form non-viable multinucleated structures (syncytia). For the construction of the virotherapeutic conjugate, called MVG-αPSMA, the anti-PSMA antibody huJ591 was coupled to a coat protein of measles virus, in which alanine substitutions of specific residues ablated the viral interaction with CD64 and SLAM. After propagation and infection, a MVG-αPSMA mediated cytopathic killing of PSMA expressing LNCaP and PC3/PIP cells was detected. Moreover, a regression or growth inhibition of tumor xenografts could be achieved (Msaouel et al., 2009). A crucial obstacle for a future clinical use of MVG-αPSMA could be pre-existing anti-viral antibodies in patients, who have been vaccinated or infected by wild type measles viruses. These antibodies might quickly neutralize the virus domain after application. Therefore, efforts are undertaken to circumvent the problem, e.g. by intratumoral application of the construct, by hiding the virus in cell carriers, or by the use of immunosuppressive drugs to dampen the patient's immune response (Liu et al., 2009a).

2.3.4 Retargeting of immune cells

The therapeutic concept of immune cell retargeting comprises the activation of T lymphocytes for the targeted cytolysis of tumor cells. For the retargeting of prostate cancer cells via PSMA, two strategies were pursued: the construction of diabodies and the generation of fusion receptors.

Generally, diabodies for T cell retargeting consist of two antibody domains. One domain binds to the tumor antigen and the other one to a T cell activating antigen. The diabody builds a bridge between the tumor cell and the immune effector cell, which then triggers the cytotoxic responses that include perforin and granzyme release.

Anti-PSMA diabodies were constructed by fusing the anti-PSMA scFvs A5 or D7 to a scFv against the CD3 T cell receptor. With these constructs, a retargeting of CD4+ and CD8+ blood lymphocytes with subsequent lysis of C4-2 cells was obtained. Moreover, a significant inhibition of C4-2 tumor growth could be achieved (Buhler et al., 2008; Buhler et al., 2009; Fortmuller et al., 2011).

A fusion receptor targeting PSMA, also referred to as chimeric antigen receptor (CAR), was generated by coupling an anti-PSMA scFv to the zeta-chain of the CD3 T-cell receptor. The CAR can be expressed at the surface of CAR-transfected T cells. Then the CAR can recruit and activate the T cell by binding to PSMA. This mechanism is independent of a human leukocyte antigen expression. Using CAR transfected peripheral blood lymphocytes, a specific killing of PSMA-expressing prostate cancer cells and an elimination of orthotopically or subcutaneously implanted PSMA-positive tumors was reached (Gade et al., 2005). In a subsequent study, the effects of CAR could be optimized by adding combined CD28 and 4-1BBL costimulatory signaling domains. With this strategy, an enhanced cytokine release, a higher *in vivo* T cell survival, and an enhanced anti-tumor activity could be measured in tumor bearing SCID mice (Zhong et al., 2010).

A similar fusion receptor against PSMA, designated as chimeric immunoglobulin T-cell receptor (IgTCR), was also used for the retargeting of immune cells. IgTCR consists of an anti-PSMA scFv from the monoclonal antibody 3D8 and a signaling portion of the CD3 zeta chain. IgTCR transfected T-cells were activated after PSMA binding, which was followed by cytokine release and specific lysis of the prostate cancer cells. Additionally, this molecule showed a high anti-tumor activity in a mouse xenograft model (Ma et al., 2004).

2.3.5 PSMA vaccination

Vaccination with PSMA peptides, which aims for boosting the patient's immune response against PSMA expressing tumor cells, represent another weapon in the battle against prostate cancer. One approach utilizes the patient's dentritic cells (DCs), to present PSMA peptides in association with the MHC class I peptide complex to naïve cytotoxic T lymphocytes (CTL) (Melief, 2008). For DC preparation, patients were leucophoresed, and peripheral blood mononuclear cells (PBMCs) were isolated. Adherent cells were differentiated with GM-CSF and IL-4. Then the obtained DCs were pulsed with recombinant PSMA peptides, which were identified in function of their ability to recruit CTLs and to be recognized as CTL targets. In a first phase I/II clinical trial involving 33 prostate cancer patients, 9 partial responders were identified with an average response duration of 225 days (Tjoa et al., 1998). In a phase II study, 2/33 patients with hormone refractory metastatic disease showed a complete response and another 6 patients a partial response (Murphy et al., 1999). In another clinical trial with 37 patients, one complete and 10 partial responses were identified (Salgaller et al., 1998; Tjoa et al., 1999).

Two subsequent protocols used DCs to present a PSMA peptide in combination with peptides from other tumor antigens to treat hormone-refractory patients. In one study, CTL responses and transient decline of serum PSA was observed in 4/8 patients, who received 4 intradermal vaccinations every other week (Fuessel et al., 2006). In the other study, 3 patients were administered with 6 vaccines intradermally at biweekly intervals and showed partial remissions. However, no CTL response against the PSMA peptide could be observed (Waeckerle-Men et al., 2006). The same PSMA peptide was loaded as a single peptide to PBMCs, which were used to treat 12 patients with hormone-resistant tumors. However, no clinical advantages were observed and no immune responses were detected in this trial (Knight et al., 2009).

A further development was the transfection of DCs with plasmids containing the extracellular domain of PSMA to activate autologous lymphocytes in an *in vitro* model. Indeed, PSMA-expressing DCs were able to generate antigen-specific cytotoxic T cell responses (Mincheff et al., 2003).

In a recent study, replication deficient adenoviruses were used to introduce a truncated form of PSMA and the T cell stimulatory molecule 4-1BBL into murine DCs. After infection of the DCs, PSMA-specific proliferative responses and an upregulation of CD80 and CD86 costimulatory molecules were detected. Moreover, vaccination of mice with the transfected DCs induced a potent protective and therapeutic anti-tumor immunity (Kuang et al., 2010).

Other strategies for PSMA vaccination are the application of DNA plasmids or viral immunizations. In a phase I study, prostate cancer patients were intradermally immunized with an expression plasmid or a replication-defective adenoviral vector bearing the PSMA gene according to six different drug regimens. All vaccinations were well tolerated and no immediate- or long-time side effects were reported (Mincheff et al., 2000). Anti-PSMA antibodies were found in 21% of patients at baseline and in 12-50% of patients at longitudinal time points ranging from 3 to 36 months after immunization (Todorova et al., 2005).

In a preclinical study it was shown that immunization of mice with xenogenic PSMA protein followed by a boosting with a vector that encoded autologous PSMA gave the best protection (Mincheff et al., 2006). These data provided the basis for a clinical study with DNA plasmid vaccines, in which 36 patients with recurrent prostate cancer received three vaccinations with mouse or human PSMA. Vaccination was well tolerated and PSA serum levels were maximally reduced at the highest dose level (Gregor et al., 2007).

2.3.6 Prodrug activation

The glutamate carboxy peptidase activity of PSMA can be used for the activation of prodrugs to a fully active compound on the surface of prostate cancer cells. Different methotrexate-based peptide analoges were screened to identify PSMA selective substrates that are stable to unspecific hydrolysis in human and mouse plasma. Analogs containing α-linked or γ-linked glutamic or aspartic acids were most efficiently hydrolyzed by PSMA to release the cytolytic anti-metabolite methotrexate. As a consequence thereof, these analoges showed the highest cytotoxicity against PSMA-expressing prostate cancer cells (Mhaka et al., 2004). In a subsequent study, these peptides were coupled to a cytotoxic analogue of the plant toxin thapsigargin that induces apoptosis by inhibition of the endoplasmatic reticulum Ca-ATPase pump. PSMA hydrolysis of these peptide prodrugs led to a cytotoxicity against PSMA-positive prostate cancer cells that was 10- to 60-fold higher than against PSMA-negative ones. One of these prodrugs was also tested in mice with CWR22H xenografts and elicited tumor growth delay or tumor regressions following a single 3-day or 10-day course of administration (Mhaka et al., 2006).

2.3.7 Photodynamic therapy

The lack of specific delivery of photosensitizers, chemical compounds that can be excited by light of a specific wavelength for the destruction of tumor tissues, represents a significant limitation for photodynamic therapies (PDT). Therefore, a conjugate was generated containing the photosensitizer pyropheophorbide-a and a PSMA inhibitor for the treatment of prostate cancer. This construct demonstrated a high and specific cytotoxicity against LNCaP cells after irradiation, whereas PSMA-negative PC-3 cells remained unaffected. PDT-mediated effects of the photodynamic conjugate were extensively studied and involved cell membrane permeabilization, rapid disruption of microtubules (α-/β-tubulin), microfilaments (actin), and intermediate filaments (cytokeratin 8/18) in the cytoplasm, activation of caspase-3, -8, and -9, Poly [ADP-ribose] Polymerase (PARP)-cleavage, and DNA fragmentation (Liu et al., 2009c; Liu et al., 2010a; Liu et al., 2010b).

2.3.8 Nanoparticles targeting PSMA

Nanotechnology represents a new alternative for the treatment of prostate cancer. The production of nanoparticles enables the targeted delivery and controlled release of thousands of drug molecules per vehicle into the tumor cells and is a promising strategy to overcome the lack of specificity and limited efficacy of conventional chemotherapeutic agents.

One of the first therapeutic nanoparticle against prostate cancer was a docetaxel-encapsulated nanoparticle formulated with biocompatible and biodegradable poly(D,L-lactic acid-co-glycolic acid)-block-poly(ethyleneglycol) copolymer (PLGA-b-PEG), which surface was derivatized with the anti-PSMA RNA-aptamer A10. With this construct, an enhanced cytotoxicity, compared to non-targeted nanoparticles that lack the aptamer, was shown. After a single intratumoral injection, the nanoparticle elicited a complete tumor reduction in 5/7 mice with LNCaP tumor xenografts of about 300 mm^3 in size. The survival rate of these mice in a 109 days study was 100%, compared to 57% of mice treated with the non-targeted nanoparticle and to 14% of mice treated with docetaxel alone (Farokhzad et al., 2006). In a subsequent study, the cisplatin prodrug Pt(IV) was encapsulated in the anti-PSMA nanoparticle. Endocytosis was detected using fluorescence microscopy by colocalization of the encapsulated green fluorescent labeled cholesterol with early endosome marker EEA-1. In a series of *in vitro* cytotoxic assays, the IC_{50} value was determined as 0.03 μM for the nanoparticele compared to 0.13 μM for the non-targeted nanoparticle and to 2.4 μM for free cisplatin on LNCaP cells. However, a high background toxicity of the nanoparticle with an IC_{50} value of 0.11 μM was also detected on PSMA-negative PC-3 cells (Dhar et al., 2008). In a recent study, the anti-PSMA aptamer based nanoparticle was optimized to a self-assembly polymeric nanoparticle carrying cisplatin and docetaxel to prostate cancer cells with synergistic cytotoxicity. The controlled released of both chemotherapeutics was observed over a time period of 48 to 72 h and formation of cisplatin 1,2d(GpG) intrastrand crosslinks could be detected. *In vitro* cytotoxicity of the targeted nanoparticle with an IC_{50} value of 0.09 μM on LNCaP cells was shown to be superior over single drug or non targeted nanoparticles (Kolishetti et al., 2010).

Epigallocatechin 3-gallate (EGCG) is a green tea catechin, which has protective effects against some common types of cancer (Yang et al., 2009). Since it was shown to be chemopreventive against prostate cancer (Bettuzzi et al., 2006; Brausi et al., 2008), an EGCG loaded nanoparticle consisting of PLGA-PEG copolymers was functionalized with an urea-based PSMA inhibitor (Sanna et al., 2011), which is capable of targeting PSMA with a similar affinity and specificity like antibodies and aptamers (Sanna et al., 2011). In *in vitro* experiments LNCaP cells were incubated for 1 or 3 h with the anti-PSMA nanoparticles. In this assay, a significant antiproliferative effect of the nanoparticles to the tumor cells, marked by a growth inhibition up to 60% after 72 h, could be measured (Sanna et al., 2011).

3. Conclusion

In the last years, PSMA arouse increasing interest as a prognostic and diagnostic biomarker as well as an attractive target antigen for new therapeutic approaches against prostate cancer.

Anti-PSMA radioimmunoconjugates demonstrated efficient targeting of soft tissue and bone metastases and led to objective anti-tumor responses in a subset of patients. Moreover, high efficacy and tolerability of anti-PSMA immunotoxins was shown in many preclinical and clinical trials. The future strategy in this field is the recombinant production of immunotoxins, by which different limitations of chemically linked immunotoxins can be overcome.

Retargeting of cytotoxic lymphocytes *in vitro* and *in vivo* led to anti-tumor activities in different preclinical studies. These effects could be enhanced by the evocation of costimulatory signaling. Additionally, early vaccination trials showed that an anti-PSMA immune response can be generated without general toxicity in prostate cancer patients.

The development of PSMA-targeted prodrugs, photosensitizers and nanoparticles is still in an early stage, but such constructs also represent alternative therapeutics in the near future.

It has to be considered that most of the discussed clinical treatments were tested in patients with advanced prostate cancer. However, as shown in preclinical trials, these new therapeutic drugs seem likely to be more effective in patients with minimal residual disease or metastases after primary therapies.

4. References

Alt, K., Wiehr, S., Ehrlichmann, W., Reischl, G., Wolf, P., Pichler, B.J., Elsasser-Beile, U. & Buhler, P. (2010). High-resolution animal PET imaging of prostate cancer xenografts with three different (64)Cu-labeled antibodies against native cell-adherent PSMA. *Prostate*, Vol. 70, No. 13, pp. 1413-1421.

Baccala, A., Sercia, L., Li, J., Heston, W. & Zhou, M. (2007). Expression of prostate-specific membrane antigen in tumor-associated neovasculature of renal neoplasms. *Urology,* Vol. 70, No. 2, pp. 385-390.

Bander, N.H., Milowsky, M.I., Nanus, D.M., Kostakoglu, L., Vallabhajosula, S. & Goldsmith, S.J. (2005). Phase I trial of 177lutetium-labeled J591, a monoclonal antibody to prostate-specific membrane antigen, in patients with androgen-independent prostate cancer. *J Clin Oncol,* Vol. 23, No. 21, pp. 4591-4601.

Behe, M., Alt, K., Deininger, F., Buhler, P., Wetterauer, U., Weber, W.A., Elsasser-Beile, U. & Wolf, P. (2011). In vivo testing of 177Lu-labelled anti-PSMA antibody as a new radioimmunotherapeutic agent against prostate cancer. *In Vivo,* Vol. 25, No. 1, pp. 55-59.

Bettuzzi, S., Brausi, M., Rizzi, F., Castagnetti, G., Peracchia, G. & Corti, A. (2006). Chemoprevention of human prostate cancer by oral administration of green tea catechins in volunteers with high-grade prostate intraepithelial neoplasia: a preliminary report from a one-year proof-of-principle study. *Cancer Res,* Vol. 66, No. 2, pp. 1234-1240.

Blechacz, B. & Russell, S.J. (2008). Measles virus as an oncolytic vector platform. *Curr Gene Ther,* Vol. 8, No. 3, pp. 162-175.

Blum, R.H., Wittenberg, B.K., Canellos, G.P., Mayer, R.J., Skarin, A.T., Henderson, I.C., Parker, L.M. & Frei, E., 3rd. (1978). A therapeutic trial of maytansine. *Cancer Clin Trials,* Vol. 1, No. 2, pp. 113-117.

Bostwick, D.G., Pacelli, A., Blute, M., Roche, P. & Murphy, G.P. (1998). Prostate specific membrane antigen expression in prostatic intraepithelial neoplasia and adenocarcinoma: a study of 184 cases. *Cancer,* Vol. 82, No. 11, pp. 2256-2261.

Brausi, M., Rizzi, F. & Bettuzzi, S. (2008). Chemoprevention of human prostate cancer by green tea catechins: two years later. A follow-up update. *Eur Urol,* Vol. 54, No. 2, pp. 472-473.

Buhler, P., Molnar, E., Dopfer, E.P., Wolf, P., Gierschner, D., Wetterauer, U., Schamel, W.W. & Elsasser-Beile, U. (2009). Target-dependent T-cell activation by coligation with a PSMA x CD3 diabody induces lysis of prostate cancer cells. *J Immunother,* Vol. 32, No. 6, pp. 565-573.

Buhler, P., Wolf, P., Gierschner, D., Schaber, I., Katzenwadel, A., Schultze-Seemann, W., Wetterauer, U., Tacke, M., Swamy, M., Schamel, W.W. & Elsasser-Beile, U. (2008). A bispecific diabody directed against prostate-specific membrane antigen and CD3 induces T-cell mediated lysis of prostate cancer cells. *Cancer Immunol Immunother,* Vol. 57, No. 1, pp. 43-52.

Burger, M.J., Tebay, M.A., Keith, P.A., Samaratunga, H.M., Clements, J., Lavin, M.F. & Gardiner, R.A. (2002). Expression analysis of delta-catenin and prostate-specific membrane antigen: their potential as diagnostic markers for prostate cancer. *Int J Cancer,* Vol. 100, No. 2, pp. 228-237.

Cao, K.Y., Mao, X.P., Wang, D.H., Xu, L., Yuan, G.Q., Dai, S.Q., Zheng, B.J. & Qiu, S.P. (2007). High expression of PSM-E correlated with tumor grade in prostate cancer: a new alternatively spliced variant of prostate-specific membrane antigen. *Prostate,* Vol. 67, No. 16, pp. 1791-1800.

Carter, R.E., Feldman, A.R. & Coyle, J.T. (1996). Prostate-specific membrane antigen is a hydrolase with substrate and pharmacologic characteristics of a neuropeptidase. *Proc Natl Acad Sci U S A,* Vol. 93, No. 2, pp. 749-753.

Chang, S.S., Reuter, V.E., Heston, W.D. & Gaudin, P.B. (2001). Metastatic renal cell carcinoma neovasculature expresses prostate-specific membrane antigen. *Urology,* Vol. 57, No. 4, pp. 801-805.

Chang, S.S., Reuter, V.E., Heston, W.D., Bander, N.H., Grauer, L.S. & Gaudin, P.B. (1999). Five different anti-prostate-specific membrane antigen (PSMA) antibodies confirm PSMA expression in tumor-associated neovasculature. *Cancer Res,* Vol. 59, No. 13, pp. 3192-3198.

Chari, R.V., Martell, B.A., Gross, J.L., Cook, S.B., Shah, S.A., Blattler, W.A., McKenzie, S.J. & Goldmacher, V.S. (1992). Immunoconjugates containing novel maytansinoids: promising anticancer drugs. *Cancer Res,* Vol. 52, No. 1, pp. 127-131.

Chu, T.C., Marks, J.W., 3rd, Lavery, L.A., Faulkner, S., Rosenblum, M.G., Ellington, A.D. & Levy, M. (2006). Aptamer:toxin conjugates that specifically target prostate tumor cells. *Cancer Res,* Vol. 66, No. 12, pp. 5989-5992.

Colombatti, M., Grasso, S., Porzia, A., Fracasso, G., Scupoli, M.T., Cingarlini, S., Poffe, O., Naim, H.Y., Heine, M., Tridente, G., Mainiero, F. & Ramarli, D. (2009). The prostate specific membrane antigen regulates the expression of IL-6 and CCL5 in prostate tumour cells by activating the MAPK pathways. *PLoS One,* Vol. 4, No. 2, pp. e4608.

Conway, R.E., Petrovic, N., Li, Z., Heston, W., Wu, D. & Shapiro, L.H. (2006). Prostate-specific membrane antigen regulates angiogenesis by modulating integrin signal transduction. *Mol Cell Biol,* Vol. 26, No. 14, pp. 5310-5324.

Davis, M.I., Bennett, M.J., Thomas, L.M. & Bjorkman, P.J. (2005). Crystal structure of prostate-specific membrane antigen, a tumor marker and peptidase. *Proc Natl Acad Sci U S A,* Vol. 102, No. 17, pp. 5981-5986.

Deb, N., Goris, M., Trisler, K., Fowler, S., Saal, J., Ning, S., Becker, M., Marquez, C. & Knox, S. (1996). Treatment of hormone-refractory prostate cancer with 90Y-CYT-356 monoclonal antibody. *Clin Cancer Res,* Vol. 2, No. 8, pp. 1289-1297.

Dhar, S., Gu, F.X., Langer, R., Farokhzad, O.C. & Lippard, S.J. (2008). Targeted delivery of cisplatin to prostate cancer cells by aptamer functionalized Pt(IV) prodrug-PLGA-PEG nanoparticles. *Proc Natl Acad Sci U S A,* Vol. 105, No. 45, pp. 17356-17361.

Elsasser-Beile, U., Reischl, G., Wiehr, S., Buhler, P., Wolf, P., Alt, K., Shively, J., Judenhofer, M.S., Machulla, H.J. & Pichler, B.J. (2009). PET Imaging of Prostate Cancer Xenografts with a Highly Specific Antibody against the Prostate-Specific Membrane Antigen. *J Nucl Med,* Vol. 50, No. 4, pp. 606-611.

Farokhzad, O.C., Cheng, J., Teply, B.A., Sherifi, I., Jon, S., Kantoff, P.W., Richie, J.P. & Langer, R. (2006). Targeted nanoparticle-aptamer bioconjugates for cancer chemotherapy in vivo. *Proc Natl Acad Sci U S A,* Vol. 103, No. 16, pp. 6315-6320.

Fortmuller, K., Alt, K., Gierschner, D., Wolf, P., Baum, V., Freudenberg, N., Wetterauer, U., Elsasser-Beile, U. & Buhler, P. (2011). Effective targeting of prostate cancer by lymphocytes redirected by a PSMA x CD3 bispecific single-chain diabody. *Prostate,* Vol. 71, No. 6, pp. 588-596.

Fracasso, G., Bellisola, G., Cingarlini, S., Castelletti, D., Prayer-Galetti, T., Pagano, F., Tridente, G. & Colombatti, M. (2002). Anti-tumor effects of toxins targeted to the prostate specific membrane antigen. *Prostate,* Vol. 53, No. 1, pp. 9-23.

Fuessel, S., Meye, A., Schmitz, M., Zastrow, S., Linne, C., Richter, K., Lobel, B., Hakenberg, O.W., Hoelig, K., Rieber, E.P. & Wirth, M.P. (2006). Vaccination of hormone-refractory prostate cancer patients with peptide cocktail-loaded dendritic cells: results of a phase I clinical trial. *Prostate,* Vol. 66, No. 8, pp. 811-821.

Gade, T.P., Hassen, W., Santos, E., Gunset, G., Saudemont, A., Gong, M.C., Brentjens, R., Zhong, X.S., Stephan, M., Stefanski, J., Lyddane, C., Osborne, J.R., Buchanan, I.M., Hall, S.J., Heston, W.D., Riviere, I., Larson, S.M., Koutcher, J.A. & Sadelain, M. (2005). Targeted elimination of prostate cancer by genetically directed human T lymphocytes. *Cancer Res,* Vol. 65, No. 19, pp. 9080-9088.

Galsky, M.D., Eisenberger, M., Moore-Cooper, S., Kelly, W.K., Slovin, S.F., DeLaCruz, A., Lee, Y., Webb, I.J. & Scher, H.I. (2008). Phase I trial of the prostate-specific membrane antigen-directed immunoconjugate MLN2704 in patients with progressive metastatic castration-resistant prostate cancer. *J Clin Oncol,* Vol. 26, No. 13, pp. 2147-2154.

Ghosh, A. & Heston, W.D. (2003). Effect of carbohydrate moieties on the folate hydrolysis activity of the prostate specific membrane antigen. *Prostate,* Vol. 57, No. 2, pp. 140-151.

Gregor, P., Wolchok, J., Pedraza, A., Orlandi, F., Jefferson, M., Rudolph, J., Curley, T., Houghton, A., Scher, H. & Slovin, S.F., 2007: A xenogeneic PSMA DNA vaccine for patients (pts) with non-castrate metastatic (NCMPC) and castrate metastatic prostate cancer (CMPC): A phase I trial of proof of principle. In 2007 Prostate Cancer Symposium (Orlando).

Henry, M.D., Wen, S., Silva, M.D., Chandra, S., Milton, M. & Worland, P.J. (2004). A prostate-specific membrane antigen-targeted monoclonal antibody-chemotherapeutic conjugate designed for the treatment of prostate cancer. *Cancer Res,* Vol. 64, No. 21, pp. 7995-8001.

Huang, X., Bennett, M. & Thorpe, P.E. (2004). Anti-tumor effects and lack of side effects in mice of an immunotoxin directed against human and mouse prostate-specific membrane antigen. *Prostate,* Vol. 61, No. 1, pp. 1-11.

Israeli, R.S., Powell, C.T., Corr, J.G., Fair, W.R. & Heston, W.D. (1994). Expression of the prostate-specific membrane antigen. *Cancer Res,* Vol. 54, No. 7, pp. 1807-1811.

Kahn, D., Austin, J.C., Maguire, R.T., Miller, S.J., Gerstbrein, J. & Williams, R.D. (1999). A phase II study of [90Y] yttrium-capromab pendetide in the treatment of men with prostate cancer recurrence following radical prostatectomy. *Cancer Biother Radiopharm,* Vol. 14, No. 2, pp. 99-111.

Kahn, D., Williams, R.D., Manyak, M.J., Haseman, M.K., Seldin, D.W., Libertino, J.A. & Maguire, R.T. (1998). 111Indium-capromab pendetide in the evaluation of patients with residual or recurrent prostate cancer after radical prostatectomy. The ProstaScint Study Group. *J Urol,* Vol. 159, No. 6, pp. 2041-2046; discussion 2046-2047.

Kahn, D., Williams, R.D., Seldin, D.W., Libertino, J.A., Hirschhorn, M., Dreicer, R., Weiner, G.J., Bushnell, D. & Gulfo, J. (1994). Radioimmunoscintigraphy with 111indium labeled CYT-356 for the detection of occult prostate cancer recurrence. *J Urol,* Vol. 152, No. 5 Pt 1, pp. 1490-1495.

Kawakami, M. & Nakayama, J. (1997). Enhanced expression of prostate-specific membrane antigen gene in prostate cancer as revealed by in situ hybridization. *Cancer Res,* Vol. 57, No. 12, pp. 2321-2324.

Knight, D., Peterson, A.C., Rini, B.I., Harlin, H., Gajewski, T.F. & Stadler, W.M. (2009). The HLA-A2-restricted PSMA peptide LLHETDSAV is poorly immunogenic in patients with metastatic prostate cancer. *Prostate,* Vol. 69, No. 2, pp. 142-148.

Kolishetti, N., Dhar, S., Valencia, P.M., Lin, L.Q., Karnik, R., Lippard, S.J., Langer, R. & Farokhzad, O.C. (2010). Engineering of self-assembled nanoparticle platform for precisely controlled combination drug therapy. *Proc Natl Acad Sci U S A,* Vol. 107, No. 42, pp. 17939-17944.

Kuang, Y., Weng, X., Liu, X., Zhu, H., Chen, Z., Jiang, B. & Chen, H. (2010). Anti-tumor immune response induced by dendritic cells transduced with truncated PSMA IRES 4-1BBL recombinant adenoviruses. *Cancer Lett,* Vol. 293, No. 2, pp. 254-262.

Kularatne, S.A., Venkatesh, C., Santhapuram, H.K., Wang, K., Vaitilingam, B., Henne, W.A. & Low, P.S. (2010). Synthesis and biological analysis of prostate-specific membrane antigen-targeted anticancer prodrugs. *J Med Chem,* Vol. 53, No. 21, pp. 7767-7777.

Kuroda, K., Liu, H., Kim, S., Guo, M., Navarro, V. & Bander, N.H. (2010). Saporin toxin-conjugated monoclonal antibody targeting prostate-specific membrane antigen has potent anticancer activity. *Prostate,* Vol. 70, No. 12, pp. 1286-1294.

Lapidus, R.G., Tiffany, C.W., Isaacs, J.T. & Slusher, B.S. (2000). Prostate-specific membrane antigen (PSMA) enzyme activity is elevated in prostate cancer cells. *Prostate,* Vol. 45, No. 4, pp. 350-354.

Liu, C., Hasegawa, K., Russell, S.J., Sadelain, M. & Peng, K.W. (2009a). Prostate-specific membrane antigen retargeted measles virotherapy for the treatment of prostate cancer. *Prostate,* Vol. 69, No. 10, pp. 1128-1141.

Liu, H., Moy, P., Kim, S., Xia, Y., Rajasekaran, A., Navarro, V., Knudsen, B. & Bander, N.H. (1997). Monoclonal antibodies to the extracellular domain of prostate-specific membrane antigen also react with tumor vascular endothelium. *Cancer Res,* Vol. 57, No. 17, pp. 3629-3634.

Liu, H., Rajasekaran, A.K., Moy, P., Xia, Y., Kim, S., Navarro, V., Rahmati, R. & Bander, N.H. (1998). Constitutive and antibody-induced internalization of prostate-specific membrane antigen. *Cancer Res,* Vol. 58, No. 18, pp. 4055-4060.

Liu, J., Kopeckova, P., Buhler, P., Wolf, P., Pan, H., Bauer, H., Elsasser-Beile, U. & Kopecek, J. (2009b). Biorecognition and Subcellular Trafficking of HPMA Copolymer-Anti-PSMA Antibody Conjugates by Prostate Cancer Cells. *Mol Pharm,* No. pp.

Liu, T., Wu, L.Y. & Berkman, C.E. (2010a). Prostate-specific membrane antigen-targeted photodynamic therapy induces rapid cytoskeletal disruption. *Cancer Lett,* Vol. 296, No. 1, pp. 106-112.

Liu, T., Wu, L.Y., Choi, J.K. & Berkman, C.E. (2009c). In vitro targeted photodynamic therapy with a pyropheophorbide--a conjugated inhibitor of prostate-specific membrane antigen. *Prostate,* Vol. 69, No. 6, pp. 585-594.

Liu, T., Wu, L.Y., Choi, J.K. & Berkman, C.E. (2010b). Targeted photodynamic therapy for prostate cancer: inducing apoptosis via activation of the caspase-8/-3 cascade pathway. *Int J Oncol,* Vol. 36, No. 4, pp. 777-784.

Ma, D., Hopf, C.E., Malewicz, A.D., Donovan, G.P., Senter, P.D., Goeckeler, W.F., Maddon, P.J. & Olson, W.C. (2006). Potent antitumor activity of an auristatin-conjugated, fully human monoclonal antibody to prostate-specific membrane antigen. *Clin Cancer Res,* Vol. 12, No. 8, pp. 2591-2596.

Ma, Q., Safar, M., Holmes, E., Wang, Y., Boynton, A.L. & Junghans, R.P. (2004). Anti-prostate specific membrane antigen designer T cells for prostate cancer therapy. *Prostate,* Vol. 61, No. 1, pp. 12-25.

Mannweiler, S., Amersdorfer, P., Trajanoski, S., Terrett, J.A., King, D. & Mehes, G. (2009). Heterogeneity of prostate-specific membrane antigen (PSMA) expression in prostate carcinoma with distant metastasis. *Pathol Oncol Res,* Vol. 15, No. 2, pp. 167-172.

McDevitt, M.R., Barendswaard, E., Ma, D., Lai, L., Curcio, M.J., Sgouros, G., Ballangrud, A.M., Yang, W.H., Finn, R.D., Pellegrini, V., Geerlings, M.W., Jr., Lee, M., Brechbiel, M.W., Bander, N.H., Cordon-Cardo, C. & Scheinberg, D.A. (2000). An alpha-particle emitting antibody ([213Bi]J591) for radioimmunotherapy of prostate cancer. *Cancer Res,* Vol. 60, No. 21, pp. 6095-6100.

Melief, C.J. (2008). Cancer immunotherapy by dendritic cells. *Immunity,* Vol. 29, No. 3, pp. 372-383.

Mesters, J.R., Barinka, C., Li, W., Tsukamoto, T., Majer, P., Slusher, B.S., Konvalinka, J. & Hilgenfeld, R. (2006). Structure of glutamate carboxypeptidase II, a drug target in neuronal damage and prostate cancer. *Embo J,* Vol. 25, No. 6, pp. 1375-1384.

Mhaka, A., Gady, A.M., Rosen, D.M., Lo, K.M., Gillies, S.D. & Denmeade, S.R. (2004). Use of methotrexate-based peptide substrates to characterize the substrate specificity of prostate-specific membrane antigen (PSMA). *Cancer Biol Ther,* Vol. 3, No. 6, pp. 551-558.

Mhaka, A., Singh, P., Rosen, M., Dionne, C.A., Christensen, S.B., Isaacs, J.T. & Denmeade, S.R. (2006). Prostate-Specific Membrane Antigen (PSMA) targeted prodrug "smartbombs" as therapy for prostate cancer. *Proc Amer Assoc Cancer Res,* Vol. 47, No. pp. 725.

Milowsky, M.I., Nanus, D.M., Kostakoglu, L., Vallabhajosula, S., Goldsmith, S.J. & Bander, N.H. (2004). Phase I trial of yttrium-90-labeled anti-prostate-specific membrane antigen monoclonal antibody J591 for androgen-independent prostate cancer. *J Clin Oncol,* Vol. 22, No. 13, pp. 2522-2531.

Milowsky, M.I., Nanus, D.M., Kostakoglu, L., Sheehan, C.E., Vallabhajosula, S., Goldsmith, S.J., Ross, J.S. & Bander, N.H. (2007). Vascular targeted therapy with anti-prostate-specific membrane antigen monoclonal antibody J591 in advanced solid tumors. *J Clin Oncol,* Vol. 25, No. 5, pp. 540-547.

Mincheff, M., Zoubak, S. & Makogonenko, Y. (2006). Immune responses against PSMA after gene-based vaccination for immunotherapy-A: results from immunizations in animals. *Cancer Gene Ther,* Vol. 13, No. 4, pp. 436-444.

Mincheff, M., Tchakarov, S., Zoubak, S., Loukinov, D., Botev, C., Altankova, I., Georgiev, G., Petrov, S. & Meryman, H.T. (2000). Naked DNA and adenoviral immunizations for immunotherapy of prostate cancer: a phase I/II clinical trial. *Eur Urol,* Vol. 38, No. 2, pp. 208-217.

Mincheff, M., Zoubak, S., Altankova, I., Tchakarov, S., Makogonenko, Y., Botev, C., Ignatova, I., Dimitrov, R., Madarzhieva, K., Hammett, M., Pomakov, Y., Meryman, H. & Lissitchkov, T. (2003). Human dendritic cells genetically engineered to express cytosolically retained fragment of prostate-specific membrane antigen prime cytotoxic T-cell responses to multiple epitopes. *Cancer Gene Ther,* Vol. 10, No. 12, pp. 907-917.

Msaouel, P., Iankov, I.D., Allen, C., Morris, J.C., von Messling, V., Cattaneo, R., Koutsilieris, M., Russell, S.J. & Galanis, E. (2009). Engineered measles virus as a novel oncolytic therapy against prostate cancer. *Prostate,* Vol. 69, No. 1, pp. 82-91.

Murphy, G.P., Elgamal, A.A., Su, S.L., Bostwick, D.G. & Holmes, E.H. (1998). Current evaluation of the tissue localization and diagnostic utility of prostate specific membrane antigen. *Cancer,* Vol. 83, No. 11, pp. 2259-2269.

Murphy, G.P., Tjoa, B.A., Simmons, S.J., Ragde, H., Rogers, M., Elgamal, A., Kenny, G.M., Troychak, M.J., Salgaller, M.L. & Boynton, A.L. (1999). Phase II prostate cancer vaccine trial: report of a study involving 37 patients with disease recurrence following primary treatment. *Prostate,* Vol. 39, No. 1, pp. 54-59.

O'Keefe, D.S., Su, S.L., Bacich, D.J., Horiguchi, Y., Luo, Y., Powell, C.T., Zandvliet, D., Russell, P.J., Molloy, P.L., Nowak, N.J., Shows, T.B., Mullins, C., Vonder Haar, R.A., Fair, W.R. & Heston, W.D. (1998). Mapping, genomic organization and promoter analysis of the human prostate-specific membrane antigen gene. *Biochim Biophys Acta,* Vol. 1443, No. 1-2, pp. 113-127.

Onda, M., Kreitman, R.J., Vasmatzis, G., Lee, B. & Pastan, I. (1999). Reduction of the nonspecific animal toxicity of anti-Tac(Fv)-PE38 by mutations in the framework regions of the Fv which lower the isoelectric point. *J Immunol,* Vol. 163, No. 11, pp. 6072-6077.

Onda, M., Nagata, S., Tsutsumi, Y., Vincent, J.J., Wang, Q., Kreitman, R.J., Lee, B. & Pastan, I. (2001). Lowering the isoelectric point of the Fv portion of recombinant immunotoxins leads to decreased nonspecific animal toxicity without affecting antitumor activity. *Cancer Res,* Vol. 61, No. 13, pp. 5070-5077.

Onda, M., Nagata, S., FitzGerald, D.J., Beers, R., Fisher, R.J., Vincent, J.J., Lee, B., Nakamura, M., Hwang, J., Kreitman, R.J., Hassan, R. & Pastan, I. (2006). Characterization of the B cell epitopes associated with a truncated form of Pseudomonas exotoxin (PE38) used to make immunotoxins for the treatment of cancer patients. *J Immunol,* Vol. 177, No. 12, pp. 8822-8834.

Pinto, J.T., Suffoletto, B.P., Berzin, T.M., Qiao, C.H., Lin, S., Tong, W.P., May, F., Mukherjee, B. & Heston, W.D. (1996). Prostate-specific membrane antigen: a novel folate hydrolase in human prostatic carcinoma cells. *Clin Cancer Res,* Vol. 2, No. 9, pp. 1445-1451.

Rajasekaran, S.A., Christiansen, J.J., Schmid, I., Oshima, E., Ryazantsev, S., Sakamoto, K., Weinstein, J., Rao, N.P. & Rajasekaran, A.K. (2008). Prostate-specific membrane antigen associates with anaphase-promoting complex and induces chromosomal instability. *Mol Cancer Ther,* Vol. 7, No. 7, pp. 2142-2151.

Rosenthal, S.A., Haseman, M.K. & Polascik, T.J. (2001). Utility of capromab pendetide (ProstaScint) imaging in the management of prostate cancer. *Tech Urol,* Vol. 7, No. 1, pp. 27-37.

Ross, J.S., Sheehan, C.E., Fisher, H.A., Kaufman, R.P., Jr., Kaur, P., Gray, K., Webb, I., Gray, G.S., Mosher, R. & Kallakury, B.V. (2003). Correlation of primary tumor prostate-specific membrane antigen expression with disease recurrence in prostate cancer. *Clin Cancer Res,* Vol. 9, No. 17, pp. 6357-6362.

Russell, P.J., Hewish, D., Carter, T., Sterling-Levis, K., Ow, K., Hattarki, M., Doughty, L., Guthrie, R., Shapira, D., Molloy, P.L., Werkmeister, J.A. & Kortt, A.A. (2004). Cytotoxic properties of immunoconjugates containing melittin-like peptide 101 against prostate cancer: in vitro and in vivo studies. *Cancer Immunol Immunother,* Vol. 53, No. 5, pp. 411-421.

Rzeszowska-Wolny, J., Przybyszewski, W.M. & Widel, M. (2009). Ionizing radiation-induced bystander effects, potential targets for modulation of radiotherapy. *Eur J Pharmacol,* Vol. 625, No. 1-3, pp. 156-164.

Sacha, P., Zamecnik, J., Barinka, C., Hlouchova, K., Vicha, A., Mlcochova, P., Hilgert, I., Eckschlager, T. & Konvalinka, J. (2007). Expression of glutamate carboxypeptidase II in human brain. *Neuroscience,* Vol. 144, No. 4, pp. 1361-1372.

Salgaller, M.L., Lodge, P.A., McLean, J.G., Tjoa, B.A., Loftus, D.J., Ragde, H., Kenny, G.M., Rogers, M., Boynton, A.L. & Murphy, G.P. (1998). Report of immune monitoring of prostate cancer patients undergoing T-cell therapy using dendritic cells pulsed with HLA-A2-specific peptides from prostate-specific membrane antigen (PSMA). *Prostate,* Vol. 35, No. 2, pp. 144-151.

Sandvig, K., Grimmer, S., Lauvrak, S.U., Torgersen, M.L., Skretting, G., van Deurs, B. & Iversen, T.G. (2002). Pathways followed by ricin and Shiga toxin into cells. *Histochem Cell Biol,* Vol. 117, No. 2, pp. 131-141.

Sanna, V., Pintus, G., Roggio, A.M., Punzoni, S., Posadino, A.M., Arca, A., Marceddu, S., Bandiera, P., Uzzau, S. & Sechi, M. (2011). Targeted biocompatible nanoparticles for the delivery of (-)-epigallocatechin 3-gallate to prostate cancer cells. *J Med Chem,* Vol. 54, No. 5, pp. 1321-1332.

Silver, D.A., Pellicer, I., Fair, W.R., Heston, W.D. & Cordon-Cardo, C. (1997). Prostate-specific membrane antigen expression in normal and malignant human tissues. *Clin Cancer Res,* Vol. 3, No. 1, pp. 81-85.

Smith-Jones, P.M., Vallabhajosula, S., Navarro, V., Bastidas, D., Goldsmith, S.J. & Bander, N.H. (2003). Radiolabeled monoclonal antibodies specific to the extracellular domain of prostate-specific membrane antigen: preclinical studies in nude mice bearing LNCaP human prostate tumor. *J Nucl Med,* Vol. 44, No. 4, pp. 610-617.

Sodee, D.B., Conant, R., Chalfant, M., Miron, S., Klein, E., Bahnson, R., Spirnak, J.P., Carlin, B., Bellon, E.M. & Rogers, B. (1996). Preliminary imaging results using In-111 labeled CYT-356 (Prostascint) in the detection of recurrent prostate cancer. *Clin Nucl Med,* Vol. 21, No. 10, pp. 759-767.

Su, S.L., Huang, I.P., Fair, W.R., Powell, C.T. & Heston, W.D. (1995). Alternatively spliced variants of prostate-specific membrane antigen RNA: ratio of expression as a potential measurement of progression. *Cancer Res,* Vol. 55, No. 7, pp. 1441-1443.

Tjoa, B.A., Simmons, S.J., Elgamal, A., Rogers, M., Ragde, H., Kenny, G.M., Troychak, M.J., Boynton, A.L. & Murphy, G.P. (1999). Follow-up evaluation of a phase II prostate cancer vaccine trial. *Prostate,* Vol. 40, No. 2, pp. 125-129.

Tjoa, B.A., Simmons, S.J., Bowes, V.A., Ragde, H., Rogers, M., Elgamal, A., Kenny, G.M., Cobb, O.E., Ireton, R.C., Troychak, M.J., Salgaller, M.L., Boynton, A.L. & Murphy, G.P. (1998). Evaluation of phase I/II clinical trials in prostate cancer with dendritic cells and PSMA peptides. *Prostate,* Vol. 36, No. 1, pp. 39-44.

Todorova, K., Ignatova, I., Tchakarov, S., Altankova, I., Zoubak, S., Kyurkchiev, S. & Mincheff, M. (2005). Humoral immune response in prostate cancer patients after immunization with gene-based vaccines that encode for a protein that is proteasomally degraded. *Cancer Immun,* Vol. 5, No. pp. 1.

Troyer, J.K., Beckett, M.L. & Wright, G.L., Jr. (1995). Detection and characterization of the prostate-specific membrane antigen (PSMA) in tissue extracts and body fluids. *Int J Cancer,* Vol. 62, No. 5, pp. 552-558.

Vallabhajosula, S., Smith-Jones, P.M., Navarro, V., Goldsmith, S.J. & Bander, N.H. (2004). Radioimmunotherapy of prostate cancer in human xenografts using monoclonal antibodies specific to prostate specific membrane antigen (PSMA): studies in nude mice. *Prostate,* Vol. 58, No. 2, pp. 145-155.

Vallabhajosula, S., Goldsmith, S.J., Hamacher, K.A., Kostakoglu, L., Konishi, S., Milowski, M.I., Nanus, D.M. & Bander, N.H. (2005). Prediction of myelotoxicity based on bone marrow radiation-absorbed dose: radioimmunotherapy studies using 90Y- and 177Lu-labeled J591 antibodies specific for prostate-specific membrane antigen. *J Nucl Med,* Vol. 46, No. 5, pp. 850-858.

Waeckerle-Men, Y., Uetz-von Allmen, E., Fopp, M., von Moos, R., Bohme, C., Schmid, H.P., Ackermann, D., Cerny, T., Ludewig, B., Groettrup, M. & Gillessen, S. (2006). Dendritic cell-based multi-epitope immunotherapy of hormone-refractory prostate carcinoma. *Cancer Immunol Immunother,* Vol. 55, No. 12, pp. 1524-1533.

Wolf, P. & Elsasser-Beile, U. (2009). Pseudomonas exotoxin A: from virulence factor to anti-cancer agent. *Int J Med Microbiol,* Vol. 299, No. 3, pp. 161-176.

Wolf, P., Gierschner, D., Buhler, P., Wetterauer, U. & Elsasser-Beile, U. (2006). A recombinant PSMA-specific single-chain immunotoxin has potent and selective toxicity against prostate cancer cells. *Cancer Immunol Immunother,* Vol. 55, No. 11, pp. 1367-1373.

Wolf, P., Alt, K., Buhler, P., Katzenwadel, A., Wetterauer, U., Tacke, M. & Elsasser-Beile, U. (2008). Anti-PSMA immunotoxin as novel treatment for prostate cancer? High and specific antitumor activity on human prostate xenograft tumors in SCID mice. *Prostate,* Vol. 68, No. 2, pp. 129-138.

Wolf, P., Freudenberg, N., Buhler, P., Alt, K., Schultze-Seemann, W., Wetterauer, U. & Elsasser-Beile, U. (2010a). Three conformational antibodies specific for different PSMA epitopes are promising diagnostic and therapeutic tools for prostate cancer. *Prostate,* Vol. 70, No. 5, pp. 562-569.

Wolf, P., Alt, K., Wetterauer, D., Buhler, P., Gierschner, D., Katzenwadel, A., Wetterauer, U. & Elsasser-Beile, U. (2010b). Preclinical evaluation of a recombinant anti-prostate specific membrane antigen single-chain immunotoxin against prostate cancer. *J Immunother,* Vol. 33, No. 3, pp. 262-271.

Wright, G.L., Jr., Grob, B.M., Haley, C., Grossman, K., Newhall, K., Petrylak, D., Troyer, J., Konchuba, A., Schellhammer, P.F. & Moriarty, R. (1996). Upregulation of prostate-specific membrane antigen after androgen- deprivation therapy. *Urology,* Vol. 48, No. 2, pp. 326-334

Yang, C.S., Wang, X., Lu, G. & Picinich, S.C. (2009). Cancer prevention by tea: animal studies, molecular mechanisms and human relevance. *Nat Rev Cancer,* Vol. 9, No. 6, pp. 429-439.

Yao, V. & Bacich, D.J. (2006). Prostate specific membrane antigen (PSMA) expression gives prostate cancer cells a growth advantage in a physiologically relevant folate environment in vitro. *Prostate,* Vol. 66, No. 8, pp. 867-875.

Yao, V., Berkman, C.E., Choi, J.K., O'Keefe, D.S. & Bacich, D.J. (2009). Expression of prostate-specific membrane antigen (PSMA), increases cell folate uptake and proliferation and suggests a novel role for PSMA in the uptake of the non-polyglutamated folate, folic acid. *Prostate,* Vol. 70, No. 3, pp. 305-316.

Zhong, X.S., Matsushita, M., Plotkin, J., Riviere, I. & Sadelain, M. (2010). Chimeric antigen receptors combining 4-1BB and CD28 signaling domains augment PI3kinase/AKT/Bcl-XL activation and CD8+ T cell-mediated tumor eradication. *Mol Ther,* Vol. 18, No. 2, pp. 413-420.

Zhou, J., Neale, J.H., Pomper, M.G. & Kozikowski, A.P. (2005). NAAG peptidase inhibitors and their potential for diagnosis and therapy. *Nat Rev Drug Discov,* Vol. 4, No. 12, pp. 1015-1026.

5

Future of Prostate Biopsy: Who Will Get It and How?

Tine Hajdinjak
Center UROL Maribor
Department of Surgery, General Hospital Murska Sobota
Medical Faculty, University of Maribor
Slovenia

1. Introduction

Prostate biopsy is a motor, driving force and entrance ticket for dealing with parade discipline in urology of recent years - prostate cancer. Therefore it receives a lot of attention and standard techniques are constantly challenged by new developments. Enormous amount of literature seem to have addressed all possible aspects regarding prostate biopsy. This chapter focuses less on historical overview but mainly on recent developments, controversies and questions.

Prostate cancer has already become leading cancer among males in developed world (Jemal et al., 2011), second reason for death due to cancer among men in US (Jemal et al., 2010) and third in Europe (Malvezzi et al., 2011). Future is looking even more serious - numbers are expected to rise much further, as recently predicted in Canadian forecast analysis (Quon et al, 2011). The authors claim expected estimates of increase in prostate cancer cases should not be limited only to aging of population, which is huge itself and is expected to cause 39% increase in prostate cancer cases. At least three further factors should be taken into account. First and most important is lowering of PSA threshold for biopsy. It seems the move of decreasing PSA cutoff from 4 to 2.5 is getting from university centers to every urologist's and generalist's office (this is especially important as they are the ones who pick and refer patients to urologists for biopsy). Increase in number of people, referred to biopsy for this reason is estimated to be much greater compared to aging of population and may increase prostate cancer incidence by 200%. If it will increase prostate cancer incidence by 200%, increase in number of biopsies should be disproportionally higher, as biopsies have lower yield for this new target population with PSA values between 2.5 and 4. PSA screening is creating at present a lot of debate, it is a very hot topic and there are very strong opponents and supporters. Introduction of formal screening would of course increase burden of cancer and burden of biopsy. It is at present unlikely to happen, probably because people who decide on health policies and their advisers do not meet, treat and care for people with advanced prostate cancer. But, call it case finding or however one prefers, a "non-formal" screening programs are actually already available in many health systems, not only in selected first adopters, like Tyrol in Austria (Oberaigner et al., 2006), but also for example in Slovenia, where every general practitioner has available extra funds for PSA measurement on all of his male patients, every two years. Extent of "non-formal" screening programs can be seen from well-known PLCO trial, where control, supposedly non-screened arm had 50% screening in comparison to intervention arm, supposedly "screened", where the rate was approximately 85% (Andriole et al., 2009). Some do not believe into usefulness of screening (Miettinen, 2010) and results of studies, which clearly show improved survival and necessity for screening, for example of European Randomized Trial of Screening for Prostate Cancer (Schröder et al., 2009). Despite those doubts, screening in one way or another is in fact increasingly taking place in every-day life. Further increase in screening is expected because recent analyzes of prostate screening studies seem to greatly reduce predicted numbers needed to screen and numbers needed to treat to save a life in prostate cancer and dispel previous doubts about usefulness of screening (Crawford et al., 2011) and treatment (Bill-Axelson et al., 2011).

Last reason for estimation of huge increase in prostate cancer cases expected in the next decade is stated (Quon et al., 2011) as "improved sensitivity of prostate biopsy". Will this really happen? This review will summarize some of the present developments in this field. If this is really the case, it may be at least one good sign, sign of relief: with improved biopsy specificity, number of repeat biopsies, which at present already represent significant burden and may also represent group of patients with higher risk for biopsy-related complications, may decrease.

Prostate biopsy aims to detect prostate cancer with as little problems and sequela as possible. Further, it aims to predict prognosis of detected cancer, therefore sampling must not only take any cancer, but representative cancer tissue samples from possibly all cancer focuses in the prostate. Third goal of modern prostate biopsy is to guide targeted therapy, which is expected to rise with increased number of lower stage cancers detected.

2. Selection of biopsy candidates

Only main criteria, which are in clinical use or are available and may be used in Europe in 2011 are included here and they are: 3 PSA's (total, free and -2proPSA), urine marker (PCA3), race, family history, previous biopsy technique and result, age and life expectancy.

There are markers, which were proposed and also used in the past, but are now outdated, like cPSA and other PSA's, not mentioned above. There are markers, which may become very useful in the future, but are at present not ready yet (for example SNP's and other genetic data or new urine markers, which may use advantage of being excreted and therefore no aggressive rectal prostate massage would be necessary (Pandha et al., 2011)).

Should we really biopsy all men with PSA above 2.5? Obviously we do not want to do that. It remains unresolved task, how should we select between those who would benefit from biopsy even earlier, at PSA 1, from those who do not need biopsy at PSA 10.

2.1 PSA's

Prostate specific antigen, during history of its discovery named with other names, for example semenogelase, is an androgen-regulated serine protease (EC 3.4.21.77), human tissue kallikrein 3 (Balk et al, 2003). Gene is located on 19q13.4. Mainly it is produced in secretory epithelial cells in prostate acini and ducts and secreted into lumen. Its function is in ejaculate liquefaction.

PSA is expressed in preproPSA form (17 aminoacid leading peptide), excreted into prostate lumen as proPSA (7 aminoacid propeptide on N-terminal) and activated by trypsine-like human kallikrein 2 (hK2), which is expressed on prostate secretory epithelial cells (Balk et.al, 2003). ProPSA can undergo cleavage at position -7, removing 7 aminoacid propeptide to form active PSA. ProPSA cleavage can also occur at positions -5 or -2. Those PSA isoforms are not catalytically active. Active PSA in part undergoes further degradation/internal cleavage by different proteases, thereby also forming inactive PSA. In seminal plasma approximately 30% of PSA is in active form. Remaining PSA represents different forms of inactive PSA. Some PSA (all forms) leaks to circulation and can be measured in serum. Active form of PSA in serum binds (complexes) to protease inhibitors, mostly to alpha1-antichymotrypsin (ACT). It represents main part of total serum PSA (70-90%) and can be measured as cPSA. Catalytically inactive PSA forms circulate freely in serum as they are not complexed to ACT or other inhibitors. This fraction represents main result of free PSA assay. Antibodies were also developed for measuring serum concentrations of specific PSA isoforms, for example [-5]pro PSA and [-2]proPSA. Assays which measure total PSA aim at detecting all isoforms, active (complexed) and inactive PSA.

As prostate cancer characteristic is disruption of basal cell layer and basement membrane, this allows increased amount of PSA and its isoforms to enter circulation (Balk et al, 2003). Free PSA fraction is decreased in serum of cancer patients. It is hypothesized there is relatively less free PSA in serum in cancer patients because more PSA enters circulation directly and complexes immediately to protease inhibitors. As there is less exposure of PSA to luminal and seminal fluid proteases, there is less chance for inactivating and producing inactive, free PSA. ProPSA isoforms are increased in serum of prostate cancer patients. Two hypotheses aim to explain this. One believes there is decreased cleavage of proPSA by hK2 in prostate cancer tissue (Balk et al., 2003). Other hypothesis believes proPSA isoforms are increased in cancer as a result of increased proPSA production from benign looking cancer associated areas in prostate gland (Makarov et al., 2009).

Higher serum PSA values were related to prostate cancer in 1980-ties. Hybritech, first commercial PSA measurement kit manufacturer, identified in a small study in 1986 in their sample 99% of tested men (different ages) had PSA below 4 and suggested this value as a cut-off. With this in hand, Catalona conducted a trial and published in 1991: 8% of tested men (mean age 68) had PSA values above 4, 22% of those with PSA between 4 and 10 had prostate cancer detected on sextant biopsy (and 67% among those with PSA above 10). Biopsy was performed using 18G needle. PSA was independent prognostic factor and positive DRE increased chance of positive biopsy (Catalona et al., 1991). 20 years later - we made a progress - now we do 12 core biopsies, use PSA cut-off 2.5 and use some other PSA derivatives to help in decisions. This modifies our outcomes a few percentages here and there, but main achievement, decrease in mortality due to prostate cancer, which was, after two decades of doubt, finally recently confirmed by a few large independent trials from both US and EU (see Introduction), was a result of a twenty years old approach, which is, with all its drawbacks and deficiencies, still valid and widely practiced around the world.

Inadequacy of PSA cut-off value of 4 was in depth explained by publication of results of control biopsies in prostate cancer prevention trial (Thompson et al., 2004). They found, among men in age range 62 to 91, median 69, 6.6% of cancers among those with PSA 0.5 or less and 12.5% among them with Gleason 7 or more (=0.8% of all men with median age 69 with PSA below 0.6 had important cancer). Among men with PSA of 1.1 to 2.0, cancer was found in 10% and 10% of those had Gleason 7 or more (=1% of all men with PSA between 1 and 2, median age 69, had Gleason 7 or higher prostate cancer). For PSA 2-3, the percentage of Gleason 7 or more among all tested was 4.6% and for PSA 3-4 it was 6.7%. Those numbers were found in a prescreened population and with sextant biopsy. Now it is believed those numbers are still accurate for overall cancer presence, but for Gleason 7 or higher cancers in general referral population, real numbers are about twice those estimates. Several thoughts follow from this data. One is related to high percentage of high grade cancers in population with median age 69 and relatively low PSA values. Once upon a time, it was suggested we should not measure PSA in men above 70. Should we now turn this completely around and biopsy all men with life expectancy of 10 yeas or more at the age of 70 irrespectively of their PSA? Or should we use other tests, like PSA isoforms derivatives?

Free PSA is measured to calculate fraction towards total PSA value, which is expressed as percentage. In PSA ranges between 4 and 10, with % free PSA below 10%, probability for biopsy detected prostate cancer in DRE negative patients was 56% and with % free PSA above 25% probability of cancer was only 8%. In PSA range between 2.5 and 4, with % free PSA below 10%, probability of cancer was 46% and with % free PSA above 20% probability of cancer was 8% (Catalona et al., 1998).

[-2]proPSA or p2PSA is new kid on the block, which is not yet universally available or accepted. It seems it will become next widely used PSA derivative, which is also used together with free PSA value (p2PSA/freePSA) or together with total and free PSA as value, calculated as p2PSA/freePSA times square root of total PSA and proprietary named by Beckman Coulter (Brea, California, USA) as PHI - prostate health index. Cut-off values for biopsy decisions using %p2PSA (p2PSA/free PSA) and PHI are not yet universally accepted and differ with regard to free PSA and total PSA calibration method (Hybritech or WHO), but it seems PHI values above 40 or 45 indicate high and below 21 low risk of prostate cancer. PHI of more than 48.5 was reported as 43% specific at 90% sensitive for detecting prostate cancer at initial prostate biopsy (Guazzoni et al., 2011). Another study reported PHI values above 34.2 to show increased probability for high risk disease (Isharwal et al., 2011). PHI was shown to indicate development of prostate cancer years before biopsy and correlated well with grade of future prostate cancer (Bektic et al., 2010). On negative side, using p2PSA compared to free PSA using ROC curves at area of high sensitivity (if we are to find cancer), increase in performance may seem marginal.

PSA density and different variants (PSA density of transitional zone etc), calculated from total PSA value and measurement of prostate volume using transrectal ultrasound, were in the past extensively evaluated. Drawback is variability of prostate volume measurements, need for this additional investigation and low sensitivity (Pepe et al., 2009). One example of cutoff value was density above 0.15 ng/ml PSA /ml prostate volume indicating higher risk of cancer. It may represent additional useful piece of information, also for example regarding prediction of disease course for patients on watchful waiting (Kotb et. al, 2011).

PSA velocity was in recent years proposed as another potentially helpful tool in picking cancers or high-risk cancers. Cutoff value of 0.35 ng/ml/year was proposed when total PSA values are less than 4. This may need adjustment for race (Tang et al., 2011). Although some doubts about value of PSA velocity in biopsy decisions were posed from analysis of PCPT trial data (Vickers et al., 2011), there are suggestions a lot of clinically important cancers in younger men may be detected by regularly and meticulously following and analyzing sequential PSA values (Bektic et al., 2011).

PSA values increase with age due to BPH. This became known early after PSA test introduction and "age-specific" PSA values were suggested. For Caucasian Americans, median, 75th and 95th percentiles of PSA were for age group 40-49 - 0.7, 1.0 and 2.1, for 50-59 age group 1.0, 1.6 and 3.6, for 60-69 age group 1.4, 2.5 and 4.3, for 70-79 decade 1.8, 3.5 and 5.8 (Morgan et al., 1996). One approach of integrating age specific PSA values in prostate biopsy decisions may be using as cutoff half of age-specific 95th percentile PSA value together with %free PSA below 18%, which was in part used in Innsbruck (Tyrol, Austria).

High increase of PSA with infection or any irritation of prostate is well known and sometimes antibiotic or anti-inflammatory treatment is suggested and repeat measurement. PSA decreases in high body-mass index-correction and decreased of cutoff values may be needed (Pater et al., 2011). Diseases (liver cirrhosis) and medications (NSAID's, thiazides and statins) may also decrease PSA values (Nieder et al., 2011). If using free PSA values as trigger for biopsy decisions, it may be important to note that use of herbal products, like Serenoa repens, may (artifically?) increase free PSA values.

2.2 Age and life expectancy

Risk of prostate cancer significantly increases with age. Age is significant independent predictor of high risk prostate cancer. Although we need age as a criterion (we do not start to think about prostate cancer before age of 40 or 35), it is clear age could not be the only factor which would preclude decisions about PSA measurement, digital rectal exam and biopsy. Age is only one parameter in estimation of life expectancy. Life expectancy, not age, is crucial factor in decisions regarding prostate cancer screening interventions. Age does increase probability of cancer and cancer related death and therefore higher age - for example 75 years or more (with additional criterion of more than 10 years life expectancy) means strong indication in-favor of PSA screening and prostate biopsy. It is true that not all men at age 75 or more have more than 10 years of life expectancy, but significant number have and for them, prostate cancer screening is most useful and fruit bearing (much higher yield compared to younger men). This thinking is in strong contrast to past belief (and even now supported by some outdated recommendations of non-urological organizations), when PSA testing was not recommended generally for all older men.

2.3 Digital rectal exam

Digital rectal exam remains important part of prostate evaluation (Gosselaar et al., 2008). Although still on occasion declined by a patient and despite hopes PSA or any other method would completely replace it (Schroder et al., 1998), one still finds from time to time a case, where PSA is low and DRE is suspicious. For such a patient, next year, when PSA has increased, may be (and cases were confirmed it was) too late. Although after many suspicious DRE's biopsy comes negative, we are more and more aware of the fact that prostate cancer may progress without PSA increase. DRE can estimate sphincter tone, in a way prepare patient for biopsy, if needed, on occasion register some other, non-urological pathology and appreciate prostate size, which may give different dimension compared to ultrasound impression. DRE is necessary for sampling prostate cells in post-massage urine - at present for PCA3 only, but in the future maybe also for other markers. DRE is necessary for clinical staging of prostate cancer. DRE is limited, it can not palpate whole gland, but at present it is here to stay (Yossepowitch, 2008).

2.4 PCA3

Comparison of mRNA expression patterns of prostate cancer and benign tissues identified significantly different expression of non-coding mRNA sequence, first called DD3 (Bussemakers et al., 1999) and later renamed PCA3. Technology (a variant of quantitative nucleic acid amplification test) was developed to identify very minute amounts of PCA3 mRNA from prostate cells shed in prostate urethra after prostatic massage and washed out immediately in first voided urine portion. Its estimated amount (number of copies) is normalized to estimated number of PSA mRNA copies in the same sample and multiplied by 1000, resulting in PCA3 score. Test is known as Progensa PCA3 Assay (Gen-Probe Inc, San Diego, USA). Higher PCA3 score values indicate greater risk of presence of prostate cancer. Values from approximately 4 to 125 can be obtained, 35 being most often suggested cut-off, which, according to package insert has 53% sensitivity and 74% specificity for detection of prostate cancer on subsequent biopsy. Other cut-off opinions are continuously evaluated (Auprich et al., 2011). Although PCA3 mRNA theoretically could be measured in urine also with standard molecular-medicine techniques, which first isolate mRNA from cells in the sample and then perform RT-PCR, is this, due to very small amounts of PCA3 mRNA, very difficult and inconsistent, therefore dedicated patented method from Gen-Probe which uses direct amplification and avoids isolation step, has become standard.

PCA3 use was suggested and marketed as help in biopsy decisions in previously negative prostate biopsies, in men with other risk factors (family history) and normal PSA values, in men with big prostates or other prostatic conditions where it is unclear whether high PSA is driven by cancer or other factor and in men on watchful waiting where high PCA3 score may indicate higher burden of disease.

Use of consecutive PCA3 tests for follow up of biopsy candidates or men on watchful waiting was questioned due to high variability of results, if test is repeated in the same individual with low risk disease (Shikanov et al., 2011).

Pre-biopsy PCA3 test results were evaluated together with PSA in relation to tumor characteristics in radical prostatectomy specimens (Vlaeminck-Guillem et al., 2011). It was found PCA3 score did not correlate with PSA and prostate volume. PCA3 score was also not related to Gleason score and pT stage. PCA3 did correlate with total tumor volume and index lesion volume. Further, multifocality was significantly correlated with PCA3. PCA3 expression can be identified on malignant and benign prostate tissue samples, only quantity varies (Quiles et al., 2011).

PCA3 test is, with many mentioned drawbacks and despite its high price, widely marketed and used in USA and EU. It seems sometimes may help in biopsy related decisions, but its role at present is still evolving.

2.5 Family history, race, previous biopsy result

Theoretically one may differentiate between familial (unpredictable clustering of disease in a family, slightly increased risk for offspring) and hereditary cancer (strong clustering pattern consistent with passage of a susceptibility gene via Mendelian inheritance) (Potter & Partin, 2000). Criteria for hereditary prostate cancer would be three or more first-degree relatives had prostate cancer, three successive generations had prostate cancer and where two relatives were affected at or before age 55. Despite identification of such families, their investigation has not resulted in such successful discoveries as in colon, ovary and breast cancers. In those classic hereditary cancers presence of a certain identifiable mutation with high probability predicts development of cancer in all affected offspring, which has resulted in formal screening programs for affected families and preventive surgery at early age. This is at present not known in prostate cancer.

Familial history of prostate cancer increases risk. In a meta-analysis brother with prostate cancer increases risk 3.3 times, father 2.2 times, two first-degree relatives 5 times (Zeegers et al., 2003).

It is accepted increased risk due to family history should result in earlier start of screening (at age 40 or 35). Some risk calculators do use family history information to modify risk estimation (increased risk for presence of cancer in first degree relatives, this means father, brother or son), which may influence biopsy decision, if based on calculated risk. But apart from this, it does not tell us anything - PSA and other cut-offs for decision about biopsy are the same as in men without family history. Also procedures for biopsy, treatment and also treatment outcomes are the same between familial, hereditary and sporadic prostate cancer. There is no known 100% risk situations, which would provoke preventive removal of prostate, as is known for breast cancer, although people sometimes do ask for this.

Recent research focused also on risk of prostate cancer in men whose family members have other forms of cancer. Men with first degree relative with breast cancer, who developed breast cancer at the age 35 or earlier, are at significantly increased risk of prostate cancer (5 to 18 times in case of BRCA mutation) (Dite et al., 2010). Other cancers in family may also increase risk of prostate cancer (Izmirlian et al., 2011).

Race is used in many prostate cancer risk calculators - African American race increases risk compared to Caucasians, Hispanic or Asian have decreased risk. But, the same as for family history, apart from earlier start of screening or a little different risk estimates from calculators, there are no other practical consequences of this fact at present.

Previous negative biopsy decreases risk of positive subsequent biopsy. There are, however, two findings, which differ: PIN (=HGPIN - high grade prostatic intraepithelial neoplasia, low grade PIN was abandoned) and ASAP (atypical small acinar proliferation). HGPIN is most probable precursor of prostate cancer. There are structurally benign ducts and acini with abnormal secretory cells with prominent nucleoli (Schoenfield et al., 2007). HGPIN is a histological entity in itself, it is not cancer. ASAP indicates finding of small focus of structure in a 2-dimensional view, which is not large enough to satisfy criteria for cancer. It may represent only specific cut of top of benign acinus or PIN. One may define different characteristics under ASAP category, like adenosis, intraductal hyperplasia... which have in common that pathologist can not say for certain, whether they represent cancer or not. As ASAP may represent cancer, is was identified as predictor of positive repeat biopsy. Identification of multiple HGPIN in a biopsy specimen was also identified as predictor of positive repeat biopsy (Akhavan et al., 2007). Therefore, ASAP and HGPIN require consideration about repeat biopsies. ASAP may require immediate scheduling for repeat biopsy. HGPIN requires careful follow up and in most cases other criteria (PSA increase) cause repeat biopsy sooner or later (for example in 1-2 years time).

2.6 Risk based strategies

Different nomograms were developed, which can predict risk of positive biopsy. They take into account risk for age, family history, race, PSA and free PSA, digital rectal exam and some also for body mass index and even new decision aids, for example PCA3 and PHI.

Nomograms have introduced new dimension in patient-physician pre-biopsy discussion. Need for individual's risk adjustment is illustrated by cardiology example. Do general practitioners and cardiologists decide whether one needs aspirin or statin on a single total cholesterol measurement (for example with result of 5.3 mmol/L, just above normal)? No. They measure HDL, LDL cholesterol, they ask for age, gender, blood pressure, smoking history. They consult nomograms and then decide whether statin drug is necessary (and reimbursed) or not. But urologists were dependent on a single PSA value? This has changed with risk calculators availability. Using single PSA cutoff value would be the same as claiming for a man, who runs marathon, has normal blood pressure, normal BMI, is a non-smoker, his parents lived till age 100 and has cholesterol of 5.3 mmol/L - to be at high risk for cardiac event because his cholesterol is elevated (above 5.2). Using single PSA value for biopsy decision would be the same as claiming for an overweight (BMI 30), sedentary man, heavy smoker, on three anti-hypertensive medications whose parents both died of cardiac event, because his cholesterol is 5.1 mmol/L (just normal) - not to be at risk for cardiac event. Everyone can clearly see ridiculosity, absurdity of such approach in cardiology - but we in urology use PSA as single dichotomous variable in our prostate biopsy decisions?! Risk calculators allow us to tell men with any PSA value their individual chances for biopsy outcome. Calculators report risk for high grade (Gleason 7 or more) and overall cancer probability. For example if calculator predicts 6% chance of significant prostate cancer (Gleason 7 or more) and 26% of overall cancer risk, we should tell patient his chance of being without cancer at present is approximately 74% (100-26), he has 6% chance of finding important high risk cancer and he has approximately 20% (26-6) chance biopsy would find cancer which may not be clinically important at present (but maybe in the future) and we would have to deal with this. If we explain this way, most men can and do take their own decision, whatever it is (to proceed with biopsy or continue PSA follow up).

Using risk calculators often surprises us with values one would not expect. For example use Sunnybroke Prostate risk calculator (see below) and take 75 years old healthy Caucasian male with PSA of 3.9, %free PSA 22%, IPSS 9, in a good health (for example upper 25% of his generation), no family history for prostate cancer and negative DRE. He has more than 15 years of life expectancy, 39% risk of prostate cancer and 20% risk of having at present high grade prostate cancer (Gleason 7 or more). 20% risk of high grade cancer and more than 15 years of life expectancy - would you suggest a biopsy?

At present (june 2011), one of the most modern (can take into account PCA3, p2PSA...) pre-biopsy nomograms is available from UT Health Science Center, San Antonio, head Ian Thompson (http://deb.uthscsa.edu/URORiskCalc/Pages/calcs.jsp). Opponents of his calculator state it has good estimation of overall cancer risk, but underestimates high risk cancers. Large urology collection of nomograms, also many pre-biopsy nomograms including estimation of biopsy risks, are available from Pierre Karakiewicz, Cancer Prognostics and Health Outcomes Unit from University of Montreal Health Centre, Canada (www.nomograms.org). Calculators derived from European Randomized study of Screening for Prostate Cancer (Fritz Schroeder) are available at SWOP Prostate Cancer Research Fundation: http://www.prostatecancer-riskcalculator.com/via.html. Useful, simple and modern (more accurate high risk cancers estimation) pre-biopsy nomogram is available from SunnyBrook Health Sciences Centre, Toronto: http://sunnybrook.ca/content/?page=OCC_prostateCalc.

Different nonograms, for example taking into account 3D biopsy approach (Sakura et al., 2011) are being developed and published constantly. Also, comparisons (Oliveira et al., 2011) and evaluations (Ngo et al., 2011) are permanently performed and published. When using nomograms, one should be aware of their limitations (Vickers & Cronin, 2010).

NCCN guidelines on prostate cancer early detection not require nomogram use, follow in part risk adapted approach, cover most "before biopsy" issues, are regularly updated and modern. They are available freely after registration from www.nccn.org.

3. Methods of biopsy

Prostate cancer was in the past diagnosed most often using histology from transurethral resection, which was performed for local complications of prostate cancer or merely BPH. As it became clear such diagnosis is most often too late, makes subsequent radical surgical treatment more difficult and as PSA become available, biopsy had become diagnostic method of choice. At first, it was finger guided, blind. With development of transrectal ultrasound (trus - transrectal ultrasound guided prostate biopsy) and coupling it to 18G needle, Pandora box of prostate cancer was opened.

3.1 Transrectal or transperineal approach?

Most prostate biopsies around the world are performed transrectally, as this naturally developed from transrectal finger guided approach, is cheaper, simpler, does not need any analgesia or anaesthesia (although it is highly recommended, see section 4.3). Transperineal approach does need at least local anaesthesia. On same occasions, like post surgical amputation of the rectum, if it is sutured, transperineal biopsy (or transgluteal) may be the only way. However, such biopsy is guided by US probe on the perineum or in the urethra or more often by CT or MRI, which is not the way transperineal biopsy is performed regularly. Regular transperineal biopsy is performed using probe in the rectum and needle is advanced through the skin above rectal opening. Transperineal approach has similarity with the way some treatments are performed (brachytherapy...). Treatment templates may be used for biopsy which may guide biopsy needle to a specific part of prostate, which is seen as potentially more effective and with better gain. Recently, stereotactic templates (even motorized and computer guided) have become available also for transrectal prostate sampling - mechanically assisted 3D TRUS guided biopsy system (Megwalu et al., 2008). Supporters of transperineal approach suggest transperineally apical and anterior parts of the prostate may be better accessed compared to transrectal approach. For those reasons, studies were designed to compare yields of transrectal versus transperineal biopsy approach in primary 12-core and saturation 20-core schemes (Hara et al., 2008; Abdollah et al., 2011). Those studies uniformly showed no difference in cancer yields. However, this has not convinced proponents of transperineal approach. In regions, where transperineal approach was used routinely and claimed to be better compared to transrectal (for example some parts of Italy), they are only lately discovering prostate biopsy with end-fire probe (Galosi et al., 2010). Due to technical development of ultrasound equipment, some manufacturers (also very respectful one), were using side-fire probe with needle "through-the-probe" technology. This was proved to be inferior (Chin et al., 2009) in comparison to end-fire biopsy approach (see below). Therefore comparison of perineal to side-fire transrectal approach is not appropriate. Combination of transrectal and transperineal approach has also been used and described, aiming at gaining best from both approaches and maximizing cancer detection rate (Kawakami et al., 2007).

Transrectal approach is recommended for routine primary and also saturation prostate biopsy. On rare occasions, where stereotactic guidance may be needed, decision on approach depends on availability of equipment. At present, equipment for transperineal stereotactic approach is more often available and more widespread, due to its use for brachytherapy (and different other new experimental approaches, such as cryotherapy or photodynamic therapy), compared to new and only limited availability of transrectal computer and motor guided tools for prostate biopsy. Therefore, transperineal biopsy may be method of choice in selected cases.

3.2 Transrectal ultrasound probe

After analogue ultrasound probes have settled to history, electronic probes prevailed. Rotating mechanical sector probes have not gained popularity in the past. Present standard is electronic multi-element transducer - array. They come in two configurations. Side-fire probes have longitudinal transducer and take biopsies in longitudinal sections - sagittal plane, while end-fire probes have curved array detector and allow biopsies to be taken also in transverse plane. In the past, Bruel and Kjaer and Kretz offered for prostate biopsy primarily side-fire probes and this was subjectively seen as better approach compared to end-fire probes (vaginal probes), used "secondarily" also for prostate biopsies. However, end-fire proponents build hypothesis better detection rate to be expected with end-fire sampling in transverse plane due to ability to direct needle more towards lateral part of the peripheral zone, where most tumors arise. This hypothesis was at first tested and confirmed for sextant biopsy in PSA range 4-10 (Paul et al., 2004). This issue was challenged again in 2009, hypothesising end-fire probe has more oblique angled trajectory allowing better peripheral sampling (Ching et al., 2009). To reach anterior gland and apex in longitudinal plane, side-fire probe should be turned a lot and moved in a way which often causes pain as moves point of entry of the needle below dentate line of the rectum. End-fire probe allows better manipulation and targeting desired areas of prostate. Hypothesis was confirmed in their study, finding significantly better detection rate overall in the end-fire group compared to side-fire group and better detection in side-fire group for biopsies with more than 8 cores (8-12, 13-19 and 20 and more) and all PSA ranges (below 2.5, 2.5-4, 4-10 and more than 10) (Ching et al., 2009)

Later, side-fire probes were often bi-planar, therefore allowing better orientation in the prostate, if one views it in two planes and offering choice between end-fire or side-fire biopsy guide. At present, interest has moved from purely end-fire or side-fire biopsy towards combined biopsy opinions and probe designs are now aiming further at 3-plane, 3D imaging and computer guidance... Biplanar probes have become standard equipment also because linear longitudinal array on the probe is necessary for transperineal prostate procedures guidance, while end-fire part is used for standard transrectal biopsy. Ideally, one should have the ability to use biplanar probe, but probably prefer end-fire setting for taking most biopsy cores.

As history is repeating and revealing again in many aspects of human life, new TargetScan device (Envisioneering Medical Technologies, St. Louis, MO, USA) uses mechanical sector probe with single rotating element, applying it in "side-fire" configuration, but with needle, which bends, thus overcoming drawbacks from side-fire systems (Taneja, 2006).

3.3 Biopsy needle

Form, length, thickness, shape of biopsy needle, as everything regarding prostate biopsy, is being constantly challenged. It seems at present thickness of the needle is settled to 18G, needles are side-notch, true-cut, straight with stroke length of 22 mm.

But it was not always so – aspiration biopsy (cytological biopsy) was around and well not so many years ago (Gustafsson et al., 1990). Length of the needle may not seem important at first sight, but for systematic sampling of all areas of big prostates, standard needle length may become limiting factor, as it may simply not be possible to advance needle from biopsy guide into the prostate enough to get sampling of all desired areas in a big or a bit

differently formed prostate. For example, TargetScan (Envisoneering) declares needle movement of 2.2 cm (standard for most biopsy guns, but not all) and possibility of needle protruding 2 cm from tip of biopsy guide before firing - together 42 mm of needle penetration. This is a description of a dedicated "robotic" system. In every day life, where ultrasound system and needle guide are one thing, hospital's supply for needles another and hospital's selection of biopsy-guns third issue, this should be considered, measured and perhaps some longer needles acquired for bigger prostates. Many other variants of needle characteristics were evaluated. Regarding stroke length, 33 mm end-cut was proposed (Dogan et al., 2005) by some, others proposed 29 mm side-notch instead of 22 mm (Fink et al., 2005). It is obvious longer is better and at least 22 mm should be used instead of old 15 mm, which was used at introduction of now obsolete sextant biopsy scheme (Hodge et al., 1989). Also thickness of needle was questioned - 18G (1.27 mm) was compared to thinner needles (0.9 mm (20G), 0.8 mm and 0.7 mm(22G)) - this old study found 0.9 mm may be acceptable (Norberg et al., 1994) - however it is not used in practice today. More recent studies evaluated thickness of needles again - non-ferromagnetic titanium needles were evaluated for quality of yield in comparison to standard needles - 16G (1.65 mm) titanium needle was found to provide samples of good quality and better compared to 18G regular (Franiel et al., 2006). However, also for MRI guided puncture, commercially available product is 18G needle (TSK, Japan) with characteristics comparable to regular needles.
Until recently, only straight needles were in wide use. This creates problem with accessibility (see section 3.2). Recent machine for stereotactic trus biopsy Targetscan aims to overcome this problem with new pliable needle, which bends and allows good approach to most sites in the prostate in side-fire configuration.

3.4 Image guidance

In the beginning of transrectal prostate ultrasound era, large efforts were made attempting to recognize cancerous areas of prostate on gray ultrasound picture. Although hypoechoic lesions were identified as important (Terris et al., 1991) and we still lean toward specifically sampling hypoechoic areas as suspect in our every-day prostate biopsy work, we can not rely on them. After color doppler ultrasound was introduced, suspect areas were proposed to be the ones, which have higher or disorganized blood flow. Many studies have confirmed better sampling with the help of doppler or color flow imaging. However, presentation of subtly disorganized prostate vasculature and blood flow in potential cancer foci is very delicate and very dependent on sonographist, so only highly specialized individuals were and are able to put theory into practice. They are still trying to improve visualization of vasculature, either with ultrasound contrast or with other pharmacological agents, but other three presently available imaging techniques seem more promising as they may be more standardized and therefore easier for every urologist or radiologist, who, in a hurry and overwhelmed with other everyday work, perform mass of prostate biopsy burden: elastography, ANNA C-TRUS and HistoScanning.

3.4.1 Role of MRI

Magnetic resonance imaging with different modalities has established its role in prostate cancer imaging. Apart from T1 and T2 weighted images (Jager et al., 1996), which are not enough, multi-modal approach, like diffusion weighted imaging and dynamic contrast enhanced imaging was found necessary to identify tumor suspicious regions. Role of endorectal coil, although sometimes debated (for example for 3T may not be so important as for 1.5T), seems also well established (Comet-Batlle et al., 2003). Tumor suspicious regions are found in different proportions, depending on criteria and number of different imaging modalities applied and can reach up to 98% even in post-trus-negative biopsy setting. After tumor suspicious regions are identified, sampling is needed.

The easiest approach would be image fusion to trus picture, which is moving from development phase (Hu et al., 2010) and in some centers already represents routine practice (for example Heidelberg, Germany). Two systems are in development: transrectal Artemis - Eigen, Grass Valley, CA, USA (Natarajan et al., 2011) and transperineal BiopSee - MedCom, Darmstadt, Germany (Hadaschik et al., 2011). Incidental reports show identification and confirmation of cancer in patients with previously negative ANNA C-TURS biopsy, however, at present there are no studies which would compare any of the mentioned techniques and show individual strengths and indications.

Some researchers perform MRI examination with plastic simulator of endorectal probe in-situ to simulate deformation expected during trus biopsy setting (Ukimura et al., 2010). Others perform 3D ultrasound imaging and use electromagnetic positioning device to perform biopsies (Turkbey et al., 2011).

Straightforward use of MRI would be MRI guided biopsy of MRI identified suspicious regions of prostate. Although at present available only in few institutions, this may very soon become more widespread as technology, procedure and equipment seem more and more ready for prime time (Roethke et al., 2011). Two independent retrospective series, performed with 1.5T or 3T magnets, from Netherlands (Hambrock et al., 2010) and from Germany (Roethke et al., 2011), report 52% and 58% (of patients with tumour suspicious regions identified) of positive MRI-guided biopsies after previous negative trus guided prostate biopsies.

3.4.2 ANNA C-TRUS and HistoScanning

Idea about reflected ultrasound wave analysis, which should reveal more data than can be seen just with naked eye, is old. There were and are still experiments taking place in developing algorithms of data analysis. Most often prostate is evaluated with transrectal ultrasound before radical prostatectomy and pictures are saved. After radical prostatectomy, histological sections of prostate with known areas of cancer and benign tissue are correlated with saved ultrasound data. Aim is to allow identification of cancer regions on ultrasound before biopsy or surgery. There may be many usages - HistoScanning is evaluated for prediction of Gleason score, volume of cancer, number and localization of cancer foci, prediction of location of cancer focus in relation to neurovascular bundle and in relation to prostate borders - all those data may be useful not only for decision to proceed or postpone biopsy and to guide biopsy, but also for pre- and peri-operative or other treatment planning.

ANNA C-TRUS is a method, which analyzes typical transrectal ultrasound pictures of prostate in transversal plane (for example 5, on sections, where one normally takes biopsy cores). Pictures can be taken with any digital US scanner. Pictures are then sent, uncompressed (using either .tif, .bmp or .png format), using internet, to the provider. After analysis, suspect areas are marked on pictures and urologist repeats examination, this time taking samples from areas marked. All data available about this method seem at present still from the inventor and copyright holder of the technique, prof. Loch from Flensburg, they seem at present not independently evaluated. From author's report in 2010, it seems C-TRUS

ANNA technique detected 66 cancers, taking up to 6 cores in a series of 132 patients with previous negative prostate biopsy. Series included 62 patients with previous 1 negative biopsy, 41 with previous 2 negative biopsies, 18 with 3 negative biopsies, 6 with 4 negative biopsies and 5 with previous more negative biopsies (5-6) (Loch, 2010). This indicates 50% positive biopsy in a setting where lower numbers would be obviously expected, but data are not clear which part of the C-TRUS ANNA positive biopsies belongs to group of only one previous negative biopsy, some of them with only 6 cores, and which was percentage in a subgroup of patients with more negative biopsies. Method is commercially available from Fresenius Kabi Deutschland, Bad Homburg and costs in 2010 without tax (VAT) approximately 378 eur per use (one set of pictures analysis - one patient).

Prostatic HistoScanning was developed proprietary by company AMD, Waterloo, Belgium in cooperation with B/K ultrasound manufacturer. According to company's web site (accessed in April 2011), it is commercially available in EU and Canada and awaits FDA approval for US. First it was aimed as "triage test for men deemed to be at risk for prostate cancer and who wish to avoid prostate biopsy" (Braeckman et al., 2008). Later it seems they realized getting rid of biopsy is at present not attainable goal and they focused on improving sampling of the prostate at biopsy (Braeckman et al., 2008). It seems method was developed by comparing raw ultrasound data from prostates before biopsy to histological results of patients, positive for cancer, who underwent radical prostatectomy. In this way it seems development was similar to ANNA C-TRUS, each using own mathematical modeling for differentiation between benign and malign areas of prostate. However, AMD's HistoScann uses in a way "more straightforward" data, in a technical sense - but it needs specific B/K ultrasound machine and specific probe and is limited regarding other US manufacturer's data. In the community, availability of proper US machines for addition of HistoScann technology is limited. Advantage, compared to C-TRUS ANNA is in data analysis and processing in a "black box", which is for AMD's HistoScanning on site, while with C-TRUS ANNA one has to send data (over internet) to central facility and wait for analysis, therefore ultrasound prostate examination and biopsy can not be performed the same day, while HistoScann allows this. How often algorithms are changed and which are better, has not been evaluated yet although both systems are already commercially available in Europe and are, as such, competitors.

Some specific claims about HistoScanning were challenged in the letter to the editor of BJU (Aigner & Frauscher, 2009), objecting name of the method and questioning resolution and ability of ultrasound to detect small tumor foci. In response, authors admit some limitations of their method, specifically lower quality of signal and therefore potentially less reliable analysis in case of dense calcifications in the prostate or for analyzing anterior component of a very large prostate. They compare it with MRI claiming there is wider availability or US compared to MRI. It is at present not true - MRI is available in a lot of hospitals, endorectal coils are single use, however, specific B/K ultrasound machine with particular probe and motorized machine for rectal probe guiding and AMD's "black box" are not available and seem at present more costly compared to MRI examination. Advantage of all ultrasound approaches compared to MRI approaches lies in assumption of ultrasound picture to be easier for use in subsequent sample acquisition. With the expected development of programs for US - MRI picture fusion, this advantage of pure-ultrasound approach may disappear. Question which is better or are all those methods (MRI (T-2, DW and spectroscopy), elastography, C-TRUS ANNA and HistoScanning) comparable or perhaps they may supplement each other, will become important source of research endeavours in the future. HistoScanning manufacturer intends to use the technology also for other cancers, like ovary, thyroid and breast, which may be advantageous as prostate diagnosis may benefit from multidisciplinary team. On the other side, C-TRUS ANNA was developed by urologists for urologists, can be used in almost any setting (any digital ultrasound machine is good) and seems to have at present more peer reviewed data. HistoScanning is not aiming only towards prostate biopsy guidance, but also aims at other potentially useful predictions regarding prostate cancer and seems to have larger research base with groups from different countries (UK, Germany) who study its potential applications. Whether one or both techniques will stand the test of time and what role they will play remains open.

3.4.3 Elastography

Real time transrectal ultrasonoelastograpy of the prostate is aimed at discrimination between harder and softer areas of prostate tissue. MRI elastography technology was also developed (S. Li et al., 2011), but here only ultrasound is described. Back-scattered ultrasound waves are displaced with compression or decompression of tissue (approximately 2%), harder areas showing less displacement compared to softer (Salomon et al., 2008). Elastography is performed in real-time, at the time of biopsy - no previous transrectal ultrasound examination (as for C-TRUS ANNA) is necessary. By subjectively observing US elastography picture, operator aims at evaluating symmetry of stiffness, focal areas of hardness and persistence of stiffness with probe tilting, aiming at stiff nodule more than 5 mm in diameter and persistence of stiffness after probe tilting (Giurgiu et al., 2011). There are different scoring systems (Salomon et al., 2009), some focus on identifying smaller lesions and potentially showing increased sensitivity (Kamoi et al., 2008). Technique of elastography is still improving, better differentiation markers are being developed constantly (Zhang et al., 2011). Further, standardization of compression with idea of leaving this part to the machine is also in testing (Tsutsumi et al., 2010). Regarding companies which provide elastography equipment, most studies have been performed using Hitachi machine, which is commercially available for prostate applications and most tested, although other manufacturers also offer this technology. Among target-biopsy techniques elastograpy seems at present most widely spread as technology is also in use for breast cancer (primarily) and investment needed is only in US machine and probe, there are no per-investigation charges as for C-TRUS ANNA. Elastography procedure is also much simpler compared to MRI-US fusion. Another advantage of elastography is in its compatibility with power/color doppler techniques for image guidance, which can be performed simultaneously, therefore gaining from two sources. There are quite a few published studies describing experience with prostate elastograpy from different parts of the world. Study results are positive and seem to support claims that elastography improves cancer detection rate. One of the very appealing studies, from USA, analyzed help of elastograpy in biopsy of men with PSA values between 1.25 and 4 and free/total PSA ratio less than 18% (Aigner et al., 2010). They were able to detect 24% of cancers using 5 cores with elastography guidance compared to 5.1% cancers using 10 systematic biopsies. Another study, from Romania, used and compared in the same set of patients gray scale, doppler and elastograpyh data (Giurgiu et al., 2011). They found, in a series of 65 patients and 43% of them with identified cancer on biopsy, sensitivity of elastograpy to be 68% and specificity 62%. Particularly promising was elastography in a subgroup of older than 70 years, where sensitivity increased above 80% and lead authors to propose, if their results are further confirmed, in case of negative elastography and doppler, biopsy in this group and in relatively stable PSA, may be avoided.

On recent demonstration of C-TRUS ANNA and elastography at the occasion of EAU Congress in Vienna (march 2011), where both techniques were exposed to a patient with 4 previous negative biopsies and rising PSA, both techniques failed to find cancer in those two patients. This shows, as one can deduce from literature cited above: in approximately 50% of patients with suspicious characteristics (PSA) and previous negative biopsy, we are unable to find cancer at present. For how long? Will they develop cancer in the future? What is the right strategy to follow them? How they end? All those questions are important and need answers in future research.

3.4.4 Color, power doppler

Angiogenesis is important in development of cancer and increased vascularity was detected in tumors in general and in radical prostatectomy specimens, therefore use of ultrasound to detect those changes was proposed. Color doppler imaging estimates mean frequency shift of doppler signal to determine velocity and direction of flow. Power doppler shows total energy of the signal by integrating it, therefore resulting in sig`nal with homogenous background and more precise detection of smaller and low flow vessels (Remzi et al., 2004). Study of usefulness of power and color doppler for evaluation of hypoechoic lesions showed 80% sensitivity and 82% specificity for detecting prostate cancer (Cho et al., 2000). Standardized criteria for scoring different degrees and distributions of prostatic vascularity were developed and also subjective scales seem to work well (Mitterberger et al., 2010), however this points to high subjectivity of the method, which is its drawback.

Power doppler was used for evaluation of peripheral prostatic capsular vessels, parenchymal vessels and vessels anastomosing with extraprostatic vessels (Sauvain et al., 2003). Criteria for suspicion of cancer in this study were increase in number of intra-lesional vessels, disoriented vessels or verticalized vessels in peripheral gland, asymmetrical blood flow, mass effect on the intraprostatic perilesional vessels and vessels in peripheral margins. Analyzing all those criteria, they aimed at estimation of prostate cancer stage by dividing lesions into three groups: absent extracapsular involvement, undetermined extracapsular involvement and presumably present extracapsular involvement. In this series, 55.7% patients had cancer and sensitivity of power doppler ultrasound was claimed to be 92%, specificity 72% (compared to 88% and 58% for ultrasound only). Group with ultrasound estimated lack of extracapsular involvement had this found in final pathology in 11%, while group with ultrasound suspicious for extracapsular involvement had it confirmed in 87%. Authors (Sauvain et al., 2003) conclude power doppler ultrasound improves accuracy of ultrasound imaging in the diagnosis of cancer, can increase detection rate, optimize number of biopsy cores and also predict extracapsular invasion by identification of capsule perforating vessels.

When using ultrasound for evaluation of minor differences in prostate blood flow between cancerous and benign areas, many factors can interfere with the results - for example position of the patient - it was shown left decubitus position caused flow asymmetry resulting in more biopsies directed toward left side without improving detection rate (Halpern et al., 2002).

Different pharmaceutical interventions were proposed to increase difference between cancer and benign tissue: improved view with contrast agent, increased flow with phosphodiesterase inhibitor (vardenafil) (Morelli et al., 2011) or decreased flow with 5-alpha reductase inhibitor or combination of 5-alpha reductase inhibitor with contrast agent (Mitterberger et al., 2008).

Contrast enhanced transrectal prostate ultrasound was extensively evaluated in multiple research projects (Wink et al., 2008). Microbubbles act as additional reflectors in bloodstream and increase sensitivity of color and power doppler imaging. Newer techniques, for example harmonic imaging, were also tested. Use of ultrasound contrast agent is associated with only minimal side effects, like alterations in taste, flush or pain at the injection site. However, it costs additional money for contrast. It should be performed in 4 minutes after contrast injection (half life of bubbles). Further drawback is strong operator-dependence of the technique. Contrast enhanced ultrasound enables visualisation of prostate cancer (in up to 78% of cases), but sensitivity and specificity are not enough to avoid systematic biopsies. Targeted biopsies using this technique are claimed to allow lower number of cores per session without decrease in detection rate (Wink et al., 2008).

Use of 5-alpha reductase inhibitor was proposed in two staged approach: first color/power doppler evaluation of prostate is followed by 1-3 week of dutasteride and than reevaluation and biopsy guided to areas, where vascular signals have not decreased after treatment. Additional sextant systematic sample was also taken. Researchers claimed increased yield in targeted cores (20%) compared to sextant cores (8%) (Ives et al., 2005).

3.5 Biopsy schemes and number of cores

After finger guided biopsy strategies were replaced with ultrasound guided, it soon became clear (group around dr. Stamey, Stanford) 6 cores, taken in a systematic fashion, finds more cancer than aiming at hypo-echoic areas or randomly (Hodge et al., 1989). Standard approach, which hold for more than 10 years, was established: six cores were taken in parasagittal plane, one at the base, one mid-gland and one at apex. However, patients with negative biopsies and still suspicious for cancer, had repeat biopsies, which were almost as often positive as first biopsy - therefore it was obvious the system was not perfect. Aim should be - perform biopsy - if it is negative, then there is no cancer. Reality was - perform classic sextant scheme biopsy - if it is negative, then there is almost the same probability for cancer as before biopsy. So - search has begun for improvement of systematic biopsy scheme (mainly searching for optimal number of cores and location of cores) and this search has not settled yet. As this text aims at the future, not past, only some examples will be pointed out. Inadequacy of sextant scheme was proven many times, for example (Norberg et al., 1997) and also recent larger and longer retrospective data analyzes still turn to this question, for example regarding sextant biopsy's ability to predict unilateral disease (Mayes et al., 2011). First it became clear biopsies should be directed more laterally in the peripheral zone of the prostate (Eskew et al., 1997). Later, it seemed transitional zone inclusion may improve cancer detection, however this was abandoned for initial biopsy, because of inferior gain from transitional zone directed cores compared to more sampling toward far lateral mid-gland and anterior-apical areas. A lot of cancers are located on anterior horn of prostate. With repeat biopsy, of course, anterior transitional zone is also sampled (Chun et al., 2010). Innumerous analyzes have shown - more cores - more cancer. Prostate size has a role (Taneja, 2006). Nomogram was developed to optimize number of cores needed in relation to prostate size - so called Vienna nomogram (Remzi et al., 2005), as it is obvious higher number of cores gives better sampling and improves detection. Later, while some still questioned Vienna nomogram's usefulness (Lecuona & Heyns, 2010), it became obvious number of biopsy detected cancers is related to sampling density, which is a quotient between prostate size and number of cores taken. A lot of nomograms, which predict probability of positive prostate biopsy, take sampling density into account (Chun et al., 2007). Regarding number of cores, it went up from six at first to eight, later ten, later twelve (a lot of us still using this number at present for majority of patients for first biopsy), fifteen, eighteen... up to twenty-one (Guichard et al., 2007) core per biopsy session. This number seems to be highest present routine extended systematic biopsy scheme, simply because twenty-four or more cores is called saturation biopsy (Ahyai et al., 2010). Many have also argued they were unable to increase their cancer detection rate after increasing number of cores from for example 12 to 18. This underscores importance not only of number, but also direction of cores.

3.6 Free hand systematic biopsy, targeted biopsy, prostatic mapping or combination

Goal of prostate biopsy is not only to find "some" cancer in the prostate, as it was in the past. Now, it has not only to provide representative sample of DIL (dominant intraprostatic lesion), but also to show all "important" cancer areas in the prostate, describe precisely where they are and ensure other regions are cancer free. This is in contrast to efforts of targeted biopsies which claim they may reduce pain and burden of biopsy by reducing number of cores.

Prostate-mapping biopsy approaches, for example TargetScann, have different approach - they aim at precisely sampling predefined sections of prostate with larger number of cores. Electronic doppler ultrasound probes are becoming increasingly complex and sensitive to detect blood flow signals in the prostate to help guiding biopsy. TargetScan's device ultrasound probe is sector and at present can not be used for image-guided approaches, but seems to provide relatively reliable results regarding prostate mapping, which is very important for all targeted therapy approaches (Andriole et al., 2007). "Robotic" probes (ultrasound systems, which are just inserted into rectum by physician and then guided by pressing buttons, are being developed also by other manufacturers.

We have therefore a mix of partly competing, some probably complementary and some excluding technologies aiming at improving prostate cancer detection and staging. Which will find its way into every-day practice and to what extent, remains open. It seems at present repeat biopsy yield is about 20%-40% and targeted biopsy methods claim, in repeat, previously negative setting, yield of 50%. All those new approaches need evaluation and confirmation. One way may be showing significantly better performance of targeted or mapping approaches compared to prediction of nomograms for repeat biopsy setting (Chun et al., 2007).

Overall, it seems at present first biopsy should be 10-18 laterally directed cores (depending on prostate size, for prostates larger than 50 ml minimum 14). Targeted biopsy only, with less than 6 cores, may generally not be appropriate for the first biopsy, as it is far from 100% and we need to assess whole prostate.

For second and later biopsies, as targeted opinions are becoming more and more widespread and therefore accessible and are not untested technical glitches any more, we may in 2011 suggest any of the recently developed opinions, depending on local availability, as follows.

1. If no targeted approach is available and also there is lack of funds (for example for C-TRUS ANNA), transrectal saturation biopsy may be performed and probably it may be useful to perform MRI or choline PET-CT to help identifying suspicious areas.
2. If equipment and local expertise allow, any of the targeted biopsy methods (for example C-TRUS ANNA or others) should be used.
3. Stereotactic biopsy (TargetScan or transperineal) is definitely better opinion compared to free-hand saturation biopsy. Stereotactic approach may also be suggested after diagnosis, regarding watchful waiting or minimally invasive therapies planning.

4. Periprocedural considerations

Prostate biopsy is potentially dangerous and painful procedure. Preparation, informed consent with explanation of possible complications, administration of proper antibiotic prophylaxis, policy on anticoagulant and antiaggregation medications and pain management should be standardized and followed in every patient.

4.1 Enema and needle handling

Although bowel preparation with enema or clear fluids are not necessary before biopsy (Zaytoun et al., 2011) or no statistically significant increase in complication rate was identified with change of regimen (Ruddick et al., 2011), some still claim less septic complications with enema use (Kanjanawongdeengam et al., 2009) or even with the way enema is properly administrated (Huang et al., 2006). In the light of modern approaches to bowel surgery, extensive enemas really look outdated, but it is obvious rectum should be empty before biopsy and suppository in the evening or morning before biopsy seems very reasonable and appropriate. The future with development of resistant bacteria may even bring back old classical methods (cleaning rectum with povidone iodine enema or simply povidone iodine suppository), but at present this is not standard.

Question of role of re-inserting "dirty" needle. Most of us use one needle for the whole procedure (all cores). Some (Kisner in Maribor, Slovenia) have insisted on using sterilized needle with every core, others studied cleaning needle with povidone iodine solution during procedure (Koc et al., 2010). No decrease in complications was shown with those techniques.

4.2 Antibiotics

Most common causative organism for infectious complications following trus prostate biopsy is E.coli. Antibiotic prophylaxis is necessary and guidelines from European and American urological societies have been issued and regulate this question, although different antibiotic regimens are used in practice. Guidelines are freely accessible on web from the issuing societies (EAU and AUA) and provide also extensive lists of literature, which will therefore not be reviewed again here.

EAU guidelines (www.uroweb.org, 2010 edition) recommend antimicrobial prophylaxis, but admit choice of regimens remains debatable. They list studies which suggest single doses for low-risk patients and remark, prolonged course should be considered for high-risk patients. Expected patogens are Enterobacteriaceae and possibly also anaerobes. Recommended antibiotics are fluoroquinolons, TMP+SMX and metronidazole with question mark (no evidence).

AUA guidelines (www.auanet.org, 2008 edition, reviewed 2010) also confirm prophylaxis is indicated in all patients as randomized controlled trials have confirmed significantly lower rates of complications in antibiotic groups. They also claim single dose may be adequate.

A lot depends on local antibiotic resistance patterns. For example, if TMP+SMX regimen is not used even for non-complicated urinary tract infections in one area, one would not use it for prostate biopsy prophylaxis either. One can never predict for sure future development of antibiotic resistance. Therefore, constant vigilance is needed and monitoring rates of infectious complications is necessary. Special attention should focus on repeat biopsies and this setting may sometimes deserve different antibiotic scheme or previous culture and susceptibility analysis. Later may be performed in two ways - patients with catheters or other urinary tract insertions may be screened using urine culture (Bruyere et al., 2010), but all who need screening should have their stools sample cultured for resistant strains. Resistant strains do occur and may significantly contribute to complications (Liss et al., 2011). Due to high probability of E.coli resistance to quinolones in cases of patients returning to hospital after prostate biopsy with quinolone prophylaxis, it is wise to use another antibiotic before cultures are known (although it seems obvious, people do often get prescribed flouroquinolone again). If there is no or low risk for ESBL, cephalosporines (probably third generation) may be the best initial guess (Zaytoun et al., 2011).

Although single dose is claimed useful, in our and many other situations most patients can be considered not low risk regarding infectious risk classifications (more than 65 years of age, concomitant diseases, like diabetes and lower urinary tract symptoms, incomplete bladder emptying). Therefore typical scheme (as we use it and others, for example (Campos-Fernandes et al., 2009), uses ciprofloxacin 500 mg twice daily started before biopsy and continued for three days. It was shown to decrease rate of complications after biopsy (Schaeffer et al., 2007). As every single infectious complication, even most minor, requiring any health-service contact, even only consultation, is seen as a big problem and aim is to avoid any complication, there are many patients who probably benefit from short course and not single dose antibiotic and this may be further reason why urologists are reluctant in accepting single dose only approach.

Metronidazol is added in some centers routinely, but most do not use it at present. However, it might be useful for specific patients, with specific predisposing conditions and in combination with other antibiotics (for example cephalosporins, although subjective experience shows more complications with their use for this purpose), when flouroquinolone resistance or intolerance is present.

Instead of 1-2 hour prior to procedure fluoroquinolone orally, same use parenteral aminogylcoside (gentamicin or amikacin) or aminopenicilline with betalactamase inhibitor (co-amoxiclav) at the time of biopsy, which is followed by oral antibiotic (often fluoroquinolone, but also others) at home. This scheme is used in some centers and may be helpful when compliance with oral regimen prior to biopsy is questionable or for allergy and non-tolerance to quinolones or in areas with high resistance to quinolones (Kehinde et al., 2008). Combination of periprocedural oral dose of ciprofloxacine with iv dose of gentamicin may be method of choice for single dose regimens.

Additional important recent problem regarding fluoroquinolones was finding significantly different serum concentrations of active drug comparing different generic manufacturers (Kehinde et al., 2010). Apart from probable reason for higher complication rate, substandard antibiotics preparations also contribute to resistance development as longer courses are needed and as a consequence low concentrations of drug are present in the environment for longer time.

4.3 Pain control

Only 11% of urologists in US used local anesthesia to reduce pain during trus biopsy in 2002 (Davis et al. 2002). At the time, a strong appeal from one of the most distinguished opinion leaders favored local anesthesia (Soloway, 2003). Thereafter, guidelines (AUA, EAU, NCCN) all recommended or even mandated (AUA) local pain medication use during this procedure. Intrarectal application of eutectic cream or lidocaine jelly may decrease pain as some anesthetic agent may reach site of pain with diffusion, but it is variable and is considered not adequate. Pain during transrectal prostate biopsy is caused by two sources.

First source of pain is probe insertion and presence and movement of probe in the anal canal during biopsy. This can be ameliorated with slow and gentle dilation and local lidocaine jelly or EMLA cream, but other measures for relaxation of sphincter were also used with success and are available – local glyceryl trinitrate oinment or spray or local 2% diltiazem or 0,2% - 0,5% nifedipine oinment. Using gylceryl trinitrate oinment, headache was noted as side effect in 10% of patients – dose was 2 mg (McCabe et al., 2007). It remains open, whether lower dose of spray (0,4 mg/activation) would reach same effect with less side effects.

Second source of pain during trus biopsy is related to nerves in prostate capsule and neurovascular bundles. After a lot of research (for example (Scattoni et al., 2010)) it seems accepted injection of 2x 5 ml (each side) of 1% lidocaine most appropriately reduces pain. Site of injection may be at the base (basolateral periprostatic nerve plexus area, described also as prostate-vesicular junction injections) or at the apex. Debate where to inject sill continues. Quality control suggested for standard technique of periprostatic block, observation of hypoechoic nodule ("wheal") formation on the site of injection is needed. It was shown least pain (best effect) was observed, when hypoechoic nodule formed after injection on both sides (Obek et al., 2006). Regarding injectable agents, for potential lidocaine allergic patients, tramadol has significant local anesthetic properties and is universally available and it has also been studied in this setting (Seckiner et al., 2011).

Addition of oral medication, either for sedation or for additional pain relief may be also helpful in selected patients.

5. Complications

Generally, complications are: hematuria (13%-74%), hemospermia (30%), blood at stools (1%), pain (4%), nausea (up to 1%), fever (up to 1%), epididymitis (up to 1%), infection which needs hospitalization (0,3%). Most feared complication is sepsis.

Another important complication is bleeding. Patients can bleed from rectum, they can observe hematuria or hemospermia. Bleeding is most often self limiting and settle in a few days. Rarely significant issues (bladder tamponade or significant rectal bleeding) would occur. Such occasions would of course necessitate hospitalization or use of appropriate standard measurements for treatment. Bleeding may be more significant with anticoagulant treatment. Warfarin is stopped well before biopsy and patient is covered with low molecular weight heparin. Low dose acetylsalicylic acid (aspirin) may be continued, although some still recommend a drug holiday for a few days (till bleeding settles). There are no experience with newer antithrombotic drugs (for example dabigatran and other factor Xa inhibitors) and it is generally suggested to be avoided during prostate biopsy (changed to low-molecular weight heparin, the same as for warfarin). Clopidogrel should also be stopped, although there is a report claiming 15% of urologists to continue with both clopidogrel or warfarin (Brewster et al., 2010). This is not advisable, except aspirin and low molecular weight haparin, all other similarly working medications should be stopped before biopsy. Regarding clopidogrel, explicit agreement and consent between patient, his cardiologist and urologist may result in exception, but extreme caution is needed.

Immediate complications, like fainting, diaphoresis should be controlled by adequate local pain control. It is also not advisable for patients to be completely fasted.

Rate of complications increases with time. Most important and frequent seem infectious complications. Reasons for increasing rates of complications may be increasing numbers of cores per procedure or increased antibiotic resistance (Nam et al., 2010).

Long term complications of prostate biopsy would be development of pain syndromes or problems with erectile function, which was described recently (Klein et al., 2010). This reminds us that indefinitely repeating biopsies and increasing number of cores per biopsy may not be the best way forward. Selective, targeted approaches must be taken seriously, as prostate biopsy is not without its consequences.

6. Chemopreventive stategies

Inhibitors of 5-alpha reductase (5ARI), finasteride or dutasteride, may be used short term to decrease blood flow in the prostate before biopsy (as described at the end of section 3.4.4). Further, it is speculated their longer term use (6 months or more) may decrease proportion of benign prostate in a whole gland and in this way increase chances for prostate cancer detection on prostate biopsy. It may also reduce development of low grade cancer. One possible strategy for use of 5ARI inhibitors is prescription of drug after first or second negative biopsy and then regular follow up of PSA. PSA is expected to decrease. Trigger for repeat biopsy is any increase of PSA above nadir or if PSA value under 5ARI is above 40% of initial PSA value. Described approach was recently retrospectively evaluated in abstract form, using REDUCE data (Roobol et al., 2011). However, a proportion of prostate cancers do progress (for example on watchful waiting) without this fact reflecting in increase of PSA. Therefore a possibility of prostate cancer progression (in patients on 5ARI treatment or without) while PSA values would not increase is a serious concern and needs further research. We should always be aware, none of our methods is 100% successful.

7. Conclusion

Future of prostate biopsy will be interesting, a lot of new ideas and technologies are competing at present and it remains open which will, in the end, dominate the market and our every-day practice.

Although new targeted technologies, either ultrasound or magnetic resonance, may improve detection and sampling and reduce need for increasing number of cores and repeat biopsy sessions, none seem at present nearing 100% sensitivity or specificity. At present, approximately 50% positive biopsy rate is expected in repeat biopsy setting using either C-TRUS ANNA or MRI-guided or MRI-US picture fusion guided biopsy.

As burden of biopsies may increase dramatically in the near future (as explained above - (Quon et al., 2011)) further increases in complexity and technological demands may not be able to satisfy mass biopsy needs. Prostate biopsy is not very demanding procedure, potential harms and problems for patients do exist, but are not nearly as large as for different forms of prostate cancer treatments. Therefore, such a breakthrough as happened in the field of prostate surgery regarding robotic assisted prostatectomy, is not expected. Perhaps we may expect in the near future coexistence of many different biopsy opinions and methods, which are showing comparable results, the same situation as developed for surgical treatment of prostate cancer, where robotic, laparoscopic and open radical prostatectomies progressed to the level, where all show same good results (Eden et al., 2011). It seems present simple system - transrectal probe with 10-20 samples per session, with some additional help of ultrasound picture analysis and systematic sampling systems or not - is here to stay and will be main working horse for enormous number of prostate biopsies which are expected to be performed in the next decade. New markers (PCA3 and p2PSA) will complement PSA and free PSA in decisions about second and further repeat biopsies. At the same time different US and MRI methods, tailored to different patients needs, wishes and different predicted treatment modalities will be available to supplement basic approach when needed and will develop further.

8. References

Abdollah, F., Novara, G., Briganti, A., Scattoni, V., Raber, M., Roscigno, M., Suardi, N., et al. (2011). Trans-rectal Versus Trans-Perineal Saturation Rebiopsy of the Prostate: Is There a Difference in Cancer Detection Rate? *Urology, 77*(4), 921-925.

Ahyai, S. A., Isbarn, H., Karakiewicz, P. I., Chun, F. K. H., Reichert, M., Walz, J., Steuber, T., et al. (2010). The presence of prostate cancer on saturation biopsy can be accurately predicted. *BJU Int, 105*(5), 636-641.

Aigner, F., & Frauscher, F. (2009). RE: Computer-aided ultrasonography (HistoScanning): a novel technology for locating and characterizing prostate cancer. *BJU Int, 103*(1), 115-116.

Aigner, F., Pallwein, L., Junker, D., Schafer, G., Mikuz, G., Pedross, F., Mitterberger, M. J., et al. (2010). Value of real-time elastography targeted biopsy for prostate cancer detection in men with prostate specific antigen 1.25 ng/ml or greater and 4.00 ng/ml or less. *J Urol, 184*(3), 913-917.

Akhavan, A., Keith, J. D., Bastacky, S. I., Cai, C., Wang, Y., & Nelson, J. B. (2007). The proportion of cores with high-grade prostatic intraepithelial neoplasia on extended-pattern needle biopsy is significantly associated with prostate cancer on site-directed repeat biopsy. *BJU Int, 99*(4), 765-769.

Andriole, G. L., Bullock, T. L., Belani, J. S., Traxel, E., Yan, Y., Bostwick, D. G., & Humphrey, P. A. (2007). Is There a Better Way to Biopsy the Prostate? Prospects for a Novel Transrectal Systematic Biopsy Approach. *Urology, 70*(6, Supplement 1), S22-S26.

Andriole, G. L., Grubb, R. L., Buys, S. S., Chia, D., Church, T. R., Fouad, M. N., Gelmann, E. P., et al. (2009). Mortality Results from a Randomized Prostate-Cancer Screening Trial. *NEJM, 360*(13), 1310-1319.

Auprich, M., van Poppel, H., Marberger, M., Stenzl, Arnulf, Mulders, P. F. A., Huland, Hartwig, Abbou, C.-C., et al. (2011). 2320 Initial and repeat prostate biopsy: comparative peerformance analysis of PSA, %FPSA, prostate volume and urinary PCA3 including development of novel PCA3 cut-off tresholds. *J Urol, 185*(4, Supplement 1), e930.

Balk, S. P., Ko, Y.-J., & Bubley, G. J. (2003). Biology of Prostate-Specific Antigen. *JCO, 21*(2), 383 -391.

Bektic, J., Darte, C., Skradski, V., Steiner, E., Schaefer, G., Bartsch, G., Horninger, W., et al. (2010). 985 Access [-2]proPSA and Beckman Coulter prostate health index (PHI) and early detection of aggressive prostate cancers. *Eur Urol Supplements, 9*(2), 309.

Bektic, J., Carroll, P. R., Cooperberg, M. R., Klocker, H., Steiner, E., Skradski, V., Horninger, W., et al. (2011). 747 The worst cancers send early PSA signals that would allow early detection if monitoring focused on increasing PSA. *Eur Urol Supplements, 10*(2), 238.

Bill-Axelson, A., Holmberg, Lars, Ruutu, M., Garmo, H., Stark, J. R., Busch, Christer, Nordling, S., et al. (2011). Radical Prostatectomy versus Watchful Waiting in Early Prostate Cancer. *NEJM, 364*(18), 1708-1717.

Braeckman, J., Autier, P., Garbar, C., Marichal, M. P., Soviany, C., Nir, R., Nir, D., et al. (2008). Computer-aided ultrasonography (HistoScanning): a novel technology for locating and characterizing prostate cancer. *BJU Int, 101*(3), 293-298.

Braeckman, J., Autier, P., Soviany, C., Nir, R., Nir, D., Michielsen, D., Treurnicht, K., et al. (2008). The accuracy of transrectal ultrasonography supplemented with computer-aided ultrasonography for detecting small prostate cancers. *BJU Int, 102*(11), 1560-1565.

Brewster, S., Turkeri, L., Brausi, M., Ravery, V., & Djavan, B. (2010). 5A prospective survey of current prostate biopsy practices among oncological urologists. *Can J Urol, 17*(2), 5071-5076.

Bruyere, F., d'Arcier, B. F., Boutin, J.-M., & Haillot, O. (2010). Is urine culture routinely necessary before prostate biopsy? *Prostate Cancer Prostatic Dis, 13*(3), 260-262.

Bussemakers, M. J., van Bokhoven, A., Verhaegh, G. W., Smit, F. P., Karthaus, H. F., Schalken, J.A., Debruyne, F. M., et al. (1999). DD3: a new prostate-specific gene, highly overexpressed in prostate cancer. *Cancer Res, 59*(23), 5975-5979.

Campos-Fernandes, J.-L., Bastien, L., Nicolaiew, N., Robert, G., Terry, S., Vacherot, F., Salomon, L., et al. (2009). Prostate cancer detection rate in patients with repeated extended 21-sample needle biopsy. *Eur Urol, 55*(3), 600-606.

Catalona, W. J., Partin, Alan W., Slawin, K. M., Brawer, M. K., Flanigan, R. C., Patel, A., Richie, J. P., et al. (1998). Use of the Percentage of Free Prostate-Specific Antigen to Enhance Differentiation of Prostate Cancer From Benign Prostatic Disease. *JAMA, 279*(19), 1542 -1547.

Catalona, W. J., Smith, D. S., Ratliff, T. L., Dodds, K. M., Coplen, D. E., Yuan, J. J. J., Petros, J. A., et al. (1991). Measurement of Prostate-Specific Antigen in Serum as a Screening Test for Prostate Cancer. *NEJM, 324*(17), 1156-1161.

Ching, C. B., Moussa, A. S., Li, J., Lane, B. R., Zippe, C., & Jones, J. S. (2009). Does transrectal ultrasound probe configuration really matter? End fire versus side fire probe prostate cancer detection rates. *J Urol, 181*(5), 2077-2082.

Cho, J. Y., Kim, S. H., & Lee, S. E. (2000). Peripheral hypoechoic lesions of the prostate: evaluation with color and power Doppler ultrasound. *Eur Urol, 37*(4), 443-448.

Chun, F. K.-H., Briganti, A., Graefen, Markus, Porter, C., Montorsi, F., Haese, A., Scattoni, V., et al. (2007). Development and external validation of an extended repeat biopsy nomogram. *J Urol, 177*(2), 510-515.

Chun, F. K.-H., Epstein, J. I., Ficarra, V., Freedland, S. J., Montironi, R., Montorsi, F., Shariat, S. F., et al. (2010). Optimizing performance and interpretation of prostate biopsy: a critical analysis of the literature. *Eur Urol, 58*(6), 851-864.

Comet-Batlle, J., Vilanova-Busquets, J. C., Saladie-Roig, J. M., Gelabert-Mas, A., & Barcelo-Vidal, C. (2003). The value of endorectal MRI in the early diagnosis of prostate cancer. *Eur Urol, 44*(2), 201-207.

Crawford, E. D., Grubb, R., Black, A., Andriole, G. L., Chen, M.-H., Izmirlian, G., Berg, C. D., et al. (2011). Comorbidity and mortality results from a randomized prostate cancer screening trial. *J Clin Oncol, 29*(4), 355-361.

Davis, M., Sofer, M., Kim, S. S., & Soloway, M. S. (2002). The procedure of transrectal ultrasound guided biopsy of the prostate: a survey of patient preparation and biopsy technique. *J Urol, 167*(2 Pt 1), 566-570.

Dite, G. S., Whittemore, A. S., Knight, J. A., John, E. M., Milne, R. L., Andrulis, I. L., Southey, M. C., et al. (2010). Increased cancer risks for relatives of very early-onset breast cancer cases with and without BRCA1 and BRCA2 mutations. *Br J Cancer, 103*(7), 1103-1108.

Dogan, H. S., Eskicorapci, S. Y., Ertoy-Baydar, D., Akdogan, B., Gunay, L. M., & Ozen, H. (2005). Can we obtain better specimens with an end-cutting prostatic biopsy device? *Eur Urol, 47*(3), 297-301.

Eden, C. G., Arora, A., & Hutton, A. (2011). Cancer Control, Continence, and Potency After Laparoscopic Radical Prostatectomy Beyond the Learning and Discovery Curves. *J Endourol.* 25(5), 815-819.

Eskew, L. A., Bare, R. L., & McCullough, D. L. (1997). Systematic 5 region prostate biopsy is superior to sextant method for diagnosing carcinoma of the prostate. *J Urol, 157*(1), 199-202.

Fink, K. G., Hutarew, G., Pytel, A., & Schmeller, N. T. (2005). Prostate biopsy outcome using 29 mm cutting length. *Urol Int, 75*(3), 209-212.

Franiel, T., Fritzsche, F., Staack, A., Rost, J., Hamm, B., & Beyersdorff, D. (2006). [Histopathologic quality of prostate core biopsy specimens: comparison of an MR-compatible biopsy needle and a ferromagnetic biopsy needle used for ultrasound-guided prostate biopsy]. *Rofo, 178*(12), 1212-1218.

Galosi, A. B., Tiroli, M., Cantoro, D., Conti, A., & Muzzonigro, G. (2010). Biopsy of the anterior prostate gland: technique with end-fire transrectal ultrasound. *Arch Ital Urol Androl, 82*(4), 248-252.

Giurgiu, C. R., Manea, C., Crisan, N., Bungardean, C., Coman, I., & Dudea, S. M. (2011). Real-time sonoelastography in the diagnosis of prostate cancer. *Med Ultrason, 13*(1), 5-9.

Gosselaar, C., Roobol, Monique J., Roemeling, S., & Schroder, Fritz H. (2008). The Role of the Digital Rectal Examination in Subsequent Screening Visits in the European Randomized Study of Screening for Prostate Cancer (ERSPC), Rotterdam. *Eur Urol, 54*(3), 581-588.

Guazzoni, G., Nava, L., Lazzeri, M., Scattoni, V., Lughezzani, G., Maccagnano, C., Dorigatti, F., et al. (2011). Prostate-Specific Antigen (PSA) Isoform p2PSA Significantly Improves the Prediction of Prostate Cancer at Initial Extended Prostate Biopsies in Patients with Total PSA Between 2.0 and 10 ng/ml: Results of a Prospective Study in a Clinical Setting. *Eur Urol, In Press,* doi: 10.1016/j.eururo.2011.03.052

Guichard, G., Larre, S., Gallina, A., Lazar, A., Faucon, H., Chemama, S., Allory, Y., et al. (2007). Extended 21-sample needle biopsy protocol for diagnosis of prostate cancer in 1000 consecutive patients. *Eur Urol,* 52(2), 430-435.

Gustafsson, O., Norming, U., Nyman, C. R., & Ohstrom, M. (1990). Complications following combined transrectal aspiration and core biopsy of the prostate. *Scand J Urol Nephrol, 24*(4), 249-251.

Hadaschik, B., Kuru, T., Tulea, C., Teber, D., Huber, J., Popeneciu, V., Pahernik, S., et al. (2011). 2304 Stereotactic prostate biopsy with pre-interventional MRI and live US fusion. *J Urol 185*(4, Supplement 1), e924.

Halpern, E. J., Frauscher, Ferdinand, Forsberg, F., Strup, S. E., Nazarian, L. N., O'Kane, P., & Gomella, L. G. (2002). High-frequency Doppler US of the prostate: effect of patient position. *Radiology, 222*(3), 634-639.

Hambrock, T., Somford, D. M., Hoeks, C., Bouwense, S. A. W., Huisman, H., Yakar, D., van Oort, I. M., et al. (2010). Magnetic resonance imaging guided prostate biopsy in men with repeat negative biopsies and increased prostate specific antigen. *J Urol, 183*(2), 520-527.

Hara, R., Jo, Y., Fujii, T., Kondo, N., Yokoyoma, T., Miyaji, Y., & Nagai, A. (2008). Optimal approach for prostate cancer detection as initial biopsy: prospective randomized study comparing transperineal versus transrectal systematic 12-core biopsy. *Urology, 71*(2), 191-195.

Hodge, K. K., McNeal, J. E., Terris, M. K., & Stamey, T. A. (1989). Random systematic versus directed ultrasound guided transrectal core biopsies of the prostate. *J Urol, 142*(1), 71-74.

Hu, Y., Ahmed, H. U., Taylor, Z., Allen, C., Emberton, M., Hawkes, D., & Barratt, D. (2010). MR to ultrasound registration for image-guided prostate interventions. *Medical Image Analysis, In Press,* doi: DOI: 10.1016/j.media.2010.11.003

Huang, Y.-C., Ho, D.-R., Wu, C.-F., Shee, J.-J., Lin, W.-Y., & Chen, C.-S. (2006). Modified bowel preparation to reduce infection after prostate biopsy. *Chang Gung Med J, 29*(4), 395-400.

Isharwal, S., Makarov, D. V., Sokoll, L. J., Landis, P., Marlow, C., Epstein, J. I., Partin, Alan W., et al. (2011). ProPSA and Diagnostic Biopsy Tissue DNA Content Combination Improves Accuracy to Predict Need for Prostate Cancer Treatment Among Men Enrolled in an Active Surveillance Program. *Urology, 77*(3), 763-763.

Ives, E. P., Gomella, L. G., & Halpern, E. J. (2005). Effect of dutasteride therapy on Doppler US evaluation of prostate: preliminary results. *Radiology, 237*(1), 197-201.

Izmirlian, G., Crawford, E. D., Grub III, R., Hsing, A., Kramer, B. S., Church, T. R., Riley, T. M., et al. (2011). 333 Family history of various cancers and the risk of incident prostate cancer in the PLCO trial. *J Urol 185*(4, Supplement 1), e134-e135.

Jager, G. J., Ruijter, E. T., van de Kaa, C. A., de la Rosette, J. J., Oosterhof, G. O., Thornbury, J. R., & Barentsz, J.O. (1996). Local staging of prostate cancer with endorectal MR imaging: correlation with histopathology. *Am J Roentgenol, 166*(4), 845-852.

Jemal, A., Siegel, R., Xu, J., & Ward, E. (2010). Cancer statistics, 2010. *CA Cancer J Clin, 60*(5), 277-300.

Jemal, A., Bray, F., Center, M. M., Ferlay, J., Ward, E., & Forman, D. (2011). Global cancer statistics. *CA Cancer J Clin, 61*(2), 69-90.

Kamoi, K., Okihara, K., Ochiai, A., Ukimura, O., Mizutani, Y., Kawauchi, A., & Miki, T. (2008). The utility of transrectal real-time elastography in the diagnosis of prostate cancer. *Ultrasound Med Biol, 34*(7), 1025-1032.

Kanjanawongdeengam, P., Viseshsindh, W., Santanirand, P., Prathombutr, P., & Nilkulwattana, S. (2009). Reduction in bacteremia rates after rectum sterilization before transrectal, ultrasound-guided prostate biopsy: a randomized controlled trial. *J Med Assoc Thai, 92*(12), 1621-1626.

Kawakami, S., Okuno, T., Yonese, J., Igari, T., Arai, G., Fujii, Y., Kageyama, Y., et al. (2007). Optimal sampling sites for repeat prostate biopsy: a recursive partitioning analysis of three-dimensional 26-core systematic biopsy. *Eur Urol, 51*(3), 675-682.

Kehinde, E. O., Sheikh, M., Anim, J., Al-Maghrebi, M., Hussein, A. Y., & John, J. S. (2008). Addition of single dose amikacin to prophylactic quinolones significantly reduces infectious complications of transrectal ultrasound guided biopsy of the prostate gland. *J Urol, 179*(4, Supplement 1), 717-718.

Kehinde, E., Abdel-Hamid, M., Philips, O., Sharaf, L., & Babu, A. (2010). 811 A comparative pharmacokinetic study of seven brands of ciprofloxacin in NZW rabbits using liquid chromatography mass spectrometry technique. *J Urol, 183*(4, Supplement 1), e316-e317.

Klein, T., Palisaar, R. J., Holz, A., Brock, M., Noldus, J., & Hinkel, A. (2010). The impact of prostate biopsy and periprostatic nerve block on erectile and voiding function: a prospective study. *J Urol, 184*(4), 1447-1452.

Koc, G., Un, S., Filiz, D. N., Akbay, K., & Yilmaz, Y. (2010). Does washing the biopsy needle with povidone-iodine have an effect on infection rates after transrectal prostate needle biopsy? *Urol Int, 85*(2), 147-151.

Kotb, A. F., Tanguay, S., Luz, M. A., Kassouf, W., & Aprikian, A. G. (2011). Relationship between initial PSA density with future PSA kinetics and repeat biopsies in men with prostate cancer on active surveillance. *Prostate Cancer Prostatic Dis, 14*(1), 53-57.

Lecuona, A., & Heyns, C. F. (2010). A prospective, randomized trial comparing the Vienna nomogram to an eight-core prostate biopsy protocol. *BJU Int. In Press.* doi: 10.1111/j.1465-410X.2010.09887.x.

Li, S., Chen, M., Wang, W., Zhao, W., Wang, J., Zhao, X., & Zhou, C. (2011). A feasibility study of MR elastography in the diagnosis of prostate cancer at 3.0T. *Acta Radiol, 52*(3), 354-358.

Liss, M. A., Chang, A., Santos, R., Nakama-Peeples, A., Peterson, E. M., Osann, K., Billimek, J., et al. (2011). Prevalence and Significance of Fluoroquinolone Resistant Escherichia coli in Patients Undergoing Transrectal Ultrasound Guided Prostate Needle Biopsy. *J Urol, 185*(4), 1283-1288.

Loch, T. (2010). [Core needle biopsy twice negative with rising PSA level. Does imaging help?]. *Urologe A, 49*(3), 369-375.

Makarov, D. V., Isharwal, S., Sokoll, L. J., Landis, P., Marlow, C., Epstein, J. I., Partin, Alan W., et al. (2009). Pro–Prostate-Specific Antigen Measurements in Serum and Tissue Are Associated with Treatment Necessity among Men Enrolled in Expectant Management for Prostate Cancer. *Clinical Cancer Research, 15*(23), 7316 -7321.

Malvezzi, M., Arfe, A., Bertuccio, P., Levi, F., La Vecchia, C., & Negri, E. (2011). European cancer mortality predictions for the year 2011. *Ann Oncol, 22*(4), 947-956.

Mayes, J. M., Mouraviev, V., Sun, L., Tsivian, M., Madden, J. F., & Polascik, T. J. (2011). Can the conventional sextant prostate biopsy accurately predict unilateral prostate cancer in low-risk, localized, prostate cancer? *Urol Oncol, 29*(2), 166-170.

McCabe, J. E., Hanchanale, V. S., Philip, J., & Javle, P. M. (2007). A randomized controlled trial of topical glyceryl trinitrate before transrectal ultrasonography-guided biopsy of the prostate. *BJU Int, 100*(3), 536-538.

Megwalu, I. I., Ferguson, G. G., Wei, J. T., Mouraviev, V., Polascik, T. J., Taneja, S., Black, L., et al. (2008). Evaluation of a novel precision template-guided biopsy system for detecting prostate cancer. *BJU Int, 102*(5), 546-550.

Miettinen, O. S. (2010). Screening for a cancer: thinking before rethinking. *Eur J Epidemiol, 25*(6), 365-374.

Mitterberger, M., Aigner, Friedrich, Pinggera, G. M., Steiner, Eberhard, Rehder, P., Ulmer, H., Halpern, E. J., et al. (2010). Contrast-enhanced colour Doppler-targeted prostate biopsy: correlation of a subjective blood-flow rating scale with the histopathological outcome of the biopsy. *BJU Int, 106*(9), 1315-1318.

Mitterberger, M., Pinggera, G., Horninger, Wolfgang, Strasser, H., Halpern, E., Pallwein, Leo, Gradl, J., et al. (2008). Dutasteride prior to contrast-enhanced colour Doppler ultrasound prostate biopsy increases prostate cancer detection. *Eur Urol, 53*(1), 112-117.

Morelli, G., Pagni, R., Mariani, C., Minervini, R., Morelli, A., Gori, F., Ferdeghini, E. M., et al. (2011). Results of Vardenafil Mediated Power Doppler Ultrasound, Contrast Enhanced Ultrasound and Systematic Random Biopsies to Detect Prostate Cancer. *J Urol*, 185(6): 2126-2131.

Morgan, T. O., Jacobsen, S. J., McCarthy, W. F., Jacobson, D. J., McLeod, D. G., & Moul, J. W. (1996). Age-Specific Reference Ranges for Serum Prostate-Specific Antigen in Black Men. *NEJM, 335*(5), 304-310.

Nam, R. K., Saskin, R., Lee, Y., Liu, Y., Law, C., Klotz, L. H., Loblaw, D. A., et al. (2010). Increasing hospital admission rates for urological complications after transrectal ultrasound guided prostate biopsy. *J Urol, 183*(3), 963-968.

Natarajan, S., Marks, L. S., Margolis, D. J. A., Huang, J., Macairan, M. L., Lieu, P., & Fenster, A. (2011). Clinical application of a 3D ultrasound-guided prostate biopsy system. *Urol Oncol, 29*(3), 334-342.

Ngo, T. C., Turnbull, B. B., Lavori, P. W., & Presti Jr., J. C. (2011). The Prostate Cancer Risk Calculator From the Prostate Cancer Prevention Trial Underestimates the Risk of High Grade Cancer in Contemporary Referral Patients. *J Urol, 185*(2), 483-488.

Nieder, C., Norum, J., & Geinitz, H. (2011). Impact of Common Medications on Serum Total Prostate-specific Antigen Levels and Risk Group Assignment in Patients with Prostate Cancer. *Anticancer Research, 31*(5), 1735 -1739.

Norberg, M., Busch, C., Stavinoha, J., Scardino, P.T., & Magnusson, A. (1994). Transrectal ultrasound-guided core biopsies of the prostate. A comparison between the standard 1.2-mm needle and three thinner needles. *Acta Radiol, 35*(5), 463-467.

Norberg, M., Egevad, L., Holmberg, L., Sparen, P., Norlen, B. J., & Busch, C. (1997). The sextant protocol for ultrasound-guided core biopsies of the prostate underestimates the presence of cancer. *Urology, 50*(4), 562-566.

Obek, C., Ozkan, B., Tunc, B., & Can, G. (2006). Hypoechoic space formation with periprostatic nerve block: myth or reality? *Urol Int, 76*(3), 236-239.

Oberaigner, W., Horninger, Wolfgang, Klocker, Helmut, Schonitzer, D., Stuhlinger, W., & Bartsch, Georg. (2006). Reduction of prostate cancer mortality in Tyrol, Austria, after introduction of prostate-specific antigen testing. *Am J Epidemiol, 164*(4), 376-384.

Oliveira, M., Marques, V., Carvalho, A. P., & Santos, A. (2011). Head-to-head comparison of two online nomograms for prostate biopsy outcome prediction. *BJU Int, 107*(11), 1780-1783.

Pandha, H., Ismail, M., Boxall, A., Bhatt, A., Langley, S., Hindley, R., & Morgan, R. (2011). 2326 Engrailed-2 (EN2): a urinary biomarker for the diagnosis of prostate cancer without DRE. *J Urol, 185*(4, Supplement 1), e932-e933.

Pater, L. E., Hart, K. W., Blonigen, B. J., Lindsell, C. J., & Barrett, W. L. (2011). Relationship Between Prostate-specific Antigen, Age, and Body Mass Index in a Prostate Cancer Screening Population. *American Journal of Clinical Oncology, In Press.*

Paul, R., Korzinek, C., Necknig, U., Niesel, T., Alschibaja, M., Leyh, H., & Hartung, R. (2004). Influence of transrectal ultrasound probe on prostate cancer detection in transrectal ultrasound-guided sextant biopsy of prostate. *Urology, 64*(3), 532-536.

Pepe, P., Candiano, G., Fraggetta, F., Galia, A., Grasso, G., Allegro, R., & Aragona, F. (2009). Is PSA density still useful in diagnosing prostate cancer? *Arch Ital Urol Androl , 81*(4), 199-202.

Potter, S. R., & Partin, A.W. (2000). Hereditary and familial prostate cancer: biologic aggressiveness and recurrence. *Rev Urol, 2*(1), 35-36.

Quiles, M. T., Arbos, M. A., de Torres, I. M., Blazquez, C., Bastaros, J. M., Placer, J., Doll, A., et al. (2011). 2321 Comparative analysis of prostate cancer antigen 3 mRNA expression in benign peripheral prostatic tissue, cancer and isolated or cancer-associated high grade prostatic intraepithelial neoplasia. *J Urol, 185*(4, Supplement 1), e930-e931.

Quon, H., Loblaw, A., & Nam, R. (2011). Dramatic increase in prostate cancer cases by 2021. *BJU Int. In Press.* doi: 10.1111/j.1464-410X.2011.10197.

Remzi, M., Dobrovits, M., Reissigl, A., Ravery, V., Waldert, Mattias, Wiunig, C., Fong, Y. K., et al. (2004). Can Power Doppler Enhanced Transrectal Ultrasound Guided Biopsy Improve Prostate Cancer Detection on First and Repeat Prostate Biopsy? *Eur Urol, 46*(4), 451-456.

Remzi, M., Fong, Y. K., Dobrovits, M., Anagnostou, T., Seitz, C., Waldert, Matthias, Harik, M., et al. (2005). The Vienna nomogram: validation of a novel biopsy strategy defining the optimal number of cores based on patient age and total prostate volume. *J Urol, 174*(4 Pt 1), 1256-1260.

Roethke, M., Anastasiadis, A. G., Lichy, M., Werner, M., Wagner, P., Kruck, S., Claussen, C. D., et al. (2011). MRI-guided prostate biopsy detects clinically significant cancer: analysis of a cohort of 100 patients after previous negative TRUS biopsy. *World J Urol. In Press* doi: 10.1007/s00345-011-0675-2.

Roobol, M.J., Van Leeuwen, P. J., & Schroder, F.H. (2011). 19 Combining screening and chemoprevention of prostate cancer. *Eur Urol Supplements, 10*(2), 34.

Ruddick, F., Sanders, P., Bicknell, S. G., & Crofts, P. (2011). Sepsis rates after ultrasound-guided prostate biopsy using a bowel preparation protocol in a community hospital. *J Ultrasound Med, 30*(2), 213-216.

Sakura, M., Kawakami, S., Ishioka, J., Fujii, Y., Yamamoto, S., Iwai, A., Numao, N., et al. (2011). A novel repeat biopsy nomogram based on three-dimensional extended biopsy. *Urology, 77*(4), 915-920.

Salomon, G., Graefen, M., Heinzer, H., Huland, H., Pallwein, L., Aigner, F., & Frauscher, F. (2009). [The value of real-time elastography in the diagnosis of prostate cancer]. *Urologe A, 48*(6), 628-636.

Salomon, Georg, Kollerman, J., Thederan, I., Chun, F. K. H., Budaus, L., Schlomm, T., Isbarn, H., et al. (2008). Evaluation of prostate cancer detection with ultrasound real-time elastography: a comparison with step section pathological analysis after radical prostatectomy. *Eur Urol, 54*(6), 1354-1362.

Sauvain, J. L., Palascak, P., Bourscheid, D., Chabi, C., Atassi, A., Bremon, J. M., & Palascak, R. (2003). Value of Power Doppler and 3D Vascular Sonography as a Method for Diagnosis and Staging of Prostate Cancer. *Eur Urol, 44*(1), 21-31.

Scattoni, V., Maccagnano, C., Zanni, G., Angiolilli, D., Raber, M., Roscigno, M., Rigatti, P., et al. (2010). Is extended and saturation biopsy necessary? *Int J Urol, 17*(5), 432-447.

Schaeffer, A. J., Montorsi, F., Scattoni, V., Perroncel, R., Song, J., Haverstock, D. C., & Pertel, P. E. (2007). Comparison of a 3-day with a 1-day regimen of an extended-release formulation of ciprofloxacin as antimicrobial prophylaxis for patients undergoing transrectal needle biopsy of the prostate. *BJU Int, 100*(1), 51-57.

Schoenfield, L., Jones, J. S., Zippe, C. D., Reuther, A. M., Klein, E., Zhou, M., & Magi-Galluzzi, C. (2007). The incidence of high-grade prostatic intraepithelial neoplasia and atypical glands suspicious for carcinoma on first-time saturation needle biopsy, and the subsequent risk of cancer. *BJU International, 99*(4), 770-774.

Schroder, F.H., van der Maas, P., Beemsterboer, P., Kruger, A. B., Hoedemaeker, R., Rietbergen, J., & Kranse, R. (1998). Evaluation of the digital rectal examination as a screening test for prostate cancer. Rotterdam section of the European Randomized Study of Screening for Prostate Cancer. *J Natl Cancer Inst, 90*(23), 1817-1823.

Schröder, F. H., Hugosson, J., Roobol, Monique J., Tammela, T. L. J., Ciatto, S., Nelen, V., Kwiatkowski, M., et al. (2009). Screening and Prostate-Cancer Mortality in a Randomized European Study. *NEJM, 360*(13), 1320-1328.

Seckiner, I., Sen, H., Erturhan, S., & Yagci, F. (2011). A Prospective, Randomized Controlled Study Comparing Lidocaine and Tramadol in Periprostatic Nerve Blockage for Transrectal Ultrasound-guided Prostate Biopsy. *Urology, In Press,* doi: 10.1016/j.urology.2011.03.010.

Shikanov, S., Jayram, G., McGuire, M. S., & Brendler, C. B. (2011). 2322 PCA3 variability in men with very low risk prostate cancer. *J Urol, 185*(4, Supplement 1), e931.

Soloway, M. S. (2003). Do unto others - why I would want anesthesia for my prostate biopsy. *Urology, 62*(6), 973-975.

Taneja, S. S. (2006). Prostate biopsy: targeting cancer for detection and therapy. *Rev Urol, 8*(4), 173-182.

Tang, P., Du, W., Xie, K., Fu, J., Chen, H., Yang, W., & Moul, J. W. (2011). Characteristics of baseline PSA and PSA velocity in young men without prostate cancer: Racial differences. *The Prostate, In Press.* doi:10.1002/pros.21418

Terris, M. K., Freiha, F. S., McNeal, J. E., & Stamey, T. A. (1991). Efficacy of transrectal ultrasound for identification of clinically undetected prostate cancer. *J Urol, 146*(1), 78-83.

Thompson, I. M., Pauler, D. K., Goodman, P. J., Tangen, C. M., Lucia, M. S., Parnes, H. L., Minasian, L. M., et al. (2004). Prevalence of Prostate Cancer among Men with a Prostate-Specific Antigen Level ≤4.0 ng per Milliliter. *NEJM, 350*(22), 2239-2246.

Tsutsumi, M., Miyagawa, T., Matsumura, T., Endo, T., Kandori, S., Shimokama, T., & Ishikawa, S. (2010). Real-time balloon inflation elastography for prostate cancer detection and initial evaluation of clinicopathologic analysis. *AJR Am J Roentgenol, 194*(6), 471-476.

Turkbey, B., Xu, S., Kruecker, J., Locklin, J., Pang, Y., Bernardo, M., Merino, M. J., et al. (2011). Documenting the location of prostate biopsies with image fusion. *BJU Int, 107*(1), 53-57.

Ukimura, O., Hirahara, N., Fujihara, A., Yamada, T., Iwata, T., Kamoi, K., Okihara, K., et al. (2010). Technique for a hybrid system of real-time transrectal ultrasound with preoperative magnetic resonance imaging in the guidance of targeted prostate biopsy. *Int J Urol, 17*(10), 890-893.

Vickers, A. J., & Cronin, A. M. (2010). Everything You Always Wanted to Know About Evaluating Prediction Models (But Were Too Afraid to Ask). *Urology, 76*(6), 1298-1301.

Vickers, A. J., Till, C., Tangen, C. M., Lilja, H., & Thompson, I. M. (2011). An Empirical Evaluation of Guidelines on Prostate-specific Antigen Velocity in Prostate Cancer Detection. *Journal of the National Cancer Institute, 103*(6), 462 -469.

Vlaeminck-Guillem, V., Devonec, M., Colombel, M., Rodriguez-Lafrasse, C., Decaussin-Petrucci, M., & Ruffion, A. (2011). Urinary PCA3 score predicts prostate cancer multifocality. *J Urol, 185*(4), 1234-1239.

Wink, M., Frauscher, Ferdinand, Cosgrove, D., Chapelon, J.-Y., Palwein, L., Mitterberger, M., Harvey, C., et al. (2008). Contrast-Enhanced Ultrasound and Prostate Cancer; A Multicentre European Research Coordination Project. *Eur Urol, 54*(5), 982-993.

Yossepowitch, O. (2008). Digital Rectal Examination Remains an Important Screening Tool for Prostate Cancer. *Eur Urol, 54*(3), 483-484.

Zaytoun, O. M., Anil, T., Moussa, A. S., Jianbo, L., Fareed, K., & Jones, J. S. (2011). Morbidity of prostate biopsy after simplified versus complex preparation protocols: assessment of risk factors. *Urology, 77*(4), 910-914.

Zaytoun, O. M., Vargo, E. H., Rajan, R., Berglund, R., Gordon, S., & Jones, J. S. (2011). Emergence of Fluoroquinolone-resistant Escherichia coli as Cause of Postprostate Biopsy Infection: Implications for Prophylaxis and Treatment. *Urology. In Press* doi: 10.1016/j.urology.2010.12.067.

Zeegers, M. P. A., Jellema, A., & Ostrer, H. (2003). Empiric risk of prostate carcinoma for relatives of patients with prostate carcinoma: a meta-analysis. *Cancer, 97*(8), 1894-1903.

Zhang, Y., Tang, J., Li, Y.-M., Fei, X., Lv, F.-Q., He, E.-H., Li, Q.-Y., et al. (2011). Differentiation of prostate cancer from benign lesions using strain index of transrectal real-time tissue elastography. *Eur J Radiol. In Press* doi: 10.1016/j.ejrad.2011.02.037.

Part 2

Surgical Treatment Options

6

Radical Prostatectomy in High Risk Prostate Cancer

Jorge Rioja, Carlos Blanco and Jorge Aranda
Dept Urology, University Hospital Miguel Servet, Zaragoza
Spain

1. Introduction

Prostate cancer is the leading cancer diagnosis in men, and the second cuase, after lung cancer, of cancer death in men in the U.S. Worldwide is the fourth most common cancer in men with variable incidence and mortality rates, based on geographic regions (1). In Europe is the most common solid tumor, with an incidence of 214 cases per 1000 men, outnumbering the lung and colorectal cancers, and is the second most common cause of cancer death in men.

In recent years, the incidence of prostate cancer is increasing in most countries due to the improvement and widespread use of PSA, aging and probably a real increase in incidence. In men after 40 years there is a progressively incidence increase, with a peak at age 80. The countries with the highest mortality rate for prostate cancer are: Switzerland, Scandinavia and the USA-adjusted death rates by age group between 15-20/100.000 inhabitants. By contrast, the Asian countries with Japan and China leading the way, have the lowest mortality rate (less than 5 per 100,000 population) (1).

The geographic incidence variations of prostate Cancer are multiple and complex, but there are genetic and environmental factors, which seem to be more involved in its genesis. African Americans are those who have higher rates of prostate ca. As mentioned above, China and Japan have lower rates in the incidence of prostate ca and USA one of the highest in the world, well, it is noteworthy that Asian Americans have lower incidence rate of prostate cancer than white Americans, the indicating that the genetic factor is crucial in the development of the disease.

The overall increase in the incidence of prostate cancer worldwide in recent decades, is justified with the development of PSA screening protocols of prostate Cancer. The diagnosis of prostate cancer is based on the determination of serum PSA. The risk of prostate cancer is depending on Serum PSA (2):

PSA 0-2 ng / ml: 15-25%.
PSA 2-4 ng / ml: 17-32%
PSA 4-10 ng / ml: 17-32%
PSA> 10 ng / ml: 43-65%.

There is still much controversy among health professionals about what is the best protocol for the screening of prostate cancer. The long awaited results of two prospective, randomised trials were published in 2009. The Prostate, Lung, Colorectal, and Ovarian

(PLCO) Cancer Screening Trial randomly assigned 76,693 men at 10 US centres to receive either annual screening with PSA and DRE or standard care as the control. After 7 years' follow-up, the incidence of prostate cancer per 10,000 person-years was 116 (2,820 cancers) in the screening group and 95 (2,322cancers) in the control group (rate ratio, 1.22) (3). The incidence of death per 10,000 person-years was 2.0 (50 deaths) in the screened group and 1.7 (44 deaths) in the control group (rate ratio, 1.13). The data at 10 years were 67% complete and consistent with these overall findings. The PLCO project team concluded that prostate cancer related mortality was very low and not significantly different between the two study groups. The European Randomized Study of Screening for Prostate Cancer (ERSPC) included a total of 162,243 men from seven countries aged between 55 and 69 years. The men were randomly assigned to a group offered PSA screening at an average of once every 4 years or to an unscreened control group. During a median follow-up of 9 years, the cumulative incidence of prostate cancer was 8.2% in the screened group and 4.8% in the control group (4). The rate ratio for death from prostate cancer was 0.80 in the screened group compared with the control group. The absolute risk difference was 0.71 deaths per 1,000 men. This means that 1410 men would need to be screened and 48 additional cases of prostate cancer would need to be treated to prevent one death from prostate cancer. The ERSPC investigators concluded that PSA-based screening reduced the rate of death from prostate cancer by 20%, but was associated with a high risk of over-diagnosis.

Both trials have received considerable attention and comments. In the PLCO trial, the rate of compliance in the screening arm was 85% for PSA testing and 86% for DRE. However, the rate of contamination in the control arm was as high as 40% in the first year and increased to 52% in the sixth year for PSA testing and ranged from 41% to 46% for DRE. Furthermore, biopsy compliance was only 40-52% versus 86% in the ERSPC. Thus, the PLCO trial will probably never be able to answer whether or not screening can influence prostate cancer mortality. In the ERSCP trial, the real benefit will only be evident after 10-15 years of follow-up, especially because the 41% reduction of metastasis in the screening arm will have an impact.

Recent sub-analysis, with longer follow up have shown a potential benefit of screening, lowering the number of men needed to screen, and the number of patients needed to treat to safe one life.

Two key items remain open and empirical:

- at what age should early detection start
- what is the interval for PSA and DRE.

A baseline PSA determination at age 40 years has been suggested upon which the subsequent screening interval may then be based (5) (GR: B). A screening interval of 8 years might be enough in men with initial PSA levels < 1 ng/mL (6) . Further PSA testing is not necessary in men older than 75 years and a baseline PSA < 3 ng/mL because of their very low risk of dying from prostate cancer (7).

D'Amico in 1998 proposed a classification according to risk group for prostate cancer based on T stage, PSA value and Gleason. This has allowed to simplify the classification of patients with prostate cancer as well as trying to unify its treatment. (Table 1)

The widespread use of PSA testing has led to a significant migration in stage and grade of prostate cancer, with > 90% of men in the current era diagnosed with clinically localised disease (8). Despite the trends towards lower-risk prostate cancer, 20-35% of patients with newly diagnosed prostate cancer are still classified as high risk, based on either PSA > 20 ng/mL, Gleason score > 8, or an advanced clinical stage (9). Patients classified with high-risk prostate cancer are at an increased risk of PSA failure, the need for secondary therapy, metastatic progression and death from prostate cancer. Nevertheless, not all high-risk patients have a uniformly poor prognosis after RP (10). There is no consensus regarding the optimal treatment of men with high-risk prostate cancer. Decisions on whether to elect surgery as local therapy should be based on the best available clinical evidence.

Low risk	**Intermediate risk**	**High risk**
T1-T2a & PSA<10 y Gleason ≤6	T2b or PSA 10-20 or Glesason 7	T2c-T3-T4 or PSA > 20 or Gleason ≥8

Table 1. D'Amico classification of patients according to risk group

As expected, survival and success of the treatment applied in prostate cancer is closely linked to the stadium and the risk presented by the patient.
In this chapter we will focus on Prostate Cancer at high risk as well as the different therapeutic options, focusing on the radical prostatectomy as an effective treatment of the disease.

2. Defining high risk prostate cancer

The factors that best define the high risk prostate cancer are those described by D'Amico (11) approved by the American Urological Association in 2007 are:

$$\text{Gleason} \geq 8 \text{ points and / or PSA} \geq 20 \text{ and / or clinical stage} \geq \text{T2c}$$

These high-risk tumors are at high risk for recurrence, either local or remote, so they are also traditionally called "locally advanced" (12) or "poorly differentiated" (13). If the patient has the 3 items they are considered "very high risk" and have a high probability to die from prostate cancer (14).
Another factor that has been added as a fourth factor is pretreatment *PSA velocity* which if greater 2ng/ml/year is included as criteria for high-risk disease (15,16).
The simplification of the term "risk" has led many doctors to select patients and improperly included in high-risk groups. Also, following the analysis of these high-risk criteria, we can not quantify the individual risk to a patient, for example, with stage T2c and Gleason 8 would have the same risk that a patient with a PSA 70 and stage T3a (17). That is why this classification system is inadequate and we must use another tool to individualize the risk of each patient; this tool are *Nomograms* which individually allow to analyze and quantify the risk presented by each patient in response to multiple risk factors or variables, integrated in a complex mathematical formula (18). There are plenty of nomograms (19) that have been designed for use in prostate cancer in recent years and could be classified into 3 groups:
Diagnostic nomograms: those who pretend to estimate the probability of a patient developing prostate cancer. For example, the Vienna nomogram (20) that analyzes the number of cylinders to take a biopsy of the prostate.
Staging nomograms: such as the Partin tables (21), which indicates the likelihood of organ-confined disease. Or A. Borque neural network for predicting pathological stage in men undergoing radical prostatectomy. (22)

Prognostic nomograms: are tools that estimate the probability of success in applying a certain treatment to analyze different variables. The most famous and globally applied is Kattan nomogram (23). It analyzes a combination of three factors to determine the probability of PSA relapse after local therapy. These factors are: PSA, Gleason score and clinical stage. They apply both to radical prostatectomy, radiotherapy and brachytherapy. Nomograms derived from the results of treating thousands of patients. The statistical probability of relapse depends on the presence of pre-existing micro metastases at the time of local therapy (23). Hence the likelihood of relapse determined by the Kattan nomograms can be taken as an indication of the presence of micro metastases at the time of local therapy, resulting in an estimate to calculate the probability of success / failure when applying a certain treatment.
In summary, nomograms are useful modern tools that exist today, which may help us making treatment decisions in patients with prostate cancer, especially those with high-risk prostate cancer. As well as providing more information to the patient.

2.1 Locally advanced prostate cancer cT3a

When the disease has overpassed the prostate capsule, it is a T3a stage. Typically, when a patient is at this stage we are advise against radical prostatectomy (24) as primary treatment based on the high rate of positive surgical margins and lymph node metastases (25,26). Numerous studies have shown that the risk/benefit of a radical prostatectomy is even more clear in the treatment of high risk prostate cancer (27-32), but unfortunately, there are not studies comparing combination therapy (radiotherapy plus hormones) with RP.
Between 13% and 27% of patients diagnosed with stage T3 are overstimated (31,32).
The development of CT imaging or MRI, as well as directed needle biopsies of lymph nodes or seminal vesicles (32), help identify patients who have less probability to benefit from a surgical treatment (33) as well as to plan surgery upon results.
Due to an increased sophistication and experience of the different surgical techniques, there has been a decreased in operative morbidity and better functional outcomes after RP in stage T3 cancer than before (31,33). Urinary incontinence and erectile dysfunction remain the two major consequences of the surgery, but due to surgical expertise and experience, as well as a proper surgical planning, an improvement in functional results has been shown (35).

2.2 High grade prostate cancer: Gleason score 8-10

Patients with high Gleason score 8-10 tumors, which are confined to the prostate on histopathological examination, they still have a good prognosis after RP (36). The differences between the Gleason score biopsy and the Gleason score regarding the surgical specimen are between 36 and 60% of cases, although a study by Dr. Grossfeld (37) shows that 39% of patients had Gleason 8-10 in the biopsy specimen, showed a Gleason score of 7 or less in the prostatectomy speciem.
In a recent publication (38) in which the outcome of 781 patients undergoing RP clinically localized stages T1-T2 was analysed, they divided into 2 groups according to Gleason: Gleason patients 2-7 and another group with Gleason 8-10. Over all, they showed a worse prognostic features and higher PSA relapse. (Table 2)
Patients with Gleason score 8-10 prostate cancer have a higher likelihood of recurrence, but due to the PSA era, many of these patients are diagnosed with an early stage and therefore a potential local curative treatment is applicable successful (38).

Various studies such as those of Mian et al (39), Lau et al (40) and Soloway et al (41) analyze and study the survival in these patients concluded similarly.
The clinical Gleason 8-10 is an independent prognostic factor for biochemical progression-free survival. The radical prostatectomy remains one of the most valid treatments for these short of patients and providing good oncological and functional outcomes.

	Group Gleason 2-7	Group Gleason 8-10	P value
N° of patients	673	108	
PSA (ng/ml)	Av 13,48 Median 9,8	Av. 16,89 Median 12	<0,01
T1c	55%	50%	<0,0001
>T1c	45%	50%	
<pT3b	69%	44%	<0,0001
pT3b	30%	56%	
Surgical Margin-	67%	48%	<0,0001
Surgical Margin +	33%	53%	
Biochemical Progression -	74,3%	52,5%	<0,0001
Biochemical Progression +	25,7%	47,5%	

Table 2.

2.3 Prostate cancer with PSA > 20

Different studies show that the RP in patients with a PSA> 20 is associated with a high recurrence rate, D'Amico and colleagues found that males with a PSA level higher than 20 ng/ml had risk recurrence of 50% at 5 years after RP (42). Similarly, Yossepowitch published the results of their series of patients with PSA> 20ng/ml who underwent radical prostatectomy, showing a PSA recurrence rate of 44 and 53% at 4 and 20 years respectively (10). It is perhaps the high preoperative PSA, the factor that best relates to a worse prognosis preoperatively.
On the other hand, Inman and colleagues, in their series of patients with PSA> 50ng/ml who underwent RP with multimodal adjuvant therapy, had biochemical progression-free survival at 10 years of 83% with a cancer-specific survival 87% (43). These highlights the potential benefit of surgery with in a multimodal approach.

3. Therapeutic options in "high risk" prostate cancer

3.1 Introduction

Localized prostate cancer

The lack of evidence regarding the effectiveness of treatment options for clinically localised prostate cancer continues to impact on clinical decision-making. The two such options are radical prostatectomy (RP) and active surveillance (AS). (44)
For the majority of men with favorable-risk localized disease, older than 65, surveillance will be an attractive option that avoids adverse effects of treatment(45). But the existing trials,

provide insufficient evidence to allow confident statements to be made about the relative beneficial and harmful effects of RP and AS for patients with localised prostate cancer.(44)
Klotz L et al. assure that active surveillance with treatment reserved for evidence of rapid PSA progression or increase in tumor volume or grade is associated with about a 3% risk of prostate cancer death at 10 years. (46)

Advanced prostate cancer

In the other hand, patients with prostate cancer continue to present with metastatic disease or to relapse following initial hormone therapy; for these men, the optimal combination and sequencing of new medical treatments must be defined. (45)

High risk prostate cancer

For these patients, (T2c-T3-T4 or PSA >20 or Gleason score ≥8) it is very important to give information about the different treatment options, and trying to adequate them to their live expectancy and quality of live.
Urologist, traditionally recommended radiotherapy or androgen deprivation therapy over RP, not because oncologic outcomes were better with radiotherapy, but because incontinence and impotence rates with RP were higher, and cure rates was discouraging. (47)
Actually, RP and radiotherapy have potential benefits and cumulative toxicities that must be matched to disease characteristics and patient expectations in selecting a treatment course. (48)

3.2 Pre-treatment management in high risk prostate cancer

A critical assessment of the location, size, and extent of the primary tumor provides prognostic information, is essential for treatment planning.
D'Amico and colleagues have defined high-risk prostate cancer as that associated with any 1 of 3 risk factors: biopsy Gleason score ≥8, PSA ≥20 ng/mL, or clinical stage ≥T2c. (11)
More recently, D'Amico and colleagues refined their high-risk definition to incorporate an absolute number of high-risk features (stage ≥T2b, biopsy Gleason score ≥7, and pre-treatment PSA >20 ng/mL). (14) Patients are classified into 1 of 3 high-risk groups, defined by the presence of 1, 2, or all 3 features. Probability of death from prostate cancer was highest among men with 3 high-risk features.
High-risk patients with aggressive tumors (PSA >20 ng/mL and Gleason sum >7), advanced local lesions (T3-T4), or patients with symptoms suggestive for metastatic disease, should have imaging studies. (17)
While not uniformly accurate, there are some imaging studies that help us to identificate the high rish disease:

- DRE provides some evidence of the cancer's size and pathologic stage.
- Transrectal ultrasonography (TRUS) is extremely useful for guiding needle biopsies.
- Computed tomography (CT) scans poorly the prostate and lack of sensitivity and specificity for detecting extraprostatic extension.
- Magnetic Resonance Imaging (MRI) provides additional information about the local lession, it has largely replaced CT in the local staging of prostate cancer.
- MRI has been used primarily to determine local disease extent. Body MRI has a role in identifying seminal vesicle involvement, but not extra capsular extension.
- Bone Scan, which is highly sensitive but relatively nonspecific because areas of increased radiotracer uptake are not always secondary to osteoblastic activity from metastases. (17)

An alternative to patients risk-grouping with similar but not identical risk features is use of multivariable models such as nomograms. These models incorporate data from all risk factors relevant to the probability of treatment failure and proportionately weigh their relative contribution in order to calculate a risk score. (48)
Eastham et al. demonstrate that high-risk patients were more likely to exhibit adverse pathologic features and to have biochemical progression. Nevertheless, roughly one-third of high-risk patients (22% to 63%, depending on the definition) had organ-confined cancers and roughly half (41% to 74%) remained progression-free 10 years after surgery alone. These results confirm that current definitions of high risk disease are unreliable in identifying patients who cannot be cured by local therapy. (48)

3.3 Objectives of treatment in high risk prostate cancer

The actual objectives of the treatment of high prostate cancer are:

1. To offer a radical treatment
2. Trying to decrease prostate cancer progression
3. To increase metastatic disease free interval
4. To provide a proper quality of life.

Men with high-volume lesions or high-stage yet clinically localized disease must receive multimodal therapy. More advances will require concerted efforts through clinical trials. (45)
Neoadjuvant Androgen Deprivation Therapy may indeed provide no additional benefit over surgery alone for patients with clinically localized prostate cancer. Recent studies have demonstrated the feasibility of neoadjuvant chemotherapy prior to RP in patients with high-risk prostate cancer. (17). If such a strategy was shown to be effective, future clinical practice could be altered significantly. A randomized phase 3 clinical trial, CALGB 90203, is currently investigating whether neoadjuvant chemo-hormonal therapy followed by RP reduces the risk of biochemical recurrence when compared to RP alone.

3.4 Actual treatment in high risk prostate cancer

Actually, the optimal treatment are:

- radical prostatectomy (RP) + radiation therapy (RT)
- radical prostatectomy + hormonotherapy
- radiation therapy + hormone therapy

There is no consensus regarding the optimal treatment of men with high-risk PCa.
Surgery is showing good results, but decisions on whether to elect surgery as local therapy should be based on the best available clinical evidence. (49)
On the other hand, it has been recently assessed the effect of RP and RT on the rate of distant metastases in patients with clinically localized prostate cancer on the study from Memorial Sloan Kettering Cancer Center comparing patients whom underwent surgery versus radiotherapy (50). Patients with clinical stages T1c-T3b prostate cancer treated with intensity-modulated RT (81 Gy) from 1998 to 2002 were compared with similar cohort of men treated with RP.
This study, showed that patients with higher-risk disease, treated with RP had a lower risk of metastatic progression and prostate cancer-specific death, than men treated with RT. The metastatic progression is infrequent in men with low-risk prostate cancer, treated with either RP or RT.
These results, despite being from retrospective review of patients treated at a single institution, certainly suggest that RP should be considered as a treatment option in men with clinically localized, high-risk prostate cancer. (50)

As mentioned above, the multimodal treatment is achieving good results, and to corroborate this, several randomised studies of radiotherapy combined with androgen-deprivation therapy (ADT) versus radiotherapy alone have shown a clear advantage for combination treatment, but no trial has ever proven combined treatment to be superior to RP.

4. Radical prostatectomy in high risk CaP

4.1 Introduction

Actually radical prostatectomy is accepted as an election treatment in both low and high risk prostate cancer with different evidence level, and even for very high risk prostate cancer. (Table 3)

INDICATIONS	LE
In patients with low and intermediate risk localised PCa (cT1a-T2b and Gleason score 2-7 and PSA ≤ 20) and a life expectancy > 10 years	1b
Optional	
Patients with stage T1a disease and a life expectancy >15 yr or Gleason score 7	3
Selected patients with low-volume high-risk localised PCa (cT3a or Gleason score 8-10 or PSA > 20)	3
Highly selected patients with very high-risk localised PCa (cT3b-T4 N0 or any T N1) in the context of multimodality treatment	3
Optional for selected patients with T3a, PSA < 20 ng/mL, biopsy Gleason score ≤ 8 and a life expectancy > 10 years.	3

Table 3.

The goals of RP are to remove the cancer completely with negative surgical margins, minimal blood loss, no serious perioperative complications, and complete recovery of potency and urinary continence. From an oncologic standpoint, obtaining negative surgical margins is paramount. A positive surgical margin has been associated with as much as 4-fold higher risk of biochemical recurrence, even after adjusting for other prognostic factors such as Gleason grade, extracapsular extension, seminal vesicle invasion, and lymph node metastasis. (48)
On the same way, there are good results in terms of morbidity and survival when radical prostatectomy is offered as a radical treatment.

4.2 Evidence of RP in HR.PC

RP in locally advanced PCa: cT3a

Is defined, as cancer that has perforated the prostate capsule. Surgical treatment has traditionally been discouraged, mainly because patients have an increased risk of positive surgical margins and lymph node metastases and/or distant relapse
In recent years, there has been renewed interest in surgery for locally advanced PCa, and several retrospective case-series have been published. In general, 33.5-66% of patients will have positive section margins, and 7.9-49% will have positive lymph nodes.
On the other hand, excellent 5-, 10- and 15-year overall survival (OS) and cancer-specific survival (CSS) rates have been published.
Therefore, it is increasingly evident that surgery has a place in treating locally advanced disease (45)

The problem remains on patient selection before surgery: Nomograms, nodal imaging with CT and seminal vesicle imaging with magnetic resonance or directed specific puncture biopsies of the nodes or seminal vesicles can help to identify those patients unlikely to benefit from a surgical approach. (17)

In addition, it is extremely important that radical prostatectomy for clinical T3 cancer requires sufficient surgical expertise to keep an acceptable morbidity level.

RP in High-grade PCa: Gleason score 8-10

In this group of patients, the incidence of organ-confined disease is around 26% to 31%. The PSA value and percentage of positive prostate biopsies may help to select men with high-grade PCa most likely to benefit from RP.

Rioja Zuazu J. et al. (38) analyzed the characteristics of the clinical Gleason 8-10 group of patients within their series of patients diagnosed with prostate cancer and treated by means of radical prostatectomy, and tried to ascertain which were the influence factors within this group, upon progression and progression free survival. They conclude, that Clinical Gleason Score 8-10 is a negative independent prognostic factor on the progression free survival, but its prognosis is better if they present a PSA prior surgery lower than 11 ng/ml and the pathological stage is a pT2. So, these kind of patients could be beneficed of RP.

RP in PCa with PSA > 20

Yossepowitch et al. (19) and D'Amico et al. (15) have investigated the results of RP in these patients. In all cases, very good results were seen, with a cancer- specific survival of up to 91% in 10 years in patients treated with RP.

More recently, Inman and co-workers (43) described the long-term outcomes of RP with multimodal adjuvant therapy in men with PSA > 50. Systemic progression-free survival rates at 10 years were 83% and 74% for PSA 50-99 and > 100, respectively, while CSS was 87% for the whole group. These results argue for aggressive management with RP as the initial step.

RP in cT3b-T4 N0

Provided that the tumour is not fixed to the pelvic wall, or that there is no invasion of the urethral sphincter, RP is a reasonable first step in selected patients with a low tumour volume.

In 2005, The Mayo Clinic reported a series of patients with seminal invasion, treated with RP + HT adjuvant. They had a progression free survival at 5, 10 and 15 years, of 85%, 73% and 67% respectively, and a cancer specific survival of 95%, 90% and 79%.

Despite this, management decisions should be made after all treatments, and should be discussed by a multidisciplinary team, and after balancing benefits and side-effects of each therapy modality by the patient, with regard to his own individual circumstances, decision has to be taken.

4.3 Optimal surgical technique for high risk cancer

Surgeons must understand the important anatomical and surgical principles that will allow them to improve their own technique, particularly when operating in the high-risk setting. Certain principles are important, and apply equally to open, laparoscopic and robotic surgical techniques.

Even in a patient with a high risk of extra prostatic disease, a portion of the neurovascular bundle can often be preserved. (17)

This approach has been facilitated by recent anatomical descriptions of the periprostatic anatomy. (51)

Dissection of the neurovascular bundles can be done in an intrafascial plane (directly adjacent to the prostatic capsule; complete nerve sparing), an interfascial plane (within the lateral prostatic fascia; partial nerve sparing) and extrafascial plane (outside the lateral prostatic fascia; nerve resection)

Deep dissection beneath Denonvilliers' fascia posteriorly should be performed routinely, as few nerves are present in this area and deep dissection will reduce the incidence of posterolateral margins.

Large, high-grade cancers, near the base of the prostate, or in the anterior transition zone often invade the bladder neck. For anterior cancers, begin division of the bladder neck a centimeter or more from its junction with the prostate. For large posterior tumors or those with seminal vesicle invasion, include the posterior bladder distal to the interureteral ridge in the specimen. (48)

5. Pelvic lymph node dissection

For patients with low risk disease, PLND is not necessary and is not recommended, because the chance of metastasis is low.

For patients with high and intermediate risk disease, extended PLND at least for external iliac, obturator and hypogastric lymph nodes should be performed during radical prostatectomy. Removing at least 10 lymph nodes is recommended to detect LNI. (52)

Prostate cancer lymphatic spread ascends from the pelvis up to the retroperitoneum invariably through common iliac lymph nodes. PC lymphatic spread can be divided in two main levels: pelvic and common iliac plus retroperitoneal lymph nodes. (53)

So the technique try to remove all lymphatic tissue between the external iliac vein and hypogastric vein above and below the obturator nerve, including the hypogastric and obturator lymph nodes.

Therefore may assert that an eLND should be performed in all high-risk cases, as the estimated risk for positive lymph nodes will be in the range 15-40%. (10)

However, despite the above, some authors like Bubley are not so categorical in affirming this.

Although it is generally accepted that eLND provides important information for prognosis (number of nodes involved, tumour volume within the lymph node, capsular perforation of the node) that cannot be matched by any other current procedure, consensus has not been reached as to when eLND is indicated and to what extent it should be performed. When making such decisions, many physicians rely on nomograms based on pre-operative biochemical markers and biopsies. (54)

5.1 Role of RT in high risk prostate cancer

Indications for RT after RP

As stated earlier, currently, a multimodal treatment is chosen to increase survival and reduce biochemical progression. In this sense the RT play an important role.

There are two important studies about this:

The EORTC Trial 22911 included 1,005 patients with positive surgical margins or pT3 disease (extracapsular extension and seminal vesicle involvement) and randomized them to adjuvant EBRT (50 Gy to the prostatic fossa and periprostatic tissue plus a 10–14 Gy boost to the prostatic fossa only) versus no immediate treatment. (55) The cumulative rate of loco regional failure was significantly lower in the irradiated group (P <0.0001). However, other clinically important endpoints were not improved. In particular, 5-year metastasis-free survival, cause-specific survival, and overall survival were not affected by adjuvant RT.

The Southwest Oncology Group (SWOG) trial 8794 included 425 patients with high-risk localized disease, who were randomized to receive either 60–64 Gy to the prostatic fossa or observation only. (56) Biochemical control, disease-free survival, cancer-specific mortality, and overall survival were significantly increased in the adjuvant irradiation arm at a median follow-up of 10.6 years.

Both the EORTC and SWOG randomized trials, provide evidence that adjuvant post-prostatectomy irradiation reduces the risk of biochemical recurrence and local clinical failure. It remains uncertain, whether administration of radiation immediately after PSA is detected, could provide equally effective long-term outcomes to patients receiving adjuvant therapy, while sparing such patients from unnecessary irradiation. (17) (48)

Salvage radiotherapy

The efficacy of radiotherapy in the setting of a rising PSA after RP is unproven, and its use is highly controversial. Stephenson et al. reported on a large retrospective analysis of salvage irradiation of 501 patients from 5 institutions. (57)

Positive surgical margins, Gleason scores <8, or PSADT >10 months. In such patients, PSA relapse-free survival outcomes were in the range of 70% to 80% at 3 years.

6. Survival

Regarding cancer-specific survival rate, and the overall survival rate, there are many studies, with different results (table 4).

First, in terms of morbidity, Berglund and colleagues (58) showed, that recovery from surgery, duration of catheterization, and the overall return of continence were essentially similar to those observed in the low-risk population.

Another important factor to consider when analyzing survival, is the overstaging sometimes happens in the T3. Therefore, Ward et al report a long-term experience with radical surgery in patients presenting with locally advanced (cT3) prostate cancer, as the best management of such patients remains a problem. They found that, significantly many patients with cT3 prostate cancer were over-staged (pT2) in the PSA era, and RP as part of a multimodal treatment strategy for patients with cT3 disease offers cancer control and survival rates approaching those achieved for cT2 disease. (31)

For short term survival, Loeb et al (35) reported a complication rate of 11% in 288 consecutive high-risk patients treated by RP, which was not different from the rate in a previous study from the same group that included 3,477 consecutive patients with prostate cancer (59) when analyzing intermediate-term cancer control, and quality-of-life outcomes after radical retropubic prostatectomy (RRP), and concluded that RRP offers excellent intermediate-term cancer control for selected men, of all ages, who present with high-risk or locally advanced disease. Both, continence and potency, were preserved in most patients, although the potency rates were significantly greater for the younger men. RRP with appropiate postoperative radiotherapy and/or hormonal therapy is a reasonable treatment option for selected men with high-risk or locally advanced disease. (35) (Table 4)

	↑Risk	Nº Patients	% 5 years BR free survival	% 10 years cancer especif survival
Van de Ouden (29)	T3 clínic	136	39	72
Hsu (26)	T3 clínic	235	60	92
Ward (20)	T3 clínic	841	58	90; 15 y 79
Lau (23)	Gleason 8-10	407	49	85
Berglund (19)	PSA ≥15 or Gleason 8-10	281	65	NR
Loeb (21)	T2 and Gleason 8-10 or PSA ≥15 o T3	288	39-53	70-93
Van Poppel (27)	T3a y PSA ≤20 and Gleason ≤7	32	3mo:90	NR

BR: Bioquimical recurrence
NR: No results.

Table 4.

For long term survival, Van Poppel (60) showed in 2006, that in patients with locally advanced disease, the cancer-specific survival rate after RP at 5- and 10-years of follow-up, was 85-100% and 57-91.6%, respectively. The overall survival rate at 5 and 10 yr was, 75% and 60%, respectively. In patients with high-grade prostate cancer (Gleason score> or =8), the biochemical recurrence-free survival, after RP at 5 and 10 yr of follow-up was, 51% and 39%, respectively.

Van Der Ouden et al. determined the progression and survival rates, and investigate subgroups of patients who may not benefit from this treatment. Defining that Radical prostatectomy as monotherapy, in patients with locally advanced non-metastatic prostate cancer (T3) produces acceptable results, in those with well or moderately differentiated tumors. The results of progression and survival, are not significantly different from those patients with organ confined prostate cancer. (29)

Yossepowitch describe the results of RP in their patient's serie, classify patients in risk groups: (61) he studied pathological and clinical outcomes among high-risk patients treated with RP. To identify high-risk subsets, eight definitions from the medical literature were applied. Depending on the criteria, high-risk patients comprised 3% to 38% of the entire study population, highlighting the immense variability among available high-risk definitions.

High-risk patients were more likely to exhibit adverse pathological features (35%-71% with extra capsular extension, 10%-33% with seminal vesicle invasion, and 7%-23% with lymph node involvement), but roughly one third (22%-63%) had organ-confined cancers and nearly half (41%-74%) remained progression-free 10 years after surgery alone. (Table 5)

More recently the group from the Mayo Clinic, has reported their long-term result after radical prostatectomy versus external bean radiotherapy for patients with high-risk prostate cancer. (62) The 10-year cancer specific survival rate was 92%, 92% and 88% after RRP, EBRT plus ADT and EBRT alone. After adjusting for case mix, no significant differences in the risks of systemic progression or prostate cancer death were observed between patients who received EBRT plus ADT and patients who underwent RRP. However, the risk of all causes of mortality was greater, and statistically significant, after EBRT plus ADT than after RRP.

Criterion ↑R	N° patients	% confined organ	% free survival in 5 years	% cancer specific survival in 10 years
Gleason 8-10	274	35	53	88
PSA > 20	275	33	56	91
T3c(*year 1992)	144	22	49	89
Nomogram PFP 5 years ≤50%	391	28	53	92
PSA velocity >2 ng/mL/year	952	63	80	97
PSA≥ 20 o ≥T2c o Gleason 8-10	957	43	68	93
PSA≥15 o T2Bc o Gleason 8-10	1752	51	73	95

Table 5.

7. Local control

Local control, main objective with both techniques, is better achieved with surgery. Local relapse rates between 3-30%(63-65) Depends on clinical stage (pT2: 2-7%; negative margins 7%; pT3-4: 40%; positive margin 27%) While with Radiotherapy, local recurrence rate is for T1: 17-22% (Standford); 4.6% (Schelhamer); T2: 19%-35%.

The rate of positive biopsies is between 20-70%, although is difficult to classify its meaning, they highlight disease and progression. It depend on clinical stage (B=17%, C=59%) and Gleason score. A valuable biopsy is at 18 months after finishing treatment.

Frequency of positive prostate biopsies on patients whom underwent radiotherapy, is around 38% on average.

In the study (66) with 100 patients, with biopsy every 6 months showed following results T-1b: 21%; en T-2a: 24%; en T-2b-c: 28%.

There is no doubt regarding its prognostic value. Although the pioneers showing these results were Rhamy (1972) and Sewel (1975) Scardino has been reporting, and highlighting its value (67). At Baylor-Collegue (Houston) 147 patients treated with Au 198 and external bean radiotherapy, clinical stage A2, B, C with pelvic lymphadenectomy. They had a positive biopsy rate of 42%, 36%, 28% at 6, 12 and 18 months. The chance of local recurrence at 5 years for positive and negative biopsies is around 52% and 12%, and at 10 years of 72% and 30%.

8. Conclusions

Many cancers, categorized clinically as high risk, are actually pathologically confined to the prostate, and most men with such cancers who undergo RP, are free of additional therapy long after surgery.

For men with high-risk, clinically localized prostate cancer, decisions on whether to elect surgery as local definitive therapy should be based on the best available clinical evidence rather than on an individual practitioner's experiences and biases.

Patients classified with high-risk prostate cancer, by commonly used definitions, are at increased risk of PSA failure, need for secondary therapy, metastatic progression, and death from systemic disease. Nevertheless, such high risk patients do not have a uniformly poor prognosis after RP.

- If the prostate cancer risk has a high probability of progression to metastasis or death, we must offer aggressive treatment, which achieves high cure rate, and eliminate the illness onset.
- Radical prostatectomy is proving a very valid option with high success rate, for which we must select patients appropriately
- The success of RP in high-risk patients, with stage T3 resection depends entirely local tissue containing the tumor and include the resection of seminal vesicles and extended lymphadenectomy.

9. References

[1] Reiter R.E., de Kernion J.K Epidemiology, etiologyand prostate cancer prevention. In Campbell-Walsh Urology, 8th ed. Volume 4, Section XI, Chapter. Pagina 328-85, Ed: Wein A.W., Kavoussi L., Novick A.C., Partin M.D. and Peters C.A. Saunders.

[2] NCCN prostate Guidelines 2011

[3] Andriole GL, Crawford ED, Grubb RL 3rd, et al; PLCO Project Team. Mortality results from a randomized prostate-cancer screening trial. N Engl J Med 2009 Mar 26;360(13):1310-9.

[4] Schröder FH, Hugosson J, Roobol MJ, et al; ERSPC Investigators. Screening and prostate-cancer mortality in a randomized European study. N Engl J Med 2009 Mar 26;360(13):1320-8.

[5] Börgermann C, Loertzer H, Hammerer P, et al. [Problems, objective, and substance of early detection of prostate cancer]. Urologe A 2010 Feb;49(2):181-9

[6] Roobol MJ, Roobol DW, Schröder FH. Is additional testing necessary in men with prostate-specific antigen levels of 1.0 ng/mL or less in a population-based screening setting? (ERSPC, section Rotterdam). Urology 2005 Feb;65(2):343-6.

[7] Carter HB, Kettermann AE, Ferrucci L, et al. Prostate specific antigen testing among the elderly; when to stop? J Urol 2008 Apr:174.

[8] Makarov DV, Trock BJ, Humphreys EB, et al. Updated nomogram to predict pathologic stage of prostate cancer given prostate-specific antigen level, clinical stage, and biopsy Gleason score (Partin tables) based on cases from 2000 to 2005. Urology 2007 Jun;69(6):1095-101.

[9] Shao YH, Demissie K, Shih W, et al. Contemporary risk profile of prostate cancer in the United States. JNatl Cancer Inst 2009 Sep 16;101(18):1280-3.

[10] Yossepowitch O, Eggener SE, Bianco FJ Jr, et al. Radical prostatectomy for clinically localized, high risk prostate cancer: critical analysis of risk assessment methods. J Urol 2007 Aug;178(2):493-9 discussion 499.

[11] D'Amico AV, Whittington R, Malkowicz SB, et al. Biochemical outcome after radical prostatectomy, external beam radiation therapy, or interstitial radiation therapy for clinically localized prostate cancer. Jama 1998;280:969-974

[12] Gerber GS, Thisted RA, Chodak GW, et al. Results of radical prostatectomy in men with locally advanced prostate cancer: multi-institutional pooled analysis. Eur Urol 1997;32:385-390

[13] Donohue JF, Bianco FJ, Jr., Kuroiwa K, et al. Poorly differentiated prostate cancer treated with radical prostatectomy: long-term outcome and incidence of pathological downgrading. J Urol 2006;176:991-995
[14] Tsai HK, Chen MH, McLeod DG, et al. Cancer-specific mortality after radiation therapy with short-course hormonal therapy or radical prostatectomy in men with localized, intermediate-risk to high-risk prostate cancer. Cancer 2006;107:2597-2603
[15] D'Amico AV, Chen MH, Roehl KA, Catalona WJ. Preoperative PSA velocity and the risk of death from prostate cancer after radical prostatectomy. N Engl J Med 2004;351:125-135
[16] Bianco FJ, Jr., Kattan MW, Scardino PT. PSA velocity and prostate cancer. N Engl J Med 2004;351:1800-1802; author reply 1800-1802
[17] Scardino P., Vicent P. Laudone. The Role of Radical Prostatectomy and pelvic lymph node dissection in an integrated program of treatment of high risk prostate cancer. Educational Course handout book. AUA, May 2011
[18] Borque A., Sanz G. Current validity of nomograms for staging of prostate cancer. Arch Esp Urol, 59, 10(989-1000), 2006.
[19] Ross, P.L; Scardino, P.T.; Kattan, M.W.: "A catalog of prostate cancer nomograms". J. Urol., 165: 1562, 2001.
[20] Remzi, M., Fong, Y.K., Dobrovits, M. y cols.: "The Vienna nomogram: validation of a novel biopsy strategy defining the optimal number of cores based on patient age and total prostate volume". J. Urol., 174: 1256, 2005.
[21] Partin, A.W.; Kattan, M.W.; Subong, E.N.P. y cols.: "Combination of prostate-specific antigen, clinical stage, and Gleason score to predict pathological stage of localized prostate cancer". JAMA, 277: 1445, 1997.
[22] Borque A., Sanz G., Allepuz C., Plaza L., Rioja LA. The use of neural networks and logistic regression analysis for predicting pathological stage in men undergoing radical prostatectomy: a population based study. J Urol 2001; 166: 1672-8
[23] Kattan, M.W.; Eastham, J.A.; Stapleton, A.M. y cols.: "A preoperative nomogram for disease recurrence following radical prostatectomy for prostate cancer". J. Natl. Cancer Inst., 90: 766,1 998.
[24] Hodgson D, Warde P, Gospodarowicz M. The management of locally advanced prostate cancer. Urol Oncol 1998;4:3-12.
[25] Fallon B, Williams RD. Current options in the management of clinical stage C prostatic carcinoma. Urol Clin North Am 1990 Nov;17(4):853-66.
[26] Boccon-Gibod L, Bertaccini A, Bono AV, et al. Management of locally advanced prostate cancer: a European Consensus. Int J Clin Pract 2003 Apr;57(3):187-94.
[27] Yamada AH, Lieskovsky G, Petrovich Z, et al. Results of radical prostatectomy and adjuvant therapy in the management of locally advanced, clinical stage TC, prostate cancer. Am J Clin Oncol 1994 Aug;17(4):277-85.
[28] Gerber GS, Thisted RA, Chodak GW, et al. Results of radical prostatectomy in men with locally advanced prostate cancer: multi-institutional pooled analysis. Eur Urol 1997;32(4):385-90.
[29] van den Ouden D, Hop WC, Schroder FH. Progression in and survival of patients with locally advanced prostate cancer (T3) treated with radical prostatectomy as monotherapy. J Urol 1998 Oct;160(4):1392-7.

[30] Isorna Martinez de la Riva S, Belón López-Tomasety J, Marrero Dominguez R, et al. Radical prostatectomy as monotherapy for locally advanced prostate cancer (T3a): 12 years follow-up. Arch Esp Urol 2004 Sep;57(7):679-92.
[31] Ward JF, Slezak JM, Blute ML, et al. Radical prostatectomy for clinically advanced (cT3) prostate cancer since the advent of prostate-specific antigen testing: 15-year outcome. BJU Int 2005 Apr;95(6):751-6.
[32] Hsu CY, Joniau S, Oyen R, et al. Outcome of surgery for clinical unilateral T3a prostate cancer: a single-institution experience. Eur Urol 2007 Jan;51(1):121-8
[33] Allepuz Losa C., Sanz Velez JI., Gil Sanz MJ., Mas LP., Rioja Sanz LA. J Urol 1995;154:1407-11
[34] Van Poppel H, Ameye F, Oyen R, et al. Accuracy of combined computerized tomography and fine needle aspiration cytology in lymph node staging of localized prostatic carcinoma. J Urol 1994 May;151(5):1310-14.
[35] Loeb S, Smith ND, Roehl KA, et al. Intermediate-term potency, continence, and survival outcomes of radical prostatectomy for clinically high-risk or locally advanced prostate cancer. Urology 2007 Jun;69(6):1170-5.
[36] Heidenreich A., Bellmunt J., Bolla M., et al. European Guidelines on prostate cancer. Part 1: Screeing, diagnosis, and treatment of clinically localised disease. Euro Urol 2011; 59: 61-71
[37] Grossfeld GD, Latini DM, Lubeck DP, Broering JM, Li YP, Mehta SS, et al. Predicting disease recurrence in intermediate and high-risk patients undergoing radical prostatectomy using percent positive biopsies: results from CaPSURE. Urology. 2002;59(4):560-565
[38] Rioja Zuazu, J. Gleason Score 8-10 prostatic adenocarcinoma: prognostic influence in the biochemical progression free survival. Actas Urol Esp. 2008;32(8):792-798
[39] Mian BM, Troncoso P, Okihara K, Bhadkamkar V, Johnston D, Reyes AO. Outcome of patients with Gleason score 8 or higher prostate cancer following radical prostatectomy alone. J Urol. 2002;167(4):1675-1680.
[40] Lau WK, Bergstralh EJ, Blute ML, Slezak JM, Zincke H. Radical prostatectomy for pathological Gleason 8 or greater prostate cancer: influence of concomitant pathological variables. J Urol. 2002;167(1): 117-122
[41] Manoharan M, Bird VG, Kim SS, Civantos F, Soloway MS. Outcome after radical prostatectomy with a pretreatment prostate biopsy Gleason score of ≥8. BJU Int. 2003;92(6):539-544.
[42] D'Amico AV, Whittington R, Malkowicz SB, et al. Pretreatment nomogram for prostate-specific antigen recurrence after radical prostatectomy or external-beam radiation therapy for clinically localized prostate cancer. J Clin Oncol 1999 Jan;17(1):168-72
[43] Inman BA, Davies JD, Rangel LJ, et al. Long-term outcomes of radical prostatectomy with multimodal adjuvant therapy in men with a preoperative serum prostate-specific antigen level >or = 50 ng/mL. Cancer 2008 Oct;113(7):1544-51
[44] Hegarty J, Beirne PV, Walsh E, Comber H, Fitzgerald T, Wallace Kazer M. Radical prostatectomy versus watchful waiting for prostate cancer. Cochrane Database Syst Rev. 2010 Nov 10;(11):CD006590.
[45] Thompson IM, Klotz L.Active Surveillance for prostate cancer. JAMA. 2010 Dec 1;304(21):2411-2.

[46] Klotz L, Zhang L, Lam A, Nam R,Mamedov A, Loblaw AClinical results of long-term follow-up of a large, active surveillance cohort with localized prostate cancer. J Clin Oncol. 2010;28(1):126–131.
[47] J.A. Eastham et al. / Urologic Oncology: Seminars and Original Investigations 28 (2010) 557–567).
[48] Eastham JA, Evans CP, Zietman A. What is the optimal management of high risk, clinically localized prostate cancer. Urol Oncol. 2010 Sep-Oct;28(5):557-67.
[49] Thompson I, Thrasher JB, Aus G, et al. Guideline for the management of clinically localized prostate cancer: 2007 update. J Urol 2007;177:2106-2131
[50] Zelefsky MJ, Eastham JA, Cronin AM, et al. Metastasis after radical prostatectomy or external beam radiotherapy for patients with clinically localized prostate cancer: A comparison of clinical cohorts adjusted for case mix. J Clin Oncol 2009.
[51] Walz J, Graefen M, Huland H. Basic principles of anatomy for optimal surgical treatment of prostate cancer. World J Urol 2007;25:31-38.
[52] Kazzazi A, Djavan B. Current status of pelvic lymph node dissection in prostate cancer: the New York PLND nomogram. Can J Urol. 2011 Apr;18(2):5585-91.
[53] Briganti A. et al. Prostate. 2011 May 2. doi: 10.1002/pros.21420.
[54] Bubley GJ, Carducci M, Dahut W, et al. Eligibility and response guidelines for phase II clinical trials in androgen-independent prostate cancer: recommendations from the Prostate-Specific Antigen Working Group. J Clin Oncol 1999 Nov;17(11):3461-7.
[55] Bolla M, van Poppel H, Collette L, et al. Postoperative radiotherapy after radical prostatectomy: a randomised controlled trial (EORTC trial 22911). Lancet 2005;366:572-578.
[56] Thompson IM, Jr., Tangen CM, Paradelo J, et al. Adjuvant radiotherapy for pathologically advanced prostate cancer: a randomized clinical trial. JAMA 2006;296:2329-2335
[57] Stephenson AJ, Scardino PT, Kattan MW, et al. Predicting the outcome of salvage radiation therapy for recurrent prostate cancer after radical prostatectomy. J Clin Oncol 2007;25:2035-2041
[58] Berglund RK, Jones JS, Ulchaker JC, et al. Radical prostatectomy as primary treatment modality for locally advanced prostate cancer: A prospective analysis. Urology 2006;67:1253- 6.
[59] Kundu SD, Roehl KA, Eggener SE, et al. Potency, continence and complications in 3,477 consecutive radical retropubic prostatectomies.J Urol 2004;172:2227–31.
[60] Van Poppel H, Vekemans K, Da Pozzo L, et al.: Radical prostatectomy for locally advanced prostate cancer: results of a feasibility study (EORTC 30001). Eur J Cancer 2006, 42:1062–1067.
[61] Yossepowitch O, Eggener SE, Serio AM, et al. Secondary therapy, metastatic progression, and cancerspecific mortality in men with clinically high-risk prostate cancer treated with radical prostatectomy. Eur Urol 2008;53:950-959.
[62] Boorjian S.A. Karnes R.J., Viterbo R., et al. Long-term survival after radical prostatectomy versus external bean radiotherapy for patients with high-risk prostate cancer. Cancer 2011; 117:2883-91
[63] Pound CR, Christens-Barry OW, Gurganus RT, Partin AW, Walsh PC. Digital rectal examination and imaging studies are unnecessary in men with undetectable prostate specific antigen following radical prostatectomy. J Urol. 1999 Oct;162(4):1337-40

[64] Petrovich Z, Lieskovsky G, Langholz B, Bochner B, Formenti S, Streeter O, Skinner DG. Comparison of outcomes of radical prostatectomy with and without adjuvant pelvic irradiation in patients with pathologic stage C (T3N0) adenocarcinoma of the prostate. Am J Clin Oncol. 1999 Aug;22(4):323-31.
[65] Obek C, Sadek S, Lai S, Civantos F, Rubinowicz D, Soloway MS. Positive surgical margins with radical retropubic prostatectomy: anatomic site-specific pathologic analysis and impact on prognosis. Urology. 1999 Oct;54(4):682-8.
[66] Crook J, Robertson S, Collin G, Zaleski V, Esche B. Clinical relevance of trans-rectal ultrasound, biopsy, and serum prostate-specific antigen following external beam radiotherapy for carcinoma of the prostate. Int J Radiat Oncol Biol Phys. 1993 Sep 1;27(1):31-7.
[67] Goad JR, Chang SJ, Ohori M, Scardino PT. PSA after definitive radiotherapy for clinically localized prostate cancer. Urol Clin North Am. 1993 Nov;20(4):727-36.

7

High-Intensity Focused Ultrasound (HIFU) - An Alternative Choice in Prostate Cancer Treatment

Umberto Maestroni and Francesco Ziglioli
Department of Urology, University Hospital of Parma, Parma
Italy

1. Introduction

Prostate cancer is considered one of the most discussed topics in male health with an important social impact on the quality of life.
In Europe, it is the most common solid neoplasm with an incidence rate of 214 cases per 100,000 men[1]. The increasing life expectancy and the more and more widespread use of Prostate Specific Antigen (PSA) are probably the two most important reasons why more patients are diagnosed with prostate cancer. In Europe, 2,6 million new cases of prostate cancer are yearly observed (11% of male cancer diagnosis), responsible for 9% of deaths for male cancer cases.
Radical surgery represents the treatment of choice in clinically localized prostate cancer and in > 10 year life expectancy prostate cancer. Nevertheless, radical surgery itself may be considered a high morbility treatment[2].
Mini-invasive procedure development, such as three-dimensional external radiotherapy, brachytherapy or cryotherapy, especially in elderly or anaesthetically high risk patients, represents a useful treatment in prostate cancer.
HIFU (High-Intensity Focused Ultrasound) is a new and alternative choice in localized and low or intermediate-risk prostate cancer treatment[3-5].
For a variety of reasons, transrectal HIFU appears highly attractive as a minimally invasive treatment for localized prostate cancer. It is a method of delivering ultrasonic energy with resultant heat and tissue destruction to a discrete point without damaging intervening tissue or cells. HIFU has been used for the management of patients diagnosed with various types of cancer, including prostate, breast, liver, pancreas, kidney, bone, and soft tissue.

2. Experimental studies

It has been shown in canines and humans that HIFU is capable of ablating prostatic tissue both contact and irradiation free[6,7].
One of the first investigators who experimented the application of the technique to human beings has been S. Madersbacher[8].
Early studies considered focused ultrasound as a potential technique for neurosurgery (Lynn, 1942; Warwick and Pond, 1968). A significant development was the construction of precision apparatus suitable for human treatment by Fry et al. in 1958.

HIFU has also been used in other clinical fields including ophthalmology (Coleman, 1985), urology (by Foster and Gelet in 1993) and oncology (Chapelon in 1992 and Prat in 1995). To date, focused ultrasound has been used successfully in the management of many tumours, including prostate cancer, in which this technique represents a good treatment option.
HIFU was also used by Madersbacher and colleagues as a treatment for Benign Prostatic Hyperplasia (BPH). To date, this technique is not still used to treat BPH, because of its side effects on bladder neck function.

3. Description of the procedure

HIFU is performed through a computerized surgical device equipped with a treatment table, an ultrasound treatment system connected to an endorectal probe, a safety infrared ray detector, a refrigeration system keeping the rectal mucosa temperature below 14°C and a monitor to set and control the treatment procedure through echographic screening (Fig. 1).
For anatomical reasons, the transrectal approach appears ideally suited to ablate prostatic tissue because the proximity of HIFU transducer and target tissue facilitates HIFU treatment from the technical standpoint.
After introducing the rectal probe, anatomic landmarks must be echographically set (apex, bladder neck, rectal side, prostate capsule), in order to make the computer able to determine the correct subdivision in different prostate portions (generally four).
The probe is equipped with a transducer that gives out a beam of high-focused convergent ultrasounds. The HIFU transducer has an aperture of 37 cm and a focal distance of 25.5 cm. The focus has a -6 dB beam width of 1.6 mm and axial length of 10 mm. In the ultrasound converging point (focal point), the ultrasound beam absorption generates an immediate growth of temperature (85-100°C), destroying prostate cells in the circumscribed area.

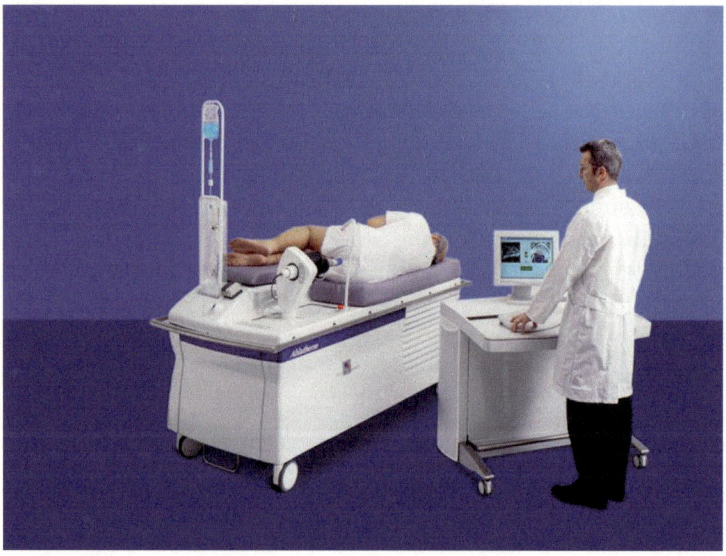

(Ablatherm®-Edap Technomed device).

Fig. 1. Overview of HIFU procedure. The bed with the High-intensity ultrasound probe can be clearly seen. On the right, the ultrasound screen and the screen to set the machine and follow the procedure

Adequately translating the focal point with a robotic and automatic device, the successive ultrasound emissions may destroy all prostate cells (Fig. 2).

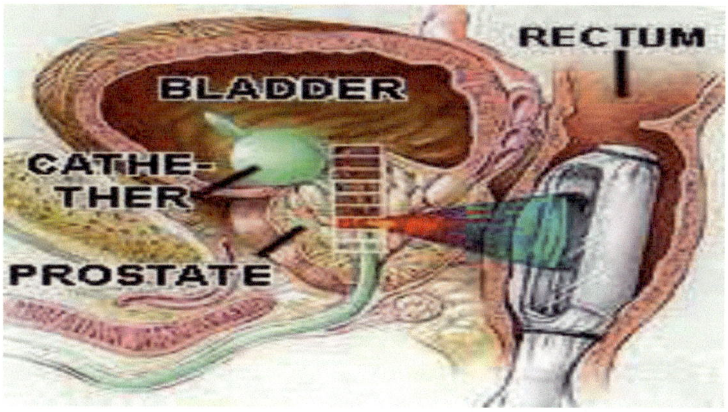

Fig. 2. Anatomical scheme of HIFU endorectal device

These lesions have a predictable size and shape, closely matching the focal region of the ultrasound source. As the lesion width is almost constant along their length, they can be placed side-by-side without leaving gaps (Fig. 3).

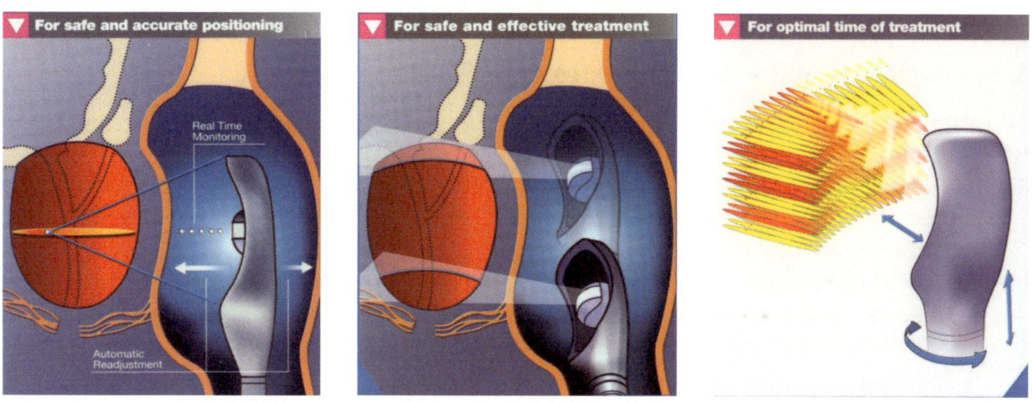

Fig. 3. HIFU mechanism scheme. On the left, ultrasound beam positioning; in the middle, the area to treat; on the right, an overall view of the sections treated by high-intensity ultrasound.

A standard procedure can be personalized in order to obtain ideal treatment settings: ultrasound frequency (standard 3 MHz), shot duration (standard 5 seconds) and waiting-time between shots (standard 5 seconds) may be modified (Fig. 4). Elementary lesion volume measures 19-24 mm and its diameter measures 1.7 mm

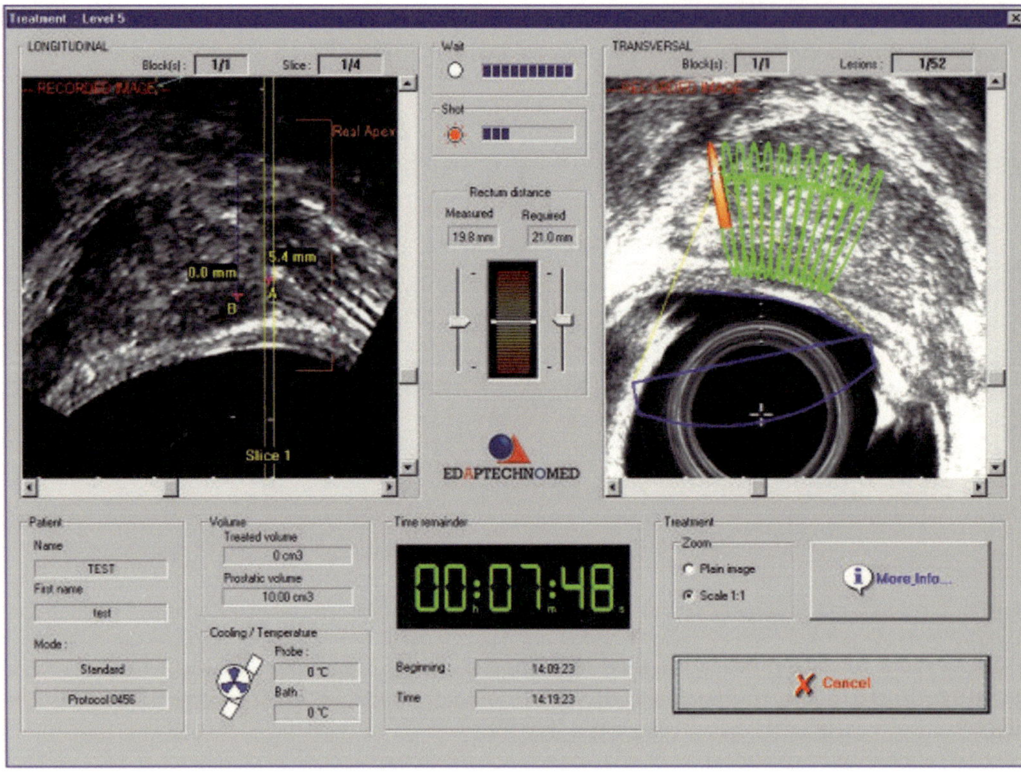

Fig. 4. On the screen, it is possible to follow the procedure and to change settings, such as ultrasound frequency and shot duration. Thus, a safe and optimal treatment can be performed.

4. Management of the patient before and after the procedure

In order to safely perform the treatment, the surgeon is advised to follow some recommendations, in accordance with the European and American guidelines:

a. Anti-trombotic prophylaxis with sodic Dalteparin 5.000 I.U. the day before the procedure. Other low molecular weight heparin (LMWH) can be administrated, according with local policies.
b. Antibiotic prophylaxis should be given in order to prevent infection. A quinolone represents a good choice, but other antibiotic can be used, according with local policies.
c. Careful intestinal toilet. This is an important key point in infection prevention. Also, it is fundamental to obtain a good view of the whole prostate on ultrasound, which is important in order to treat the target area properly. This will also prevent some side effects of the treatment, such as bladder neck irritation, reduces the risk of rectum fistulisation, and improves the erectile function outcome.

All patients undergo intra-spinal block with Chirocaine®.

Marcaine® can be used instead of Chirocaine.

If Marcaine is administrated, it is important to begin the procedure from the left lobe of the prostate, because this lobe is above due to the left decubitus of the patient on the device.

In order to make the procedure more bearable and to obtain the best cooperation from the patient, Midazolam 0,03 mg/kg administration during the procedure is recommended.

Other benzodiazepine can be used, according with their pharmacocynetic and pharmacodynamic features.
Reportedly, patients have no postoperative pain, except in case of complication. Just in the first two hours after the treatment the patient might complain of confusion and dazzling, but these are considered common consequences of the anaesthetic treatment.
The anaesthetist should be involved pre-operatively, intra-operatively and post-operatively, in order to manage the patient properly before and during the treatment and in order to relieve post-operative pain and anaesthetic side-effects and/or complications.

5. Mechanism

Conceptually, a piezoelectric transducer generates a high intensity converging ultrasound beam that destroys local tissues through three mechanisms:
1. Coagulative necrosis;
2. Cavitation;
3. Heat damage.

These three key-points are discussed below.

5.1 Coagulative necrosis

Coagulative necrosis, is due to hyperthermia (85-100°C) generated in the focal point.
Elementary lesion has ellipsoidal shape. The short length of the shot limits heat diffusion around the focal point. Shot by shot, it is possible to generate a plethora of elementary lesions until all prostate tissue is destroyed.
Coagulative necrosis is a non-reversible phenomenon (Fig. 5).

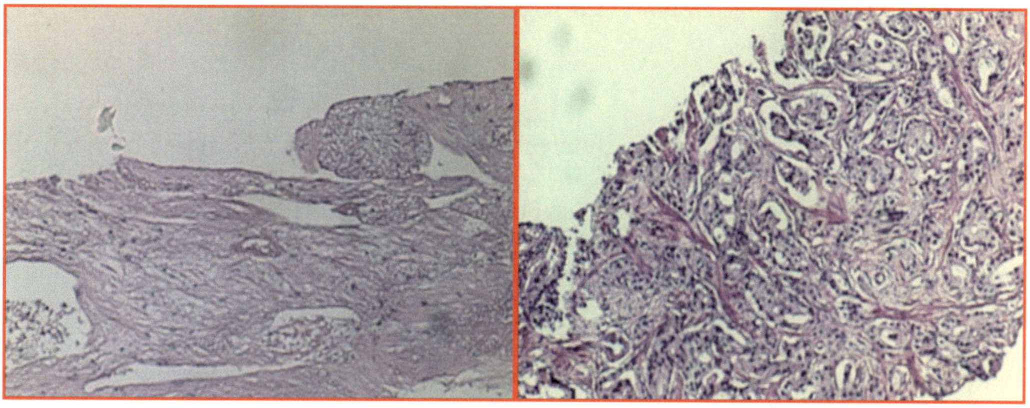

Fig. 5. On the left, pre-HIFU histology aspect; on the right, post-HIFU histology change

This kind of lesion can be clearly seen on optical microscopy. Its effectiveness in cancer treatment is demonstrated by the absence of cell functional structures, such as membranes, active nuclei, and organelles.
After the treatment, glandular structures cannot be seen any longer, thus demonstrating that the HIFU technique provides a lack of function in the treated prostate.
Also liquefactive necrosis and apoptotic necrosis are reported as a common consequence of HIFU treatment (see § 6.1), but these kinds of necrotic lesions do not affect the whole amount of necrotic areas.

5.2 Cavitation

Cavitation is due to the gas microbubble (bubble clouds) vibration dissolved in prostate tissue. Lindau and Lauterborn investigated the collapse and rebound of a cavitation bubble near a flat rigid wall using a high-speed camera[9].

Due to the depression caused by the negative part of the ultrasound wave, intracellular water may enter the gaseous phase.

That would lead to the development of microbubbles.

When they reach the size of resonance, these bubbles suddenly collapse and produce high-pressure shock waves, destroying adjacent tissue.

In a study carried out by Chen H and colleagues[10], the dynamics of cavitation bubble clouds generated at the tissue boundary in continuous HIFU fields has been experimentally investigated by a high-speed photography method.

The experimental results revealed that the cavitation bubble clouds organize into two shapes, which were named ''cone-shape" bubble cloud structure and ''crown-shape" bubble cloud structure.

The cavitation bubble cloud is visible at the tissue surface at 200 μs; then a tiny tip becomes obvious at 600 μs. The elongated tip leads to the formation of a cone-shape bubble cloud structure.

After 1.8 ms, the cone-shape bubble cloud attaines a dynamically stable state.

The bubble cluster grows larger and developes a crown-like shape. Meanwhile, it moves forward and finally hits the tissue boundary forming the crown-shape cavitation bubble cloud structure.

Among the 171 image series recorded in the study carried out by Chen H et al, 85% showed the evolution of the cone-shape bubble cloud structure. Another 11% of the image series showed the dynamics of the crown-shape bubble cloud structure.

The remaining 4% exhibited the interchanging of these two structures.

5.3 Heat damage

The tissue ablation induced by high-intensity ultrasound results primarily from bulk heating, with possible contributions from boiling and acoustic cavitation. Bubbles, when present, may enhance local absorption (Fig. 6).

The position and shape of the heated region are determined by the intensity of the field near the focus, the attenuation and the effects of diffusion.

The rate of change of temperature at any point is proportional to the absorbed power density and hence to the incident beam power and attenuation[11].

The irreversible changes in proteins associated with tissue denaturation and coagulation start at low temperature.

When temperatures of approximately 60°C are approached, the rate of denaturation becomes so great that irreversible changes can occur in seconds.

Temperature reached during HIFU treatment is clearly higher, as reported above: When lesioning occurs, the attenuation within the treated volume increases[12], thus altering the absorbed power distribution, depending on the biologic feature of the prostate.

Consequently, the region in which heat is deposited may be expected to change during the heating process.

By a macroscopic point of view, we can say that heat growth is maximal in the middle of the treated volume and minimal in the external area of the treated volume.

This difference allows to surely set the treatment outlines and save the prostate apex, and the striated sphincter and vasculo-nervous bundles.

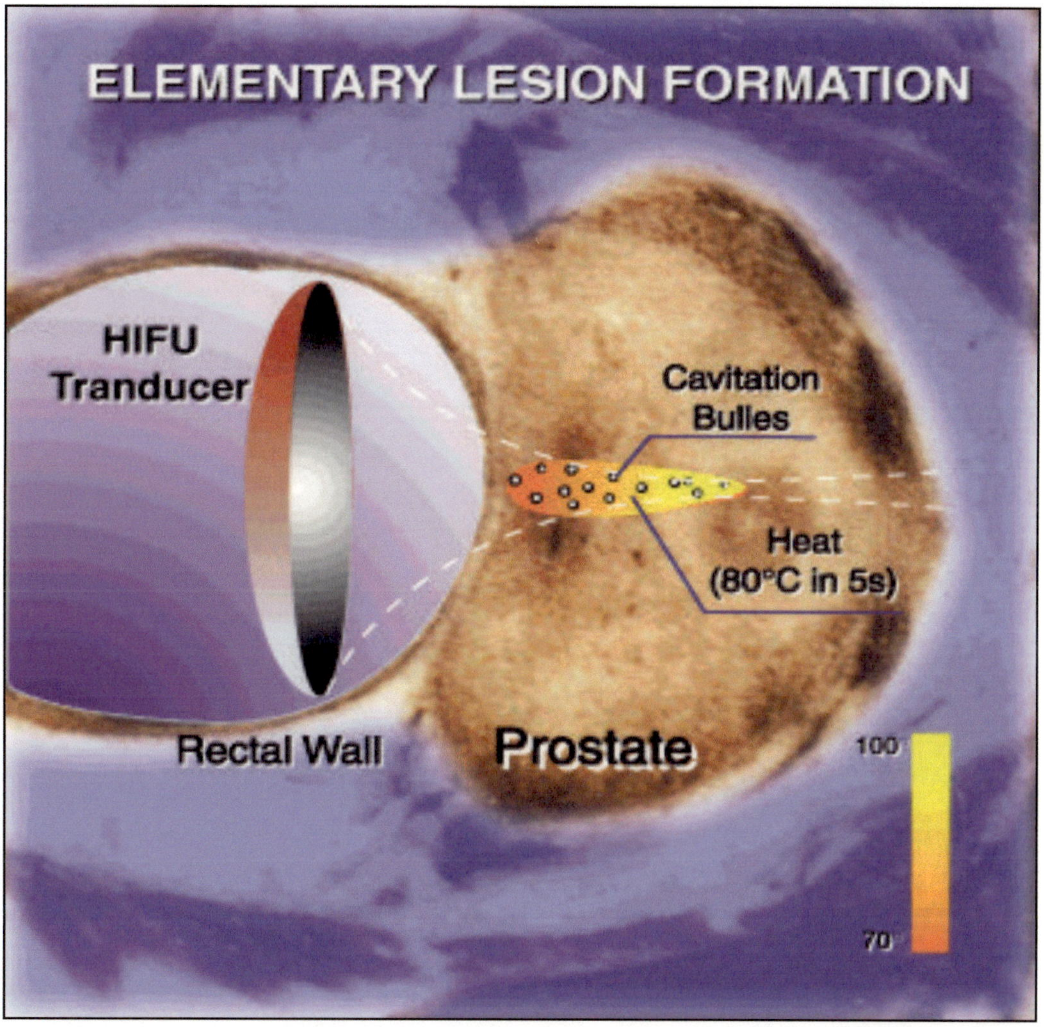

Fig. 6. Elementary lesion formation and its effects on prostate parenchyma, due to heat and mechanical damage.

6. HIFU-induced histopathological changes

HIFU-induced histopathological changes can be studied thanks to light microscopy, immunoistochemistry and electron microscopy.

6.1 Light microscopy

At light microscopy, we can say that the prostatic structure is completely disrupted and hardly recognizable. Three different types of cellular necrosis are generally found:

a. liquefactive necrosis;
b. coagulative necrosis;
c. apoptotic necrosis.

Cell death is generally due to a mixture of the three with liquefactive necrosis being the least common and coagulative necrosis the most common.

Histological findings show consistent coagulative necrosis with precisely defined, sharp margins to normal tissue.

Lesion size and position correlates well with the assumed target zones, thus demonstrating that HIFU permits therapeutic tissue ablation.

Strictly speaking, HIFU treatment induces a spectrum of morphological changes ranging from apparent light microscopic necrosis to more subtle ultrastructural cell damage (see below).

Necrotic tissue in the coagulative necrosis areas consists of homogenously stained eosinophilic fragments (Fig. 7a).

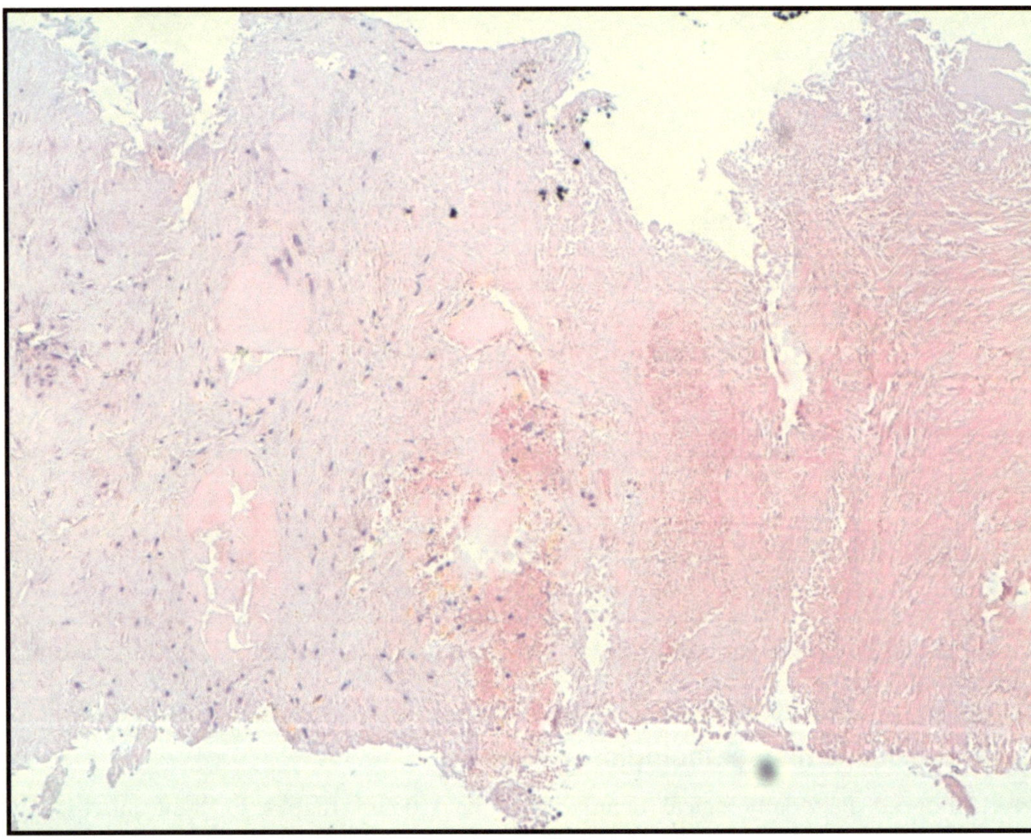

Fig. 7a. Areas of coagulative necrosis can be clearly seen, thus demonstrating the effectiveness of HIFU treatment.

Little structure is apparent aside from some faintly staining collagenous bands and rare indications of the former glandular epithelium. In some cases, necrotic tissue expelled from the coagulative necrosis areas is visible in prostatic ductules of the margin area. Brightly staining blood droplets can be observed on the hematoxylin-eosin slide, of which most are concentrated in the coagulative necrosis area.

The nuclei of epithelial and stromal cells are either pyknotic or totally absent, corresponding to cell necrosis. The nuclei are of normal size with a fine chromatin structure and sporadically small nucleoli.

This epithelial cells also contain pale to eosinophilic cytoplasm, with few vacuoles. Although cell borders are not discernable in most of these cells, they can be identified locally.

Every so often, extended haemorragic areas are found (Fig. 7b).

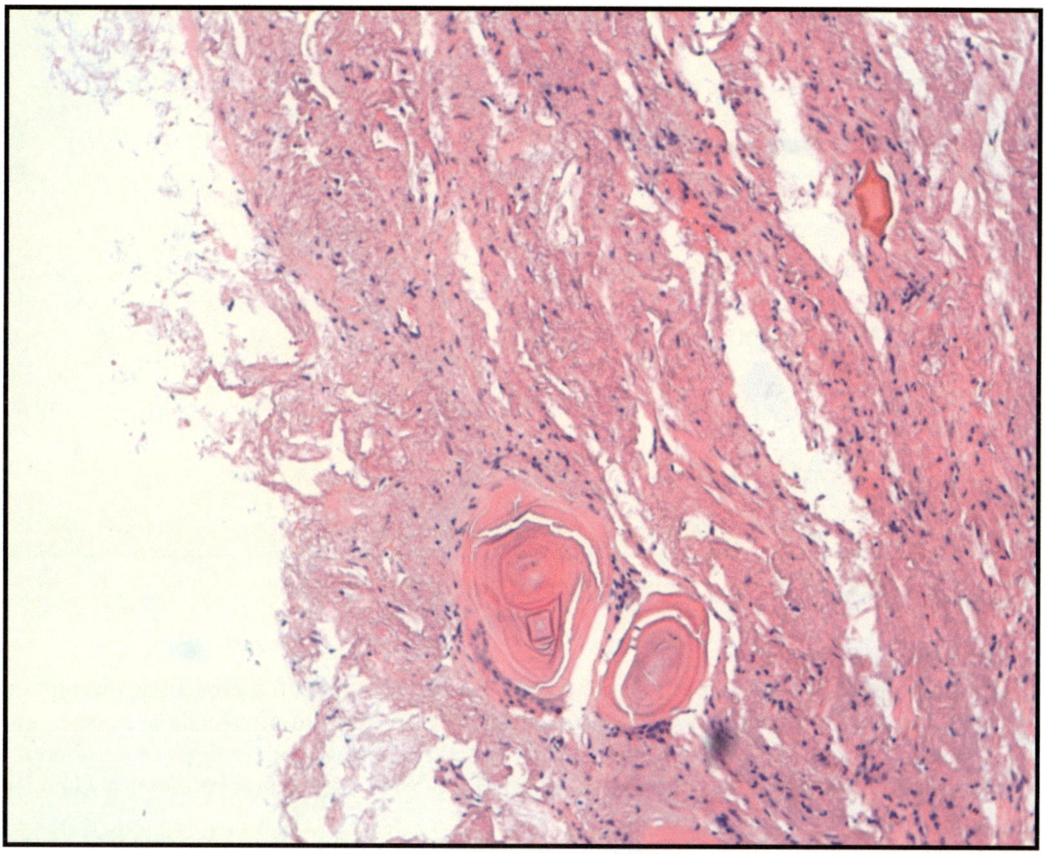

Fig. 7b. Areas of tissue damage, including haemorragic areas

Also, HIFU causes injuries to small vessels, with considerable oedema and swelling of endothelial cells in the margin between the treated and untreated areas. However, in the centre of treated tumor tissue, severely damaged tumor vessels show pyknotic nuclei and debris of nuclei, which indicated endothelial cell death.

Endothelial cells exhibited an irreversible cell death. Almost all of the endothelial cell nuclei disappear, cellular margins were not distinct and junctions between individual cells were disrupted.

The repair of lesions appears to have slow processes of damaged tissue absorption and granulation tissue replacement (Fig. 8).

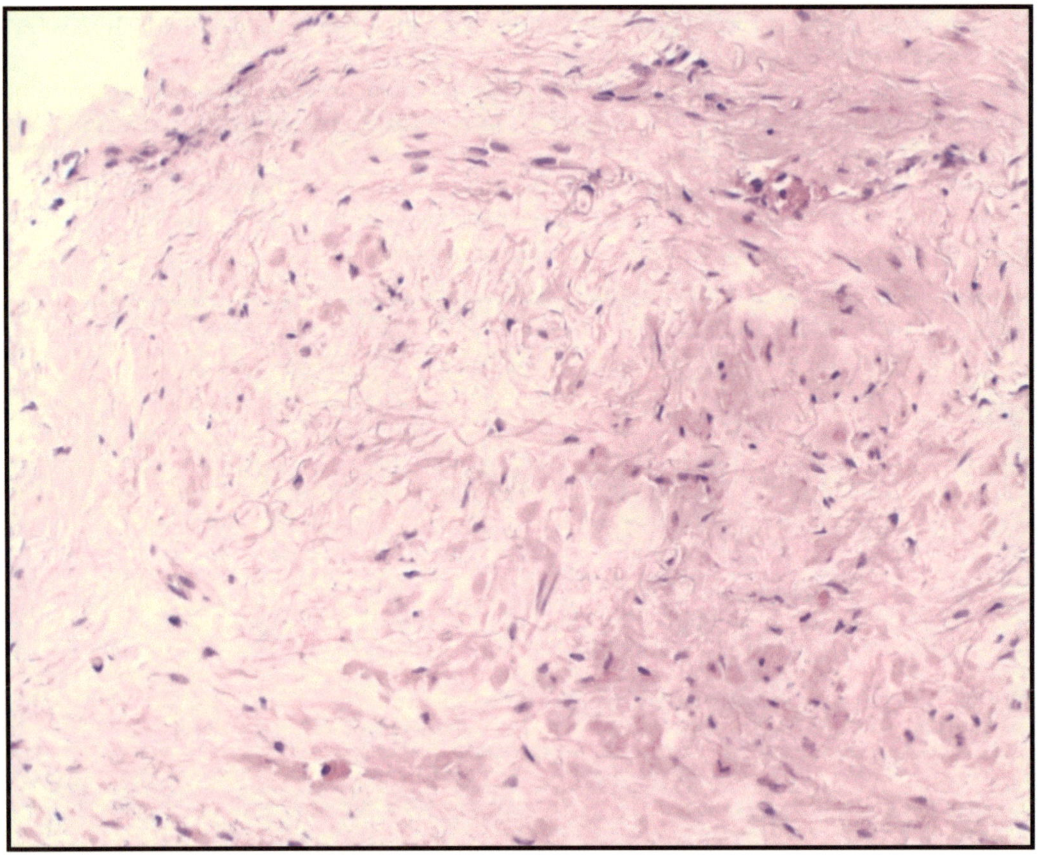

Fig. 8. Granulation tissue and fibrosis 6 months after HIFU treatment.

6.2 Immunoistochemistry

The expression of PSA, panCK, and Ki67 in non-treated regions of the prostate is marginally stronger than in the HIFU region. CK8 is strongly expressed in luminal cells of normal and malignant glands outside the HIFU lesion, but pre-existing and malignant epithelium within the HIFU lesion does not express CK8, regardless of the histomorphological changes in conventional light microscopy.

The hyperplastic epithelium at the periphery of the HIFU lesions reacts with the basal cell antibody 34βE12.

In summary, we can say that prostate glandular epithelium after HIFU treatment reacts with antibodies to pancytokeratin, prostate specific antigen (PSA), and Ki67, but does not express cytokeratin 8, which is indicative of severe cellular damage.

6.3 Electron microscopy

Ultrastructural examination after HIFU reveals disintegration of cellular membranes and cytoplasmic organelles consistent with cell necrosis.

Electron microscopy is not routinely performed. When performed, it confirms submicroscopical cellular damage in the centre of the HIFU lesion.

Electron microscopy is capable to demonstrate cell necrosis also in areas that show no apparent morphological cell necrosis by conventional light microscopy.
Treated areas lack nuclear membranes, but show a fine chromatin pattern that is clumped at the periphery of the nuclei, and conspicuous nucleoli.
The cytoplasm contain some vacuoles, but organelle structures and cell membranes are not generally identified.

7. Immunologic response after HIFU

T-lymphocytes appear in granulation tissue along the ablation margin in all HIFU-treated neoplasms, with no infiltration in those showing typical signs of coagulation necrosis.
The tumor-infiltrating lymphocytes are found mainly in granulation tissue along with immature fibroblasts, new capillaries, and other inflammatory cells.
This observation suggest that their infiltration occurs after HIFU ablation and that these tumor-infiltrating lymphocytes are new lymphocytes moving into the ablated neoplasms from peripheral blood.
As it has been reported by Hartveit and colleagues, this is a typical findings in all tissues treated with HIFU[13].
HIFU treatment may definitively increase the local infiltration of tumor infiltrating lymphocytes in the ablation area, including activated cytotoxic T-Cells and Natural-Killer cells[14].

8. The role of heat-shock proteins (HSP)

Heat shock proteins (HSPs) were first discovered in 1962 as a group of highly conserved proteins that are induced by hyperthermia and other kinds of cellular insults.
There are four principal HSP: HSP-90, HSP-70, HSP-60 and the subgroup of small HSPs including HSP27.
Benign and malignant human prostatic cells respond to heat by increased expression of HSP *in vitro* and *in vivo*.
To obtain a more detailed insight on the effect of heat on prostatic cells, heat shock protein expression of normal and malignant prostatic cells has been studied.
Transrectal HIFU therapy induces intraprostatic necrosis surrounded by a zone characterized by a massive up-regulation of HSP expression.
Recently, several molecular heat shock proteins have been reported to be involved in development and progression of hormone-refractory prostate cancer.
HSP27 and HSP70 are the most strongly induced heat shock proteins during cellular stress (Fig. 9).
HSPs are not all of prognostic value, however some have been demonstrated to have clinical utility as prognostic markers: among this group of heat shock proteins, the most important one is HSP-27, which particularly plays a role in many immunological processes and might stimulate immune defence responses against tumour cells[15].
Accumulating evidence suggests that HSP27 levels correlate with both hormone-refractory prostate cancer and development of resistance to heat. Nevertheless, the functional significance of changes in HSP27 expression associated with heat-resistant prostate cancer remains undefined.

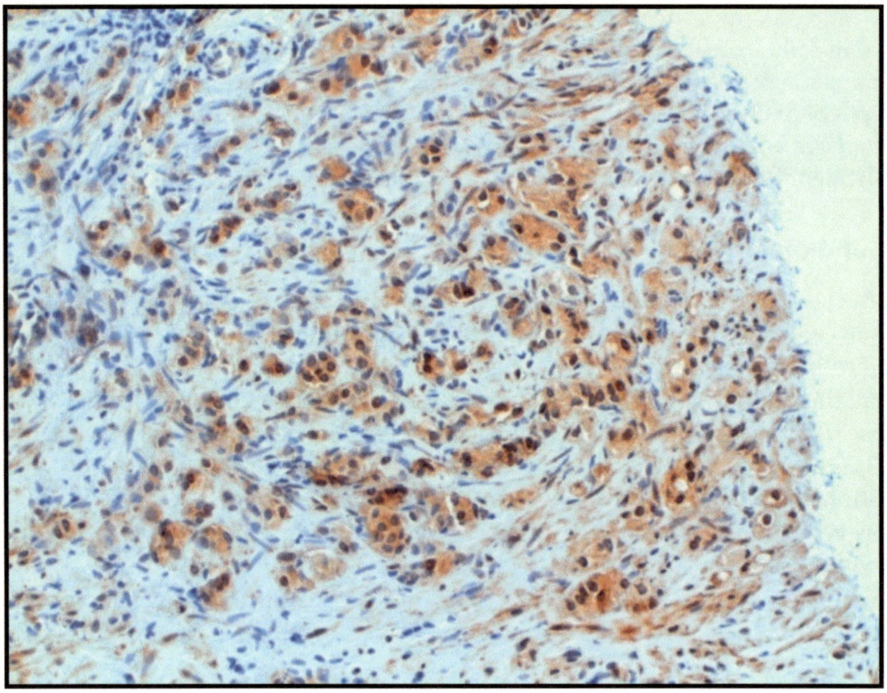

Fig. 9. HSP-70 expression in prostate tissue after HIFU treatment in a case of recurrence

9. Long-term results of HIFU treatment

Many authors have reported their series after HIFU treatment.
One of the most recent is the multicentric study carried out by Crouzet et al[16], who reported a series of 803 patients with a mean follow-up of 43 months. The results of this study are excellent, showing that local control and disease-free survival rate achieved with HIFU were similar to those expected with conformal external-beam radiation therapy (EBRT).
The excellent cancer-specific survival rate reported in this study is also explained by the possibility to repeat HIFU and use salvage EBRT.
The first UK series was reported by Ahmed et al and published on the British Journal of Cancer. 172 men were treated with HIFU with excellent result: 92.4% of patients had no recurrence after a mean follow-up of 346 days[17].
Blana et al published a series of 140 men treated with HIFU, reporting good oncological outcome in long-term follow-up (6.4 years), demonstrating the effective long-term cancer control achieved with HIFU in patients with low- or intermediate-risk localised prostate cancer[18].
Finally, it is correct to cite the negative results reported by Challacombe et al, who interrupted the treatment because of the poor oncological outcome[19].
From all the studies presented, there is clear evidence that the treatment could affect prostate cancer, as shown by both a substantial decrease in serum PSA and negative biopsies after therapy there is clear evidence that the treatment could affect prostate cancer.
The effect has also been demonstrated on radical prostatectomy specimens examined 2 weeks after HIFU.

There are no randomized controlled studies available to compare the outcome of these therapies with each other, other therapies, or watchful waiting.
The combination of a TURP performed just before an HIFU seems to reduce the complications but without affecting the oncologic outcome negatively.
As of today, it is not possible to compare the outcome of HIFU with other treatment modalities for localized prostate cancer.

10. Complications and side effects of HIFU treatment

HIFU is a minimally invasive treatment for prostate cancer, thus resulting in a low complication rate.
Sometimes, minor complications can occour, in the vast majority of cases related to lower urinary tract.
The first one is urinary retention, commonly treated with longer catheterism. The most common is urge incontinence, due to the irritative effect of high-focused ultrasound on the bladder neck. Generally, it disappears in a couple of month, and only in rare cases anticolinergic treatment is required.
Lower urinary tract symptoms, such as frequency, nocturia, weak urinary stream, and so on, are prevented by Trans-Urethral Resection of Prostate (TUR-P), that is recommended to be done 6-8 weeks before HIFU treatment. Anyway, the surgeon is advised to administrate IPSS questionnaire (or equivalent) before the treatment end 3 months after the treatment, in order to assess persistent lower urinary tract symptoms, that should be treated pharmacologically or surgically, if needed.
Infection is another possible complication of this treatment. Antibiotic prophylaxis should prevent this complication, if administrated in accordance with guidelines on infection prevention.
Among the major complications, the most important is recto-vesical or recto-urethral fistula. Only few cases are reported in literature. This complication can be initially treated with longer catheterization, but in some cases surgical repair is required. A common tip to avoid this complication is to safely set the target area on the ultrasound screen, as the slight wall of the rectum can easily lead to fistulization. Also, patients previously diagnosed with ulcerative recto-colitis must not be treated with high-intensity focused ultrasound.
The most important side-effect of HIFU treatment is erectile disfunction and impotency, due to the effect of high intensity ultrasound on the neural bundle. This effect is well known and must be discussed with the patient before the treatment.
Color-doppler-combined technique is reported in literature in order to perform a sort of vessel-sparing procedure, thus resulting in a better outcome by the andrological point of view. However, there is not common agreement among the investigators about the effectiveness and the feasibility of this technique. For this reason, it cannot be recommended at the present time (Fig. 10).
The best management of the patient should include IIEF questionnaire (or equivalent) to be giver before the treatment and 6 months after the treatment in order to assess the sexual outcome.
Patients who are keen on having sexual activity should receive a proper treatment.

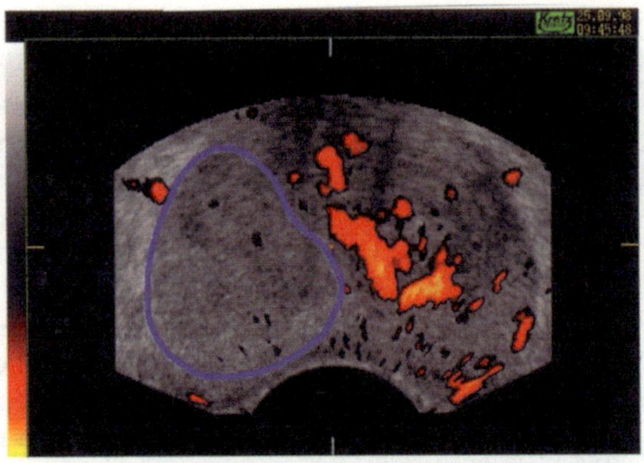

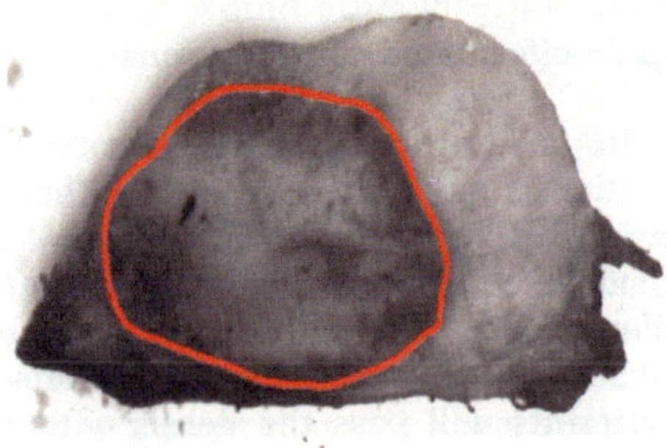

not affected by tumor (red line).

Fig. 10. Color-doppler device for HIFU treatment. Thanks to this additional equipment, it is possible to perform a highly selective treatment (blu line). This can preserve vascular bundle or a portion of prostate

11. Summary

At the time of diagnosis, prostate cancer is organ-confined in 70% of the cases.

The choice of the appropriate treatment for localized prostate cancer is one of the most controversial issues in urologic oncology. Approximately, the most majority of these patients undergo local therapy: surgery or external beam radiation. The rest of the remaining patients do not fit this treatment and are scheduled for Androgen Depriving Therapy (ADT) or watchful waiting.

Besides these treatments, other mini-invasive procedures have emerged in the last few years, such as Brachytherapy, Cryosurgical Ablation, Radiofrequency Interstitial Tumour Ablation and High-Intensity Focused Ultrasound (HIFU).

HIFU represents an alternative choice in mini-invasive treatment of prostate cancer. The treatment is performed under regional anaesthesia and is generally preceeded by limited Trans-Urethral Resection of Prostate (TUR-P).

It is a transrectal procedure: after introducing the rectal probe, anatomic limits must be echographically set (apex, bladder neck, rectal side, prostate capsule), in order to make the computer able to determine the correct subdivision in different prostate portions (generally four).

An absolute contraindication to the procedure is every rectal anatomic or pathologic condition that excludes the transrectal approach.

The technology of the device used to perform the treatment allows to exactly destroy a pre-selected area and to save all the tissues around it.

Conceptually, a piezoelectric trasducer generates a high intensity converging ultrasound beam that destroys local tissues through three mechanisms:

1. *coagulative necrosis*, due to hyperthermia (85-100°C) generated in the focal point. Elementary lesion is ellipsoidal and the short length of the shot limits heat diffusion around the focal point. Shot by shot, it is possible to generate a plethora of elementary lesions until all prostate tissue is destroyed;
2. *cavitation*, due to the gas microbubble vibration dissolved in prostate tissue;
3. *heat growth*, maximal in the middle of the treated volume and minimal in the external area of the treated volume.

This difference allows to surely set the treatment outlines and save the prostate apex (and the striated sphincter) and vasculo-nervous bundles.

HIFU is a minimally invasive ablative technology for managing localized prostate cancer in both the primary and salvage setting. It is a single-session procedure with the possibility of a re-treatment if required.

The advantage of this technique are short hospital stay, reduced convalescence, low morbidity and preservation of continence and erectile function.

As reported in literature, HIFU demonstrated a good oncologic outcome.

The PSA nadir is a major predictive factor for HUFU success and it is generally reached within 6 months after the treatment in all patients.

The most recent results are reported in a study carried out by Crouzet et al. In this multicentric study the mean PSA nadir was 1.0±2.8 ng/mL with a median of 0.25 ng/mL. The 5-year and 7-year Disease Free Survival Rate (DFSR) for low, intermediate-, and high-risk patients (according to D'Amico risk stratification criteria) were, respectively, 83-75%, 72-63% and 68-62%.

As expected by most investigators, the development of more sophisticated technologies should improve these results and lead to a widespread use of this technique. Focal treatment or doppler-combined devices for nerve- or vessel- sparing procedures will be available in the next years.

12. References

[1] Steinberg GD, Carter BS, Beaty TH, et al. Family history and the risk of prostate cancer. Prostate 1990;17:337-47

[2] European Association of Urology. Guidelines 2011 Edition.

[3] Gelet A, Chapelon JY, Bouvier R, Pangaud C, Lasne Y. Local control of prostate cancer by transrectal high intensity focused ultrasound therapy: preliminary results. *J Urol* 1999; 161: 156-62.

[4] Gelet A, Chapelon JY, Bouvier R, Rouviere O, Lyonnet D, Dubernard JM. Transrectal high intensity focused ultrasound of localized prostate cancer: factos influencing the outcome. *Eur Urol* 2001; 40: 124-9

[5] Rebillard X, Gelet A, Davin JL, et al. Transrectal high intensity focused ultrasound in the treatment of localized prostate cancer. *Journal of Endourology* 2005, 19, 6:693-701.

[6] Foster RS, Bihrle R, Sanghvi N, Fry F, Kopecky K, et al. Production of prostatic lesions incanines using transrectally administered high-intensity focused ultrasound. Eur. Urol., 23: 330-336, 1993.
[7] Susani M, Madersbacher S, Kratzik C, Vingcrs L, Marberger M. Morphology of tissue destruction induced by focused ultrasound. Eur. Urol., 23 (Suppl. I): 34-38, 1993.
[8] Madersbacher S, Pedevilla M, Vingers L, et al., Martin Susani, and Michael Marberger. Effect of High-Intensity Focused Ultrasound on human prostate cancer in vivo. Cancer Research 1995; 55: 3346-3351
[9] Lindau O, Lauterborn W., Cinematographic observation of the collapse and rebound of a laser-produced cavitation bubble near a wall, J. Fluid Mech. 479, (2003) 327–348.
[10] Chen H, Li X, Wan M, Wang S. High-speed observation of cavitation bubble clouds near a tissue boundary in high-intensity focused ultrasound fields. Ultrasonics 49 (2009) 289–292.
[11] Clarke RL, Ter Haar GR. Temperature rise recorded during lesion formation by high-intensity focused ultrasound. Ultrasound in Med e Biol 1997;23:299-306.
[12] Bush N. Rivens I, Ter Haar GR, Bamber JC. Acoustic properties of lesions generated with an ultrasound therapy system. Ultrasound Med Biol 1993; 19:789-801.
[13] Hartveit F. Breast cancer: poor short-term prognosis in cases with moderate lymphocyte infiltration at the tumour edge: a preliminary report. Oncol Rep 1998;5:423-6.
[14] Lu P, Zhu XQ, Xu ZL, Zhou Q, Zhang J, Wu F. Increased infiltration of activated tumor-infiltrating lymphocytes after high intensity focused ultrasound ablation of human breast cancer. Surgery 2009; 145: 286-93.
[15] Srivastava, P. Roles of heat-shock proteins in innate and adaptive immunity. *Nat. Rev. Immunol.* 2002, *2*(3): 185-194.
[16] Crouzet S, Rebillard X, Chevallier D, Rischmann P, Pasticer G, Garcia G, et al. Multicentric oncologic outcome of High-Intensity Focused Ultrasound for localized prostate cancer in 803 patients. Eur Urol 2010;58:559-66
[17] Ahmed U, Zacharakis E, Dudderidge T, Armitage JN, Scott R, Calleary J. High-intensity-focused ultrasound in the treatment of primary prostate cancer: the first UK series. Br J Cancer 2009;101:19-26
[18] Blana A, Murat F, Walter B, Thuroff S, Wieland WF, Chaussy C. First analysis of the long-term results with transrectal hifu in patients with localised prostate cancer. Eur Urol 2008;53:1194-203
[19] Challacombe B, Murphy DG, Zakri R, Cahill DJ. High-intensity focused ultrasound for localized prostate cancer: initial experience with a 2-year follow-up. BJU Int 2009;104: 200-4

Part 3

Radiation Therapy and Its Potential Sequelae

8

Radiotherapy in Prostate Cancer

Tatjana Arsenijević, Kata Dabić Stanković,
Miodrag Aćimović and Ljiljana Radošević Jelić
*Institute for Oncology and Radiology of Serbia, Institute for Urology
Serbia*

1. Introduction

Therapeutic management of prostate cancer has become complex, multidisciplinary and stage-specific. (Heidenereich et al., 2011) Based on PSA level, histopathological grading and clinical staging, prostate cancer is classified as low-, intermediate- and high risk for disease recurrence. The risk status often plays a major role in deciding further therapy. (Kirby & Madhavan, 2010) It is usually impossible to state that one therapy is superior to another because of the lack of randomized controlled trials. However some recommendations can be made. (Heidenereich et al., 2011, Aus et al. 2001) Based on European Association of Urology recommendations in 2010, patients with low-risk (PSA ≤10 ng/ml, Gleason score <6 and cT1c-cT2a) or intermediate risk prostate cancer (PSA 10.1-20 ng/ml, Gleason score 7 or cT2b-c) are to be treated interdisciplinary with an urologist and a radiation oncologist. Treatment options for these patients vary from watchful waiting and active surveillance to radical prostatectomy or definitive radiotherapy. Multidisciplinary tumor board is needed when discussing neoadjuvant and adjuvant treatment options in high-risk prostate cancer patients (PSA>20ng/ml, Gleason score 8-10 or ≥cT3a) (Heidenereich et al., 2011, Choe & Liauw, 2010).

Radiotherapy is widely used as curative treatment modality for prostate cancer. There is a diverse array of radiotherapeutic strategies that can be effectively used to treat both organ-confined and locally advanced disease, alone or in combination with androgen-deprivation therapy. Furthermore, it has also a significant role in post-prostatectomy setting, as adjuvant or salvage radiotherapy.

In recent decades, radiotherapy in prostate cancer has undergone significant clinical and technological advances that aim to optimize cancer control outcomes while minimizing treatment morbidity. (Choe & Liauw, 2010, Hayden et al., 2010)

2. External-beam radiotherapy in prostate cancer

External-beam radiotherapy has a very long history in the curative treatment of prostate cancer. It is proven and most extensively used radiation modality. As a flexible, noninvasive, outpatient therapy, external-beam radiotherapy can be used in all stages of prostate cancer. (Hayden et al., 2010) It is based on daily delivery of radiation to a target volume using high-energy radiation beams from linear accelerators (or cobalt machines) over a course of 7 to 9 weeks.

In the last 30 years it has undergone a long, improving path from conventional, two-dimensional radiotherapy to intensity-modulated and image-guided radiotherapy and onwards. In low-risk prostate cancer its efficacy appears to be comparable to that of radical prostatectomy but with different toxicities (Choe & Liauw, 2010). For patients not suitable for surgery, external-beam radiotherapy will be the treatment of choice in most cases, alone or combined with androgen-deprivation therapy.

2.1 Conventional radiotherapy

Introducing high-energy radiotherapy machines it become possible to deliver tumoricidal doses to target volume while minimizing damage to the skin and adjacent organs. Historically, various techniques have been used, ranging from parallel anteroposterior-/posteroanterior (AP/PA) portals to lateral portals (box technique) or rotational fields to irradiate or supplement the dose to the prostate. (Chao et al, 2002) Due to the difficulty of localizing the prostate gland, a large volume was treated to ensure proper coverage. More of the surrounding tissues were included in the treated volume so the safely applicable dose was limited to 60-65Gy. (Choe & Liauw, 2010)

The treatment fields for prostate cancer were simulated and designed on plane films and using bony markers with the patient in the supine position. Rectum and bladder were marked by intraluminal injection of iodinated contrast. Small intestine was marked with barium contrast ingested per os one hour prior to simulation.

If the external-beam radiotherapy was applied to the prostate only (local technique), the field size was approximately 8x10 cm for T1 and T2 tumors, 10x12 cm or 12x14 cm for T3 and T4 prostate cancer. Patients younger than 71 years of age with clinical T1c, T2a, and Gleason score more than 7 and PSA 20ng/ml or more, as well as patients with T2b, c T3 and T4 were treated to the whole pelvis with the field size of 15x15 cm, or 15x18 cm to cover the common iliac nodes. The inferior margin of the field usually was 1.5 cm distal to the junction of the prostatic and membranous urethra that is at or caudal to the bottom of the ischial tuberosities. The lateral margins were approximately 1 to 2 cm from the lateral bony pelvis.

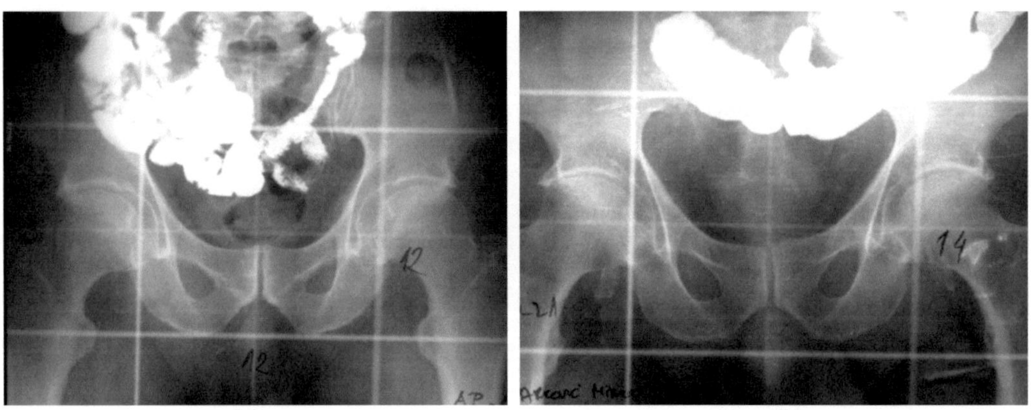

(a) (b)

Fig. 1. Simulation AP radiograph for field verification (a) size 12x12 cm and (b) 14x14 cm Low field border is on the lower border of ishiadic bone and the field centre on the symphisis. Barium contrast in bowels (With thanks to the Institute for oncology and radiology of Serbia, Belgrade)

The initial lateral fields included a volume similar to that treated with AP/PA portals. The anterior margin was 1.5 cm posterior to the projection of the anterior cortex of the pubic symphisis. Posteriorly, the fields included the pelvic and presacral lymph nodes above the S3 segment, which allowed some sparing of posterior rectal wall distal to this level.

Large treated volume was obtained since the average variation of prostate position relative to bony markers was approximately 8 mm in the superior and posterior positions, 7 mm in the inferior, 5 mm in the lateral and 4 mm in anterior position. The seminal vesicles are located high in the pelvis, and posterior to the bladder, which was very critical when reducing treated volume in T3 patients.

When indicated, the periaortic lymph nodes could be treated through extended AP/PA portals or separate periaortic fields placed above the pelvic fields. The superior margin of the periaortic field was at the Th12-L1 vertebral interspace with the width usually above 10 cm (determined by lymphangiogram or CT scan). (Chao et al., 2002, Dobbs et al., 1999)

Conventional external-beam radiotherapy required daily radiation delivery to target volume using high-energy beams (more than 10MV). In most institutions a standard fractionation was used with 1.8 to 2Gy per day. In radical approach, initially a dose of 45-50Gy was applied to the whole pelvis or to the prostate through two parallel opposed fields (AP/PA). Than addition of a boost dose was delivered, up to a total dose of 65-66Gy through lateral opposed fields, two anterior or two posterior oblique fields. (Chao et al., 2002, Dobbs et al., 1999)

2.2 Two-dimensional radiotherapy (2D-RT)

Once a decision is being made to treat prostate cancer with external-beam radiotherapy, the radiotherapy plan is defined either to limit treatment to the gland or to extend treatment field to include the periprostatic tissues, seminal vesicles and pelvic lymph nodes. (Hayden et al. 2010) CT or MRI of the abdomen and pelvis is used to assess the involvement of surrounding structures. MRI is particularly useful for distinguishing capsular invasion, seminal vesicle involvement and periapical extension. CT scanning for treatment planning is performed to every patient, which means that two-dimensional (2D) radiotherapy is a step forward comparing to conventional radiotherapy.

The patient is immobilized in supine position with skin tattoos over the pubic symphisis and laterally over the iliac crests to prevent lateral rotation. CT scans of pelvis are obtained with slice thickness of 4-5 mm. No oral, rectal or intravenous contrast is used. The CT section at the centre of the volume is used as the main planning slice to outline patient contour, target volume, rectum, and bladder. The margins of the target volume are determined by the tumor extent. The gross tumor volume contains entire prostate gland, but if there is a risk of seminal vesicles involvement, they must be included in target volume too. The gross tumor volume is outlined on the central slice only. To allow position variation, an additional margin is added to gross tumor volume (1-1.5 cm in all directions) defining planning target volume (PTV). For two-dimensional planning, PTV is outlined on multiple sections to ensure that the entire tumor is encompassed. The rectal outline must be transposed on to the central section so that the dose can be adequately calculated. Shaping the target volume by shielding blocks or multileaf collimators reduces the dose to normal tissues.

Treatment technique depends on the target volume size and shape. Three-field technique using an anterior and two posterior oblique or opposed lateral fields give a high dose to the prostate but spare the posterior rectal wall. Four-field (box) technique may result in better dose distribution when seminal vesicles are included in target volume, but increases the dose posteriorly.

The patient is than treated daily, 1.8 to 2Gy per fraction, on linear accelerator. The correct position is assured with skin tattoos. The field centre is marked with a tattoo also. All fields are treated isocentrically with shielding as instructed. The recommended dose is 64Gy in 32 fractions given in 6.5 to 7 weeks. (Dobbs et al., 1999)

2.3 Three-dimensional conformal radiotherapy (3D-CRT)

Introducing CT-based radiotherapy simulations by the mid 1980s and multileaf collimator in new aged linear accelerators, it became possible to arrange treatment fields to individually match prostate target volume minimizing high dose exposure to adjacent normal tissues. This led to dose escalation without inducing more toxicity and implementing three-dimensional conformal radiotherapy in clinical practice as a gold standard in prostate cancer radiotherapy treatment. Practically, the aim is to minimize treatment toxicity for patients with more favorable disease, and to maximize locoregional tumor control for those with less favorable disease. (Hayden et al., 2010, Dearnaley, 2001, Gazdda et al., 1996/97)

For 3D-CRT treatment planning a multi-slice CT scan and 3D planning system is used. In order to minimize random and systemic setup error, prior to CT scan, patient should be positioned and immobilized in a fashion that position obtained can be maintained and reproduced. This is secured by the use of alpha cradles, shells or by positioning the patient in supine position with leg restraints. In all this cases a midline and lateral laser lights are used for set up. These markers are tattooed on the skin over the pubic symphisis and laterally over the iliac crests. This is very important for daily positioning of the patient and prevention of lateral rotation. The position is later verified by portal image. (Dobbs et al., 1999, Hayden et al., 2010, Malone et al., 2000)

CT scan of pelvis is performed in a treatment position. Patient should empty the rectum and the bladder should be comfortably full both on the simulation and on the radiation. This standard should be followed because the variation in bladder and rectum distension results in significant prostate displacement. A great controversy still remains regarding prostate apex. MRI of pelvis and CT/MRI fusion is recommended to reduce inter-observer variability in contouring, improving target delineation accuracy, particularly the prostate apex. This fusion is also recommended were significant CT artifact is present i.e. from hip prosthesis.

Once the CT and/or MRI scans are obtained on each slice a target volume and organs at risk are delineated. Organs at risk are adjacent structures endangered by high radiation dose delivered to treated volume. These organs include bladder, rectum, femoral heads and small bowel when it is in the treatment field. (Fiorino et al., 2009)

In 3D-CRT of prostate cancer target volume consists of clinical target volume (CTV) and planning target volume (PTV). CTV includes prostate only, or prostate with seminal vesicles and lymph nodes depending on risk category of the disease. In low-risk prostate cancer, the risk of seminal vesicles involvement is less than 5%, so the CTV should be restricted to prostate only. But, for intermediate risk patients the risk of seminal vesicle involvement is higher (over 15%) hence the proximal third of the seminal vesicles (1 cm) should be included in CTV. For high-risk patients proximal 2 cm of seminal vesicles should be in encompassed with CTV. In cases were seminal vesicle involvement is proven, whole of them should be included in CTV. Any extracapsular extension is also delineated under the CTV, and even a margin of 2-5 mm (excluding rectum) should be considered in high-risk and T3 disease. (Hayden et al., 2010, Koh et al., 2003, Boehmer et al., 2006) According to RTOG guidelines in 2009, pelvic lymph node irradiation may be considered in high-risk patients judged by the treating clinician. The risk of lymph node involvement approaches the risk of distant metastases so the benefit of lymph node irradiation remains controversial. (Lawton et al., 2009)

PTV is a margin added to CTV to reduce the impact of set-up error and organ motion on CTV displacement. PTV also covers inter-observer variability in both delineating of mentioned structures and verification process. According to RTOG recommendation, a PTV is determined by institutional set-up and verification protocol, and measurement of institutional random and systemic errors of prostate position. (Lawton et al., 2009) In many institutions the acceptable CTV-PTV margin ranges from 5 do 10 mm. (Hayden et al., 2010) (Figure 2.)

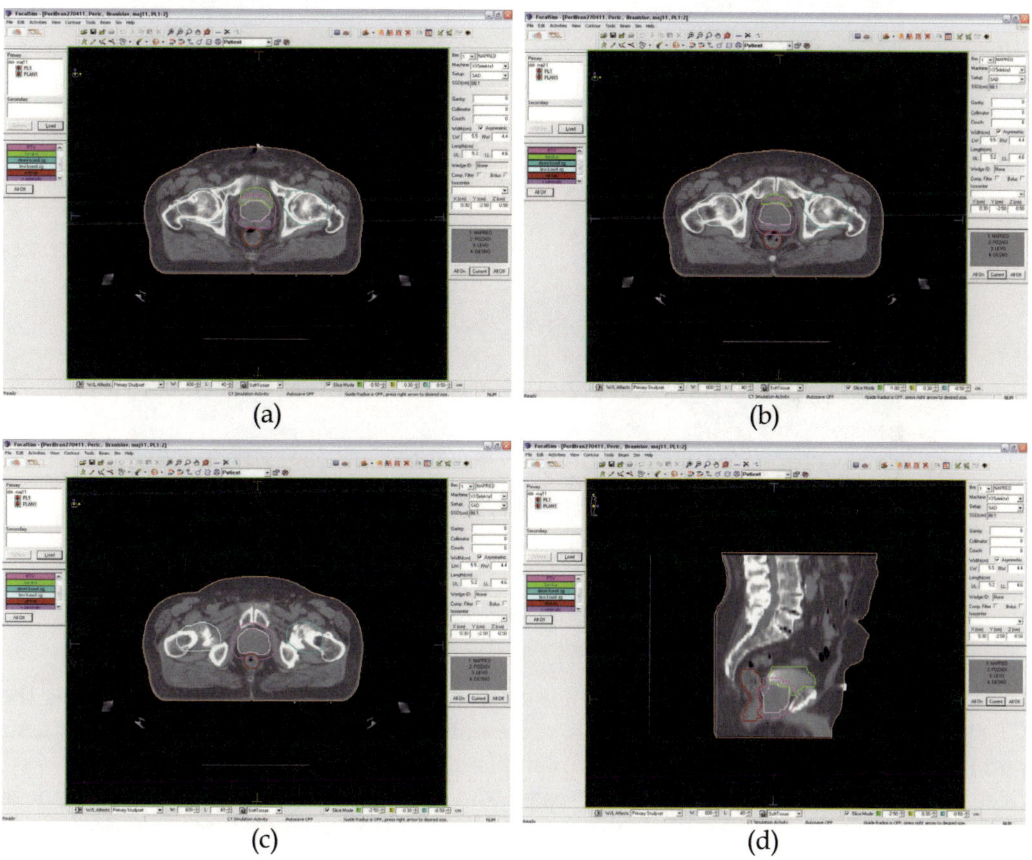

Fig. 2. Delineation of target volume (prostate-pink and seminal vesicles-purple) and organs at risk (bladder-green, rectum-red and femoral heads-light green and dark green) delineation. PTV margin-magenta (a, b, c). Sagital reconstruction (d). (With thanks to the Institute for oncology and radiology of Serbia, Belgrade)

When the delineation process is completed, the medical physicists arrange beam angles and adjust them to maximize target coverage and minimize high-dose exposure to normal organs. (Choe & Liauw, 2010) (Figure 3.)

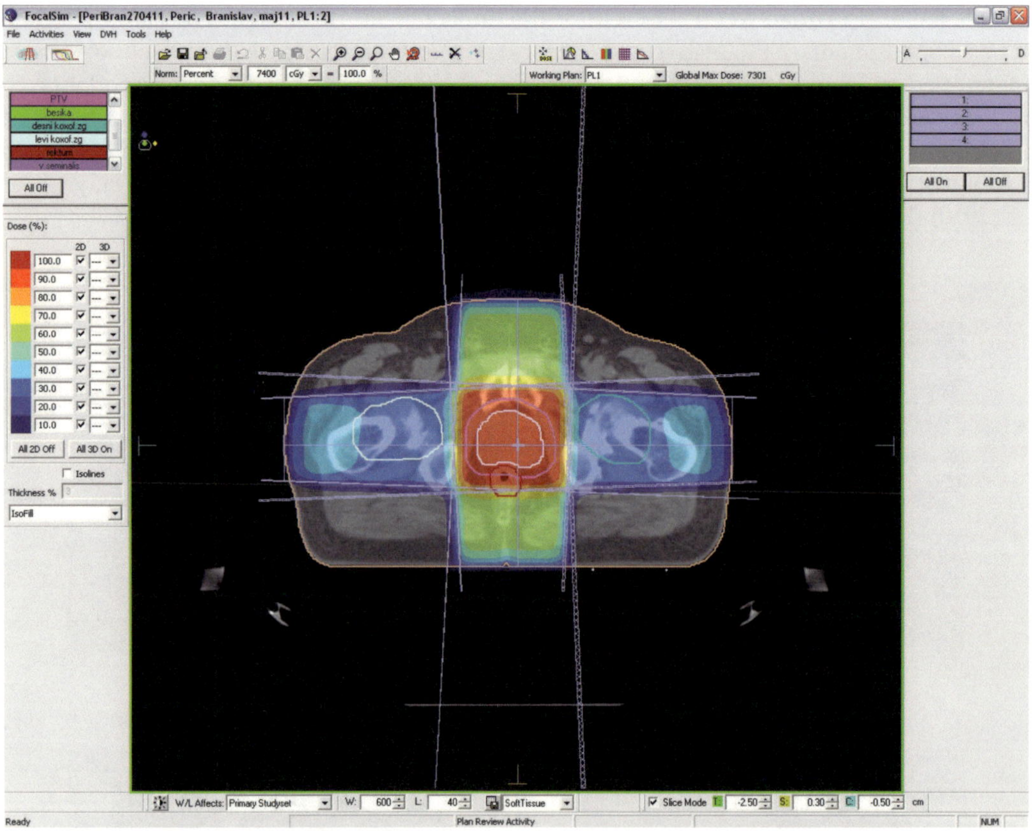

Fig. 3. Field arrangement for four-field (box) treatment (With thanks to the Institute for oncology and radiology of Serbia, Belgrade)

Digitally reconstructed radiograph (DRR) is created by computer program transforming the CT slices into a radiograph image. DRR represents the referent image to which the later portal films of treatment field position are compared. (Figure 4.)

Dose-volume-histogram (DVH) is also created and it shows the percent of prescribed dose to every delineated structure. For organs at risk the ALARA principle (as low as reasonably achievable) is recommended following the tolerant dose of each organ. But, although DVH gives valuable information on the dose to each structure, it is calculated on a single pretreatment pelvic organs position, and they are mobile. That is the reliability on a single pretreatment DVH is limited, and does not have to correlate with late toxicity (Fiorino et al., 2009) (Figure 5.)

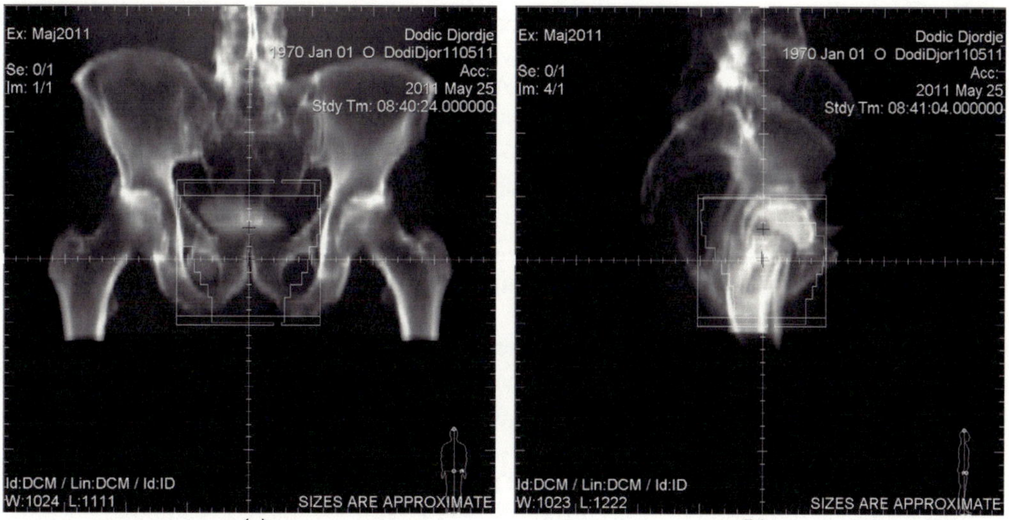

(a) (b)

Fig. 4. Digitaly reconstructed radiographs (DRR) for AP (a) and right lateral (b) field (With thanks to the Institute for oncology and radiology of Serbia, Belgrade)

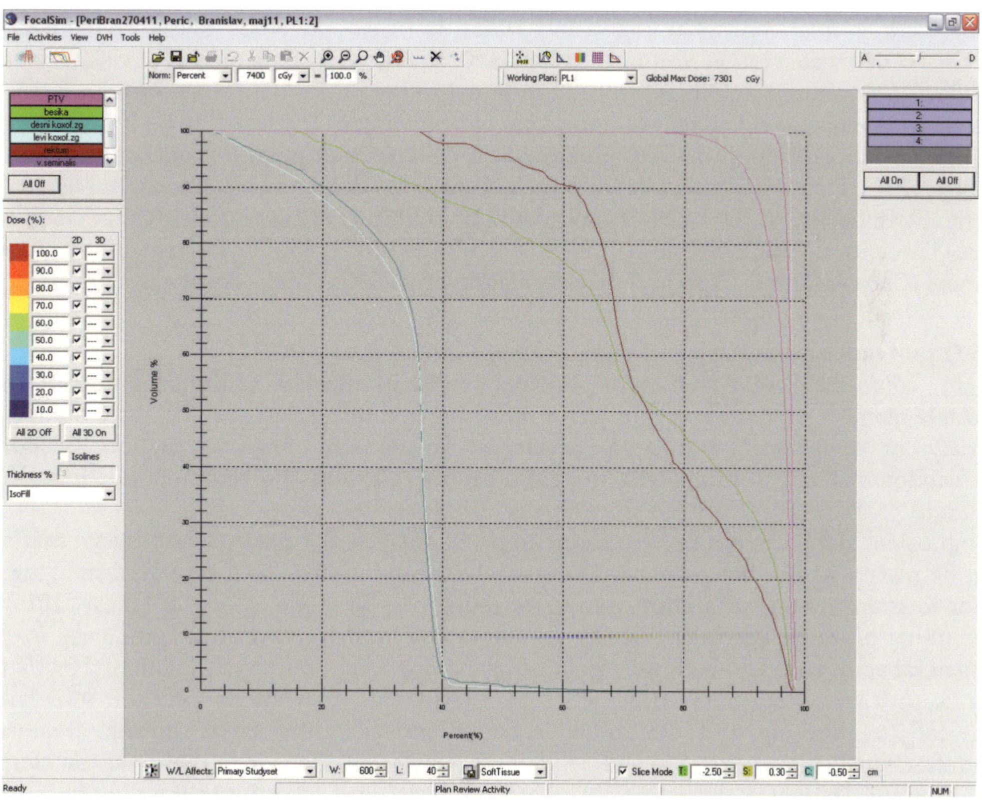

Fig. 5. Dose-volume-histogram (DVH) showing the doses delivered to each delineated structure (With thanks to the Institute for oncology and radiology of Serbia, Belgrade)

According to EAU guidelines in prostate cancer in 2010, for external radiotherapy, a dose of at least 74Gy to PTV is recommended for low-risk prostate cancer because the biochemical disease-free survival is significantly higher when compared to a dose of under 72Gy (69% vs. 63%; P=0.046). For intermediate-risk prostate cancer the dose is ranging from 76Gy to 81Gy, and for high-risk prostate cancer a combination with androgen deprivation is recommended regardless dose escalation since the risk of systemic relapse has to be covered. (Heidenereich et al., 2011)

The patient is treated daily, 1.8 to 2Gy per fraction, on linear accelerator in a position that matches the position taken during CT simulation. The correct position is obtained by immobilizing devices and by setting up the skin tattoo markers to treatment room wall lasers. Once the radiotherapy has started, portal films of arranged fields are taken on the accelerator, in treatment position and compared with digitally reconstructed radiograph (DRR) for set-up or other errors several times during radiotherapy course.

2.4 Intensity-modulated radiotherapy (IMRT)

Intensity-modulated radiotherapy is considered a grate improvement in radiation oncology. It is a form of 3D-CRT in which the optimization of the dose prescribed to the target volume is achieved by x-ray beam intensity changes. By using computer algorithms the intensity of the beam is changed in order to increase the dose difference between the target volume and organs at risk.

Radiotherapy treatment planning using IMRT is based on a CT slices on which the physician delineates target volumes as for the 3D-CRT, as well as organs at risk. For each delineated structure the tolerant dose in imputed in the mathematical algorithms and than the beam intensity is calculated as a function of beam angle. The beam angle is individually adjusted by inclination of the radiotherapy bed, collimator or gentry. (Valicenti et al., 2000)

Unlike 3D-CRT, in IMRT the dose from each beam is not delivered all at once. At each beam angle, the intensity of the beam is modulated by multiple smaller subfields that change in time. This allows a high degree of dose conformity around complex and irregularly shaped tumors (Choe & Liauw, 2010) and dose escalation up to 86Gy. (Zelefsky et al., 2002)

2.5 Organ motion tracking and image-guided radiotherapy (IGRT)

Highly conformal radiation therapy requires precise localization of the prostate. Since the prostate gland is a movable organ due to breathing and distention of rectum and bladder, a variety of strategies have been developed to account prostate motion including transabdominal ultrasound-based imaging, on-line CT and implantation of radiopaque markers.

The prostate gland can not be visualized on portal images, but radiopaque fiducial markers can be placed within the prostate. These markers can be visualized on portal imaging so prior to every treatment a correction of targeting can be made. (Choe & Liauw, 2010) A minimum of three markers should be implanted under ultrasound guidance in the ipsilateral apex, base and contra-lateral mid-gland one week prior to simulation. (Hayden et al., 2010) This technique is used to track interfraction movement (prostate movement between treatments), but it cannot account prostate movement during treatment (intrafractional movement). Nowadays there is a growing interest in real-time tracking of the prostate. There is a special system that uses a real-time tracking of the radiofrequency transponders implanted into the prostate and if they present outside of the predetermined margins the radiation stops.

These new technologies are still under investigation, but first results are optimistic. (Choe & Liauw, 2010) When IGRT is used prostate displacement caused by rectal distension is largely corrected. (Hayden et al., 2010)

2.6 Acute and late toxicity of external-beam radiotherapy in prostate cancer

Radiation-induced complications can be acute and late. Acute adverse events occur during treatment and late may develop months to years after treatment. When we irradiate the prostate, acute and late toxicity are a consequence of high dose given to the surrounding organs i.e. bladder, rectum and skin. The severance of these side-effects largely depends on the tissue volume irradiated and relates to the treatment technique.

During conventional radiotherapy of the prostate acute toxicity include acute proctitis followed by rectal discomfort, tenesmus and diarrhea, and rarely rectal bleeding. It is mostly mild and resolves after symptomatic therapy with hydration and antidiarrheal and anti-inflammatory medication. Skin reactions include erythema, dry and humid desquamation. According to RTOG scale (RTOG, 1999) acute toxicity has four grades of severity stated in table 1.

Grade	0	1	2	3	4
Dermatitis	No complications	Mild erythema or dry desquamation	Moderate erytherma or incipient moist desquamation, mild skid edema	Confluent moist desquamation more than 1.5 cm of the skin, moderate edema	Ulcerations or skin necrosis
Colitis	No complications	Asymptomatic	Abdominal pain, mucus and/or blood in stool	Abdominal pain, fever, peritoneal signs or ileus	Perforation
Diarrhea	No complications	Up to 4 stools per day	4-6 stools per day, night stools	More than 7 stools per day and/or incontinency or parentheral substitution due to dehydrations	Hemodynamic collapse
Cystitis, dysuria	No complications	Mild dysuria	Moderate dysuria that need symptomatic therapy	Symptoms not relieved on symptomatic therapy	

Table 1. Acute toxicity in radical radiotherapy of prostate cancer-RTOG scale

The most frequent adverse event on the urinary tract is radiation cystitis producing dysuria, nocturia, frequency and urgency. It is low graded in most cases (7.7%) while severe urinary complications are seen in less than 0.5% of patients. According to RTOG study on over 1000 prostate cancer patients treated with external-beam radiotherapy, acute toxicity occurs in 70-90% of the patients with mild symptoms. Moderate symptoms are developed in 20-45% of the patients while 1-4% has severe or prolonged reactions. (Dearnaley, 2001)
Although acute toxicity is very unpleasant for the patient it usually resolves after the treatment. Late toxicity is of much more concern since it is unpredictable and very often irreversible. According to RTOG, late toxicity also has four grades of severity (table 2).
Mostly it is mild and does not influence quality of life, but sever late toxicity is reported in 4-8% of patients. Most common genitourinary side effects are chronic cystitis (5%), incontinency, urethral stricture (5%, mostly patients with previous transurethral resection of the prostate), bladder ulceration and impotency (30-40%). Late toxicity on rectum affects 3% of the patients and includes tenesmus, sphincter dysfunction, occasional bleeding, strictures or ulcerations. (Dearnaley, 2001)

Grade	0	1	2	3	4
Bladder	No complications	Mild epithelia atrophy, discreet teleangiectasia	Diffuse teleangiectasia, macroscopic hemathuria	Frequent urinating, dysuria and hemathuria, bladder capacity less than 150 ml	Bladder necrosis, capacity less than 100 ml, hemorrhagic cystitis
Skin	No complications	Mild skin atrophy, hyperpigmentation, hair loss	Moderate skin atrophy, teleangiectasis, total hair loss	Severe skin atrophy, severe teleangiectasia	Ulceration
Bowels	No complications	Mild diarrhea or increased bowel motion, or mild rectal bleeding	Moderate diarrhea, abdominal pain, rectal mucus or harder bleeding	Ileus or bleeding that requires surgical treatment	Necrosis, perforation, fistula

Table 2. Late toxicity in radical radiotherapy of prostate cancer-RTOG scale

Introducing 3D-CRT and IMRT the volume of bladder and rectum irradiated is limited, but the dose escalation can still induce significant toxicity. In trials of dose escalation, reported rates of acute toxicity are very similar to those of conventional radiotherapy. Late toxicity however is still considered high. MD Anderson trial has shown a significant gastrointestinal toxicity (grade 2 or more) in 25% of patients with escalated dose comparing to 13% in low dose group (78Gy vs. 70Gy). (Kuban et al., 2008) The Dutch trial reported 26% of late rectal toxicity grade 2, and Medical research council 33% in dose escalated group. (Al-Mamgani et al., 2008, Dearnaley et al., 2007) These results compare with reports of IMRT treatment with 81Gy (3% of patients experienced late rectal toxicity at grade 2 or grater) and treatment with IGRT with 79.8Gy (12% of patients with grade 2 rectal toxicity). (Hayden et al. 2010) For urinary toxicity none of these trials found significant correlation between late adverse events and radiation dose. Although improved radiotherapy techniques appear to enable dose escalation with less toxicity, the optimal dose that can eradicate the disease without the risk of toxicity is jet to be defined. (Choe & Liauw, 2010)

2.7 Results of external-beam radiotherapy of prostate cancer

Following external-beam radiotherapy, long-term clinically assessed local tumor control is good for patients with stage T1 cancers (83% at 15 years), but it is falling to 65-68% for T2 and 44-75% for T3 cancers. Reported incidence of positive biopsy after external-beam radiotherapy vary from 18 to 45% and increases with disease bulk from 15% for T1 disease, to 68-79% for men with T2 and T3 cancers. Regarding biochemical control, Hanks et al. reported a long-term biochemical control in 72% of T1 cancers, falling to 22% and 28% for bulky T2 and T3 cancers in a mean follow-up of 12.6 years.

PSA level and Gleason score are powerful predictors of outcome. In patients with low Gleason score the rate of biochemical control ranges about 75%, compared to only 18% for Gleason score 7 and 0% for Gleason score 8 or 9. In patients with pretreatment PSA more than 20 ng/ml only 28% remained biochemically free of progression at 4 years in the results of Hanks et al (Dearnaley, 2001)

Several randomized controlled trials and one meta-analysis shown that improved biochemical outcomes (biochemical failure free survival) are associated with dose escalation. (Kuban et al., 2008, Al-Mmgani et al., 2008, Dearnaley et al., 2007, Zietman et al., 2010, Viani et al., 2009). Radiation Therapy Oncology Group trials have even shown that higher radiation dose improves disease-specific and overall survival in high-grade prostate cancer. (Valicenti et al., 2000) Despite promising results of dose escalation there are still uncertainties regarding routine application of dose escalation especially. The subgroup of patients that will benefit the most from dose escalation is not clearly defined. These trials enrolled men in all risk groups of localized prostate. Only U.K. Medical Research Council trial divided patients in risk groups showing the benefit of dose escalation in all groups. But statistically significance was reached only in high-risk group. In the Dutch trial the benefit from dose escalation from 68 to 78Gy was also registered in intermediate and high-risk patients. These results led to a question whether a higher dose is required for low-risk prostate cancer. Although MD Anderson trial shown the benefit form dose escalation in high-risk group of patients, it also reported longer follow-up of 8.7 years that can indirectly demonstrate a benefit of dose escalation even in the low-risk group. While the improved biochemical outcomes are practically proven with dose escalation, there is still no sufficient evidence of improvement in cancer-specific survival and overall survival. (Choe & Liauw, 2010)

Regarding overall survival, radiotherapy is efficient method for many cases of localized prostate cancer. Five-year overall survival for T1 and T2 stage ranges about 70-80%, and 90% of local tumor control. Locally advanced stages have poorer prognosis with 5-year overall survival of 40-50%. High Gleason score is the most significant negative prognostic marker since it is associated with higher malignant potential. Cancer related death for high Gleason score tumors (8-10) is about 60-80% in 15 years. (Hadzi-Djokic, 2005)

3. Brachytherapy in prostate cancer

In the age of the developed imaging technology (CT, MRI, PET, US), and advanced biochemical markers (tumor-specific and nonspecific), a large number of tumors, including prostate cancer, are being diagnosed in the early stages. In early stages of prostate cancer (T1-T2 N0 M0, PSA <10ng/ml, Gleason Score <6, prostate volume <50ml, maximum urinary flow>15ml/s), in addition to the conventional, laser and robotic prostatectomy, hyperthermia, hormone therapy and brachytherapy is often applied.

In brachytherapy sealed sources of radiation are placed either in direct contact or in proximity of the tumor, so the interstitial brachytherapy for localized prostate cancer often represents the method of choice, and its efficiency is not far behind the effectiveness of surgery, with less morbidity. Brachytherapy allows local application of extremely high doses (up to 160Gy, even more). The effectiveness of prostate cancer brachytherapy is directly correlated with the total dose and precision of administration, which represents its advantage over transcutaneous radiotherapy.

Prostate cancer is usually multicentric, so the brachytherapy target is the entire prostate, and the total dose has to cover the area of about 2-5 mm beyond the prostate capsule. From the point of radiotherapy, particularly brachytherapy, the initial prostate cancer (prostate itself, with or without vesicles involved) represents the ideal target, with adequate spare of the urethra, rectum, bladder and perineal area. Moreover, brachytherapy can be applied within a combined radiotherapy (brachytherapy + transcutaneous radiotherapy) by the additional dose (*boost*), as well as in the case of local recurrence or rest after prostatectomy or transcutaneous radiotherapy.

Brachytherapy for prostate cancer is not a new therapy method, though in the history of medicine it experienced its ups and downs, mainly due to the previous imperfections of visualization techniques and applications, as well as, imperfection in radiation and dosimetric characteristics of the radiation sources, while today it is a routine method of treatment. With the introduction of transrectal ultrasound (TRUS), CT and development of new sources of radiation (^{103}Pd, and ^{192}Ir), techniques of radioisotope implantation (loading and afterloading) and computer systems for brachytherapy planning in routine clinical practice, interstitial brachytherapy for prostate cancer began to experience another upswing, but with markedly better results and lower morbidity.

Today, two modalities for interstitial brachytherapy are applied:

1. **low dose rate (LDR)**, about 2Gy/day, with low activity ^{125}I sources (from 0.03 to 1.5GBq per seed, max. photon energy of 35.5 keV, the half-life about 60 days in the form of cylinders /height 4.5 mm, 0.8 mm diameter, encapsuled in titanium sleeve/) or ^{103}Pd (Blasko et al., 2000) (dose rate to about 5Gy/day; activity around 0.07GBq per source, the maximum photon energy of 21 keV, the half-life 17 days in the form of cylinder/ height 4.5 mm, 0.8 mm diameter /or spheres/ diameter of about 1 mm /) - a permanent implant;
2. **(high) dose rate (HDR)** about 0.2 to 3Gy / min with radioactive ^{192}Ir source in the form of cylinder /dimensions around 0.6 x3,5 mm / (initial activity of about 370GBq; time

half-life of 74.2 days, mean photon energy of about 380keV,) - a temporary implantation.

3.1 Low dose rate brachytherapy

Strictly speaking, from the point of view of radiobiology, the only differences (not great) in the indications for applying permanent (LDR) or temporary implantation (HDR) are mostly related to tumor grade. For example, with low-grade and low-risk tumors (eg Stage<T2a, PSA<10, Gleason Score 2-4) and slow-growing tumors, we expect greater efficiency in the application of permanent implants, while with tumors of high grade and higher risk, higher efficiency is expected from temporary implantation. Although there are relative differences in the indications for application of LDR or HDR brachytherapy, it seems that the predominant technique is the one with permanent implants (LDR). Selection of isotopes (^{125}I or ^{103}Pd) is in the favor of the cheaper iodine, so if otherwise not indicated it's considered that radioisotope ^{125}I is being used in LDR brachytherapy for treating prostate cancer. Permanent implants are rarely used in cases of rest or local recurrence after prostatectomy or transcutaneous radiotherapy. In this case a HDR brachytherapy with ^{192}Ir of initial activity over 370 GBq, by using afterloading device, is applied.
Prostate brachytherapy requires a multidisciplinary approach, which assumes collaboration between urologists, radiation oncologists (brachytherapists), anesthesiologists and brachytherapy physicists. Regardless of which brachytherapy modality is implemented in prostate brachytherapy, and with the aim to providing a top quality treatment, all steps are strictly determined:

1. Assessing the stage and spread of the disease (laboratory-biochemical, prostate morphology / palpatory findings, prostate size - US and TRUS /, histopathological verification and determination of Gleason Score, a CT/MRI, scintigraphy, determination of TNM disease stage)
2. Assessing the possibility of applications (talk with the patient, the patient's state, maximum urinary flow rate, the presence of residual urine, previous TUR, assessment of cardiovascular conditions, the possibility of implanting, anatomy of the pelvis, prostate size, type of implant LDR vs. HDR)
3. Preparing the patient prior to implantation - 24 hours in advance (admission of the patient, medical therapy, anti-coagulant and antibiotic, preparation of the patient, rectum cleaning)
4. Preparation of instrumentarium (selection and sterilization of instruments, calibration of stepper, network and TRUS) (Figure 6.)
5. Patient's positioning and anesthesia (in lithotomic position on the movable therapy table; spinal or general anesthesia)
6. Placing markers of critical radiosensitive structures (Folly catheter for marking the bladder and urethra)
7. Setting TRUS probes, template and steper, and prostate visualisation, and visualisation of urethra and rectum (in steps of max. 5 mm from base to apex (Grey et al., 2000), (Figure 7. a, c)
8. Pre-planning (determinatuion of the number and location of radiation sources and methods of implantation)
9. The application (placing the radiation source guides/needles; in the LDR technique inserting a radiation source - seeds) - TRUS-guided (Figure 8. b)

10. Verification and correction (cistoscopic, fluoroscopic, x-ray (Figure 7. c) - optional CT and/or MRI; in case of LDR brachytherapy adding of seeds, if necessary)
11. Computer reconstruction (seeds / LDR / - needles / HDR /, prostate capsule, the position of the urethra and rectum), optimization, plan analysis (the determination of DVH - Dose Volume Histogram, ie. minimum volume of prostate receiving 90%, 100%, 150% and 200% of the total dose, and the dose and volumes that receive critical radiosensitive structures), (Figure 7. d, e);
12. Irradiation; for HDR brachytherapy: deapplication of needles or observation of the patient (LDR)
13. Transport of patient to the patient room
14. Patient care (analgesic and antibiotics therapy, toilet)
15. Check-up (of dysuric problems and estimate the degree of proctitis) and discussion with the patient, the patient's discharge
16. Regular checks (during treatment /HDR/ and in 2, 3, 6, 12 and 18 months, then annually - the level of PSA, rectal examination, assessing the level of dysuric problems and evaluation of potency)

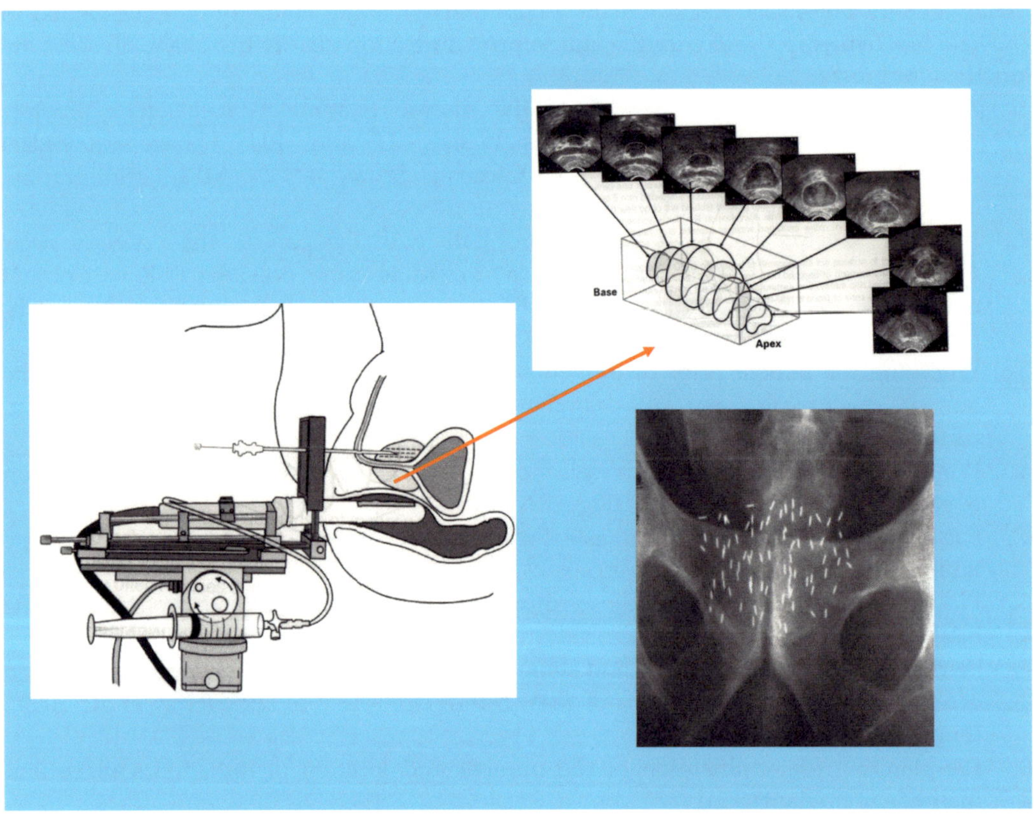

Fig. 6. Schematic representation of TRUS-guided brachytherapy with radioactive seeds.

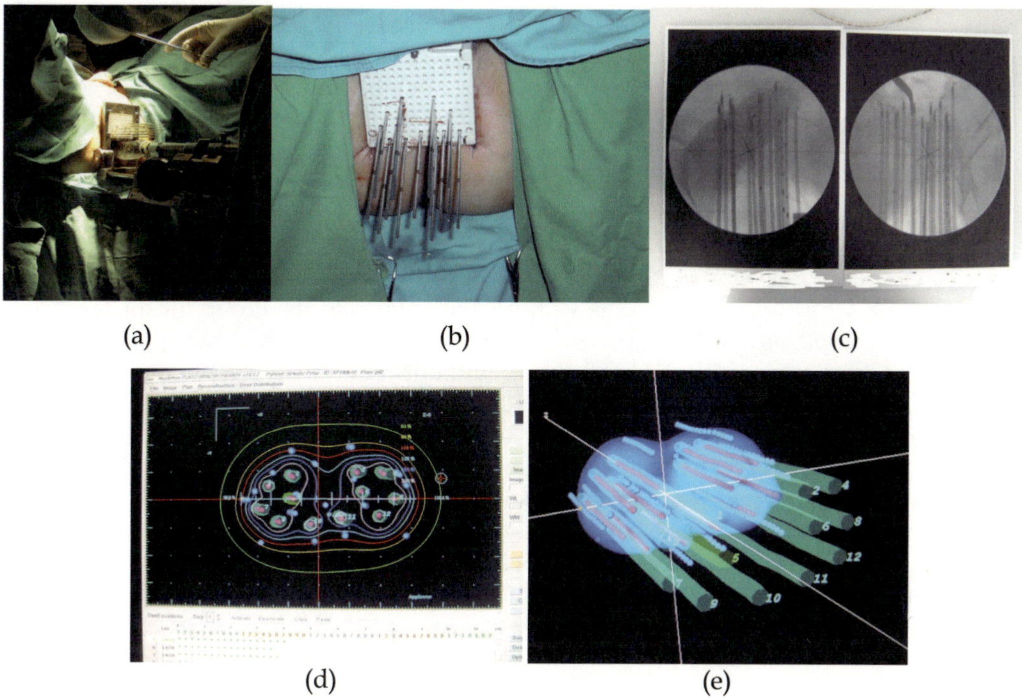

(a) TRUS guided needles application
(b) Administrated needles / guides of ^{192}Ir source
(c) Radiographic verification of the needles' positions
(d) Isodose transversal view
(e) 3D treatment volume
(With the thanks of the General Hospital Medical System, Belgrade)

Fig. 7. Steps in HDR prostate cancer brachytherapy - real patient

When using permanent implantation (monotherapy) radiation sources (seeds) remain in the prostate of the patient. It is therefore recommended to the patient a minimal two-week sexual abstinence and avoidance of contact with pregnant women and small children for a minimum of 2 months. A typical therapeutic dose of radiation, when ^{125}I is implanted, is in the range 140-160Gy, and when ^{103}Pd is implanted to about 125Gy. In a case of a "boost" dose, for ^{125}I a somewhat lower dose of 80-120 is applied or to about 90-100Gy for ^{103}Pd. (Blasko et al., 2000, Beyer, 2001)

3.1.1 Results of low dose rate brachytherapy

Prostate cancer with its characteristics and different biological behavior represents a problem in the analysis of brachytherapy final outcomes in terms of overall survival or local control. We are aware that many patients with untreated prostate cancer can survive tens of years, ie. do not die from prostate cancer. Therefore to evaluate the effectiveness of treatment of patients with prostate cancer, as for overall survival and local control, the PSA level was adopted.

Greem and associates (Greem et al., 1997)provide representation of the results of treatment of patients with permanent implants (monotherapy), showing a five-year survival of NED (no evidence of disease) of 94%, 84% and 54% for low risk, medium risk and higher risk group of 403 patients, respectively . Blasko and associates (Blasko et al, 2000) show the results of a five-year biochemical PSA control: 94%, 82% and 65% for low risk, medium risk and higher risk respectively. Slightly worse, but comparable results are displayed by other authors: 85-94%, 33-82% and 5-65% for low risk, medium risk and high-risk group, respectively (Beyer, 2001). Based on these results, most urologists and brachytherapists exclude a group of patients at high risk from the LDR brachytherapy and consider them patients with advanced disease in which the tumor penetrated the prostate capsule. Association of American Brachytherapy Society has established a Low Dose-Rate Task Group (Merrick, G., Zelefsky, M., Sylvester, E., Nag, S., Bice, W) with the task of defining the general criteria for inclusion of patients with prostate cancer in the group for the treatment by permanent implants (LDR): expected survival > 5 years, clinical stage T1b-T2c and selected T3, Gleason Score<10, PSA<50ng/ml, without involved lymph nodes, no distant metastases, Karnofsky performance status> 70%. Criteria for exclusion are: inflammatory prostate disease, severe urinary obstruction, the middle lobe hyperplasia, extensive TUR defects, a prostate size greater than 60x50 mm, the extension of disease to the seminal vesicles and bladder, involved lymph nodes, previously conducted EBRT. Absolute contraindications are distant metastatic disease, the inability of anesthesia (general, spinal, epidural), no possibility of peaceful lying, expected survival <5 years.

It is obvious that the consistent application of these criteria for inclusion and exclusion would ensure consistent application of LDR brachytherapy in this roup of patients, with the results of treatment (five-and even ten-year PSA control NED> 85%).

3.1.2 Toxicity of low dose rate brachtherapy

Mild and transient acute urinary symptoms (LENT SOMA, 1995) (hematuria and dysuria grade G1-G2) often accompany LDR brachytherapy, while the acute symptoms on the rectum (proctitis, tenesms and bleeding) are rare and mainly a result of edema and hematoma. All of the symptoms can be associated to radiation or trauma during the application procedure.

As late symptoms of bladder neck irradiation, chronic irritative urinary symptoms may occur and in a small number of cases due to urethral scarring, obstruction or incontinence may occur. Late effects on the rectum are mild, and manifested by periodic bleeding and proctitis. Erectile function was preserved for over 70% of treated patients whose erectile function was satisfactory before the implementation of brachytherapy. In order to preserve erectile function, it is important to avoid positioning of seeds in the perineal area, outside the prostate apex, which prevents the occurrence of fibrosis and consequent devascuralisation of this region. Most patients (over 2/3) treated with permanent implants, estimate their quality of life as good, which is just as important as biochemical and clinical course of disease.

However, due to the relatively limited fixation of radioactive seeds (which are smooth on the surface) there is a possibility of their inter-prostate migration and the creation of "hot" and "cold" zones, as well as, their migration to other organs (rectum, bladder and pelvic veins and even lungs), which sometimes requires serious surgical treatment and drastically reduces the quality of patient's life.

3.2 High dose rate brachytherapy

HDR temporary prostate cancer brachytherapy with ^{192}Ir entered into clinical practice mainly in combination with transcutaneous radiotherapy about 20 years ago. Obviously, it was necessary to acquire certain technical and technological advances for its application

Soon, the advantages of HDR regime compared to LDR brachytherapy of prostate cancer were noticed, which are reflected in: the high precision of application, the possibility of subsequent dose optimization, more accurate dose planning and application, sparing the surrounding tissues and organs, more favorable radiobiological effect, the fact that after treatment there are no sources of radiation in the patient and therefore no possibility of source "seeds" migration into the bladder, rectum or surrounding larger blood vessels, there is no irradiation of staff, there is the possibility of extending indicational scope of application and easier possibility of combination with transcutaneous radiotherapy. However, when it comes to temporary HDR brachytherapy of prostate cancer as monotherapy, less obvious results and experiences are presented in the literature, so one can get the wrong impression that this modality of brachytherapy is either less efficient or at very least, least mystified. To clarify this problem to an extent, if not totally resolve, the association of American Brachytherapy Society has formed a High-Dose Rate Task Group (Hsu, C., Yamada, Y., Vigneaut, E., Pouliout, J.) with the aim to define general criteria for inclusion of patients with prostate cancer in the treatment group Temporary implants (HDR), which was formed following the general criteria for inclusion: clinical stageT1-T3 and selected T4, Gleason Score any, PSA no upper limit, no distant metastases (T1-3N0M0). Criteria for relative exclusion are: severe urinary obstruction, extensive TUR defects, the TUR within 6 months, vascular disease. Absolute contraindications are impossibility to anesthesia and no possibility of peaceful lying

Given all the above-mentioned recommendations, for inclusion and exclusion, and in particular those given by the American Brachytherapy Society, extended operational criteria and opinions can be formed related to the application of HDR brachytherapy in different patient groups, including recommendations on the total dose and method of its fractions, and as:

- monotherapy - with tumor stage T1-T2 N0 M0, Gleason Score <7 and prostate volume to 70 cc and T3 confined to the prostate (TD - 31.5 Gy/3 fr. To TD45/6 hypofractioned (Duchesne & Peters, 1999) or hyperfractioned / pause between the fraction of at least 6 hours or even up to 54Gy/9 fr./5 days (Yoshioka et al., 2006) (where the stage T3 N0 M0 may include seminal vessicles);
- boost in the combined radiotherapy approach (TD - 12 (Mate et al., 1998) -24 (Demanes et al., 2009) Gy/1-4 fr. EBRT ± 36-50Gy or 9-15Gy/1-2 fr. EBRT ± 65Gy);
- for recurrent disease confined to the prostate (depending on the previousl therapy TD> Gy/1-2 7-14 fr. to 8Gy/4 fr.)
- further: to have no contraindications (no indication for exclusion).

3.2.1 Results of high dose rate brachytherapy

Yoshioka et al (Yoshioka et al., 2006) presented the results of 111 patients (15 low, 28 medium and 68 high risk, according to the ASTRO criteria (ASTRO, 1997) treated with HDR temporary implantation (monotherapy), showing a three year and five-year survival without signs of biochemical disease of 83% and 70%, and overall survival of 100% and 97%, respectively. For the 17 patients from high risk groups, in which biochemical relapse was observed, in 9 patients the presence of distant metastases were confirmed, of which 4 patients died. Given that this group of patients is not stratified based on risk, it is clear that the shown results after the HDR brachytherapy are comparable or even better than in patients treated with permanent implants (monotherapy) (Blasko et al., 2000, Beyer, 2001, Greem et al., 1997).

3.2.2 Toxicity of high dose rate brachytherapy

Mild and transient acute urinary symptoms (dysuria and hematuria of grade G1) followed HDR brachytherapy in about 50% of patients in the first week or two, and persist for up to 6 months in less than 35% of treated patients, while grade G2 symptoms occurred in about 11 % of patients in the first weeks after treatment and after 6 months they completely disappeared. Pronounced symptoms of grade G3 (urethral stricture at the level of bladder base) are very rare (less than 2%), and they require a retention of urinary catheter, and usually occur immediately after irradiation, and disappear within ten days. Acute symptoms of grade G1 rectum (proctitis, tenesma and bleeding) are rare and mainly are result of edema and hematoma, and occur in less than 25% of patients in the first weeks and decrease to about 8% in the 6-month after conducted therapy. Acute complications of grade G3 were not observed.

All listed acute symptoms may be connected to radiation and trauma during application procedure, although problems have not been noted during the application itself.

The frequency and severity of late complications after HDR brachytherapy is similar to the permanent implant brachytherapy (LDR), except that complications associated with the migration of radiation sources do not occur.

When HDR brachytherapy (22-24 Gy/5-6 fr.) is applied in combination with transcutaneous radiotherapy (EBRT to 40Gy), the results of treatment (five-year survival NED/biochemical/and overall survival) of 63% in patients with high risk are comparable and slightly better than with the application of brachytherapy (LDR and HDR) as a monotherapy. (Deamens et al., 2009) In the same paper, the authors conclude that no benefit was noted when applying deprivate androgen therapy in relation to combined radiotherapy.

Acute and late effects on the bladder and rectum are more pronounced in cases of combined radiotherapy, which can be expected.

4. Postoperative radiotherapy in prostate cancer

Radical prostatectomy is proven treatment modality for prostate cancer control for a long time. Some authors report 10-year cancer-specific survival of 85-90% in localized prostate cancer after radical prostatectomy, and 82% at 15 years. Survival is better if the tumor is low grade i.e. low Gleason score and low stage.

The risk of surgical margins positivity is of great concern after radical prostatectomy. Positive margins are noticed in 28% of patients with T1-T2 prostate cancer and prostate apex is the most common site. For T3 cancers this percent is even higher-up to 52%.

High tumor stage (T3a and T3b) and a positive surgical margin are strong predictors of local recurrence, biochemical and clinical failure. In general, it is considered that the percent of local recurrence after radical prostatectomy ranges about 15% for T2 prostate cancers, and 50-70% for T3 tumors.

In order to analyze the impact of predictive factors on development of local recurrence, univariate and multivariate analyzes were performed. In univariate analyzes strong predictors of local relapse are high-grade cancer, positive surgical margins and involvement of seminal vesicles. In multivariate analyzes these predictors are high-grade tumor, positive surgical margin and elevate prostatic phosphatase.

Identification of patients that are candidates for adjuvant therapies after radical prostatectomy is still a great issue. The adequate treatment modality for these patients is an open question too. There is no consensus yet.

After radical prostatectomy, the application of radiotherapy can lower the incidence of local relapses, but its effect on distant metastases appearance is not confirmed. Alternative regimen is the use of androgen-deprivation therapy alone or in combination with radiotherapy which can also improve local control and eradication of distant metastases. (Hadzi-Djokic, 2005)

Three randomized trials (Bolla, Wiegel & Thompson), have shown an advantage in biochemical relapse-free survival with postoperative radiotherapy for men with positive surgical margins or pT3 disease. These trials compared postoperative radiotherapy with 60-Gy to the prostatic fossa to radical prostatectomy alone in men with high-risk prostate cancer. With the use of postoperative irradiation the 5-year biochemical progression-free survival was significantly improved, as well as clinical progression-free survival. Thompson's trial has also show an advantage of overall survival (10.3 years for irradiated patients after prostatectomy to 3.1 year for prostatectomy only). Bolla failed to demonstrate this advantage. That means that not all men with adverse prognostic factors will relapse. Also, not all men treated with postoperative radiotherapy will be cured. Combined treatment is also associated with greater toxicity than radiotherapy or prostatectomy alone. So what will the optimal treatment be? (Hayden et al., 2010, Bolla et al., 2005, Wiegel et al., 2009, Thompson et al., 2009) Eastham et al. managed to give actually 4 possible scenarios for post-prostatectomy setting: (1) there is no residual disease and adjuvant radiation is not necessary; (2) persistent disease is present in the prostatic fossa only and adjuvant irradiation may provide long-term cure; (3) there is a residual local disease as well as microscopic disseminated disease and adjuvant irradiation may eradicate local disease but will have no impact on the systemic component; (4) disease is only systemic and adjuvant local irradiation is not necessary.

Salvage radiotherapy in the setting of a rising PSA after prostatectomy is unproven and still controversial. This is most likely the result of inadequately selected patients for post-prostatectomy irradiation. Many of them already have systemic recurrence so a detail diagnostic workout is necessary. (Eastham et al., 2010)

The special issue is the use of adjuvant hormone therapy. Some studies show that the application of adjuvant hormone therapy reduces the risk of positive surgical margins, improves local disease control, eradicates micro metastases and prolongs time to progression and overall survival. On the other hand, neoadjuvant hormone therapy, prior to surgery, in order to downstage the disease, has not been proven for successes neither in preventing biochemical or clinical relapse nor in improving survival so in most centres it is deserted. (Dearnaley, 2005)

5. Androgen-derprivation therapy combined with radiotherapy of the prostate cancer

Radiotherapy is traditionally the treatment of choice in locally advanced prostate cancer. Unfortunately the results of radical radiotherapy regarding 10-years and 15-years overall survivals are not satisfactory (Zlotecki, 2001) (Table 3.)

Androgen deprivation therapy is used routinely in combination with radiotherapy for locally advanced prostate cancer, but recent studies show that it improves treatment result is localized and intermediate-risk disease.(Milecki et al., 2010).

Hormone therapy, that is in fact androgen deprivation, can be realized in several ways: orchyectomy, blockade of the hypothalamus-hypophysis-gonade path (with gonadothropin realizing hormone agonist) or by direct blockade of androgen receptors with androgen antagonists. (Anderson, 2003) Although, it is generally thought that androgen deprivation combined with radiotherapy influence the results of treatment in local and systemic way, it is uncertain whether that action is the result of radiosensitizing, systemic micro metastases eradication or both. Androgen deprivation leads to the shrinkage of the entire prostate gland reducing the irradiated volume to which the higher dose can be applied. In several studies this prostate shrinkage is ranging form 30% to 40%. Some authors say that it improves radiotherapy effectiveness by oxygenation of hypoxic cancer cells and that it even induces apoptosis and tumoricidal immune system response.

Study/Institution	Clinical T stage	10 Year Survival (%)	15 Year Survival (%)
Pattern of Care	T3-T4	33	23
RTOG 75-06	T3-T4	38	No results
Mallinckrodt	T3	38	No results
Stanford	T3	35	18
Stanford	T4	15	15
M.D. Anderson	T3	45	31

Table 3. 10 and 15-year survival rate for patients with locally advanced prostate cancer treated with radical RT

The role of androgen deprivation therapy is unclear in men with low risk prostate cancer but some patients still received it as primary or neoadjuvant treatment. The Radiation Therapy Oncology Group (RTOG) 94-08 randomized trial included almost 2000 men with T1b-T2 prostate cancer and PSA less than 20ng/ml. Androgen deprivation therapy was administered 4 months prior or concomitantly with radiotherapy. Overall survival at 8 years was 76% vs. 73% for combined treatment and radiotherapy only, respectively. The disease-specific survival was 98% for hormone and irradiation vs. 99% for radiotherapy alone. This study did not bring solid results, as well as many others, because some patients were clinically in a higher risk stage than deemed low risk according to National Comprehensive Network classification. Retrospective studies of Bolla et al. and Cietzki at al. are among few that have shown the advantage of radiotherapy combine with androgen-deprivation in low risk prostate cancer (Milecki et al., 2010)

For intermediate and high-risk patients many randomized studies were performed such as RTOG 85-31 (977 patients T1-T2, T3, N+, adjuvant hormone therapy vs. radiotherapy alone), RTOG 86-10 (456 patients, T2-T4, neoadjuvant/concomitant hormone therapy for 4 months vs. radiotherapy alone), EORTC 22863 (415 patients, T1-T4 prostate cancer, concomitant/adjuvant hormone therapy for 36 months vs. radiotherapy alone). In 5-years follow-up all of them have shown a statistically significant difference in improved local disease control, reduction of distant metastases and longer progression free survival in hormone therapy-radiotherapy group. (Jelić et al., 2005) (Table 4.)

	N	Stage	Therapy	Therapy duration	Local control	PFS (%)	OS (%)	Follow-up
RTOG 85-31	977	T1-T2, N+,T3	Adj vs. only RT	>24m vs. 0	+	53 vs. 20 p<0.0001	Gs 8-10 66 vs. 55 p=0.03	5 years
RTOG 86-10	456	T2-T4	Neoadj/conc vs. only RT	4m vs. 0	+	33 vs. 21 p=0.004	Gs 2-6 70 vs. 52 p=0.015	5 years
EORTC 22863	415	T1-T4	conc/adj vs. only RT	36m vs. 0	+	85 vs. 48 p<0.001	79 vs. 62 p=0.01	5 years
RTOG 92-02	1554	T2c-T4	Neoadj/conc /adj vs. Neoadj/conc	28m vs. 0	+	46.4 vs. 28.1 p<0.001	Gs 8-10 81 vs. 70.7 p=0.044	5 years
RTOG 94-13	1323	T1c-T4	Neoadj vs. adj	4m vs. 4m	+	NA	NA	4 years

Table 4. Hormone therapy and RT. Randomized studies

Bolla M. recommends concomitant and adjuvant hormone therapy for three years in combination with radiotherapy for patients with locally advanced, intermediate or high-risk prostate cancer. (Bolla, 2003)

Although it is shown that androgen deprivation before, concomitantly and/or after radiotherapy significantly improves local disease control, minimizes progression and prolongs overall survival in locally advanced prostate cancer on intermediate and high-risk, there is not enough evidence for recommendation of optimal time to start hormone therapy, the type of hormones and the duration of the treatment which in clinical trials lasts from 3 months to 3 years. (ESMO, 2003)

6. Radiotherapy In metastatic prostate cancer

For patients in which prostate cancer develops quickly with bony and/or other metastases and elevation of PSA, androgen deprivation is considered a therapeutic method of choice. It includes orchyectomy or TAB. Radiotherapy is considered only as palliative for painful bony metastases or threatening pathological fracture.

Radiotherapy of bony metastases is mostly performed as local therapy to involved bones but sometimes it can be applied as half-body or total-body irradiation. For solitary or localized bony metastases radiotherapy is applied through simple fields (two opposed fields, single direct field etc). A higher daily dose of 2.5 Gy or 3 Gy is given. Single dose of 8 Gy (single shoot), 20 Gy in 5 fractions or 30Gy in 10 fractions are considered to have the same results regarding pain relief and survival.

Half-body irradiation is performed when there are many disseminated bony metastases and probably as many occult. The dose of 8 Gy is applied to lower half, and 6 Gy to upper half of the body. If we treat the whole body, the gap between irradiation of upper and lower half of the body is four weeks. (Samija et al., 1996)

On the other hand, for patients with extensive locoregional prostate cancer, radiotherapy can be applied to pelvis with a total dose of 50-60Gy in order to reduce pain, hemathuria, urethral obstruction or lymphedema (Jelić, 2005)

7. New radiation techniques

The biological effect of ionizing radiation to cancer cells and normal tissues it based on the fact that the cancer cells are more susceptible to radiation because the lack of normal repair mechanism. Hypofractionated radiotherapy can reduce the duration of treatment since larger dose is given per day and the cumulative dose is adjusted to a lower dose. The randomized trials that compared hypofractionation with conventional RT did not have long enough follow-up and used to low total dose for current standards. But the investigation is still on. The extreme form of hypofractionation is stereotactic body radiotherapy (radiosurgery). This method uses only few fractions but with very high doses applied to a target volume in a very precise fashion. Although these techniques are attractive for theoretical advantage in radiobiology, the risk of late toxicity is considerable.

Another possible radiotherapy approach to enhance radiotherapeutic ratio for prostate cancer is to utilize charged particles such as protons and carbon ions. The clinical benefit is still unclear but the optimism is based upon the fact that charged particles deposit most of their energy at a given depth followed by a dose fall-of with almost no dose deposition beyond the point of maximal dose called Bragg peak which can lead to increased normal tissue sparing. For proton therapy, a dosimetric analysis did not show a significant improvement in conformity to spare normal tissues over photon IMRT. Clinical outcome and toxicity is also similar. Carbon ion has the same dose distribution as proton beams with Bragg peak and following dose fall-of. But the relative biological effectiveness of carbon ion is four times higher than protons and photons that can lead to improved local tumor control without causing more toxicity. However these technologies are still developing and results are yet to be seen. (Choe & Liauw, 2010)

8. Conclusion

Radiotherapy is widely used as curative treatment modality for many cases of prostate cancer. There is a diverse array of radiotherapeutic strategies that can be effectively used to treat both organ-confined and locally advanced disease, alone or in combination with androgen-deprivation therapy. In recent decades it has undergone significant clinical and technological advances that aim to optimize cancer control outcomes while minimizing treatment morbidity.

9. References

Al-Mamgani, A., Van Putten, WL., Heemsbergen, WD. et al. (2008). Update of Dutch multicenter dose-escalation trial of radiotherapy for localized prostate cancer. *International Journal of Radiation Oncology Biology Physics*, vol. 72, pp. (980-988)

American Society for Theapeutic Radiology and Oncology Consensus Panel, Consensus statement: Guidelines for PSA following radiation therapy. (1997). *International Journal of Radiation Oncology Biology Physics*, vol. 37, pp. (1035-1041)

Anderson, J. (2003). Treatment of Prostate Cancer. The Role of Primary Hormonal Therapy. *EAU Update Series*, vol. 1, pp. (32-39)

Aus, G., Abbou, C., Bolla, M. et al. (2001). Guidelines on prostate cancer. *European Urology*, vol. 40, no. 2, pp. (97-101)

Beyer, D. (2001). The evolving role of prostate brachytherapy. *Cancer Control*, vol. 8, pp. (163-170)

Blasko, J., Grimm, D., Sylvester, E. et al. (2000). Paladium 103 brachytherapy for prostate carcinoma. *International Journal of Radiation Oncology Biology Physics*, vol. 46, pp. (839-850)

Blasko, J., Grimm, D., Sylvester, E. et al. (2000). The role of external beam radiotherapy with I-125/Pd-103 brachytherapy for prostate carcinoma. *Radiotherapy and Oncology*, vol. 57, pp. (273-278)

Boehmer, D., Maingon, P., Poortman, P. et al. (2006). Guidelines for primary radiotherapy of patients with prostate cancer. *Radiotherapy and Oncology*, vol. 79, pp. (259-269)

Bolla, M. (2003). Treatment of Locally Advanced Prostate Cancer. The Clinical Use of Radiotherapy. *EAU Update Series*, vol. 1, pp. (23-31)

Bolla, M., van Poppel, H., Collette, L. et al. (2005). Postoperative radiotherapy after radical prostatectomy: a randomized controlled trial (EORTC trial 22911). *Lancet*, vol. 366, pp. (572-578)

Chao, KSC., Perez, C., & Brady, LW. (2002). Prostate, In: *Radiation oncology management decision*, pp. (447-467), Lippincot-Williams&Wilkins, ISBN 0-7817-3222-0, Philadelphia

Choe, KS., & Liauw, SL. (2010). Radiotherapeutic strategies in the management of low-risk prostate cancer. *The Scientific World JOURNAL: TSW* Urology, vol. 10, pp. (1854-1869)

Common Toxicity Criteria Version 2.0, DCTD, NCI, NIH, DHHS. (1999). Cancer Therapy Graduation Programme. RTOG: Late radiation morbidity scoring system.

Deamens, J., Brandt, D., Schour, L. et al. (2009). Excellent results from high dose rate brachytherapy and external beam for prostate cancer are not improved by androgen deprivation. *American Journal of Clinical Oncology*, vol. 32, pp. (342-347)

Dearnaley, DP., (2001). Radiotherapy and combined modality approaches in localized prostate cancer. *Prostate Cancer. Educational Book. ECCO 11*, pp. (137-140), Lisbon

Dearnaley, DP., (2005). Radiotherapy in locally advanced prostate cancer. *EJC Education Book. ECCO 13*, pp. (317-330), Paris

Dearnaley, DP., Sydes, MR., Graham, JD. et al. (2007). Escalated-dose versus standard-dose conformal radiotherapy in prostate cancer: first results from MRC RT01 randomized controlled trial. *Lancet Oncology*, vol. 8, pp. (475-487)

Dobbs, J., Barrett, A., & Ash, D., (1999). Prostate, In: *Practical radiotherapy planning*, pp. (271-280), Arnold, ISBN 0-340-70-631-7, Great Britain

Duchesne, G., & Peters, L. (1999). What is the alpha/beta ratio for prostate cancer? Rationale for hypofractionated high-dose-rate brachytherapy. *International Journal of Radiation Oncology Biology Physics*, vol. 44, pp. (747-748)

Eastham, JA., Chirstopher, PE., & Zietman, A. (2010). What is the optimal management of high risk, clinically localized prostate cancer? *Urologic Oncology*, vol. 28, pp. (557-567)

ESMO Minimum Clinical Recommendations for Diagnosis, Treatment and Follow up of Prostate Cancer. (2003). *Annals of Oncology*, vol. 14, pp. (1010-1011)

Fiorino, C., Valdagni, R., Rancati, T. et al. (2009). Dose-volume effects for normal tissues in external radiotherapy: pelvis. *Radiotherapy and Oncology*, vol. 93, pp. (153-167)

Gazdda, MJ., Lawrence, R., & Coia, MD. (1996/97). *Radiation treatment planning and techniques. Cancer Management: A Multidisciplinary Approach. Medical, Surgical & Radiation Oncology*, pp. (593-604), Huntington, New York

Greem, P., Blasko, J., Ragde, H. et al. (1997). Transperineal ultrosund guided 1251/103Pd brachytherapy for early stage prostate cancer: Update on clinical experience at seven years. *International Journal of Radiation Oncology Biology Physics*, vol. 39, pp. (219)

Grey, J., Merricks, S., Beyer, D. et al. (2000). Comparartive analysis of prostate brachytherapy pre-planing. *Radiotherapy and Oncology*, vol. 55, pp. (42-43)

Hadži-Đokić, J. (2005). *Lokalizovani karcinom prostate*, Elit. Medica, Beograd

Hayden, AJ., Catton, C., & Pickles, T. (2010). Radiotherapy in prostate cancer: a risk risk-adapted strategy. *Urologic Oncology*, vol. 17, no. 2, pp. (18-24)

Hayden, AJ., Martin, JM., Kneebone, AB. et al. (2010). Australian & New Zealand faculty of radiation oncology genito-urinary group; 2010 consensus guidelines for definitive external beam radiotherapy for prostate carcinoma. *Journal of Medical Imaging and Radiation Oncology*, vol. 54, pp. (513-525)

Heidenereich, A., Bellmunt, J., Bolla, M. et al. (2011). EAU guidelines on prostate cancer. Part 1: screening, diagnosis and treatment of clinically localized prostate cancer. *European Urology*, vol. 59, pp. (61-71)

Jelić, Lj., Stojanović, S., & Popov, I. (2005). Radiotherapy in prostate cancer treatment. *Acta Chirurgica Iugoslavica*, vol. 2, no. 4, pp. (93-102)

Jelić, Lj., & Stojanović, S. (2005). Radioterapija karcinoma prostate, In: *Lokalizovani karcinom prostate*, Hadži-Đokić J., pp. (109-118), Elit. Medica, Beograd

Kirby, R., & Madhavan, SG. (2010). Prostate cancer. Renal and urology II, In: *Surgery*, vol. 28, no. 12, pp. (594-598)

Koh, H., Kattan, MW., Scardino, PT. et al. (2003). A nomogram to predict seminal vesicles invasion by the extent and location of cancer in systemic biopsy results. *Journal of Urology*, vol. 170, pp. (1203-1208)

Kuban, DA., Tucker, SL., Dong, L. et al. (2008). Long-term results of the M. D. Anderson randomized dose escalation trial for prostate cancer. *International Journal of Radiation Oncology Biology Physics*, vol. 70, pp. (67-74)

Lawton, CA., Michalski, J., El-Naqa, I. et al. (2009). RTOG GU radiation oncology specialists reach consensus on pelvic lymph node volumes for high risk prostate cancer. *International Journal of Radiation Oncology Biology Physics*, vol. 74, pp. (383-387)

LENT SOMA scales for all anatomic sites. (1995). *International Journal of Radiation Oncology Biology Physics*, vol. 31, pp. (1049-1091)

Malone, S., Szanto, J., Perry, G. et al. (2000). A prospective comparison of three systems of patient immobilization for prostate radiotherapy. *International Journal of Radiation Oncology Biology Physics*, vol. 48, pp. (657-665)

Mate,T., Gottesman, J., Hatton, J. et al. (1998). High-dose-rate afterloading Ir-192 brachytherapy: Feasibility report. *International Journal of Radiation Oncology Biology Physics*, vol. 41, pp. (522-533)

Milecki, P., Martenka, P., Antczak, A. et al. (2010). Radiotherapy combined with hormonal therapy in prostate cancer: the state of art. *Cancer Management and Research*, vol. 2, pp. (243-253)

Thompson, IM., Tangen, CM., Paradelo, J. et al. (2009). Adjuvant radiotherapy for pathological T3N0M0 prostate cancer significantly reduces risk of metastases and improves survival: long term follow-up of a randomized clinical trial. *Journal of Urology*, vol. 181, pp. (956-962)

Valicenti, R., Lu, J., Pilepich, M. et al. (2000). Survival advantage from higher-dose radiation therapy for clinically localized prostate cancer treated on Radiation Oncology Group trials. *Journal of Clinical Oncology*, vol. 18, pp. (2740-2749)

Viani, GA., Stefano, EJ., & Alfonso, SL. (2009). Higher than conventional radiation doses in localized prostate cancer treatment: a meta-analysis of randomized controlled trials. *International Journal of Radiation Oncology Biology Physics*, vol. 74, pp. (1405-1418)

Wiegel, T., Bottke, D., Steiner, U. et al. (2009). Phase III postoperative adjuvant radiotherapy after radical prostatectomy compared with radical prostatectomy alone in T3 prostate cancer with postoperative undetectable prostate-specific antigen: ARO 96-02/AUO AP 09/95. *Journal of Clinical Oncology*, vol. 27, pp. (2924-2930)

Zelefsky, MJ., Fuks, Z., Hunt, M. et al. (2002). High-dose intensity modulated radiation therapy for prostate cancer: early toxicity and biochemical outcome in 772 patients. *International Journal of Radiation Oncology Biology Physics*, vol. 53, pp. (1111-1116)

Zietman, AL., Bac, K., Slater, JD. et al. (2010). Randomized trial comparing conventional-dose with high-dose conformal radiotherapy in early-stage adenocarcinoma of the prostate: long-term results from photon, radiation oncology group/American college of radiology. *Journal of Clinical Oncology*, vol. 28, pp. (1106-1111)

Zivkovic, M., & Deponte, V. (1996.) Palijativna radioterapija, In: *Radioterapija*, Samija, M., Krajina, Z., Purisic, A., pp. (363-378), Nakladni zavod Globus, Zagreb

Zlotecki, RA. (2001). External-Beam Radiation in the Management of Carcinoma of the Prostate. *Cancer Control*, vol. 8, pp. (503-510)

Yoshioka, Y., Konishi, K., Oh, R-J. et al. (2006). High-dose-rate brachytherapy without external beam irradiation for locally advanced prostate cancer. *Radiotherapy and Oncology*, vol. 80, pp. (62-68)

9

Combination of Immunotherapy & Radiotherapy for the Treatment of Prostate Cancer

Zsuzsanna Tabi, Lisa K. Spary and John Staffurth
Department of Oncology, School of Medicine, Cardiff University, Cardiff United Kingdom

1. Introduction

There are around 35,000 new cases of prostate carcinoma (PCa) in the UK per annum, making it the most common solid malignancy. Approximately 10,000 men die of PCa each year in the UK (http://infocancerresearchukorg/cancerstats/). Disease incidence is increasing partly due to earlier detection and the increasing age of the population. Environmental causes especially dietary factors have been postulated but this is still an area of research. At presentation ~60% of patients have localised, ~30% locally advanced and 10% metastatic disease.

Radical radiotherapy (RT) can be used as part of curative therapy for both localised and locally advanced disease but has no proven role in the metastatic setting. Recently, radiation has been shown to cause immunogenic tumour cell death and to modify immunosuppression in the tumour environment. Importantly, reduction of tumour burden by RT, in an ablative setting, has been shown to depend largely on T cell responses (Lee et al., 2009). Combination of ionising radiation (IR) and immunological approaches in pre-clinical models of PCa has also proved to be synergistic. Immunotherapy offers a unique co-treatment that enables the patients' own immune cells to contribute to the success of RT. Immunological memory, developing as the result of the combination treatment, may provide long-term protection from tumour recurrence. There are however very few clinical trials addressing how immunotherapy and RT can be best combined for clinical efficiency.

2. Radiotherapy of prostate cancer

There are four major treatment approaches for localised prostate cancer: active surveillance, radical prostatectomy, external beam radiotherapy (EBRT) and low-dose rate (LDR) brachytherapy. RT is conventionally delivered with photons with delivery systems that have developed considerably over the past decade, leading to lower toxicity and allowing safe dose escalation. Higher doses have been demonstrated to improve tumour control outcomes in several large Phase III trials (Viani et al., 2009). Present trials are evaluating the role of intensity modulated radiotherapy (IMRT), hypofractionation (treatment in ~4 weeks) and improved imaging during treatment with image-guided radiotherapy (IGRT) (Khoo & Dearnaley, 2008). Further developments in EBRT delivery systems allow highly targeted treatment in 5-7 fractions, called stereotactic body radiotherapy (SBRT), although tumour control outcomes are not yet known (King et al., 2011; Madsen et al., 2007).

Proton therapy is the delivery of EBRT using protons instead of photons. Protons have a different pattern of dose delivery within tissue, with energy deposited in a very tightly defined area as the protons slow. This results in less radiation being delivered beyond the target, and has become the radiotherapeutic modality of choice for childhood cancers and several other tumors. The evidence base for proton therapy for prostate cancer is less established, but its use in some countries has become widespread partly due to the results of a dose escalation trial using protons (Coen & Zietman, 2009). Proton therapy has not been compared to dose-equivalent photon-RT. LDR brachytherapy, which uses multiple permanently planted radioactive seeds, can be used to deliver a very high radiation dose to a highly targeted volume in a single treatment with equivalent outcomes to EBRT and surgery.

Locally advanced disease is usually treated with a combination of EBRT and androgen deprivation therapy (ADT) (Shelley et al., 2009; Shelley et al., 2009; Warde et al., 2010). However, the outcome is still relatively poor. Recent and ongoing UK-based trials are currently exploring the potential advantage of dose escalation in either systemic therapies (James et al., 2009; Guerrero Urbano et al., 2010). High dose rate (HDR) brachytherapy, which uses a single high-intensity radiation source that is temporarily inserted into multiple positions in the prostate, may also have a role in locally advanced disease as a single agent or in combination with ADT and/or RT (Hoskin, 2008). EBRT has a proven role as adjuvant or salvage therapy after radical prostatectomy. In the adjuvant setting, it has been shown to reduce the rate of relapse in high risk patients by approximately 50% in three randomised trials (Bolla et al., 2007; Thompson et al., 2006; Wiegel et al., 2009).

The commonest site of metastases in castrate refractory metastatic PCa is bone, with 80% of patients dying with prostate cancer dying with bone metastases. They can cause one of several skeletal-related events, but pain is the predominant problem. Palliative EBRT is highly efficacious for single sites of disease. An alternative approach is the use of therapeutic bone-targeted radioisotopes. The interim results of a trial with a novel alpha-emitting isotope, Radium-223, have reported a 3-month overall survival advantage, (http://www.algeta.com) suggesting that these drugs will be used more widely in the future. Radioimmunotherapy (RIT) refers to the use of antibody labelled with a therapeutic radionuclide, with the aim of delivering a cytotoxic radiation dose specifically to the tumour. The concept is equivalent to bone-targeted radioisotopes, but with the targeting of tumour-associated antigens (TAA) rather than osteoblastic metastases. The same principle can be used for imaging of micrometastatic disease if radionuclides of different properties (radiation type and energy) are used. There is much research in this field over recent years (Bouchelouche et al., 2011), partly due to the increasing number of PCa-specific TAA, as discussed later in this chapter.

3. Immunological aspects of PCa

PCa is an immunogenic cancer, as evidenced by a positive correlation between the frequency of $CD8^+$ tumour-infiltrating T cells and prostate-specific antigen (PSA) recurrence-free survival (Kärjä et al., 2005). Immune cell behaviour towards tumour cells has been described by three stages: (1) elimination of tumour cells, (2) equilibrium between tumour, and immune cells - maintained by active immunological control of the tumour - and (3) escape of tumour cells from immunological control. Apart from evidence from animal models underpinning this theory (Teng et al., 2008), clinical observations of donor-derived melanoma developing in immunosuppressed organ transplant recipients provide indirect evidence about the immune system's role in tumour-control (Strauss & Thomas, 2010). Overcoming anti-tumour immune responses is described as an emerging hallmark of cancer (Hanahan & Weinberg, 2011). Further observations and experiments are accumulating in order to provide firm evidence about the role of anti-tumour immune responses in the control of cancer.

3.1 Tumour-associated antigens in PCa

The specificity of tumour-infiltrating T cells reflects engagement with TAA. The presence of TAA-specific T cells in the TIL pool results in longer median survival compared to those patients whose TIL did not contain tumour-specific T cells, as observed in melanoma (22.5 months vs. 4.5 months) (Haanen et al., 2005). There is no such prognostic correlation for the frequency of TAA-specific T cells in the peripheral blood of patients. TAA-specific T cell infiltration is likely to be important in PCa too.

PCa-associated antigens include prostate-specific differentiation antigens, expressed both on healthy and malignant prostate epithelial cells, such as kallikrein-4, PAP (prostatic acid phosphatase) and PSA. Tumour antigens that are overexpressed on malignant cells (not all specific for PCa) compared to healthy epithelial cells are: PSMA (prostate specific membrane antigen), PSCA (prostate stem cell antigen), Her-2, MUC-1, survivin, STEAP (six transmembrane epithelial antigen of the prostate) and telomerase. Cancer-germline or cancer-testis oncofoetal antigens observed in PCa are not expressed on normal cells, but may be expressed by placental trophoblasts and testicular germ cells, such as NY-ESO, MAGE-C1, MAGE-C2 and 5T4 (Chen et al., 1997; Hudolin et al., 2006; Southall et al., 1990).

More recent additions to the list of potential TAAs in PCa are; AMACR (Honma et al., 2009), WT-1 (Nakatsuka et al., 2006), ADAM-17 (Sinnathamby et al., 2011), RHAMM (CD168) (Gust et al., 2009), SIM2 (Arredouani et al., 2009), TARP (Epel et al., 2008), SH3GLB2 (Fassò et al., 2008) and the androgen receptor (Olson & McNeel, 2011). T cells specific for some of these antigens have been identified in PCa patients and T cell clones or lines killed PCa cells, confirming the suitability of most of these TAA-antigens for targeted therapies.

3.2 Tumour-infiltrating immune cells in PCa

Prostate cancer has a complex microenvironment which develops during the course of tumour development. Tumour cells are surrounded by endothelial cells of blood vessels, stromal fibroblasts, bone marrow-derived cells and lymphocytes. These cells produce growth factors and enzymes that enhance tumour growth and survival, aid stroma-remodelling and recruit further immune cells into the tumour. The two main immune cell types infiltrating the tumour are lymphocytes and myeloid cells.

3.2.1 Lymphocytes

The presence of activated T and/or natural killer (NK) cells in the tumour tissue is a positive prognostic factor in several solid cancers, including PCa (Kärjä et al., 2005; Gannon et al., 2009). $CD8^+$ T cells are responsible for direct killing of target cells which express appropriate peptides on MHC Class I molecules, while NK cells play a role in killing tumour cells which downregulate MHC Class I molecules as an evasion mechanism from T cell recognition. Target cell killing occurs via delivering perforin and apoptosis-inducing granzyme complexes into the target cell (Thiery et al., 2011). $CD4^+$ T cells, depending on their subtype: Th1, Th2, Th17 or T regulatory cells (Treg) produce cytokines which support pro- or anti-inflammatory responses, respectively. CD4+, CD8+ and regulatory T cells are all present in PCa tumour tissue, with CD8+ T cells being predominant, unlike in the peripheral blood where CD4+ T cell frequencies are higher (Bronte et al., 2005). The majority of tumour-infiltrating CD8+ T cells are memory or terminally differentiated cells but their ability to upregulate activation markers is impaired (Bronte et al., 2005; Drake, 2010). In radical prostatectomy specimens of PCa, IFN-γ and perforin expression is lower than in T cells in healthy prostate tissue (Ebelt et al., 2008). Lymphocytes can mainly be observed in clusters in peritumoural areas while only a few infiltrate the tumour areas (Fig. 1).

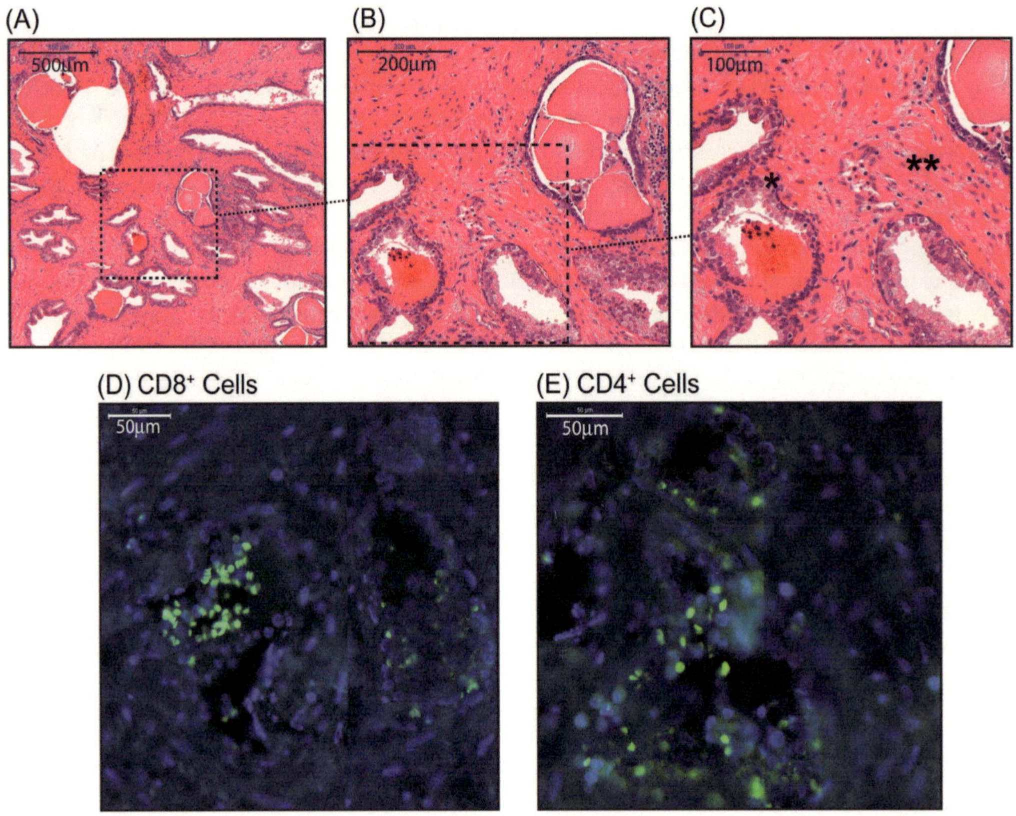

Fig. 1. (A-C) PCa prostatectomy sections stained with haematoxylin and eosin shown at increasing magnifications; (C) a region with glandular (★) and stromal areas (★★). (D) peritumoural CD8+ T lymphocyte cluster, identified by fluorescence microscopy. (E) CD4+ cells are also present in this region.

T cells with regulatory function (CD4+CD25+Foxp3+) are present at higher frequencies in PCa than in healthy tissue. They can be found mainly in T cell clusters surrounding prostate cancer lesions or in the stroma (Ebelt et al., 2009; Miller et al., 2006; Sfanos et al., 2008). Some of these Treg cells express the glucocorticoid-induced TNF-receptor (GITR) and ICOS (a CD28-superfamily costimulatory molecule) at higher levels than in blood, indicating recent activation. They also express CCL22 which mediates Treg cell trafficking into the tumour (Miller et al., 2006). T cell clusters infiltrated by Treg cells often express high levels of PD-1 and B7-H1 markers (Ebelt et al., 2008) which indicates T cell exhaustion and functional impairment.

3.2.2 Myeloid cells

$CD68^+$ monocytes and macrophages have been observed at higher frequencies in PCa compared to benign prostate tissues in a Gleason-score and disease stage-associated manner (Lindholm et al., 2010). $CD68^+$ monocytes and less differentiated $CD11b^+CD33^+$ myeloid cells have been shown by immunohistochemistry to be present in PCa stroma (Sorrentino et al., 2011). There is no information available as to whether these cells function as tumour-associated macrophages (TAM) or myeloid-derived suppressor cells (MDSC). Monocytic MDSC have been characterised as $CD11b^+$, $CD14^+$, $CD15^{+/-}$, $CD16^-$, $CD33^+$, $CD66b^+$, $CD124^+$, $VEGFR1^-$ and $HLA\text{-}DR^{low}$ cells (Gabrilovich & Nagaraj, 2009; Marigo et al., 2008). More work is needed to establish if immunosuppressive MDSC are present in the microenvironment in PCa. Myeloid-derived dendritic cells (DC) have also been documented in PCa tissues although at relatively low frequencies and in a minimally activated state (Troy et al., 1998).

3.3 Immune evasion in PCa

The most common immunosuppressive factors in the tumour tissue include vascular endothelial growth factor (VEGF), transforming growth factor beta (TGF-β), interleukin (IL)-10 and adenosine which inhibit proliferation, differentiation and activation of T lymphocytes and DC.

VEGF supports tumour growth and metastasis by initiating endothelial cell proliferation and the formation of new blood vessels, thus providing a continuous blood supply to the tumour (Carmeliet & Jain, 2000). Increased angiogenesis has been observed in PCa tissue compared to benign prostatic hyperplasia (BPH) (Jackson et al., 1997). VEGF production by PCa cells in vitro is enhanced by addition of IL-1 and tumour necrosis factor alpha (TNF-α), both of which are found in the tumour microenvironment in PCa (Ferrer et al., 1997). VEGF is also important in immune suppression not only by inhibiting DC maturation and T cell development but also by acting as a chemoattractant for MDSC (Gabrilovich et al., 1996; Ohm et al., 2003; Oyama et al., 1998).

TGF-β is a pleiotropic cytokine. During PCa development it first acts as a tumour suppressor and later switches roles to become a tumour promoter and immunosuppressor in the tumour environment. TGF-β regulates immune cells by inhibiting cytotoxic T cell function, supporting the development of Treg cells and interfering with DC differentiation (Wan & Flavell, 2007; Wrzesinski et al., 2007). PCa-derived TGF-β has been shown to convert $CD4^+CD25^-$ T cells into $CD4^+$ $CD25^+$ $Foxp3^+$ Treg cells (Liu et al., 2007).

The anti-inflammatory cytokine IL-10 secreted by tumour and stromal cells can inhibit proliferation, differentiation and activation of T lymphocytes via impaired DC (Sato et al., 2002). In the presence of IL-10, alternatively activated DC maintain an immature phenotype in the tumour microenvironment and induce tolerance rather than immune activation and support Treg cell development (H Huang et al., 2010).

Extracellular adenosine is generated from ATP or ADP via the combined action of CD39 and CD73. These are ecto-nucleoside triphosphate diphosphohydrolases which, in the tumour tissue, are predominantly expressed on Treg cells while CD73 is also expressed on CD8+ T cells and tumour cells (CD73) (Stagg & Smyth, 2010). CD39 and CD73 are also expressed on tumour-derived exosomes, thus potentially extending the immunosuppressive tumour microenvironment (Clayton et al., 2010). Adenosine, generated by CD39 (ATP to ADP) and CD73 (ADP and AMP to adenosine) engage androgen receptors on effector T cells, monocytes and DC. As a consequence, pro-inflammatory cytokine production (IL-2, IL-4, IFNγ, TNFα, IL-12) and co-stimulatory molecule expression (e.g. CD86) decreases and cyclic AMP (cAMP) accumulates in these cells. cAMP further amplifies anti-inflammatory responses (Ernst et al., 2010).

Cytokines, such as monocyte chemotactic protein-1 (MCP-1) and stromal-derived factor-1 alpha (SDF-1α) secreted by tumour cells and tumour-associated stromal cells have been associated with enhanced prostate epithelial cell proliferation and migration (Begley et al., 2005; Lu et al., 2006). They also induce the recruitment of myeloid cells at the tumour site and suppress immune responses (Allavena et al., 2008; Loberg et al., 2007). TAM also produce MCP-1 resulting in an amplification loop for further monocyte recruitment (Allavena et al., 2008).

4. Immunological aspects of radiation therapy

The effects of IR on human tissue have been studied for decades. The key therapeutic effect is thought to be via direct killing of tumour cells by initiating irreparable double-stranded DNA breaks. However, the consequences of RT are much more complex than that, as radiation also affects tumour stroma, including tumour-resident immune cells, and results in the re-modelling of the tumour microenvironment. One of the consequences is the reduction of immunosuppression in the tumour tissue.

4.1 IR-mediated release of cellular tumour antigens

The details of the multiple cellular events downstream of radiation-induced DNA damage are beyond the scope of this chapter. The damage results in activation of damage recognition pathways and proliferative arrest, which can ultimately be repaired (fully or partially), or lead to cell death. RT-induced apoptotic and necrotic tumour cell death provide a cellular source of tumour antigens. The tissue damage attracts phagocytic cells to the site of radiation. Monocytes, macrophages and dendritic cells (DC) phagocytose and process dead tumour cells and carry TAA into draining lymph nodes where antigen presentation and T cell stimulation occur. Contrary to natural cell death which occurs without generating an inflammatory response, IR-treated tumour cells express heat shock proteins, translocate antigens such as calreticulin (CR) from the endoplasmic reticulum to the cell surface and passively release high mobility group protein B1 (HMGB1). DNA, RNA and ATP release are also observed at the site of radiation damage. Phagocytosis and simultaneous signalling in DC by HMGB1 via Toll-like receptors (TLR) such as TLR4 and TLR2, or via RAGE (receptor for advanced glycan end products) trigger DC to release IL-1β and present TAA in an immunogenic manner to T cells and B cells (Ma et al., 2011). ATP, released by damaged cells, also contributes to DC maturation via stimulating purinergic P2RX7 receptors and driving IL-1β secretion (Aymeric et al., 2010). Local radiation of mouse B16 tumour has generated DC efficiently cross-present tumour antigens in a Type I interferon (IFN)-dependent manner (Burnette et al., 2011). Single nucleotide polymorphisms (SNP) of TLR4 (Asp299Gly and Thr399Ilr) or P2RX7 (Glu496Ala) (Sluyter et al., 2004; Arbour et al., 2000), which affect the function of these molecules, may be associated with worse prognosis, as shown in breast cancer patients undergoing chemotherapy (Apetoh et al., 2007).

4.2 Chemokine and cytokine induction by IR

Tumour cells, not killed by IR, respond to radiation by increasing the production of pro-inflammatory cytokines that include TNFα, IL-1α/β, IL-6 and IL-8 (Shiao & Coussens, 2010; Formenti & Demaria, 2009; Van Der Meeren et al., 1999; Matsumura & Demaria, 2010). The main effect of these cytokines is an inflammatory response and the recruitment of activated T cells and macrophages to irradiated tumours (Formenti & Demaria, 2009). The widely used PCa cell line, LNCaP, is extremely sensitive to TNFα (Chopra et al., 2004). TNFα-treatment results in growth-arrest and apoptosis of LNCaP cells but not of normal prostate epithelial cells, suggesting that IR-induced TNFα expression may selectively induce apoptosis of tumour cells without affecting normal prostate epithelial cells. Immune cell recruitment is further enhanced by the production of the chemokine CXCL16 which is induced by IL-1β and TNFα, both upregulated by IR (Lu et al., 2008). PCa cell lines (LNCaP, DU145, C4-2B and PC3) produce CXCL16 in culture without IR treatment (Lu et al., 2008).

4.3 Irradiated tumour cells become sensitive to immune cell attack

In tumour cells, not killed by IR, surface molecules such as MHC, the death receptor Fas and heat-shock proteins become upregulated (Shiao & Coussens, 2010; Garnett et al., 2004; Lugade et al., 2008). IR-induced upregulation of MHC Class I molecules, on both tumour cells and APC, improves antigen presentation and may enhance tumour cell recognition by activated $CD8^+$ cells that infiltrate the tumour at an enhanced rate following radiation (Reits et al., 2006; Lugade et al., 2005).

Adhesion molecules, such as intracellular adhesion molecule (ICAM)-1, vascular cell adhesion molecule (VCAM)-1 and platelet endothelial cell adhesion molecule (PECAM)-1, along with integrins, selectins and cadherins are also upregulated in the tumour tissue by IR (Baluna et al., 2006; Lugade et al., 2008). ICAM-1 is known to be upregulated by inflammatory cytokines such as TNFα, IL-1α/β and IL-6 thus resulting in lymphocyte and macrophage accumulation in inflamed tissues. As previously discussed, these cytokines are upregulated in the tumour tissue as a response to IR. ICAM-1 has an important role in enhancing T cell killing via cell-cell adhesion to lymphocyte function-associated antigen (LFA)-1 and by directly co-stimulating activated T cells (Garnett et al., 2004; Baluna et al., 2006). PCa cells express ICAM-1 and VCAM-1 and in tissue areas of high lymphocyte and neutrophil accumulation the expression of ICAM-1 is significantly elevated (Fujita et al., 2008; Rokhlin & Cohen, 1995). These data suggest that ICAM-1 upregulation by IR may facilitate immune responses by recruiting lymphocytes and macrophages to the tumour site. Increased adhesion between tumour cells with upregulated ICAM-1 and activated $CD8^+$ T cells expressing $LFA\text{-}1^+$ may result in more powerful cytotoxic T cell activity.

4.4 Direct effect of IR on immune cells

Immune cells are highly susceptible to IR-induced damage and readily undergo apoptosis. Therapeutic doses of RT often result in lymphopenia. One of the potential immunologically positive effects of direct IR on tumour-infiltrating immune cells is the depletion of Treg cells. However, there is some controversy regarding this question. Cao et al. observed that the proportion of $Foxp3^+$ cells within purified $CD4^+CD25^+$ T cell population decreased significantly (48.2% to 23.3%) following irradiation with 1.8 Gy in vitro and was abolished (1.2%) by 30 Gy. The suppressive function of these Treg cells was also impaired by IR probably due to loss of membrane-bound TGF-β (Cao et al., 2009). Tregs were especially sensitive to low-dose radiation compared to effector T cells (Cao et al., 2011). Another study, in TRAMP mice, had the opposite findings: Treg cell numbers increased in immune organs after local or whole body irradiation without changes to their functional activity (Kachikwu et al., 2010), indicating relative resistance to 0-20 Gy radiation. It remains to be seen what happens to Tregs in situ during RT of PCa.

We showed recently that lymphopenia following prostate and pelvic RT causes preferential death of naïve or unstimulated T-cells (Tabi et al., 2010). Elevated frequencies of Treg cells were observed in the circulation following 44 Gy radiation in 20 fractions to the pelvic nodes and 55 Gy to the prostate (Fig.2). T cell proliferative function was also impaired (Tabi et al., 2010) but it was restored in vitro with exogenous IL-2 without increasing Treg frequencies (Fig. 2). This indicates that IL-2 maybe used to support T cell function after patients completed standard RT.

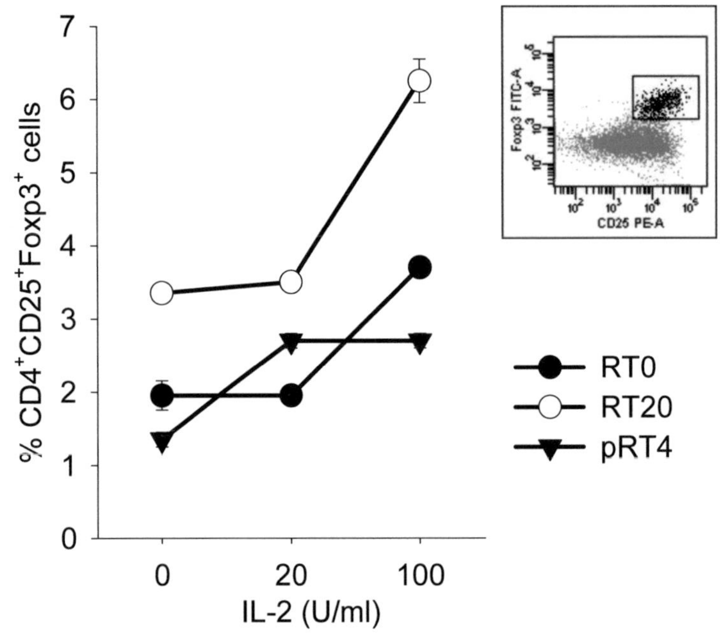

Fig. 2. IL-2 response of Treg cells from the peripheral blood of PCa patients undergoing standard RT. Frequencies of $CD4^+CD25^+Foxp3^+$ T cells (see gate in insert) were measured before (RT0), immediately after radical radiation in 20 fractions (RT20) and 4 weeks after the last fraction (pRT4). Means and SD of triplicates are shown from a representative patient. Frequencies of Tregs were elevated at RT20, but returned to pre-radiation (RT0) level at pRT4. Unlike at RT0 or RT20, exogenous IL-2, added to the cells in vitro, did not increase Treg frequencies at pRT4.

Most importantly, we identified novel TAA-specific T-cell responses post-RT (Tabi et al., 2010), which were not present before RT. Similar findings were observed by others (Nesslinger et al., 2007; Schaue et al., 2008), indicating the ability of radiation to shift the balance between tumour-specific regulatory and effector immune mechanisms.

5. RT and immunotherapy combination modalities

5.1 Pre-clinical models

The use of IL-2 as a monotherapy in cancer has been extensively researched but due to issues with toxicity its clinical use has been limited. In the murine renal adenocarcinoma model, IR was found to augment the response of pulmonary metastases to IL-2 therapy (Younes et al., 1995). Following IR to one lung, plus systemic IL-2 treatment, a reduction in tumour size was observed in both lungs. The effect is dose-dependent and immunohistological studies show significant infiltration of T cells and macrophages at the tumour site. IL-2 is capable of rescuing T cells from IR-induced apoptosis and restores T cell proliferation after RT (Tabi et al., 2010). Its use in combination with RT may minimise the immunosuppressive effects of RT and enhance tumour cell killing via T cells (Mor & Cohen, 1996). In PCa, the combination of IL-2 and radiation in a mouse bone metastases model demonstrated a ~50% inhibition of tumour growth (Hillman et al., 2003). There was a greater degree of tumour destruction in IL-2-treated irradiated tumours than in irradiated tumours alone and the histology revealed increased fibrosis and elevated numbers of infiltrating inflammatory immune cells.

Antitumour effects were also observed in a model utilising IL-12 and RT. IL-12 is secreted by mature DC and macrophages and required for IFNγ and TNFα production from T cells and mediates a Th1-type immune response. Adenovirus-derived IL-12 plus RT significantly increased local antitumour and systemic antimetastatic effects in a preclinical model of metastatic PCa when compared to either treatment alone (Fujita et al., 2008). This antimetastatic activity is due to the antitumoural activities of natural killer (NK) cells. These results were also observed in the 4T1 mammary carcinoma. The combination of RT and an adenoviral vector encoding IL-12 and the co-stimulatory molecule CD80 resulted in a significant reduction in tumour growth (Lohr et al., 2000). The antitumour effect observed in the combination therapy group was far superior if the IL-12 and CD80-expressing adenovirus was administered after the final fraction of radiation.

Further cytokine studies have evaluated the combined effect of IL-3 and RT. IL-3 differentiates haematopoietic stem cells into myeloid progenitor cells and stimulates the proliferation of myeloid-derived cells such as DC and monocytes. In mouse models of fibrosarcoma and PCa, IL-3 was found to increase the tumour response to radiation. Combining adenoviral-IL-3 and radiation in the TRAMP-C1 mouse prostate model caused significant delays in tumour growth. Further reports indicated that adenoviral-IL-3 plus radiation enhanced IFNγ-producing $CD4^+$ and $CD8^+$ T cell responses in the spleen (Oh et al., 2004). This shifted the immune response to a Th1-type response from a suppressive Th2-type response (Tsai et al., 2006).

The combination of the pro-inflammatory cytokine TNFα and RT in mouse mammary carcinoma delayed tumour growth at a greater extent than either treatment alone (Nishiguchi et al., 1990). Similar synergistic effects have also been observed in mouse melanoma, lung adenocarinoma and brain tumours. The combined effects were attributed to increased recruitment and enhanced activation of lymphocytes and neutrophils (Gridley et al., 1996; Gridley et al., 2002; Gridley et al., 2000; Jin et al., 2005; Li et al., 1998).

Adoptive-cell-transfer (ACT) therapy is the passive transfer of tumour-specific T cells that have been expanded ex vivo. Local tumour irradiation can enhance the therapeutic efficacy of ACT therapy (Teitz-Tennenbaum et al., 2009). Combination of RT with ACT of carcinoembryonic antigen (CEA)-specific $CD8^+$ T cells in a mouse colon carcinoma

demonstrated increased tumour rejection, that could be attributed to the upregulation of the death receptor Fas on the surface of irradiated tumour cells (Chakraborty et al., 2003).
The anti-tumour effect can be further enhanced by intratumoural administration of DC. In a murine metastatic melanoma model reduction in the size of tumour and extent of spontaneous metastasis and prolonged survival were observed after irradiation and intratumoural DC administration. This was associated with an increase in proliferation, accumulation and cytokine production of $CD4^+$ cells. Similar results were observed in DC plus irraditation in melanoma and sarcoma models (J. Huang et al., 2007). Kjaergaard et al. (2005) reported a method of fusing DC with tumour cells via an electric field resulting in a TAA-DC primed vaccine. These DC/tumour cell fusions induce a potent immune response in combination with local cranial RT in mouse glioma. Both $CD4^+$ and $CD8^+$ T cells infiltrate the tumours, leading to complete tumour regression. Tumour rejection was also observed after subsequent tumour challenge, indicating the presence of immunological memory.
Vaccines containing either modified tumour cells that are more immunogenic than the "native" tumour cells or TAA-vaccines have been tested extensively in preclinical models. Combination of cytokine-producing vaccines with local RT in mouse glioma demonstrated that IL-4 and GM-CSF vaccines alone were capable of curing 20-40% of mice but in combination with local RT 80-100% of the mice were cured. The brain tumours were heavily infiltrated with $CD4^+$ T cells (Lumniczky et al., 2002). The increased anti-tumour effect of GM-CSF and RT was also demonstrated in mouse glioma using a vaccine which contained GM-CSF-secreting tumour cells (Newcomb et al., 2006).
Strategies using RT in combination with monoclonal antibodies that are specific for TAA are now commonly used in clinical oncology (reviewed by Drake, 2010). In a mouse lung cancer model, monoclonal antibody to OX40 (a secondary co-stimulatory molecule expressed on activated $CD4^+$ and $CD8^+$ T cells) and RT resulted in a synergistic effect on survival compared to either treatment alone (Yokouchi et al., 2008). The effect was $CD8^+$ T cell dependent. Antibody-based immunotherapy strategies aiming to neutralise molecules implied in immune tolerance have also been examined. Antibodies for the cytotoxic T lymphocyte antigen (CTLA)-4 (a CD28-superfamily molecule causing T cell functional inhibition) have been shown to induce effective anti-tumour responses via lowering the threshold of tumour-specific T cell activation (reviewed by Drake, 2010). Based on the preclinical findings, CTLA-4 inhibition by the antibody Ipilimumab is now an FDA approved treatment of metastatic melanoma (Chambers et al., 2001). Its combination with RT is being tested in animal models (Dewan et al., 2009) and in clinical trials (see next section).

5.2 Clinical trials

There is huge potential for augmentation of the radiation response with the use of immunotherapy but as yet there are only a few clinical trials published. These were carried out in PCa patients at the National Cancer Institute, using a recombinant viral vaccine consisting of recombinant vaccinia virus (rV) encoding PSA, admixed with rV encoding the co-stimulatory molecule B7.1, followed by booster vaccinations with recombinant fowlpox (rFP) vector expressing PSA prior to RT. The product has been further developed and is presently marketed as Prostvac® which encodes ICAM-1 and LFA-3 in addition to B7.1 (PSA-TRICOM). This agent has been shown to improve median overall survival from 16.6 months to 25.1 months in a phase II multi-centre randomized controlled trial in 125 men with asymptomatic or minimally symptomatic metastatic castrate refractory prostate cancer (Kantoff et al., 2010). There was similar progression-free survival in the two arms of the trial, but the hazard ratio for death was 0.56 (95% CI 0.37 to 0.85) in the PSA-TRICOM arm and the treatment was generally well tolerated.

The initial results of the phase II trial in combination with radiation were highly encouraging. Thirty patients were randomised in a 2:1 ratio to receive vaccine plus EBRT or EBRT alone. In this trial the vaccine consisted of a priming vaccine with rV-PSA plus rV-B7.1 followed by monthly booster vaccines with rFP-PSA. The immunological adjuvants used were GMCSF and high dose IL-2. PSA-specific T cell responses generated prior to RT were not adversely affected by RT, confirming our observation (Tabi et al., 2010). In total, 13 of the 17 patients in the combination arm had increases in PSA-specific T cells and epitope spreading to 4 other prostate cancer TAA (PSMA, PAP, PSCA and MUC-1) was noted (Gulley et al., 2005), possibly due to cross-presentation of a mix of TAA from dying tumour cells by DC (Obeid et al., 2007). There was some IL-2 toxicity, which was reduced in a single-arm follow-up study using lower doses but longer durations of IL-2; immunological effects were equivalent (Gulley et al., 2005; Lechleider et al., 2008).

There is one other reported ongoing work of immunotherapy-radiotherapy combination with intraprostatic injections of autologous DC. The first report confirms the safety of this approach in 5 HLA-A2$^+$ patients with high risk, localised disease, also treated with ADT, EBRT to 45 Gy and LDR brachytherapy. Autologous intraprostatic DC injections were given at four timepoints during EBRT. Measurable, induced increases in TAA-specific T cell frequencies in peripheral blood using ELISPOT were observed in some patients. The pattern of distribution of CD8$^+$ cells in tissue was consistent with PCa TAA-targeting, rather than non-specific organ infiltration (Finkelstein et al., 2011).

There are no other published studies in PCa patients of EBRT in combination with cytokines, antibodies, immune modulators or immunologically relevant gene therapy. However, there are a few prostate cancer clinical trials combining RT and immunotherapy currently recruiting according to the ClinicalTrials.gov website, such as anti-CTLA-4 (Ipilimumab) antibody therapy in castration-resistant prostate cancer following RT (Phase III trial, Bristol-Myers Squibb; NCT00861614) and treatment with anti-OX40 and cyclophosphamide in combination with RT in metastatic prostate cancer (Providence Health & Services, Oregon USA, Phase I/II trial; NCT01303705).

5.3 Designs of combination clinical trials

Clinical trial design, investigating the benefit of immunotherapy in addition to EBRT is challenging in PCa, as long-term tumour control outcome is already good in both localised (assuming dose escalated image-guided IMRT) and locally advanced disease (assuming combination of long term ADT and EBRT). Phase III trials, adequately powered to show a clinically relevant improvement, would need to address biochemical relapse-free survival or overall survival, both of which require prolonged follow-up of many hundreds and perhaps thousands of patients. Before such trials were undertaken, it is important to optimise the immunotherapy-RT schedules. Reliable biomarkers of treatment-efficacy are needed and this is difficult, especially if neoadjuvant or adjuvant ADT is used, as changes in PSA-kinetics become redundant in these patients. Therefore, development of reliable immunological biomarkers is crucial. We believe that the presence of systemic TAA-specific T cell responses is likely to be the most reliable and easily detectable indicator of a sustainable immunological effect. It may also assist patient selection for optimised treatment of those patients who are most likely to benefit from combination therapies.

The successful result of the IMPACT trial showing the survival advantage with Sipuleucel-T is expected to lead to a dramatic increase in the use of systemic immunotherapy for prostate cancer (Sonpavde et al., 2011). Presently there are only production facilities within the USA and the cost is likely to remain prohibitive for many healthcare systems. Radiation has great potential to augment the effect of systemic immunotherapy and we can expect many combination trials in the future. Clinical trial design in this setting will remain challenging as immunotherapy appears to improve overall survival but demonstrable tumour or biochemical responses are often delayed. Augmenting immunotherapy with radiation may improve overall advantage further.

6. Conclusions

PCa has become a huge burden on the health and wealth of Western societies. It is now the commonest solid malignancy and in spite of an excellent general outcome it is expected to become the main cause of cancer-related death in men. There is therefore an urgent need for improved therapies. Sipuleucel-T for PCa was the first immunotherapy to show a survival advantage in cancer, and it has been quickly followed by ipilimumab in melanoma. Radiotherapy has many applications for PCa and it is clear that there are many interactions between immunotherapy and radiation. In general these are positive such that immunotherapy may improve outcomes for those being irradiated and vice versa. The challenge is to move the science into the clinical setting, optimising combinations and sequences, identification of appropriate biomarkers and designing appropriate trials.

7. Acknowledgements

Experimental work presented in this chapter was supported by Cancer Research Wales (Cardiff UK) to ZT, LKS and JS and by Velindre NHS Trust R&D (Cardiff, UK) to JS.

8. References

Allavena, P., Sica, A., Solinas, G., Porta, C. & Mantovani, A. (2008). The inflammatory micro-environment in tumor progression: the role of tumor-associated macrophages. *Critical Reviews in Oncology/Hematology* 66, 1, (Apr), 1-9.

Apetoh, L., Ghiringhelli, F., Tesniere, A., Criollo, A., Ortiz, C., Lidereau, R., Mariette, C., Chaput, N., Mira, J.P., Delaloge, S., Andre, F., Tursz, T., Kroemer, G. & Zitvogel, L. (2007). The interaction between HMGB1 and TLR4 dictates the outcome of anticancer chemotherapy and radiotherapy. *Immunol Rev* 220, (Dec), 47-59.

Arbour, N., Lorenz, E., Schutte, B., Zabner, J., Kline, J., Jones, M., Frees, K., Watt, J. & Schwartz, D. (2000). TLR4 mutations are associated with endotoxin hyporesponsiveness in humans. *Nat Genet* 25, 2, 187-191.

Arredouani, M., Lu, B., Bhasin, M., Eljanne, M., Yue, W., Mosquera, J., Bubley, G., Li, V., Rubin, M., Libermann, T. & Sanda, M. (2009). Identification of the transcription factor single-minded homologue 2 as a potential biomarker and immunotherapy target in prostate cancer. *Clin Cancer Res* 15, 18, 5794-5802.

Aymeric, L., Apetoh, L., Ghiringhelli, F., Tesniere, A., Martins, I., Kroemer, G., Smyth, M. & Zitvogel, L. (2010). Tumor cell death and ATP release prime dendritic cells and efficient anticancer immunity. *Cancer Res* 70, 3, 855-858.

Baluna, R.G., Eng, T.Y. & Thomas, C.R. (2006). Adhesion molecules in radiotherapy. *Radiat Res* 166, 6, (Dec), 819-831.

Begley, L., Monteleon, C., Shah, R.B., Macdonald, J.W. & Macoska, J.A. (2005). CXCL12 overexpression and secretion by aging fibroblasts enhance human prostate epithelial proliferation in vitro. *Aging Cell* 4, 6, (Dec), 291-298.

Bolla, M., Van Poppel, H. & Collette, L. (2007). [Preliminary results for EORTC trial 22911: radical prostatectomy followed by postoperative radiotherapy in prostate cancers with a high risk of progression]. *Cancer Radiother* 11, 6-7, (Nov), 363-369.

Bouchelouche, K., Tagawa, S.T., Goldsmith, S.J., Turkbey, B., Capala, J. & Choyke, P. (2011). PET/CT imaging and radioimmunotherapy of prostate cancer. *Semin Nucl Med* 41, 1, (Jan), 29-44.

Bronte, V., Kasic, T., Gri, G., Gallana, K., Borsellino, G., Marigo, I., Battistini, L., Iafrate, M., Prayer-Galetti, T., Pagano, F. & Viola, A. (2005). Boosting antitumor responses of T lymphocytes infiltrating human prostate cancers. *J Exp Med* 201, 8, 1257-1268.

Burnette, B.C., Liang, H., Lee, Y., Chlewicki, L., Khodarev, N.N., Weichselbaum, R.R., Fu, Y.X. & Auh, S.L. (2011). The efficacy of radiotherapy relies upon induction of type I interferon -dependent innate and adaptive immunity. *Cancer Res* 71, 7, (Apr 1), 2488-2496.

Cao, M., Cabrera, R., Xu, Y., Liu, C. & Nelson, D. (2009). Gamma irradiation alters the phenotype and function of CD4+CD25+ regulatory T cells. *Cell Biol Int* 33, 5, (May), 565-571.

Cao, M., Cabrera, R., Xu, Y., Liu, C. & Nelson, D. (2011). Different radiosensitivity of CD4+CD25+ regulatory T cells and effector T cells to low dose gamma irradiation in vitro. *Int J Rad Biol* 87, 1, 71-80.

Carmeliet, P. & Jain, R.K. (2000). Angiogenesis in cancer and other diseases. *Nature* 407, 6801, (Sep 14), 249-257.

Chakraborty, M., Abrams, S.I., Camphausen, K., Liu, K., Scott, T., Coleman, C.N. & Hodge, J.W. (2003). Irradiation of tumor cells up-regulates Fas and enhances CTL lytic activity and CTL adoptive immunotherapy. *J Immunol* 170, 12, (Jun 15), 6338-6347.

Chambers, C., Kuhns, M., Egen, J. & Allison, J. (2001). CTLA-4-mediated inhibition in regulation of T cell responses: mechanisms and manipulation in tumor immunotherapy. *Ann Rev Immunol* 19, 565-594.

Chen, Y., Scanlan, M., Sahin, U., Türeci, O., Gure, A., Tsang, S., Williamson, B., Stockert, E., Pfreundschuh, M. & Old, L. (1997). A testicular antigen aberrantly expressed in human cancers detected by autologous antibody screening. *Proc Natl Acad Sci USA* 94,5,1914-1918.

Chopra, D.P., Menard, R.E., Januszewski, J. & Mattingly, R.R. (2004). TNF-alpha-mediated apoptosis in normal human prostate epithelial cells and tumor cell lines. *Cancer Lett* 203, 2, (Jan 20), 145-154.

Clayton, A., Al-Taei, S., Webber, J., Mason, M.D. & Tabi, Z. (2011). Cancer exosomes express CD39 and CD73, which suppress T cells through adenosine production. *J Immunol* 187, 2, (July 15) 676-683.

Coen, J. & Zietman, A. (2009). Proton radiation for localized prostate cancer. *Nat Rev Urol* 6, 6, 324-330.

Dewan, M., Galloway, A., Kawashima, N., Dewyngaert, J., Babb, J., Formenti, S. & Demaria, S. (2009). Fractionated but not single-dose radiotherapy induces an immune-mediated abscopal effect when combined with anti-CTLA-4 antibody. *Clin Cancer Res* 15, 17, 5379-5388.

Drake, C.G. (2010). Prostate cancer as a model for tumour immunotherapy. *Nat Rev Immunol* 10, 8, (Aug), 580-593.

Ebelt, K., Babaryka, G., Figel, A., Pohla, H., Buchner, A., Stief, C., Eisenmenger, W., Kirchner, T., Schendel, D. & Noessner, E. (2008). Dominance of CD4+ lymphocytic infiltrates with disturbed effector cell characteristics in the tumor microenvironment of prostate carcinoma. *Prostate* 68, 1, 1-10.

Ebelt, K., Babaryka, G., Frankenberger, B., Stief, C., Eisenmenger, W., Kirchner, T., Schendel, D. & Noessner, E. (2009). Prostate cancer lesions are surrounded by FOXP3+, PD-1+ and B7-H1+ lymphocyte clusters. *Eur J Cancer* 45, 9, 1664-1672.

Epel, M., Carmi, I., Soueid-Baumgarten, S., Oh, S., Bera, T., Pastan, I., Berzofsky, J. & Reiter, Y. (2008). Targeting TARP, a novel breast and prostate tumor-associated antigen, with T cell receptor-like human recombinant antibodies. *Eur J Immunol* 38, 6, 1706-1720.

Ernst, P.B., Garrison, J.C. & Thompson, L.F. (2010). Much ado about adenosine: adenosine synthesis and function in regulatory T cell biology. *J Immunol* 185, 4, (Aug 15) 1993-1998.

Fassò, M., Waitz, R., Hou, Y., Rim, T., Greenberg, N., Shastri, N., Fong, L. & Allison, J. (2008). SPAS-1 (stimulator of prostatic adenocarcinoma-specific T cells)/SH3GLB2: A prostate tumor antigen identified by CTLA-4 blockade. *Proc Natl Acad Sci USA* 105, 9, 3509-3514.

Ferrer, F.A., Miller, L.J., Andrawis, R.I., Kurtzman, S.H., Albertsen, P.C., Laudone, V.P. & Kreutzer, D.L. (1997). Vascular endothelial growth factor (VEGF) expression in human prostate cancer: in situ and in vitro expression of VEGF by human prostate cancer cells. *J Urol* 157, 6, (Jun), 2329-2333.

Finkelstein, S.E., Gabrilovich, D., Rodriguez, F.A., Chuang, T., Kang, L., Torres-Roca, J., Heysek, R., Pow-Sang, J.M., Antonia, S., Fishman, M.N. & Immunotherapy Research Group. (2011). Know when to say when: Serial assessment of apoptosis and lymphocyte infiltrates with combined intraprostatic autologous dendritic cell immunotherapy radiation therapy in high-risk prostate cancer. *ASCO Meeting Abstracts* 29, 7S, 149.

Formenti, S.C. & Demaria, S. (2009). Systemic effects of local radiotherapy. *Lancet Oncol* 10, 7, (Jul), 718-726.

Fujita, K., Ewing, C.M., Sokoll, L.J., Elliott, D.J., Cunningham, M., De Marzo, A.M., Isaacs, W.B. & Pavlovich, C.P. (2008). Cytokine profiling of prostatic fluid from cancerous prostate glands identifies cytokines associated with extent of tumor and inflammation. *Prostate* 68, 8, (Jun 1), 872-882.

Gabrilovich, D.I., Chen, H.L., Girgis, K.R., Cunningham, H.T., Meny, G.M., Nadaf, S., Kavanaugh, D. & Carbone, D.P. (1996). Production of vascular endothelial growth factor by human tumors inhibits the functional maturation of dendritic cells. *Nat Med* 2, 10, (Oct), 1096-1103.

Gabrilovich, D.I. & Nagaraj, S. (2009). Myeloid-derived suppressor cells as regulators of the immune system. *Nat Rev Immunol* 9, 3, (Mar), 162-174.

Gannon, P., Poisson, A., Delvoye, N., Lapointe, R., Mes-Masson, A. & Saad, F. (2009). Characterization of the intra-prostatic immune cell infiltration in androgen-deprived prostate cancer patients. *J Immunol Methods* 348, 1-2, 9-17.

Garnett, C.T., Palena, C., Chakraborty, M., Tsang, K.Y., Schlom, J. & Hodge, J.W. (2004). Sublethal irradiation of human tumor cells modulates phenotype resulting in enhanced killing by cytotoxic T lymphocytes. *Cancer Res* 64, 21, (Nov 1), 7985-7994.

Gridley, D.S., Andres, M.L., Garner, C., Mao, X.W. & Slater, J.M. (1996). Evaluation of TNF-alpha effects on radiation efficacy in a human lung adenocarcinoma model. *Oncol Res* 8, 12, 485-495.

Gridley, D.S., Li, J., Kajioka, E.H., Andres, M.L., Moyers, M.F. & Slater, J.M. (2000). Combination of pGL1-TNF-alpha gene and radiation (proton and gamma-ray) therapy against brain tumor. *Anticancer Res* 20, 6B, (Nov-Dec), 4195-4203.

Gridley, D.S., Baer, J.R., Cao, J.D., Miller, G.M., Kim, D.W., Timiryasova, T.M., Fodor, I. & Slater, J.M. (2002). TNF-alpha gene and proton radiotherapy in an orthotopic brain tumor model. *Int J Oncol* 21, 2, (Aug), 251-259.

Guerrero Urbano, T., Khoo, V., Staffurth, J., Norman, A., Buffa, F., Jackson, A., Adams, E., Hansen, V., Clark, C., Miles, E., McNair, H., Nutting, C., Parker, C., Eeles, R., Huddart, R., Horwich, A. & Dearnaley, D.P. (2010). Intensity-modulated Radiotherapy Allows Escalation of the Radiation Dose to the Pelvic Lymph Nodes in Patients with Locally Advanced Prostate Cancer: Preliminary Results of a Phase I Dose Escalation Study. *Clin Oncol* 22, 3, 236-244.

Gulley, J.L., Arlen, P.M., Bastian, A., Morin, S., Marte, J., Beetham, P., Tsang, K.Y., Yokokawa, J., Hodge, J.W., Menard, C., Camphausen, K., Coleman, C.N., Sullivan, F., Steinberg, S.M., Schlom, J. & Dahut, W. (2005). Combining a recombinant cancer vaccine with standard definitive radiotherapy in patients with localized prostate cancer. *Clin Cancer Res* 11, 9, (May 1), 3353-3362.

Gust, K., Hofer, M., Perner, S., Kim, R., Chinnaiyan, A., Varambally, S., Moller, P., Rinnab, L., Rubin, M., Greiner, J., Schmitt, M., Kuefer, R. & Ringhoffer, M. (2009). RHAMM (CD168) is overexpressed at the protein level and may constitute an immunogenic antigen in advanced prostate cancer disease. *Neoplasia* 11, 9, 956-963.

Haanen, J., Baars, A., Gomez, R., Weder, P., Smits, M., de Gruijl, T., von Blomberg, B., Bloemena, E., Scheper, R., van Ham, S., Pinedo, H. & van den Eertwegh, A. (2005). Melanoma-specific tumor-infiltrating lymphocytes but not circulating melanoma-specific T cells may predict survival in resected advanced-stage melanoma patients. *Cancer Immunol Immunother* 1-8.

Hanahan, D. & Weinberg, R. (2011). Hallmarks of cancer: the next generation. *Cell* 144, 5, 646-674.

Hillman, G.G., Maughan, R.L., Grignon, D.J., Yudelev, M., Che, M., Abrams, J., Wang, Y., Layer, A., Wright, J.L., Rubio, J. & Forman, J.D. (2003). Responsiveness of experimental prostate carcinoma bone tumors to neutron or photon radiation combined with cytokine therapy. *Int J Radiat Oncol Biol Phys* 56, 5, (Aug 1), 1426-1437.

Honma, I., Torigoe, T., Hirohashi, Y., Kitamura, H., Sato, E., Masumori, N., Tamura, Y., Tsukamoto, T. & Sato, N. (2009). Aberrant expression and potency as a cancer immunotherapy target of alpha-methylacyl-coenzyme A racemase in prostate cancer. *J Transl Med* 7, 103.

Hoskin, P. (2008). High dose rate brachytherapy for prostate cancer. *Cancer Radiother* 12, 6-7, (Nov), 512-514.

Huang, H., Dawicki, W., Zhang, X., Town, J. & Gordon, J. (2010). Tolerogenic dendritic cells induce CD4+CD25hiFoxp3+ regulatory T cell differentiation from CD4+CD25-/loFoxp3- effector T cells. *J Immunol* 185, 9, 5003-5010.

Huang, J., Wang, Y., Guo, J., Lu, H., Lin, X., Ma, L., Teitz-Tennenbaum, S., Chang, A.E. & Li, Q. (2007). Radiation-induced apoptosis along with local and systemic cytokine elaboration is associated with DC plus radiotherapy-mediated renal cell tumor regression. *Clin Immunol* 123, 3, (Jun), 298-310.

Hudolin, T., Juretic, A., Spagnoli, G., Pasini, J., Bandic, D., Heberer, M., Kosicek, M. & Cacic, M. (2006). Immunohistochemical expression of tumor antigens MAGE-A1, MAGE-A3/4, and NY-ESO-1 in cancerous and benign prostatic tissue. *Prostate* 66, 1, 13 - 18.

Jackson, M.W., Bentel, J.M. & Tilley, W.D. (1997). Vascular endothelial growth factor (VEGF) expression in prostate cancer and benign prostatic hyperplasia. *J Urol* 157, 6, (Jun), 2323-2328.

James, N.D., Sydes, M.R., Clarke, N.W., Mason, M.D., Dearnaley, D.P., Anderson, J., Popert, R.J., Sanders, K., Morgan, R.C., Stansfeld, J., Dwyer, J., Masters, J. & Parmar, M.K.B. (2009). Systemic therapy for advancing or metastatic prostate cancer (STAMPEDE): a multi-arm, multistage randomized controlled trial. *BJU Internatl* 103, 4, 464-469.

Jin, G.H., Jin, S.Z., Liu, Y., Xu, R.M., Yang, J.Z., Pan, X.N. & Liu, S.Z. (2005). Therapeutic effect of gene-therapy in combination with local X-irradiation in a mouse malignant melanoma model. *Biochem Biophys Res Commun* 330, 3, (May 13), 975-981.

Kachikwu, E., Iwamoto, K., Liao, Y., Demarco, J., Agazaryan, N., Economou, J., McBride, W. & Schaue, D. (2010). Radiation enhances regulatory T Cell representation. *Int J Radiat Oncol Biol Phys* Epub ahead of print Nov 17.

Kantoff, P.W., Higano, C.S., Shore, N.D., Berger, E.R., Small, E.J., Penson, D.F., Redfern, C.H., Ferrari, A.C., Dreicer, R., Sims, R.B., Xu, Y., Frohlich, M.W. & Schellhammer, P.F. (2010). Sipuleucel-T Immunotherapy for castration-resistant prostate cancer. *N Engl J Med* 363, 5, 411-422.

Kärjä, V., Aaltomaa, S., Lipponen, P., Isotalo, T., Talja, M. & Mokka, R. (2005). Tumour-infiltrating lymphocytes: A prognostic factor of PSA-free survival in patients with local prostate carcinoma treated by radical prostatectomy. *Anticancer Res* 25, 6C, 4435-4438.

Khoo, V.S. & Dearnaley, D.P. (2008). Question of dose, fractionation and technique: ingredients for testing hypofractionation in prostate cancer--the CHHiP trial. *Clin Oncol* 20, 1, (Feb), 12-14.

King, C.R., Brooks, J.D., Gill, H. & Presti, J.C., Jr. (2011). Long-Term Outcomes from a Prospective Trial of Stereotactic Body Radiotherapy for Low-Risk Prostate Cancer. *Int J Radiat Oncol Biol Phys*, (Feb 5).

Kjaergaard, J., Wang, L.X., Kuriyama, H., Shu, S. & Plautz, G.E. (2005). Active immunotherapy for advanced intracranial murine tumors by using dendritic cell-tumor cell fusion vaccines. *J Neurosurg* 103, 1, (Jul), 156-164.

Lechleider, R., Arlen, P., Tsang, K., Steinberg, S., Yokokawa, J., Cereda, V., Camphausen, K., Schlom, J., Dahut, W. & Gulley, J. (2008). Safety and immunologic response of a viral vaccine to prostate-specific antigen in combination with radiation therapy when metronomic-dose interleukin 2 is used as an adjuvant. *Clin Cancer Res* 14, 16, 5284-5291.

Lee, Y., Auh, S.L., Wang, Y., Burnette, B., Wang, Y., Meng, Y., Beckett, M., Sharma, R., Chin, R., Tu, T., Weichselbaum, R.R. & Fu, Y.-X. (2009). Therapeutic effects of ablative radiation on local tumor require CD8+ T cells: changing strategies for cancer treatment. *Blood* 114, 3, (July 16), 589-595.

Li, J., Andres, M.L., Fodor, I., Nelson, G.A. & Gridley, D.S. (1998). Evaluation of pGL1-TNF-alpha therapy in combination with radiation. *Oncol Res* 10, 7, 379-387.

Lindholm, P., Lu, Y., Adley, B., Vladislav, T., Jovanovic, B., Sivapurapu, N., Yang, X. & Kajdacsy-Balla, A. (2010). Role of monocyte-lineage cells in prostate cancer cell invasion and tissue factor expression. *Prostate* 70, 15, 1672-1682.

Liu, V.C., Wong, L.Y., Jang, T., Shah, A.H., Park, I., Yang, X., Zhang, Q., Lonning, S., Teicher, B.A. & Lee, C. (2007). Tumor evasion of the immune system by converting CD4+CD25- T cells into CD4+CD25+ T regulatory cells: role of tumor-derived TGF-beta. *J Immunol* 178, 5, (Mar 1), 2883-2892.

Loberg, R.D., Ying, C., Craig, M., Yan, L., Snyder, L.A. & Pienta, K.J. (2007). CCL2 as an important mediator of prostate cancer growth in vivo through the regulation of macrophage infiltration. *Neoplasia* 9, 7, (Jul), 556-562.

Lohr, F., Hu, K., Haroon, Z., Samulski, T.V., Huang, Q., Beaty, J., Dewhirst, M.W. & Li, C.Y. (2000). Combination treatment of murine tumors by adenovirus-mediated local B7/IL12 immunotherapy and radiotherapy. *Mol Ther* 2, 3, (Sep), 195-203.

Lu, Y., Cai, Z., Galson, D.L., Xiao, G., Liu, Y., George, D.E., Melhem, M.F., Yao, Z. & Zhang, J. (2006). Monocyte chemotactic protein-1 (MCP-1) acts as a paracrine and autocrine factor for prostate cancer growth and invasion. *Prostate* 66, 12, (Sep 1), 1311-1318.

Lu, Y., Wang, J., Xu, Y., Koch, A.E., Cai, Z., Chen, X., Galson, D.L., Taichman, R.S. & Zhang, J. (2008). CXCL16 functions as a novel chemotactic factor for prostate cancer cells in vitro. *Mol Cancer Res* 6, 4, (Apr), 546-554.

Lugade, A., Moran, J., Gerber, S., Rose, R., Frelinger, J. & Lord, E. (2005). Local radiation therapy of B16 melanoma tumors increases the generation of tumor antigen-specific effector cells that traffic to the tumor. *J Immunol* 174, 12, 7516-7523.

Lugade, A., Sorensen, E., Gerber, S., Moran, J., Frelinger, J. & Lord, E. (2008). Radiation-induced IFN-gamma production within the tumor microenvironment influences antitumor immunity. *J Immunol* 180, 5, 3132-3139.

Lumniczky, K., Desaknai, S., Mangel, L., Szende, B., Hamada, H., Hidvegi, E.J. & Safrany, G. (2002). Local tumor irradiation augments the antitumor effect of cytokine-producing autologous cancer cell vaccines in a murine glioma model. *Cancer Gene Therapy* 9, 1, (Jan), 44-52.

Ma, Y., Aymeric, L., Locher, C., Kroemer, G. & Zitvogel, L. (2011). The dendritic cell-tumor cross-talk in cancer. *Current Op Immunol* 23, 1, 146 - 152.

Madsen, B.L., Hsi, R.A., Pham, H.T., Fowler, J.F., Esagui, L. & Corman, J. (2007). Stereotactic hypofractionated accurate radiotherapy of the prostate (SHARP), 33.5 Gy in five fractions for localized disease: first clinical trial results. *Int J Radiat Oncol Biol Phys* 67, 4, (Mar 15), 1099-1105.

Marigo, I., Dolcetti, L., Serafini, P., Zanovello, P. & Bronte, V. (2008). Tumor-induced tolerance and immune suppression by myeloid derived suppressor cells. *Immunol Rev* 222, (Apr), 162-179.

Matsumura, S. & Demaria, S. (2010). Up-regulation of the pro-inflammatory chemokine CXCL16 is a common response of tumor cells to ionizing radiation. *Radiat Res* 173, 4, (Apr), 418-425.

Miller, A., Lundberg, K., Ozenci, V., Banham, A., Hellström, M., Egevad, L. & Pisa, P. (2006). CD4+CD25high T cells are enriched in the tumor and peripheral blood of prostate cancer patients. *J Immunol* 177, 10, 7398-7405.

Mor, F. & Cohen, I.R. (1996). IL-2 rescues antigen-specific T cells from radiation or dexamethasone-induced apoptosis. Correlation with induction of Bcl-2. *J Immunol* 156, 2, (Jan 15), 515-522.

Nakatsuka, S., Oji, Y., Horiuchi, T., Kanda, T., Kitagawa, M., Takeuchi, T., Kawano, K., Kuwae, Y., Yamauchi, A., Okumura, M., Kitamura, Y., Oka, Y., Kawase, I., Sugiyama, H. & Aozasa, K. (2006). Immunohistochemical detection of WT1 protein in a variety of cancer cells. *Mod Pathol* 19, 6, 804-814.

Nesslinger, N.J., Sahota, R.A., Stone, B., Johnson, K., Chima, N., King, C., Rasmussen, D., Bishop, D., Rennie, P.S., Gleave, M., Blood, P., Pai, H., Ludgate, C. & Nelson, B.H. (2007). Standard treatments induce antigen-specific immune responses in prostate cancer. *Clin Cancer Res* 13, 5, (March 1, 2007), 1493-1502.

Newcomb, E.W., Demaria, S., Lukyanov, Y., Shao, Y., Schnee, T., Kawashima, N., Lan, L., Dewyngaert, J.K., Zagzag, D., McBride, W.H. & Formenti, S.C. (2006). The combination of ionizing radiation and peripheral vaccination produces long-term survival of mice bearing established invasive GL261 gliomas. *Clin Cancer Res* 12, 15, (Aug 1), 4730-4737.

Nishiguchi, I., Willingham, V. & Milas, L. (1990). Tumor necrosis factor as an adjunct to fractionated radiotherapy in the treatment of murine tumors. *Int J Radiat Oncol Biol Phys* 18, 3, (Mar), 555-558.

Obeid, M., Tesniere, A., Ghiringhelli, F., Fimia, G.M., Apetoh, L., Perfettini, J.L., Castedo, M., Mignot, G., Panaretakis, T., Casares, N., Métivier, D., Larochette, N., van Endert, P., Ciccosanti, F., Piacentini, M., Zitvogel, L. & Kroemer, G. (2007). Calreticulin exposure dictates the immunogenicity of cancer cell death. *Nat Med* 13, 1, 54-61.

Oh, Y.T., Chen, D.W., Dougherty, G.J. & McBride, W.H. (2004). Adenoviral interleukin-3 gene-radiation therapy for prostate cancer in mouse model. *Int J Radiat Oncol Biol Phys* 59, 2, (Jun 1), 579-583.

Ohm, J.E., Gabrilovich, D.I., Sempowski, G.D., Kisseleva, E., Parman, K.S., Nadaf, S. & Carbone, D.P. (2003). VEGF inhibits T-cell development and may contribute to tumor-induced immune suppression. *Blood* 101, 12, (Jun 15), 4878-4886.

Olson, B. & McNeel, D. (2011). CD8+ T cells specific for the androgen receptor are common in patients with prostate cancer and are able to lyse prostate tumor cells. *Cancer Immunol Immunother* 60, 6, 781-792.

Oyama, T., Ran, S., Ishida, T., Nadaf, S., Kerr, L., Carbone, D.P. & Gabrilovich, D.I. (1998). Vascular endothelial growth factor affects dendritic cell maturation through the inhibition of nuclear factor-kappa B activation in hemopoietic progenitor cells. *J Immunol* 160, 3, (Feb 1), 1224-1232.

Reits, E., Hodge, J., Herberts, C., Groothuis, T., Chakraborty, M., Wansley, E., Camphausen, K., Luiten, R., de Ru, A., Neijssen, J., Griekspoor, A., Mesman, E., Verreck, F., Spits, H., Schlom, J., van Veelen, P. & Neefjes, J. (2006). Radiation modulates the peptide repertoire, enhances MHC class I expression, and induces successful antitumor immunotherapy. *J Exp Med* 203, 5, 1259-1271.

Rokhlin, O.W. & Cohen, M.B. (1995). Expression of cellular adhesion molecules on human prostate tumor cell lines. *Prostate* 26, 4, (Apr), 205-212.

Sato, K., Yamashita, N. & Matsuyama, T. (2002). Human peripheral blood monocyte-derived interleukin-10-induced semi-mature dendritic cells induce anergic CD4(+) and CD8(+) T cells via presentation of the internalized soluble antigen and cross-presentation of the phagocytosed necrotic cellular fragments. *Cell Immunol* 215, 2, (Feb), 186-194.

Schaue, D., Comin-Anduix, B., Ribas, A., Zhang, L., Goodglick, L., Sayre, J., Debucquoy, A., Haustermans, K. & McBride, W. (2008). T-cell responses to survivin in cancer patients undergoing radiation therapy. *Clin Cancer Res* 14, 15, 4883-4890.

Sfanos, K., Bruno, T., Maris, C., Xu, L., Thoburn, C., DeMarzo, A., Meeker, A., Isaacs, W. & Drake, C. (2008). Phenotypic analysis of prostate-infiltrating lymphocytes reveals TH17 and Treg skewing. *Clin Cancer Res* 14, 11, 3254-3261.

Shelley, M.D., Kumar, S., Coles, B., Wilt, T., Staffurth, J. & Mason, M.D. (2009). Adjuvant hormone therapy for localised and locally advanced prostate carcinoma: A systematic review and meta-analysis of randomised trials. *Cancer Treatment Reviews* 35, 7, 540-546.

Shelley, M.D., Kumar, S., Wilt, T., Staffurth, J., Coles, B. & Mason, M.D. (2009). A systematic review and meta-analysis of randomised trials of neo-adjuvant hormone therapy for localised and locally advanced prostate carcinoma. *Cancer Treatment Reviews* 35, 1, 9-17.

Shiao, S.L. & Coussens, L.M. (2010). The tumor-immune microenvironment and response to radiation therapy. *J Mammary Gland Biol Neoplasia* 15, 4, (Dec), 411-421.

Sinnathamby, G., Zerfass, J., Hafner, J., Block, P., Nickens, Z., Hobeika, A., Secord, A., Lyerly, H., Morse, M. & Philip, R. (2011). ADAM metallopeptidase domain 17 (ADAM17) is naturally processed through major histocompatibility complex (MHC) class I molecules and is a potential immunotherapeutic target in breast, ovarian and prostate cancers. *Clin Exp Immunol* 163, 3, 324-332.

Sluyter, R., Shemon, A. & Wiley, J. (2004). Glu496 to Ala polymorphism in the P2X7 receptor impairs ATP-induced IL-1 beta release from human monocytes. *J Immunol* 172, 6, 3399-3405.

Sonpavde, G., Agarwal, N., Choueiri, T. & Kantoff, P. (2011). Recent advances in immunotherapy for the treatment of prostate cancer. *Expert Opin Biol Ther* 11, 8, 997-1009.

Sorrentino, C., Musiani, P., Pompa, P., Cipollone, G. & Di Carlo, E. (2011). Androgen deprivation boosts prostatic infiltration of cytotoxic and regulatory T lymphocytes and has no effect on disease-free survival in prostate cancer patients. *Clin Cancer Res* 17, 6, 1571-1581.

Southall, P., Boxer, G., Bagshawe, K., Hole, N., Bromley, M. & Stern, P. (1990). Immunohistological distribution of 5T4 antigen in normal and malignant tissues. *Br J Cancer* 61, 1, 89-95.

Stagg, J. & Smyth, M.J. (2010). Extracellular adenosine triphosphate and adenosine an cancer. *Oncogene* 29, (Sept 30), 5346-5358.

Strauss, D. & Thomas, J. (2010). Transmission of donor melanoma by organ transplantation. *Lancet Oncol* 11, 8, 790-796.

Tabi, Z., Spary, L., Coleman, S., Clayton, A., Mason, M.D. & Staffurth, J. (2010). Resistance of CD45RA- T cells to apoptosis and functional impairment, and generation of tumor-antigen specific T cell responses during radiation therapy of prostate cancer. *J Immunol* 185, 2, (Jul 15), 1330-1339.

Teitz-Tennenbaum, S., Li, Q., Davis, M.A., Wilder-Romans, K., Hoff, J., Li, M. & Chang, A.E. (2009). Radiotherapy combined with intratumoral dendritic cell vaccination enhances the therapeutic efficacy of adoptive T-cell transfer. *J Immunother* 32, 6, (Jul), 602-612.

Teng, M., Swann, J., Koebel, C., Schreiber, R. & Smyth, M. (2008). Immune mediated dormancy: an equilibrium with cancer. *J Leukocyte Biol* 84, 4, 988-993.

Thiery, J., Keefe, D., Boulant, S., Boucrot, E., Walch, M., Martinvalet, D., Goping, I., Bleackley, R., Kirchhausen, T. & Lieberman, J. (2011). Perforin pores in the endosomal membrane trigger the release of endocytosed granzyme B into the cytosol of target cells. *Nat Immunol*, 19 Jun, Epub ahead of print.

Thompson, I.M., Jr., Tangen, C.M., Paradelo, J., Lucia, M.S., Miller, G., Troyer, D., Messing, E., Forman, J., Chin, J., Swanson, G., Canby-Hagino, E. & Crawford, E.D. (2006).

Adjuvant radiotherapy for pathologically advanced prostate cancer: a randomized clinical trial. *Jama* 296, 19, (Nov 15), 2329-2335.

Troy, A., Davidson, P., Atkinson, C. & Hart, D. (1998). Phenotypic characterisation of the dendritic cell infiltrate in prostate cancer. *J Urol* 160, 1, (Jul), 214-219.

Tsai, C.H., Hong, J.H., Hsieh, K.F., Hsiao, H.W., Chuang, W.L., Lee, C.C., McBride, W.H. & Chiang, C.S. (2006). Tetracycline-regulated intratumoral expression of interleukin-3 enhances the efficacy of radiation therapy for murine prostate cancer. *Cancer Gene Therapy* 13, 12, (Dec), 1082-1092.

Van Der Meeren, A., Squiban, C., Gourmelon, P., Lafont, H. & Gaugler, M.H. (1999). Differential regulation by IL-4 and IL-10 of radiation-induced IL-6 and IL-8 production and ICAM-1 expression by human endothelial cells. *Cytokine* 11, 11, (Nov), 831-838.

Viani, G., Stefano, E. & Afonso, S. (2009). Higher-than-conventional radiation doses in localized prostate cancer treatment: a meta-analysis of randomized, controlled trials. *Int J Radiat Oncol Biol Phys* 74, 5, 1405-1418.

Wan, Y. & Flavell, R. (2007). 'Yin-Yang' functions of transforming growth factor-beta and T regulatory cells in immune regulation. *Immunol Rev* 220, 199-213.

Warde, P., Mason, M., Sydes, M., Gospodarowicz, M., Swanson, G., Kirkbride, P., Kostashuk, E. & al., e. (2010). Intergroup randomised phase III study of androgen deprivation therapy (ADT) plus radiation therapy (RT) in locally advanced prostate cancer (CaP) (NCIC-CTG, SWOG, MRC-UK, INY: T94-0110; NCT00002633). *J Clin Oncol* 28, 18s, CRA 4504.

Wiegel, T., Bottke, D., Steiner, U., Siegmann, A., Golz, R., Storkel, S., Willich, N., Semjonow, A., Souchon, R., Stockle, M., Rube, C., Weissbach, L., Althaus, P., Rebmann, U., Kalble, T., Feldmann, H.J., Wirth, M., Hinke, A., Hinkelbein, W. & Miller, K. (2009). Phase III postoperative adjuvant radiotherapy after radical prostatectomy compared with radical prostatectomy alone in pT3 prostate cancer with postoperative undetectable prostate-specific antigen: ARO 96-02/AUO AP 09/95. *J Clin Oncol* 27, 18, (Jun 20), 2924-2930.

Wrzesinski, S., Wan, Y. & Flavell, R. (2007). Transforming growth factor-beta and the immune response: implications for anticancer therapy. *Clin Cancer Res* 13, 18 Pt 1, 5262-5270.

Yokouchi, H., Yamazaki, K., Chamoto, K., Kikuchi, E., Shinagawa, N., Oizumi, S., Hommura, F., Nishimura, T. & Nishimura, M. (2008). Anti-OX40 monoclonal antibody therapy in combination with radiotherapy results in therapeutic antitumor immunity to murine lung cancer. *Cancer Sci* 99, 2, (Feb), 361-367.

Younes, E., Haas, G.P., Dezso, B., Ali, E., Maughan, R.L., Kukuruga, M.A., Montecillo, E., Pontes, J.E. & Hillman, G.G. (1995). Local tumor irradiation augments the response to IL-2 therapy in a murine renal adenocarcinoma. *Cell Immunol* 165, 2, (Oct 15), 243-251.

10

Bone Seeking Radiopharmaceuticals for Metastatic Bone Pain

Marnix G.E.H. Lam[1] and Bernard A. Zonnenberg[1,2]
[1]*Department of Radiology and Nuclear Medicine*
[2]*Department of Internal Medicine*
University Medical Center Utrecht
The Netherlands

1. Introduction

Prostate cancer is the most common malignancy in men in the Netherlands. The majority of patients with advanced prostate cancer develop skeletal metastases, with bone pain as a frequent symptom. This poses a significant medical problem. Amongst other treatments, bone seeking radiopharmaceuticals are used to palliate painful metastatic bone disease. Efficacy has been sufficiently proven, as well as safety and feasibility. Practical issues as well as new developments and future prospects will be discussed.

This chapter will discuss the treatment of metastatic bone pain in hormone-refractory prostate cancer patients with bone seeking radiopharmaceuticals. Two main issues will be discussed:

1. Bone seeking radiopharmaceuticals in clinical practice. Issues regarding radiation safety and a protocol for routine use of bone seeking radiopharmaceuticals will be discussed in order to improve routine clinical care.
2. Enhancement of efficacy of bone seeking radiopharmaceuticals.

But first a short introduction will be given on clinical relevance and bone seeking radiopharmaceuticals in general.

2. Prostate cancer and skeletal metastases

The incidence of malignancy in the Netherlands was 74.500 patients in 2005. This will increase to approximately 95.000 new cases in 2015. Because malignancy related death is decreasing and it is likely to decrease further the prevalence of cancer patients will increase to an estimated 692.000 patients in 2015, compared to 366.000 in 2000 (an estimated doubling time of 15 years) (Coebergh, van de Poll-Franse, and Alers 2004; Visser and van Noord 2005). One of the major causes of cancer related death in men is prostate cancer. These patients will be the focus of this chapter.

The incidence of prostate cancer is high worldwide. It is the most common malignancy in men in the Netherlands. Approximately 9000 men are being diagnosed with prostate cancer each year (Figure 1). The rising incidence may be attributed to the incremental use of screening methods using prostate specific antigen (PSA) to detect prostate cancer. This hypothesis is supported by the growing number of patients being diagnosed with early stages of prostate cancer. The incidence also increases with age. Consequently, with a growing number of old men in our society the incidence of prostate cancer will further increase. Fortunately mortality from prostate cancer is decreasing due to better diagnostic methods and treatments (Dijkman and Debruyne 1996).

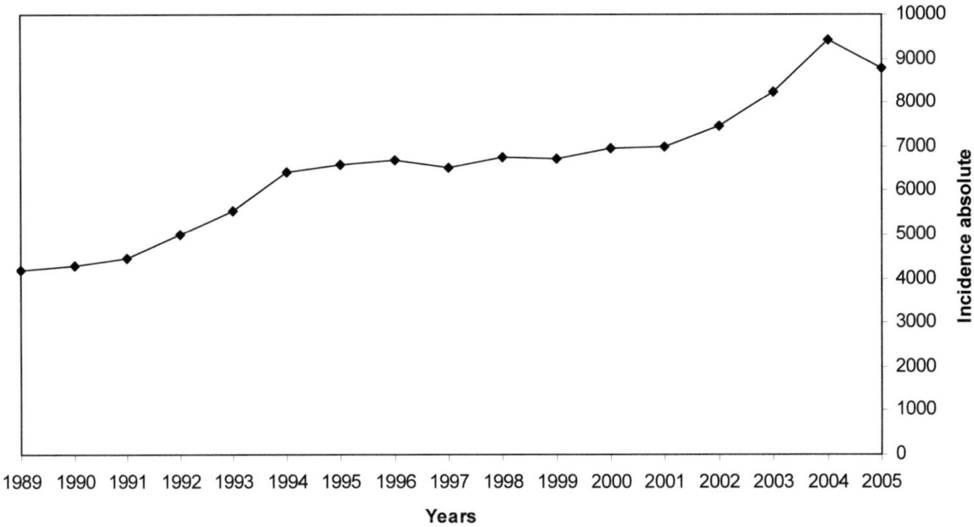

Fig. 1. Prostate cancer incidence between 1989 - 2005 derived from data on www.ikcnet.nl

A hallmark of metastatic prostate cancer is the development of osteoblastic bone metastases. Almost all patients with advanced prostate cancer eventually develop osseous metastases. In a majority of patients with prostate cancer, bone is the only site of clinical metastases. Many of the established prognostic factors for advanced prostate cancer (eg, performance status, alkaline phosphatase level, and haemoglobin level) reflect the clinical consequences of bone metastases. Hence, patients who develop widespread, progressive, or early bone metastases tend to suffer more from their symptoms and fare worse. Conversely, patients who develop limited, stable, or delayed bone metastases tend to experience less morbidity and have a less dismal clinical outcome. Conceivably, targeting the relevant bone metastases-associated factors may improve therapeutic results (Tu and Lin 2008). These factors consist of the main cells involved in bone metastasis (cancer cells, osteoblasts, osteoclasts, endothelial cells and stromal cells) and the numerous communicating substances (eg, interleukins, VEGF, RANKL, TNF-alfa, endothelins). They form a complex interaction and a microenvironment in which cancer cells may flourish (Tu and Lin 2008).

Frequently these skeletal metastases cause pain. Less common complications include myelum compression and pathological fractures (Dijkman and Debruyne 1996). Besides hormonal treatment most other treatment modalities in advanced prostate cancer patients are intended to palliate bone pain. Metastatic bone pain is a nociceptive somatic pain, initiated and maintained through local tissue injury. It is well recognized that chronic pain (including cancer pain) is a multidimensional phenomenon consisting of five dimensions (pathophysiological, sensory, emotional, cognitive, and behavioural). These five dimensions together form a complex pattern of relations (Quirijnen et al. 1996). Stress is a well known stimulus for nociceptive pain. The impression that pain may be uncontrollable produces stress for patients, which may lead to increased suffering and despair, and decreases the patient's performance (Chapman and Gavrin 1999). An effective pain management strategy requires breaking off this cycle using all available means. An effective pain control strategy, however, requires patients to take large quantities of opioids, often as much as 60 - 200 mg/day. This large dose may cause considerable side effects, including nausea, vomiting, constipation, and central sedation, all of which combine to a decrease in quality of life. Patients will have to take large doses of anti-emetics and laxatives to counteract nausea and constipation, respectively. Central sedation increases drowsiness, resulting in frequent falls, bone fractures, and driving accidents (Etches 1999). Supplemental therapy with local radiation, wide-field radiation, bisphosphonates, or bone seeking radiopharmaceuticals can significantly reduce the dose of opioids for most patients or may even completely eliminate the need for the medications in a few patients (Krishnamurthy and Krishnamurthy 2000).

Metastatic disease in prostate cancer may be treated first with hormonal therapy such as bilateral orchidectomy or medical first line hormone treatment (luteinizing hormone-releasing hormone agonist therapy). This androgen-deprivation therapy may be extended to maximal androgen blockade by adding anti-androgens (bicalutamide, flutamide, nilutamide). High risk prostate cancer patients may benefit from such a regimen even in the early stages of the disease (Klotz 2008). It is also recognized that discontinuation of an anti-androgen once hormone-refractory biochemical progression occurs is associated with a biochemical response in many patients. Anti-androgens may become agonistic due to a combination of androgen receptor over-expression and mutation (Kelly and Scher 1993; Small and Srinivas 1995). After a median of two years the prostate cancer cells generally become insensitive for hormonal treatment. In the case of hormone-refractory disease the patient may be treated by chemotherapy, local radiotherapy, systemic radiopharmaceuticals, bisphosphonates and analgesics, depending on the clinical status (Auclerc et al. 2000).

The clinical benefit of chemotherapy in hormone-refractory prostate cancer patients is limited. Some drugs showed potential as first-line treatment in hormone-refractory prostate carcinoma but were not sufficiently tested in clinical trials (Berthold, Sternberg, and Tannock 2005). Patients however may benefit from docetaxel chemotherapy in combination with prednisone. In a landmark study treatment with 75 mg/m^2 docetaxel i.v. every three weeks with 5 mg prednisone twice daily p.o. was compared with mitoxantrone 12 mg/m^2 every three weeks (Tannock et al. 2004). The median survival increased from 16.3 months in the mitoxantrone-group to 19.2 months in the docetaxel-group (Berthold et al. 2008). The group receiving docetaxel three weekly had a hazard ratio for death of 0.79 (95 percent confidence interval, 0.67 to 0.93; $p=0.004$) compared to the mitoxantrone-group (Berthold et al. 2008). Pain and quality of life improved significantly better in the docetaxel group and more patients (45% versus 32%; $p<0.001$) showed a 50% reduction of serum PSA levels (Tannock et al. 2004). However, docetaxel nor any other treatment will be curative in an advanced stage of prostate cancer.

Patients with hormone-refractory prostate cancer who have progressive disease after first-line chemotherapy may still benefit from several treatment options. At this stage of disease, patients can expect only a short duration of survival, and most patients become

symptomatic. Most patients will cease docetaxel treatment because of progressive disease or unacceptable adverse events. To control symptoms after the cessation of chemotherapy should rely on optimizing medical therapy for palliation. This may be combined with radiotherapy applied to dominant painful bone lesions. External beam radiotherapy for painful skeletal metastases leads to a decrease of pain in 60 – 65% of the patients. In 33% of the patients a total remission of pain symptoms was observed (McQuay et al. 2008). Patients may be treated in one fraction (8 Gray). No difference has been found between such a single-dose regimen and multiple fractions (Hartsell et al. 2005; Kaasa et al. 2006; Roos et al. 2005). Furthermore, when needed, patients may be treated a second time with a reported response rate between 66% and 84% (Mithal, Needham, and Hoskin 1994; Van der Linden et al. 2004).
Besides chemotherapy further hormonal manipulation with prednisone or dexamethasone may have some benefit as well. Glucocorticoids may lead to PSA response and/or relief of symptoms in patients with late-stage prostate cancer (Tannock et al. 1989). Some investigators have suggested that the superior results of regimens with taxanes may be due in part to the dexamethasone that is administered to avoid toxic reactions to these drugs. However, most patients have already received substantial treatment with glucocorticoids concurrent with first-line chemotherapy, so their potential benefit in later stages is probably minimal.
Other treatment options in the advanced stage of prostatic cancer include ketoconazole and estrogens. Inhibition of steroid synthesis by ketoconazole may increase the probability of an anti-androgen withdrawal response, although this did not translate into improved survival (Small et al. 2004). Estrogens may improve symptoms but caution must be used because of their ability to stimulate thrombosis and cardiovascular events. Estrogens were found to be equivalent to estramustine (which contains estrogen), probably as its activity is largely due to the estrogen component (Small et al. 2000). Transdermal administration of oestrogens through a patch avoids the entero-hepatic circulation and therefore it should not be associated with the same level of cardiovascular toxicity. Early data confirm the safety and efficacy of oestrogen patches as hormonal treatment in prostate cancer patients (Langley et al. 2008).
Currently new non chemotherapeutic options are studied such as endotheline antagonists (James et al. 2008) and abiraterone acetate, a potent, selective, small-molecule inhibitor of cytochrome P (CYP) 17, a key enzyme in androgen synthesis (Attard et al. 2008). Many other agents are being developed (Tu and Lin 2008).

3. Bone seeking radiopharmaceuticals

Bone seeking radiopharmaceuticals have proven to be useful for treatment of more generalized bone pain. All patients will finally progress to end stage disease with multiple skeletal metastases. These patients may receive bone seeking radiopharmaceuticals for generalized painful disease (Berthold, Sternberg, and Tannock 2005). The association of integrated cancer centres in the Netherlands (VIKC) developed an evidence based guideline on the diagnosis and treatment of pain in cancer patients. Radionuclide treatment of cancer patients with metastatic bone pain (so called bone seeking radiopharmaceuticals) was evaluated using all available literature (VIKC 2008). The conclusions are stated together with their level of evidence in Table 1.
Most of the patients who have participated in the mentioned trials were heavily pre-treated patients with previous radiotherapy, chemotherapy and/or hormone therapy. It was recommended that radionuclide treatment with bone seeking radiopharmaceuticals is indicated in patients with multifocal pain originating from osteoblastic skeletal metastases.

Repeated treatments are indicated after an initial response to treatment. The committee had the opinion that combined multimodality treatment should be performed in a trial setting. Further research in that field is warranted (VIKC 2008).
Radionuclide therapy with bone seeking radiopharmaceutical agents has been long used. It evolved from agents like ^{32}P-phosphate to newer agents like ^{188}Re-HEDP or ^{223}Ra (Table 2). Bone seeking radiopharmaceuticals consist of a radionuclide for the therapeutic effect and a carrier to reach the target site at the bone matrix level. Sometimes the carrier and the radionuclide are one and the same. This is the case for ^{32}P-phosphate, ^{223}Ra and ^{89}Sr. These radiopharmaceuticals behave as physiologic phosphate (^{32}P-phosphate) or Ca^{2+}-analogues (^{223}Ra and ^{89}Sr). They do not need a non-radioactive substance as a carrier to reach the target. Carriers like hydroxyethylenediphosphonic acid (HEDP in ^{186}Re-HEDP) and ethylenediaminetetramethylenephosphonic acid (EDTMP in ^{153}Sm-EDTMP) are being used in other bone seeking radiopharmaceuticals. They behave as bisphosphonates. These differences influence the biodistribution and pharmacokinetics of the pharmaceutical. Other differences between these agents include the radiation type, the radiation energy and the radionuclide half-life.
One thing that never changed during the last decades and stimulated the search for new agents was the conflict between efficacy and toxicity. The latter consisting of bone marrow suppression in particular. This has even led to a change of indication for the use of ^{32}P-phosphate. It is not used anymore for the palliation of metastatic bone pain but instead for the treatment of myeloproliferative diseases, making use of its bone marrow suppressive potential (Berlin 2000; Cheung and Driedger 1980). Fortunately newer agents have proved to be feasible and relatively safe for the palliative treatment of osseous metastases with acceptable and reversible bone marrow toxicity.

Conclusion	Evidence [a]	Study type [b]
It has been proven that treatment with bone seeking radiopharmaceuticals yields a better pain response than treatment with placebo in patients with painful osseous metastases from diverse cancers including prostate, breast and lung cancer.	Level 1	A1 (Bauman et al. 2005; Finlay, Mason, and Shelley 2005; McQuay et al. 2008; Roque i Figuls et al. 2008) A2 (Han et al. 2002; Lewington et al. 1991; Maxon, III et al. 1991; Sartor et al. 2004; Serafini et al. 1998)
It has been proven that no difference exists with regard to local pain response between treatment with ^{89}Sr-Chloride or external beam radiotherapy in patients with painful osseous metastases from a prostate carcinoma.	Level 1	A2 (Oosterhof et al. 2003; Quilty et al. 1994)
It is likely that no difference exists with regard to pain response between treatment with ^{89}Sr-Chloride and ^{186}Re-HEDP in patients with painful osseous metastases.	Level 2	A2 (Sciuto et al. 2001) B (Piffanelli et al. 2001)

Conclusion	Evidence [a]	Study type [b]
It is likely that the onset of the pain response of ^{186}Re-HEDP is faster than the onset of the pain response of ^{89}Sr-Chloride in patients with painful osseous metastases from a breast carcinoma.	Level 2	A2 (Sciuto et al. 2001)
It is likely that combined treatment with ^{89}Sr-Chloride and chemotherapy (platinum based) yields a better pain response than treatment without chemotherapy in patients with painful osseous metastases from a prostate carcinoma.	Level 2	A2 (Sciuto et al. 2002) C (Sciuto et al. 1996)
It has been suggested that adding ^{89}Sr-Chloride to chemotherapy may lead to improved survival and a longer duration of the pain response compared to treatment with chemotherapy alone.	Level 3	B (Tu et al. 2001)
It has been suggested that no difference exists with regard to the pain response after treatment with chemotherapy or ^{89}Sr-Chloride in patients with painful osseous metastases from a prostate carcinoma.	Level 3	B (Nilsson et al. 2005)
No conclusions can be drawn on the value of adding ^{89}Sr-Chloride to external beam radiotherapy in patients with painful osseous metastases from a prostate carcinoma because of conflicting results.		A2 (Porter et al. 1993; Smeland et al. 2003)

[a] Level of evidence: 1) A1 or at least two independent and consistent A2 studies; 2) One A2 study or at least two independent and consistent B studies; 3) One B or C study; 4) Professional opinion.
[b] Quality and methodology of studies: A1) Systemic review of at least two independent A2 trials; A2) Double-blind randomized trial of sufficient size and quality (comparison with a reference test ('gold standard'), defined endpoints, independent evaluation of both tests, no confounding); B) Comparative trial not meeting A2 criteria;
[c] Non-comparative trial; D) Professional opinion.

Table 1. Evidence based conclusions on treatment with bone seeking radiopharmaceuticals (VIKC 2008).

Radiopharmaceutical	Half-life (days)	β-emission MeV max (mean)	γ-emission keV (%)
^{188}Re-HEDP	0.7	2.12 (0.76)	155 (15%)
^{153}Sm-EDTMP	1.93	0.81 (0.23)	103 (29%)
^{186}Re-HEDP	3.7	1.07 (0.35)	137 (9%)
^{177}Lu-EDTMP	6.7	0.497 (0.15)	208 (11%)
^{223}Ra	11.4	Emits alfa-particles of circa 5.7 MeV	
^{117m}Sn-DTPA	13.6	Emits conversion electrons 127 - 152 keV	
^{32}P-Phosphate	14.3	1.71 (0.70)	None
^{89}Sr	50.5	1.46 (0.58)	910 (0.01%)

Table 2. Bone seeking radiopharmaceuticals categorized by half-life.

All patients with proven osteoblastic (or mixed type) skeletal metastases that accumulate ^{99m}Tc-HDP on skeletal scintigraphy may be candidates for treatment with bone seeking radiopharmaceuticals. They may be cancer patients with advanced disease originating from prostate cancer, breast cancer, lung cancer, medullary thyroid carcinoma, or other tumors (i.e. bronchial carcinoid tumors, medulloblastoma). In routine clinical practice the vast majority of patients are prostate cancer patients. In these patients the incidence of skeletal metastases is very high. They cause high morbidity and mortality (DePuy et al. 2007; Saarto et al. 2002). Metastases originating from prostate cancer are pure osteoblastic with relatively high radionuclide uptake, resulting in high tumor to non-tumor ratio's. And last but not least other treatment options are limited in advanced stages of this disease.

In the growing field of radionuclide therapy many new radiopharmaceuticals are being developed. At the moment $^{89}SrCl_2$ (Metastron®) and ^{153}Sm-EDTMP (Quadramet®) are both FDA approved. Together with ^{186}Re-HEDP (registered in some countries, not in the Netherlands) these bone seeking radiopharmaceuticals are mostly used today.

4. Bone seeking radiopharmaceuticals in clinical practice

4.1 Radiation safety considerations

Patients treated with any kind of radionuclide treatment must be regarded as a potential risk for public health because of a potential radiation hazard. Good understanding of the radionuclide used, its physical characteristics, its biodistribution and its pharmacokinetics, will allow us to draw proper guidelines for this kind of treatment. Does the patient need to be confined after treatment? Are we able to identify the radiation hazard from a qualitative and quantitative perspective? What does that mean for an individual patient in relation to its environment?

Patients treated with 89SrCl2, 186Re-HEDP or 153Sm-EDTMP are a source of radiation, including beta-radiation that has proven to be measurable outside the patient. Beta-particles in superficial tissue (such as in bones, blood vessels) cross the skin and contribute to the ambient equivalent dose. This aspect must be considered when using beta-emitting radiopharmaceuticals in general. The calculated effective doses for bystanders are well below the recommended values and do not lead to unacceptable additional radiation burden to health care workers and patients' families. The mean total effective doses absorbed by bystanders at 30 cm distance from a patient are approximately 0.02 mSv for 89SrCl2, 0.3 mSv for 186Re-HEDP, and 1.6 mSv for 153Sm-EDTMP (Lam et al. 2009b). These observations however should be placed in some perspective. First the

individual variation in effective dose to bystanders and second the potential risk of internal contamination of bystanders.
The total effective dose, as given above, is estimated for bystanders who reside at exactly 30 cm from the patient for an indefinite time. Because this is never the case, these estimations must be corrected for variations in time and distance between bystanders and patients. In a Dutch Ministry of Housing, Spatial Planning and Environment publication accurate calculations were made to cover the various persons who may have contact with patients (VRO92; VROM 2005). These calculations are based on residence times T (in fractions of days) with the patient and distances R (in meters) from the patient. The actual effective doses for bystanders will depend on residence times and distances in relation to the patient. Estimations were made for residence times and distances during a 24-hour period. This was done in the case of an elderly patient in relation to his or her partner and in the case of a patient in relation to his or her child (Tables 3 and 4).

	Without instruction			With instruction		
	Residence time (hrs/24hrs)	Distance (m)	Correction factor [a]	Residence time (hrs/24hrs)	Distance (m)	Correction factor [a]
outdoors activities	3/24	-	0	3/24	-	0
watching TV	5/24	0.5	0.075	5/24	2	0.0047
dinner	2/24	1	0.0075	2/24	1	0.0075
sleeping	8/24	0.7	0.061	8/24	2	0.0075
other	6/24	3	0.0025	6/24	3	0.0025
total			0.15			0.02
	Mean effective dose (mSv)			Mean effective dose (mSv)		
^{153}Sm-EDTMP	0.24			0.03		
^{186}Re-HEDP	0.05			< 0.01		
^{89}Sr-Chloride	< 0.01			< 0.01		

[a] Correction factor applicable for measurements at 30 cm from the patient using the inverse-square law

Table 3. Effective dose (external radiation) of *an elderly partner* with and without instructions.

Assuming that the estimated distances and times are a reflection of reality, corrections were made for these circumstances. Estimations of the effective doses for these persons (partner and child) are given for the three most used radiopharmaceuticals. In the case of a patient and his or her partner, without instructions a correction factor of 0.15 (15%) was applied. This is explained by the fact that bystanders do not stay within 30 cm of patients 24 hours a day. Because of work and other activities a correction factor should be applied. As an example a correction factor of 0.15 may be applied. The effective dose may be further reduced by instructing the patients and their families to keep distance as much as reasonably possible (e.g. watching TV and sleeping apart). With proper instructions to family, residence times may be reduced and distances increased, lowering the correction factor to as low as 0.02 (2%), an almost eight-fold decrease in radiation burden to bystanders (Table 3). In the case of a patient and his or her child an estimated correction factor of about 0.43 (43%) should be applied without instructions and 0.11 (11%) with instructions. In all instances effective doses will be < 1 mSv and with proper instructions they will be < 0.1 mSv or even < 0.01 mSv (Tables 3 and 4). It may be concluded that patients treated with bone seeking radiopharmaceuticals do not pose any threat to others.

	Without instruction			With instruction		
	Residence time (hrs/24hrs)	Distance (m)	Correction factor [a]	Residence time (hrs/24hrs)	Distance (m)	Correction factor [a]
playing	8/24	4	0.0019	8/24	4	0.0019
close contact	1/24	0.1	0.375	0.25/24	0.1	0.094
dinner	2/24	0.5	0.03	2/24	2	0.0019
sleeping	10/24	-	-	10/24	-	-
other	3/24	2	0.0094	3/24	2	0.0094
total			0.43			0.11
	Effective dose (mSv)			Effective dose (mSv)		
^{153}Sm-EDTMP	0.69			0.18		
^{186}Re-HEDP	0.13			0.03		
^{89}Sr-Chloride	< 0.01			< 0.01		

[a] Correction factor applicable for measurements at 30 cm from the patient using the inverse-square law

Table 4. Effective dose (external radiation) of *a young child* with and without instructions.

However, an exception has to be made considering urinary excretion of activity and the possible internal contamination of bystanders. Besides radiation exposure to non-patients from direct emission by the patient, another potential radiation hazard is formed by excreted radioactivity. The calculated mean total urinary excretion percentage of ^{89}Sr during the first 3 days after administration was 16% (Lam et al. 2009b). Using a hypothetical contamination scenario, that is used in radiation protection evaluation (VROM 2005), that 0.01% of the excreted amount of radioactivity will cause internal contamination to non-patients closely related to the patient, an internal dosage of 0.0024 MBq for $^{89}SrCl_2$ therapy (administered dose of 150 MBq) was calculated. For ^{186}Re-HEDP therapy (administered dose of 1295 MBq), the corresponding amount of radioactivity will be 0.064 MBq (49% of the injected dose is excreted (de Klerk et al. 1992)). After treatment with 37 MBq/kg ^{153}Sm-EDTMP 53.1% ± 15.1% of the administered dose was excreted in urine during the first 48 hours (Lam et al. 2007). Potential contamination with 0.01% of the excreted radioactivity will lead to an internal dosage of 0.15 MBq ^{153}Sm-EDTMP. The dose conversion coefficient for ingestion of ^{89}Sr is (e_{ing}) = 2.6 x 10^{-9} Sv/Bq, of ^{186}Re (e_{ing}) = 1.5 10^{-9} Sv/Bq, and of ^{153}Sm (e_{ing}) = 7.4 10^{-10} Sv/Bq. The present data show that the effective radiation absorbed dose, caused by a potential internal contamination (0.01% of the administered dose), is 6.2 microSv for ^{89}Sr, 96 microSv for ^{186}Re and 111 microSv for ^{153}Sm. These numbers are in the same order of magnitude as the numbers given for external exposure (Table 3 and 4).

The total effective dose for non-patients may be caused by both external radiation exposure and internal contamination. In contrast to the mean effective dose caused by external radiation, the effective dose after ingestion of 0.01% of the administered dose is hypothetical and may be much higher or much lower. In the case of ^{131}I it proved to be less. The uptake of ^{131}I in the thyroid of family members was measured (Buchan and Brindle 1970). A maximum uptake of 3.8 Bq per MBq administered was found. So on one hand it must be considered that 0.01% is a hypothetical figure, while the external radiation exposure is a fact. On the other hand, internal contamination poses a real threat to non-patients. Patients that were treated with bone-seeking radiopharmaceuticals are often severely disabled (in contrast to ^{131}I patients). Especially in the case of prostate cancer patients, they often have dysurea. Personal hygiene is not as obvious as it is to others. It is therefore advisable to give the patients simple, easy-to-follow instructions, in order to reduce the risk for non-patients. Using a separate toilet, sitting while urinating and washing hands afterwards, are highly recommended. In the case of incontinence, patients must be catheterized for a certain time depending on urinary excretion of the administered activity. Due to fast renal excretion this may be 12 hours after injection of ^{186}Re-HEDP and ^{153}Sm-EDTMP. $^{89}SrCl_2$ is being administered in relatively low doses and therefore has a relatively low risk for high effective dose due to ingestion of this radiopharmaceutical (6.2 microSv for ^{89}Sr). These patients do not have to be catheterized. The risk for significant internal contamination of non-patients is much lower and acceptable for this radiopharmaceutical.

In general it is advised to hospitalize patients treated with ^{186}Re-HEDP and ^{153}Sm-EDTMP for at least 8 hours. This is mostly based on urinary excretion and the risk for internal contamination, because the radiation exposure to non-patients is < 20 microSv/hour (1 meter from the patients) directly or within a few hours after administration in all cases. In the case of incontinence it is advised to treat patients with either ^{186}Re-HEDP or ^{153}Sm-EDTMP with a urinary catheter for 12 hours after administration. Patients treated with $^{89}SrCl_2$ may return home directly.

After discharge it is advisable to keep distance where possible (Table 3 and 4), following the ALARA ('as low as reasonably achievable') principles. This means, for example, that older patients (> 60 years) may still sleep close to their older partner, while being more stringent towards younger relatives to avoid any unnecessary radiation dose. The ICRP has proposed an effective dose limit of 1 mSv per year for individuals. In special circumstances a higher value may be allowed in a single year provided that the average over 5 years does not exceed 1 mSv per year. In clinical practice, the use of bone-seeking radiopharmaceuticals will give rise to a degree of radiation exposure to all those in contact with patients, albeit in very low doses. The present results further confirm the safety of treatment with bone-seeking radiopharmaceuticals.

4.2 Treatment recommendations

$^{89}SrCl_2$ (Metastron®) and ^{153}Sm-EDTMP (Quadramet®) are both FDA approved and registered in the Netherlands. Together with ^{186}Re-HEDP (registered in some countries, not in the Netherlands) these bone seeking radiopharmaceuticals are mostly used. Most of the randomized double-blind placebo controlled trials have been performed using $^{89}SrCl_2$ or ^{153}Sm-

EDTMP. An evidence based approach would be a choice between these radiopharmaceuticals. One of the differences between these two is the magnitude and rate of renal excretion. Both may be used without confining a patient to the hospital but from a radiation safety perspective it is advised to keep the patient in a controlled setting for at least 8 hours after injection in the case of ^{153}Sm-EDTMP. This could influence the choice on practical grounds in favour of $^{89}SrCl_2$. Not all nuclear medicine departments have such facilities.

Other differences include the longer half-life and higher energy (with higher range in tissue) of $^{89}SrCl_2$ compared to ^{153}Sm-EDTMP. ^{153}Sm-EDTMP and ^{186}Re-HEDP are highly comparable with regard to energy and half-life. Most comparative randomized studies have been performed using $^{89}SrCl_2$ and ^{186}Re-HEDP. It was found that no difference exist with regard to pain response between treatment with ^{89}Sr-Chloride and ^{186}Re-HEDP in patients with painful osseous metastases (Piffanelli et al. 2001; Sciuto et al. 2001). And that the onset of the pain response of ^{186}Re-HEDP is faster than the onset of the pain response of ^{89}Sr-Chloride in patients with painful osseous metastases from a breast carcinoma (Sciuto et al. 2001). So one might argue that when a faster pain response is indicated one should use ^{186}Re-HEDP or ^{153}Sm-EDTMP. Other differences are the longer duration of response of ^{89}Sr-Chloride on one hand, and the prolonged bone marrow toxicity of ^{89}Sr-Chloride on the other hand. These differences were not investigated in direct comparative studies but should be considered nevertheless. In summary: in favour of ^{89}Sr-Chloride are:

- No confinement necessary
- Longer duration of response (suitable in relatively good clinical condition in which a prompt response is not warranted)

In favour of ^{186}Re-HEDP or ^{153}Sm-EDTMP are:

- Fast response (suitable in bad clinical condition in which immediate response is wanted)
- Favourable toxicity profile (suitable in heavily pre-treated patients, in wide spread metastatic disease and possibly in combination with other myelotoxic treatments)

In most cases today a fast response is needed. Besides that most patients, including prostate cancer patients, are heavily pre-treated. They have end stage disease with minimal bone marrow reserve. And last but not least short-living bone seeking radiopharmaceuticals like ^{186}Re-HEDP, ^{153}Sm-EDTMP and others may prove to be more suitable in combination with other treatment modalities, not just because of their toxicity profile but also because of their high dose rate, offering an effective treatment with fast recovery.

5. Enhancement of efficacy

A major concern in the treatment of prostate cancer patients in the more advanced stage of the disease is the delicate balance between efficacy and toxicity. Treatment of metastatic bone pain with analgesics or localized external beam radiotherapy is relatively safe and easy. Treatment with bone seeking radiopharmaceuticals may be more appropriate in selected cases but efficacy is sometimes disappointing and bone marrow toxicity may be high in individual patients. Enhancement of overall efficacy without increasing toxicity could push the clinical decision algorithm in a positive direction with regard to the use of bone seeking radiopharmaceuticals.

One way of improving overall efficacy is combined treatment. Combined treatment regimens may deliver the beneficial effect of two different treatment modalities. These combinations may not only be additive but possibly synergistic to each other, leading to enhancement of overall efficacy with acceptable toxicity.

5.1 Multimodality treatment

The propensity of prostate cancer to metastasize to bone and the prognostic significance of bone metastases suggest that effective treatment of bone metastases may provide clinical benefits (DePuy et al. 2007; Sabbatini et al. 1999). With regard to the 'seed' and 'soil' theory on bone metastases the seed may comprise the so-called cancer stem cells. Whereas the soil may comprise a unique microenvironment, that facilitate the growth and survival of cancer stem cells. Targeting the microenvironment may offer another way to improve treatment of prostate cancer bone metastases. The microenvironment consists of osteoclasts, osteoblasts, endothelium and stroma. In the presence of cancer stem cells they interact leading to a disruption in normal coupling between osteoclasts and osteoblasts. An improved understanding of this process will influence how we select agents to target bone metastases and how we design strategies to treat prostate cancer bone metastases. Treatments may be directed to the cancer stem cells, the osteoblasts, the osteoclasts, the endothelium or the stroma (Tu and Lin 2008).

Osteoblasts may be targeted by several pharmaceuticals including bone seeking radiopharmaceuticals. Other osteoblast directed treatments include endothelin-1-antagonists (atrasentan) (Carducci et al. 2003), vitamin D analogs (1,25-hydroxyvitamin D_3) (Beer et al. 2007), monoclonal IGF-1R (insulin-like growth factor-1-receptor) antibodies (Boyle et al. 2001) and CXRC4 (G-protein-coupled receptor) inhibitors (MSX-122), which inhibit the homing behaviour of cancer stem cells. Osteoclast activity may be inhibited by bisphosphonates (zolendronate) (Saad et al. 2002), RANK ligand inhibitors (denosumab) (Lewiecki 2006), tyrosine kinase inhibitors (dasatinib) or IL-6 antagonists (CNTO328) (Nam et al. 2005). And the endothelium and/or stroma may be targeted by anti-angiogenesis therapies. These include the vascular endothelial growth factor (VEGF) receptor antagonists bevacizumab, thalidomide and lenalidomide (Dahut et al. 2004). They reduce VEGF levels and basic fibroblast growth factor, inhibit growth and survival of tumor cells by modulation of adhesion molecules and mediate various cytokines. Also targeted to the endothelium are platelet-derived growth factor receptor (PDGFR) tyrosine kinase inhibitors (imatinib, sunitinib and tandutinib) (Ko et al. 2001). They may also have anti-angiogenetic potential. Most of these agents are under investigation. Many clinical studies in prostate cancer patients are ongoing (Tu and Lin 2008).

Combining different treatment modalities may be interesting because of additive effects or synergy effects. In the case of bisphosphonates and bone seeking radiopharmaceuticals the combined use has always been contra-indicated because of presumed interaction at the bone matrix level. It was shown that the combined use of ^{153}Sm-EDTMP and bisphosphonates in patients with hormone-refractory prostate carcinoma is feasible. The combined treatment regimen is safe and may prove to be an effective long-term treatment regimen (Lam et al. 2007).

Another combined treatment regimen would be a combination of bone seeking radiopharmaceuticals and chemotherapy. It is likely that combined treatment with ^{89}Sr-Chloride and chemotherapy (platinum based) yields a better pain response than treatment without chemotherapy in patients with painful osseous metastases from a prostate carcinoma (Sciuto et al. 2002), (Sciuto et al. 1996). And it has been suggested that adding

^{89}Sr-Chloride to chemotherapy may lead to improved survival and a longer duration of the pain response compared to treatment with chemotherapy alone (Tu et al. 2001). Studies are yet limited but they are encouraging. Most of them have been performed using ^{89}Sr-Chloride and some using ^{153}Sm-EDTMP (Ricci et al. 2007). Patients may possibly have an improved pain response and longer survival. In prostate cancer patients a most interesting choice would be combining docetaxel and a bone seeking radiopharmaceutical. These studies, using ^{153}Sm-EDTMP or ^{186}Re-HEDP, are underway. Our group investigated the combination of ^{188}Re-HEDP and capecitabine (Xeloda®) (Lam et al. 2009a). This treatment regimen proved to be feasible and safe. Phase II efficacy testing using the maximum tolerable dose of 2500 mg/m^2/day capecitabine is underway. Capecitabine is primarily used as a radiation sensitizer. It offers a convenient therapy with acceptable toxicity, ease of use as oral tablets and low costs. The same is true for ^{188}Re-HEDP. It is homemade on demand and has favourable physical characteristics with a short half-life (16.9 hours) and high beta-energy ($E_{\beta\ max}$ 2.12 MeV; $E_{\beta\ mean}$ 0.76 MeV). In theory, this high dose rate could lead to improved efficacy with rapid recovery. This is ideal for combined treatment regimens and for repeated treatment, which has already shown to be favourable with regard to pain response and survival (Palmedo et al. 2003).

Several other combinations using bone seeking radiopharmaceuticals are under investigation. Currently, a randomized phase III study (MDA-3410/CTSU in M.D. Anderson Cancer Center, Houston, Texas) combining weekly doxorubicin (20 mg/m^2) with ^{89}Sr-Chloride after response to induction chemotherapy is underway, as well as another phase I trial combining docetaxel/prednisone and ^{153}Sm-EDTMP, also at M.D. Anderson (Tu and Lin 2008). It remains to be established whether targeting both the tumor (chemotherapy) and bone compartments will improve therapeutic efficacy. This concept is also being tested in multiple other trials, mostly combining docetaxel/prednisone with bone environment directed treatments, like the agents described above (Tu and Lin 2008). The described studies add to this search for optimized treatment regimens in hormone-refractory prostate cancer patients.

5.2 Predictions of efficacy and toxicity

Most patients with advanced prostate cancer have disease limited to the bone, which is notoriously difficult to assess for response, with a small subset having soft tissue lesions. To limit response evaluation to only patients with bidimensionally measurable disease would eliminate 70% to 80% of patients who would otherwise be evaluable (Figg et al. 1996). With regard to prostate cancer patients efficacy of treatment has been monitored by PSA in a majority of studies. However it is doubtful whether PSA changes correlate with clinical benefit (Bubley et al. 1999). A 50% decrease in PSA level seems a reasonable predictor of a favourable outcome, but this was certainly not the case in all studies (Bauer et al. 1999; Sridhara et al. 1995). It was advised not to use PSA level drops as a surrogate marker for survival (Bubley et al. 1999).

In patients with advanced disease, survival and quality of life, including pain palliation, are the most important criteria of clinical response. Besides survival these parameters are difficult to measure and subject to errors. With an attempt to standardize treatment response monitoring in cancer patients the European Organization for Research and Treatment of Cancer (EORTC) has developed quality of life questionnaires (EORTC QLQ-C30 version 3.0). They were validated in many clinical trials (Aaronson et al. 1993). They include questions on global health status / quality of life, functional scales and symptom scales. The functional scales are subdivided in physical functioning, role functioning, emotional functioning, cognitive functioning and social functioning. The symptom scales are subdivided in fatigue, nausea and vomiting, pain, dyspnoea, insomnia, appetite loss, constipation, diarrhoea and financial difficulties. Each domain was scored on a scale of 0 – 100, according to the EORTC scoring manual (Fayers et al. 2001). The changes in scores may be used to monitor clinical effect.

Other often used clinical monitoring tools include the visual analogue scales (VAS) to monitor pain, changes in analgesic intake and, more basic, the physician's assessment based on anamnesis and physical examination. A matter of debate is the frequency of evaluation. It seems that daily assessment is necessary to appreciate the wide variation in clinical status that patients may experience from day to day (Han et al. 2002). In all cases it is difficult to find a good balance between accuracy and compliance. PSA is therefore still popular to measure an objective level of response (Bubley et al. 1999; Scher et al. 2008).

However, other predictors of response may prove to be much more reliable than PSA. In hormone-refractory prostate cancer patients in advanced stages of their disease the extent of metastatic disease in the skeleton is of high prognostic significance (Sabbatini et al. 1999). Furthermore it was shown that patients with advanced disease who had experienced a so-called Skeletal Related Event (defined as: pathologic fracture, spinal cord compression with vertebral compression fracture, the need for surgery to treat or prevent pathologic fractures or spinal cord compression, or the need for radiation to bone) had a significantly worse survival and poorer quality of life, in comparison with patients who had not experienced a Skeletal Related Event (DePuy et al. 2007). These results further confirm the importance to treat skeletal metastases adequately. Markers of skeletal metabolism were found to be related to outcome and survival. In several clinical studies in prostate cancer patients it was observed that markers of bone metabolism were able to predict outcome, both as absolute levels pre-treatment and as changes after treatment (Jung et al. 2004; Lein et al. 2007). In large series of cancer patients, including a majority of prostate cancer patients, treated with zoledronic acid, it was found that baseline levels of the bone marker urinary N-terminal type I collagen peptide [NTX], as well as changes of NTX after treatment were able to predict improved survival (Coleman et al. 2005; Lipton et al. 2008). Other studies emphasized the importance of the bone marker serum bone specific alkaline phosphatase [BAP] as a predictor of outcome (Cook et al. 2006; Smith et al. 2007). Most of these studies used the same bone markers as we did in the study on the combined treatment of prostate cancer patients with ^{153}Sm-EDTMP and zoledronic acid (i.e. NTX, BAP and serum procollagen type I N propeptide [PINP],). Although this study comprised a small patient population the results are of interest because they confirm the utility of these markers as predictors of clinical outcome, even in small numbers (Lam et al. 2007). Besides, they were first tested in the treatment monitoring of bone seeking radiopharmaceuticals. The bone formation markers BAP and PINP were in agreement with the clinical effect of the combined treatment regimen evaluated by EORTC questionnaires. The bone resorption marker NTX and PSA were not in agreement with the clinical effect. This supports the hypothesis that the extent of osteoblastic metastasis in hormone-refractory prostate cancer patients is an important parameter for clinical outcome. Both treatment itself and treatment monitoring should be directed to these osteoblastic metastases. Bone markers may well prove to be very useful predictors of clinical effect in the treatment with bone seeking radiopharmaceuticals. They should be used in future trials.

Last but not least the importance of imaging modalities should be mentioned with regard to individualized treatment monitoring. Functional rather than anatomical imaging techniques may be used to predict response. Several PET (Positron Emission Tomography) techniques are being developed for this purpose (John et al. 2008; Price et al. 2002). In fact, functional imaging will prove to be one of the major contributions of nuclear medicine to clinical oncology in the future. Does the treatment work? That question needs to be answered for each oncologic treatment on an individual basis. Nuclear imaging and PET in particular may be helpful.

Besides predictors of efficacy, predictors of toxicity are equally important for individualized patient management. Radiopharmaceuticals are important resources in the management of bone pain, but they need to be utilized in a manner that does not prevent other systemic therapy (Rago 1998). Thrombocytopenia is the dose limiting factor in treatment of painful bone metastases with bone seeking radiopharmaceuticals. De Klerk *et al* evaluated thrombocytopenia in patients with hormone refractory prostate carcinoma, treated with ^{186}Re-HEDP (de Klerk et al. 1994). As an index of the extent of bone involvement, the bone scan index (BSI) was determined from the pre-treatment ^{99m}Tc-HDP scintigram. The BSI is a tool to describe the extent of skeletal metastases on a scale from 0 to 100% (Blake et al. 1986). They described a functional relation ($r = 0.78$; $p < 0.001$) of the percentage of platelet decrease after treatment with the extent and distribution of skeletal metastases (BSI) and administered activity, normalized to standard body surface area. Using this relation, it is possible to predict thrombocytopenia by pre-treatment skeletal scintigraphy and to adjust the dosage for each patient to avoid unacceptable toxicity (de Klerk et al. 1994).

However, more sophisticated indices of bone marrow function might also be of paramount importance. Recently, some very interesting reports have been published on 'reticulated platelets' (Briggs et al. 2004; Wang et al. 2002). In systemic radionuclide therapy, the megakaryocyte seems to be most vulnerable to radiation. It is of great interest to gain more knowledge of bone marrow function pre-treatment using 'biological' parameters like 'reticulated platelets'. These newly released platelets are larger and contain RNA. They were suggested to be the platelet analogue of the red cell reticulocyt. Assessment of platelet production using 'reticulated platelets' would distinguish between thrombocytopenia due to bone marrow failure and impending bone marrow recovery after cytotoxic therapy or thrombocytopenia due to increased peripheral platelet destruction and turnover. In both cases platelet levels are low, but in the latter 'reticulated platelet' levels will be high due to increased production (Wang et al. 2002). This non-invasive measurement could further increase our knowledge of platelet production and the influence of radiation on this process.

By adding hematological, chemical and biological parameters, combined with the bone scan index, body surface area, administered activity and retained activity, an extended version of 'De Klerk's formula' may be developed. This is probably best done as a so called nomogram. Smaletz *et al* developed a nomogram to predict survival for patients with hormone refractory prostate carcinoma (Smaletz et al. 2002). A nomogram is a model in which individual parameters lead to a chance (from 0 to 100%) to experience a pre-defined outcome. The outcome may be defined as survival or for example toxicity. Such a model can be made to predict hematological toxicity (thrombocytopenia, leucopenia) after treatment with bone seeking radiopharmaceuticals to improve individualized patient management.

6. Future prospects

Several future implications have already been discussed above. One of the most important developments for bone seeking radiopharmaceuticals will be individualized medicine. The search for an optimized balance between efficacy and toxicity will be found rather in an individualized treatment plan than in new agents. Good predictors of efficacy and toxicity are needed for treatment monitoring. Several potential candidates were described above. They may be found in clinical evaluation, imaging and several laboratory parameters. A combination of these parameters may lead to a prediction model which may be used in daily practice.

Multimodality treatment has also been described above. Many combinations have potential. It has to be investigated which regimen will be most effective. Besides a direct anti-tumor effect which may be reached with chemotherapy (i.e. docetaxel), it is recognized that treatment directed to the bony environment may add to the overall efficacy of the treatment regimen. Bone seeking radiopharmaceuticals are bone-directed and may be of value in combination with other treatment modalities. Besides combinations with chemotherapy or bisphosphonates other interesting combinations may include for example atrasentan, or denosumab.

An important other issue is the timing of treatment with bone seeking radiopharmaceuticals. The frequency and interval of sequential treatment should be considered. Bone seeking radiopharmaceuticals are mostly used as a single shot treatment. When patients respond to the treatment repeated treatment is considered. In most instances this does not happen with a planned interval in mind but rather when symptoms reappear after an initial response. In fact this might be too late. It seems better to treat patients sequentially before symptoms reoccur. This was confirmed in a randomized controlled trial in prostate cancer patients treated with two dosages of 1.1 mCi ^{188}Re-HEDP with an interval of eight weeks compared to single shot treatment. They did not only find an improved pain response with longer duration but surprisingly an improved survival as well (Palmedo et al. 2003). Safety of repeated treatment with bone seeking radiopharmaceuticals was also confirmed (Sartor et al. 2007). This enhancement of efficacy may be attributed to chronic inhibition of osseous metabolism preventing cancer cells to thrive in the bony environment. Most other oncologic compounds are used in a repeated fashion using several cycles to reach sufficient effect. It should be investigated which multiple treatment regimen is most suitable for bone seeking radiopharmaceuticals, and whether it is safe and more effective. It may be suggested that the best result in hormone-refractory will be reached using a multimodality treatment regimen with fractionation of all treatments to be effective over a prolonged period of time.

7. Conclusion

Treatment with bone seeking radiopharmaceuticals in patients with multiple painful skeletal metastases is safe and effective when proper protocols are being used. Important improvements may be found in multimodality treatment in long-term treatment regimens and in individualized patient management. Identification of powerful indicators of toxicity and efficacy may guide patient selection and therapy monitoring to optimize the patient's outcome. This may possibly lead us beyond pain palliation towards improvement of survival.

8. References

Aaronson NK et al (1993) The European Organization for Research and Treatment of Cancer QLQ-C30: a quality-of-life instrument for use in international clinical trials in oncology. *J.Natl.Cancer Inst.* 85 (5):365-376.

Attard G et al (2008) Phase I clinical trial of a selective inhibitor of CYP17, abiraterone acetate, confirms that castration-resistant prostate cancer commonly remains hormone driven. *J.Clin.Oncol.* 26 (28):4563-4571.

Auclerc G et al (2000) Management of advanced prostate cancer. *Oncologist.* 5 (1):36-44.

Bauer KS et al (1999) A pharmacokinetically guided Phase II study of carboxyamido-triazole in androgen-independent prostate cancer. *Clin.Cancer Res.* 5 (9):2324-2329.

Bauman G et al (2005) Radiopharmaceuticals for the palliation of painful bone metastasis-a systemic review. *Radiother.Oncol.* 75 (3):258-270.

Beer TM et al (2007) Double-blinded randomized study of high-dose calcitriol plus docetaxel compared with placebo plus docetaxel in androgen-independent prostate cancer: a report from the ASCENT Investigators. *J.Clin.Oncol.* 25 (6):669-674.

Berlin NI (2000) Treatment of the myeloproliferative disorders with 32P. *Eur.J.Haematol.* 65 (1):1-7.

Berthold DR et al (2008) Docetaxel plus prednisone or mitoxantrone plus prednisone for advanced prostate cancer: updated survival in the TAX 327 study. *J.Clin.Oncol.* 26 (2):242-245.

Berthold DR, Sternberg CN, and Tannock IF (2005) Management of advanced prostate cancer after first-line chemotherapy. *J.Clin.Oncol.* 23 (32):8247-8252.

Blake GM et al (1986) Sr-89 therapy: strontium kinetics in disseminated carcinoma of the prostate. *Eur.J.Nucl.Med.* 12 (9):447-454.

Boyle BJ et al (2001) Insulin-like growth factor binding protein-3 mediates 1 alpha,25-dihydroxyvitamin d(3) growth inhibition in the LNCaP prostate cancer cell line through p21/WAF1. *J.Urol.* 165 (4):1319-1324.

Briggs C et al (2004) Assessment of an immature platelet fraction (IPF) in peripheral thrombocytopenia. *Br.J.Haematol.* 126 (1):93-99.

Bubley GJ et al (1999) Eligibility and response guidelines for phase II clinical trials in androgen-independent prostate cancer: recommendations from the Prostate-Specific Antigen Working Group. *J.Clin.Oncol.* 17 (11):3461-3467.

Buchan RC and Brindle JM (1970) Radioiodine therapy to out-patients - the contamination hazard. *Br.J.Radiol.* 43 (511):479-482.

Carducci MA et al (2003) Effect of endothelin-A receptor blockade with atrasentan on tumor progression in men with hormone-refractory prostate cancer: a randomized, phase II, placebo-controlled trial. *J.Clin.Oncol.* 21 (4):679-689.

Chapman CR and Gavrin J (1999) Suffering: the contributions of persistent pain. *Lancet* 353 (9171):2233-2237.

Cheung A and Driedger AA (1980) Evaluation of radioactive phosphorus in the palliation of metastatic bone lesions from carcinoma of the breast and prostate. *Radiology* 134 (1):209-212.

Coebergh, J. W. W., van de Poll-Franse, L. V., and Alers, J. C. Kanker in Nederland, Trends, prognoses en implicaties voor zorgvraag. Amsterdam. KWF , 65-73. 2004.

Coleman RE et al (2005) Predictive value of bone resorption and formation markers in cancer patients with bone metastases receiving the bisphosphonate zoledronic acid. *J.Clin.Oncol.* 23 (22):4925-4935.

Cook RJ et al (2006) Markers of bone metabolism and survival in men with hormone-refractory metastatic prostate cancer. *Clin.Cancer Res.* 12 (11 Pt 1):3361-3367.

Dahut WL et al (2004) Randomized phase II trial of docetaxel plus thalidomide in androgen-independent prostate cancer. *J.Clin.Oncol.* 22 (13):2532-2539.

de Klerk JM et al (1994) Evaluation of thrombocytopenia in patients treated with rhenium-186-HEDP: guidelines for individual dosage recommendations. *J.Nucl.Med.* 35 (9):1423-1428.

de Klerk JM et al (1992) Pharmacokinetics of rhenium-186 after administration of rhenium-186-HEDP to patients with bone metastases. *J.Nucl.Med.* 33 (5):646-651.

DePuy V et al (2007) Effects of skeletal morbidities on longitudinal patient-reported outcomes and survival in patients with metastatic prostate cancer. *Support.Care Cancer* 15 (7):869-876.

Dijkman GA and Debruyne FM (1996) Epidemiology of prostate cancer. *Eur.Urol.* 30 (3):281-295.

Etches RC (1999) Patient-controlled analgesia. *Surg.Clin.North Am.* 79 (2):297-312.

Fayers, P. M., Aaronson, N. K., Bjordal, K., Groenvold, M., Curran, D., and Bottomley, A. The EORTC QLQ-C30 Scoring Manual. 3rd ed. Brussels: European Organization for Research and Treatment of Cancer . 2001. Brussels. Ref Type: Generic

Figg WD et al (1996) Lack of correlation between prostate-specific antigen and the presence of measurable soft tissue metastases in hormone-refractory prostate cancer. *Cancer Invest* 14 (6):513-517.

Finlay IG, Mason MD, and Shelley M (2005) Radioisotopes for the palliation of metastatic bone cancer: a systematic review. *Lancet Oncol.* 6 (6):392-400.

Han SH et al (2002) The PLACORHEN study: a double-blind, placebo-controlled, randomized radionuclide study with (186)Re-etidronate in hormone-resistant prostate cancer patients with painful bone metastases. Placebo Controlled Rhenium Study. *J.Nucl.Med.* 43 (9):1150-1156.

Hartsell WF et al (2005) Randomized trial of short- versus long-course radiotherapy for palliation of painful bone metastases. *J.Natl.Cancer Inst.* 97 (11):798-804.

James ND et al (2008) Safety and Efficacy of the Specific Endothelin-A Receptor Antagonist ZD4054 in Patients with Hormone-Resistant Prostate Cancer and Bone Metastases Who Were Pain Free or Mildly Symptomatic: A Double-Blind, Placebo-Controlled, Randomised, Phase 2 Trial. *Eur.Urol.*

John SS et al (2008) Newer imaging modalities to assist with target localization in the radiation treatment of prostate cancer and possible lymph node metastases. *Int.J.Radiat.Oncol.Biol.Phys.* 71 (1 Suppl):S43-S47.

Jung K et al (2004) Comparison of 10 serum bone turnover markers in prostate carcinoma patients with bone metastatic spread: diagnostic and prognostic implications. *Int.J.Cancer* 111 (5):783-791.

Kaasa S et al (2006) Prospective randomised multicenter trial on single fraction radiotherapy (8 Gy x 1) versus multiple fractions (3 Gy x 10) in the treatment of painful bone metastases. *Radiother.Oncol.* 79 (3):278-284.

Kelly WK and Scher HI (1993) Prostate specific antigen decline after antiandrogen withdrawal: the flutamide withdrawal syndrome. *J.Urol.* 149 (3):607-609.

Klotz L (2008) Maximal androgen blockade for advanced prostate cancer. *Best.Pract.Res.Clin.Endocrinol.Metab* 22 (2):331-340.

Ko YJ et al (2001) A multi-institutional phase ii study of SU101, a platelet-derived growth factor receptor inhibitor, for patients with hormone-refractory prostate cancer. *Clin.Cancer Res.* 7 (4):800-805.

Krishnamurthy GT and Krishnamurthy S (2000) Radionuclides for metastatic bone pain palliation: a need for rational re-evaluation in the new millennium. *J.Nucl.Med.* 41 (4):688-691.

Lam MG et al (2009a) (188)Re-HEDP combined with capecitabine in hormone-refractory prostate cancer patients with bone metastases: a phase I safety and toxicity study. *Eur.J.Nucl.Med.Mol.Imaging* 36 (9):1425-1433.

Lam MG et al (2007) Combined use of zoledronic acid and 153Sm-EDTMP in hormone-refractory prostate cancer patients with bone metastases. *Eur.J.Nucl.Med.Mol.Imaging*.

Lam MG et al (2009b) Radiation safety considerations for the bone seeking radiopharmaceuticals. 89SrCl2, 186Re-HEDP and 153Sm-EDTMP. *Nuklearmedizin* 48 (1):37-43.

Langley RE et al (2008) Early hormonal data from a multicentre phase II trial using transdermal oestrogen patches as first-line hormonal therapy in patients with locally advanced or metastatic prostate cancer. *BJU.Int.* 102 (4):442-445.

Lein M et al (2007) Serial markers of bone turnover in men with metastatic prostate cancer treated with zoledronic Acid for detection of bone metastases progression. *Eur.Urol.* 52 (5):1381-1387.

Lewiecki EM (2006) RANK ligand inhibition with denosumab for the management of osteoporosis. *Expert.Opin.Biol.Ther.* 6 (10):1041-1050.

Lewington VJ et al (1991) A prospective, randomised double-blind crossover study to examine the efficacy of strontium-89 in pain palliation in patients with advanced prostate cancer metastatic to bone. *Eur.J.Cancer* 27 (8):954-958.

Lipton A et al (2008) Normalization of bone markers is associated with improved survival in patients with bone metastases from solid tumors and elevated bone resorption receiving zoledronic acid. *Cancer* 113 (1):193-201.

Maxon HR, III et al (1991) Rhenium-186(Sn)HEDP for treatment of painful osseous metastases: results of a double-blind crossover comparison with placebo. *J.Nucl.Med.* 32 (10):1877-1881.

McQuay, H. J., Collins, S., Carroll, D., and Moore, R. A. Radiotherapy for the palliation of painful bone metastases. The Cochrane Database of Systemic Reviews Issue 4, 1-22. 2008.

Mithal NP, Needham PR, and Hoskin PJ (1994) Retreatment with radiotherapy for painful bone metastases. *Int.J.Radiat.Oncol.Biol.Phys.* 29 (5):1011-1014.

Nam S et al (2005) Action of the Src family kinase inhibitor, dasatinib (BMS-354825), on human prostate cancer cells. *Cancer Res.* 65 (20):9185-9189.

Nilsson S et al (2005) Palliation of bone pain in prostate cancer using chemotherapy and strontium-89. A randomized phase II study. *J.Pain Symptom.Manage.* 29 (4):352-357.

Oosterhof GO et al (2003) Strontium(89) chloride versus palliative local field radiotherapy in patients with hormonal escaped prostate cancer: a phase III study of the European Organisation for Research and Treatment of Cancer, Genitourinary Group. *Eur.Urol.* 44 (5):519-526.

Palmedo H et al (2003) Repeated bone-targeted therapy for hormone-refractory prostate carcinoma: tandomized phase II trial with the new, high-energy radiopharmaceutical rhenium-188 hydroxyethylidenediphosphonate. *J.Clin.Oncol.* 21 (15):2869-2875.

Piffanelli A et al (2001) Radionuclide therapy for painful bone metastases. An Italian multicentre observational study. Writing Committee of an Ad Hoc Study Group. *Q.J.Nucl.Med.* 45 (1):100-107.

Porter AT et al (1993) Results of a randomized phase-III trial to evaluate the efficacy of strontium-89 adjuvant to local field external beam irradiation in the management of endocrine resistant metastatic prostate cancer. *Int.J.Radiat.Oncol.Biol.Phys.* 25 (5):805-813.

Price DT et al (2002) Comparison of [18 F]fluorocholine and [18 F]fluorodeoxyglucose for positron emission tomography of androgen dependent and androgen independent prostate cancer. *J.Urol.* 168 (1):273-280.

Quilty PM et al (1994) A comparison of the palliative effects of strontium-89 and external beam radiotherapy in metastatic prostate cancer. *Radiother.Oncol.* 31 (1):33-40.

Quirijnen JM et al (1996) Efficacy of rhenium-186-etidronate in prostate cancer patients with metastatic bone pain. *J.Nucl.Med.* 37 (9):1511-1515.

Rago R (1998) Management of Hormone-Sensitive and Hormone-Refractory Metastatic Prostate Cancer. *Cancer Control* 5 (6):513-521.

Ricci S et al (2007) Clinical benefit of bone-targeted radiometabolic therapy with 153Sm-EDTMP combined with chemotherapy in patients with metastatic hormone-refractory prostate cancer. *Eur.J.Nucl.Med.Mol.Imaging* 34 (7):1023-1030.

Roos DE et al (2005) Randomized trial of 8 Gy in 1 versus 20 Gy in 5 fractions of radiotherapy for neuropathic pain due to bone metastases (Trans-Tasman Radiation Oncology Group, TROG 96.05). *Radiother.Oncol.* 75 (1):54-63.

Roque i Figuls, M., Martinez-ZApata, M. J., Alonso-Coello, P., Catala, E., Garcia, J. L., and Ferrandiz, M. Radioisotopes for metastatic bone pain. The Cochrane Database of Systemic Reviews Issue 4, 1-36. 2008.

Saad F et al (2002) A randomized, placebo-controlled trial of zoledronic acid in patients with hormone-refractory metastatic prostate carcinoma. *J.Natl.Cancer Inst.* 94 (19):1458-1468.

Saarto T et al (2002) Palliative radiotherapy in the treatment of skeletal metastases. *Eur.J.Pain* 6 (5):323-330.

Sabbatini P et al (1999) Prognostic significance of extent of disease in bone in patients with androgen-independent prostate cancer. *J.Clin.Oncol.* 17 (3):948-957.

Sartor O et al (2007) Safety and efficacy of repeat administration of samarium Sm-153 lexidronam to patients with metastatic bone pain. *Cancer* 109 (3):637-643.

Sartor O et al (2004) Samarium-153-Lexidronam complex for treatment of painful bone metastases in hormone-refractory prostate cancer. *Urology* 63 (5):940-945.

Scher HI et al (2008) Design and end points of clinical trials for patients with progressive prostate cancer and castrate levels of testosterone: recommendations of the Prostate Cancer Clinical Trials Working Group. *J.Clin.Oncol.* 26 (7):1148-1159.

Sciuto R et al (2001) Metastatic bone pain palliation with 89-Sr and 186-Re-HEDP in breast cancer patients. *Breast Cancer Res.Treat.* 66 (2):101-109.

Sciuto R et al (2002) Effects of low-dose cisplatin on 89Sr therapy for painful bone metastases from prostate cancer: a randomized clinical trial. *J.Nucl.Med.* 43 (1):79-86.

Sciuto R et al (1996) Radiosensitization with low-dose carboplatin enhances pain palliation in radioisotope therapy with strontium-89. *Nucl.Med.Commun.* 17 (9):799-804.

Serafini AN et al (1998) Palliation of pain associated with metastatic bone cancer using samarium-153 lexidronam: a double-blind placebo-controlled clinical trial. *J.Clin.Oncol.* 16 (4):1574-1581.

Smaletz O et al (2002) Nomogram for overall survival of patients with progressive metastatic prostate cancer after castration. *J.Clin.Oncol.* 20 (19):3972-3982.

Small EJ et al (2000) Prospective trial of the herbal supplement PC-SPES in patients with progressive prostate cancer. *J.Clin.Oncol.* 18 (21):3595-3603.

Small EJ et al (2004) Antiandrogen withdrawal alone or in combination with ketoconazole in androgen-independent prostate cancer patients: a phase III trial (CALGB 9583). *J.Clin.Oncol.* 22 (6):1025-1033.

Small EJ and Srinivas S (1995) The antiandrogen withdrawal syndrome. Experience in a large cohort of unselected patients with advanced prostate cancer. *Cancer* 76 (8):1428-1434.

Smeland S et al (2003) Role of strontium-89 as adjuvant to palliative external beam radiotherapy is questionable: results of a double-blind randomized study. *Int.J.Radiat.Oncol.Biol.Phys.* 56 (5):1397-1404.

Smith MR et al (2007) Predictors of skeletal complications in men with hormone-refractory metastatic prostate cancer. *Urology* 70 (2):315-319.

Sridhara R et al (1995) Evaluation of prostate-specific antigen as a surrogate marker for response of hormone-refractory prostate cancer to suramin therapy. *J.Clin.Oncol.* 13 (12):2944-2953.

Tannock I et al (1989) Treatment of metastatic prostatic cancer with low-dose prednisone: evaluation of pain and quality of life as pragmatic indices of response. *J.Clin.Oncol.* 7 (5):590-597.

Tannock IF et al (2004) Docetaxel plus prednisone or mitoxantrone plus prednisone for advanced prostate cancer. *N.Engl.J.Med.* 351 (15):1502-1512.

Tu, S. and Lin, S. Current trials using bone-targeting agents in prostate cancer. Cancer J. 14, 35-39. 2008.

Tu SM et al (2001) Bone-targeted therapy for advanced androgen-independent carcinoma of the prostate: a randomised phase II trial. *Lancet* 357 (9253):336-341.

Van der Linden YM et al (2004) Single fraction radiotherapy is efficacious: a further analysis of the Dutch Bone Metastasis Study controlling for the influence of retreatment. *Int.J.Radiat.Oncol.Biol.Phys.* 59 (2):528-537.

VIKC. Richtlijn 'diagnostiek en behandeling van pijn bij patiënten met kanker' Utrecht. 2008.

Visser, O. and van Noord, K. J. Feiten en fabels over kanker in Nederland. Utrecht. VIKC , 8-9. 2005.

VRO92. Min. VROM, Publicatiereeks Stralenbescherming nr. 1992/55, mei 1992.

VROM. Recommendations: working with therapeutical doses of radionuclides, The Hague. 2005.

Wang C et al (2002) Reticulated platelets predict platelet count recovery following chemotherapy. *Transfusion* 42 (3):368-374.

11

Use of Radiobiological Modeling in Treatment Plan Evaluation and Optimization of Prostate Cancer Radiotherapy

Panayiotis Mavroidis[1], Dimos Baltas[2],
Bengt K. Lind[1] and Nikos Papanikolaou[3]
[1]*Department of Medical Radiation Physics*
Karolinska Institutet and Stockholm University
[2]*Department of Medical Physics & Engineering, Strahlenklinik,*
Klinikum Offenbach GmbH
[3]*Department of Radiological Sciences*
University of Texas Health Science Center, San Antonio, Texas
[1]*Sweden*
[2]*Germany*
[3]*USA*

1. Introduction

There are many tools available that are used to evaluate a radiotherapy treatment plan, such as isodose distribution charts, dose volume histograms (DVH), maximum, minimum and mean doses of the dose distributions as well as DVH point dose constraints. All the already mentioned evaluation tools are dosimetric only without taking into account the radiobiological characteristics of tumors or OARs. It has been demonstrated that although competing treatment plans might have similar mean, maximum or minimum doses they may have significantly different clinical outcomes (Mavroidis et al. 2001). For performing a more complete treatment plan evaluation and comparison the complication-free tumor control probability (P_+) and the biologically effective uniform dose ($\bar{\bar{D}}$) have been proposed (Källman et al. 1992a, Mavroidis et al. 2000). The $\bar{\bar{D}}$ concept denotes that any two dose distributions within a target or OAR are equivalent if they produce the same probability for tumor control or normal tissue complication, respectively (Mavroidis et al. 2001).
In this chapter, the importance of the $P - \bar{\bar{D}}$ diagrams is illustrated. These diagrams provide important information by combining the radiobiological data of the organs involved with the dosimetric information of the delivered dose distribution (Mavroidis et al. 2010). It would increase the flexibility and clinical application of the P_+ index if in its original definition the different terms related to the tumor control and normal tissue complication probabilities were accompanied by some weighting factors, which could be adjustable by the clinicians depending on the important of the different clinical endpoints used (Mavroidis et al. 2011). In practice the P_+ index finds the pure benefit from the treatment by subtracting the normal tissue complication probabilities from the tumor control probability.

In clinical practice, there are not different weighting factors that are applied but there are risk thresholds (usually 5-10%) for every organ at risk, which should not be exceeded (Mavroidis et al. 2011). So, in order to classify the different treatment plans one can select the dose level that satisfies these demands imposed by the normal tissues risk thresholds and compare the expected tumor control rates at this dose level.

By using the $\bar{\bar{D}}$ concept on the dose axis, the control and complication probabilities of the target and OARs can be examined individually. Due to the fact that different plans generally deliver different mean doses to the target for the same control rate, the use of the target mean dose as a dose scaling basis is not suitable since the expected response rates induced by the treatment to the rest of the involved organs cannot be easily compared using this scale. The major advantage is that the $\bar{\bar{D}}$ concept forces the total control probabilities of different plans to coincide and the comparison of the response curves becomes much simpler than when the mean target dose is used (Mavroidis et al. 2001).

The results and conclusions of this chapter are strongly dependent on the accuracy of the radiobiological models and the parameters describing the dose-response relation of the different tumours and normal tissues (Mavroidis et al. 2007). However, it is known that all the existing models are based on certain assumptions or take into account certain only biological mechanisms. Furthermore, the determination of the model parameters expressing the effective radiosensitivity of the tissues is subject to uncertainties imposed by the inaccuracies in the patient setup during radiotherapy, lack of knowledge of the inter-patient and intra-patient radiosensitivity and inconsistencies in treatment methodology (Buffa et al. 2001, Fenwick & Nahum 2001). Consequently, the determined model parameters and the corresponding dose-response curves are characterized by confidence intervals. In the present analysis, most of the tissue response parameters have been taken from recently published clinical studies, where these parameter confidence intervals has been reduced significantly (e.g. uncertainty of around 5% in the determination of D_{50}). So, the expected response of a tissue is known with some uncertainty, which can be considered clinically acceptable (Mavroidis et al. 2007).

In this chapter, the treatment plans were optimized using conventional physical criteria like dose volume histograms, isodose charts, DVH point constraints, target prescribed doses and OAR tolerance doses. However, the developed treatment plans were evaluated radiobiologically using the radiation sensitivities of the respective organs involved in each case. The expected normal tissue complications were estimated against the optimum target dose using radiobiological plots. Just as a dose volume histogram is a good illustration of the volumetric dose distribution delivered to the target and OAR in the patient, so is the radiobiological evaluation plot as a measure of the expected clinical outcome. The dose-response diagrams in conjunction with the dosimetric diagrams provide a more thorough viewpoint of the examined treatment plans.

2. Organ delineation and treatment planning using CT vs. CT-MRI images during in prostate cancer radiotherapy

Traditionally, targets and organs-at-risk (OAR) are anatomically delineated on computed tomography (CT)-images in prostate cancer treatment planning. However, in CT the sensitivity of visualizing extracapsular involvement is lower than in magnetic resonance imaging (MRI), which provides much more detailed information. MRI can superbly demonstrate the internal prostatic anatomy, prostatic margins and the extent of prostatic tumors (Chen et al. 2004, Parker et al. 2003, Rørvik et al. 1993, Villeirs et al. 2007). It has been shown that an important decrease in the inter-observer delineation variation, as well as a significant decrease in the clinical target volume (CTV) may be resulted in by the use of fused MRI-CT images (Villeirs et al. 2005). Using MRI for delineation, the reduced prostate-target volume is associated with a reduction of the rectal wall being irradiated, which may result in fewer rectal and urological complications (Rasch et al. 1999). More specifically, the use of axial and coronal MR scans, in localized prostate carcinoma treatment planning results in a better coverage of the prostate and a reduction of the volume of the rectum irradiated to high doses (Debois et al. 1999).

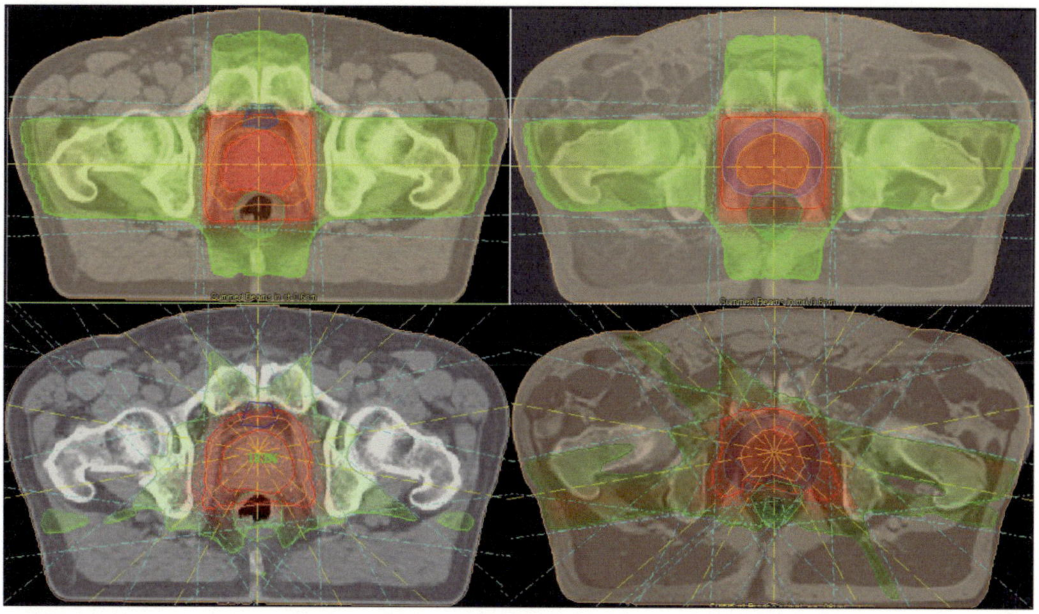

Fig. 1. The reference CT (left) and fused CT-MRI (right) slices of a prostate cancer patient is shown for the 3D-CRT (upper) and MLC-based IMRT (lower) treatment plans in the transverse plane. The delineations of the anatomical structures involved were performed based on the CT and MRI images and they are illustrated together with the dose distributions delivered to the patient (Tzikas et al. 2011) (published with permission from: Tzikas et al. Investigating the clinical aspects of using CT vs. CT-MRI images during organ delineation and treatment planning in prostate cancer radiotherapy. Technology in Cancer Research and Treatment, Vol.10, pp. 235 and 236, 2011, Adenine Press, http://www.tcrt.org).

In the present analysis, the respective CT and MRI images at treatment position were acquired for 10 prostate cancer patients (Tzikas et al. 2011). For each patient the separate CT and MRI images were used to delineate the Clinical Target Volume (CTV), which includes the prostate gland and the seminal vehicles. During treatment planning, the MRI and CT images were fused. The PTV was produced by adding to the CTV 1.0 cm margin in all directions apart from that towards rectum, which was 0.6 cm. So, 2 PTVs were produced for each patient based on the CT and MRI images. The comparison of the prostate cancer treatment plans in terms of isodose lines and dose volume histograms (DVH) is shown in

Figs. 1 and 2. Furthermore, individual dose-response curves and P_+ - $\bar{\bar{D}}_B$ plots of the CT and CT-MRI based treatment plans are presented in Fig. 3 for the CRT (left) and IMRT (right) radiation modalities, respectively.

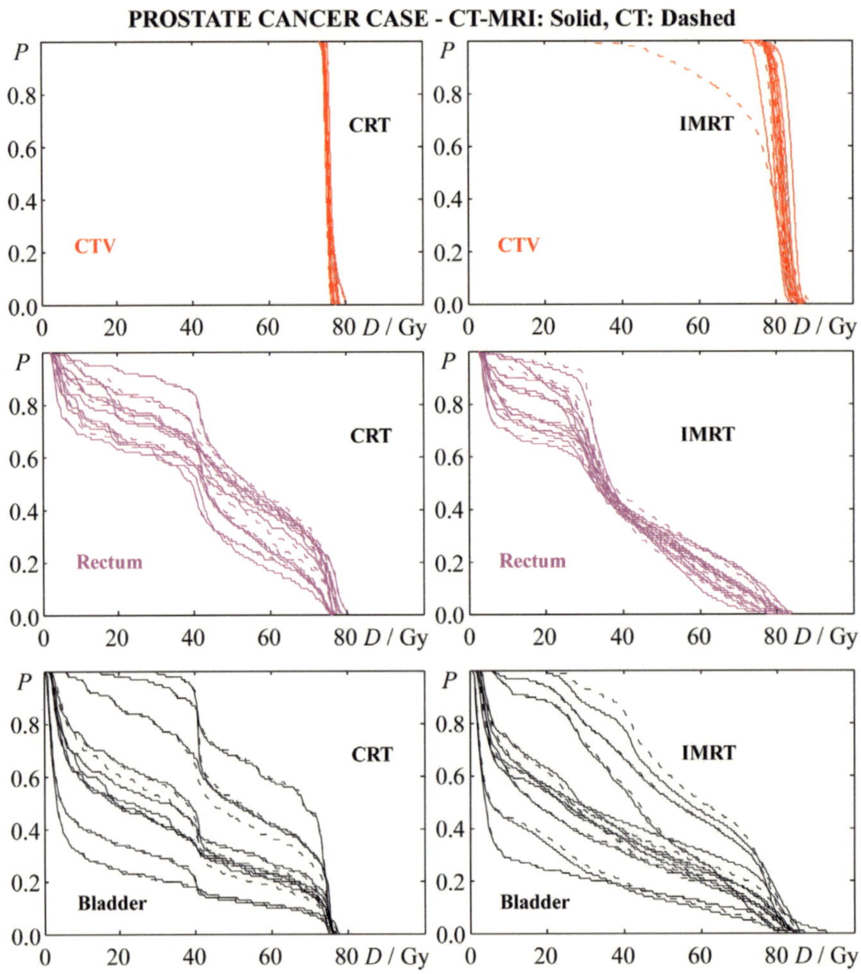

Fig. 2. The dose volume histograms (DVHs) of the CTV, rectum and bladder are presented in the upper, middle and lower diagrams, respectively for the CRT (left) and IMRT (right) treatment plans, which were optimized based on the CT and fused CT-MRI images, separately.

For the treatment plans of the CRT treatment modality, which were produced based on the CT images, at the clinical dose prescription the average P_+ value is 15.9% for a mean dose ($\bar{D}_{CTV}$) and a biologically effective uniform dose ($\bar{\bar{D}}_B$) to the CTV of 75.5 Gy. The average total control probability, P_B is 26.5% and the average total complication probability, P_I is 10.5%. Similarly, for the treatment plans that were produced based on the fused CT-MRI images, the average P_+ value is 17.5% for the same $\bar{D}_{CTV}$ and $\bar{\bar{D}}_B$. The average P_B the same with that of the treatment plans that were produced using CT images alone (26.5%) and the average P_I is 8.9%. However, at the dose level of the individual dose distributions that the complication-free tumor control gets optimum, for the CT-based treatment plans, the P_+ value becomes 42.5% for a $\bar{\bar{D}}_B$ of 86.4 Gy having average P_B = 80.0% and average P_I = 37.4%, whereas for the CT-MRI-based treatment plans, the P_+ value becomes 46.7% for a $\bar{\bar{D}}_B$ of 86.7 Gy having an average P_B = 80.6% and an average P_I by 33.8%.

For the treatment plans of the IMRT treatment modality, which were produced based on the CT images, at the clinical dose prescription, the P_+ value is 52.5% for $\bar{D}_{CTV}$ = 81.0 Gy and $\bar{\bar{D}}_B$ = 80.8 Gy. The average P_B is 57.1% and the average P_I is 4.7%. Similarly, for the CT-MRI-based treatment plans, the P_+ value is 53.4% for $\bar{D}_{CTV}$ = 80.8 Gy and $\bar{\bar{D}}_B$ = 80.5 Gy. The average P_B = 58.6% and the average P_I = 5.2%. However, at the dose level that maximizes the complication-free tumor control for the CT-based plans, the P_+ value becomes 74.7% for a $\bar{\bar{D}}_B$ of 91.5Gy having P_B = 90.0% and P_I = 15.3%, whereas for the CT-MRI-based plans, the P_+ value remains the same for a higher $\bar{\bar{D}}_B$ by 0.6 Gy. The corresponding average P_B = 90.2%, whereas the average P_I = 15.4%.

If the CT-based treatment plans were applied to calculate the dose in target and OARs that were produced using the fused CT-MRI images then the average differences would be almost zero in the case of CRT radiation modality, whereas in the case of IMRT radiation modality the P_+ value would become 2.1% lower, the average P_B would be lower by 2.1% while the average P_I would remains the same.

Observing the diagrams in Fig. 3 it is apparent that the clinically established dose prescription, which corresponds to a certain uniform dose in the CTV deviates from the optimal dose level that is indicated by the radiobiological evaluation. For example, the clinically prescribed dose level is lower than the optimum level by $\Delta\bar{\bar{D}}$ = 8-14 Gy. According to these findings, it is expected that a small increase in the dose prescription will slightly increase the complication rate but it will also be accompanied by a significant increase in the control rate. As shown in Fig. 3, a margin of improvement can be observed while the individual normal tissue responses are kept below the limit of 10% as indicated by the horizontal crossed bar.

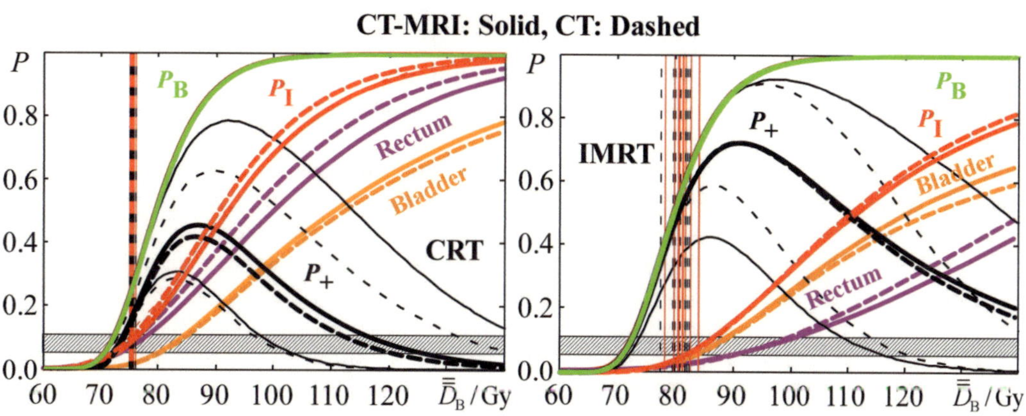

Fig. 3. The dose-response curves of the CTV / total control probability, P_B, bladder, rectum, total complication probability, P_I and complication-free tumor control probability, P_+ are presented for the CRT and IMRT treatment plans, which were optimized based on the CT and fused CT-MRI images, separately. The horizontal crossed bar indicates the 5-10% response probability region. The vertical lines represent the prescribed dose levels of the individual patients.

It is worth of noticing that the OAR with the highest risk for complications is rectum in the case of CRT and bladder in the case of IMRT (Fig. 3). This observation confirms previous reports that one of the most important advantages of IMRT over 3D-CRT is the ability of sparing the rectal wall reducing the development of late toxicity. In Fig. 3, it is shown that the results vary considerably among the patients as indicated by the thin P_+ lines.

For the CRT treatment plans, the response probabilities of CTV and bladder from the CT and fused CT-MRI based treatment plans do not differ significantly (p=0.87 and p=0.49, respectively), whereas those of rectum differ significantly (p=0.02) (Tzikas et al 2011). On the other hand, for the IMRT treatment plans, the response probabilities of all the structures (CTV, bladder and rectum) do not differ significantly between the two sets of plans (p=0.68, p=0.59 and p=0.34, respectively). The improvement that results in by the use of fused CT-MRI images in the overall effectiveness of the CRT plans is statistically significant (p=0.03), which is mainly caused by the statistically significant sparing of the OARs (p=0.03 for P_I). In the IMRT treatment plans this improvement does not get statistically significant. This stems from the fact that IMRT radiation has to capability of producing highly conformal dose distributions that can spare already from the beginning very well the OARs.

In the future, target volumes could be reduced by both CT/MRI co-registration and dose painting using MR spectroscopy (Claus et al. 2004, Hou et al. 2009, Scheidler et al. 1999, Weinreb et al. 2009). These ongoing improvements and developments in radiotherapy treatment planning are leading to treatments which offer both better tumour volume coverage, and are minimizing the risk of treatment-related complications (Beasley et al. 2005). These changes should allow the escalation in dose delivered to the tumour volume with the potential for increased cure rates.

3. Daily megavoltage CT registration on adaptive Helical Tomotherapy

In treatments where the organs-at-risk (OARs) are close to the clinical target volume (CTV), the accuracy of the delivered dose is critical. The existence of an accurate patient positioning process is a prerequisite for ensuring agreement between planned and delivered dose distributions (Creutzberg et al. 1993, Mitine et al. 1991). Patient setup inaccuracies can lead to variations in dose delivery and under-dosage of tumors or over-dosage of normal tissues, which can result in a considerable reduction of local tumor control and/or increase of side effects, respectively (Mavroidis et al. 2011).

Helical Tomotherapy (HT) is characterized by dose distributions of high dose conformity (Mackie et al. 1999, Webb 2000). Presently, the Planned Adaptive module of the Tomotherapy software is used to correct dose discrepancies that may occur during treatment delivery. The comparison of the delivered and planned fractional dose distributions can be made in several treatment fractions. To measure the extent of the patient setup deviation on a helical tomotherapy machine, a megavoltage computed tomography (MVCT) scan has been developed for daily correction of patient positioning (Boswell et al. 2006, Meeks et al. 2005, Welsh et al. 2006). Due to the highly conformal distributions that can be obtained with HT any discrepancy between the planned and delivered dose distributions may result in the degradation of the curative power and effectiveness of the treatment (Löf et al. 1995). Consequently, there is a need to measure those differences in terms of a change in the expected clinical outcome. The present analysis performs assessment of the clinical effectiveness of the delivered treatment by interpreting the dosimetric characteristics of the different dose distributions and translating them into expected rates of tumor control and normal tissue complications.

For each of the examined patients, a Helical Tomotherapy plan was developed and subsequently the calculated dose distributions with and without patient setup correction were compared by using physical and radiobiological measures (Mavroidis et al. 2011). The corresponding cumulative dose distributions, which are determined by adding the delivered fractional dose distributions, are calculated for the entire course of radiation therapy (Fig. 4).

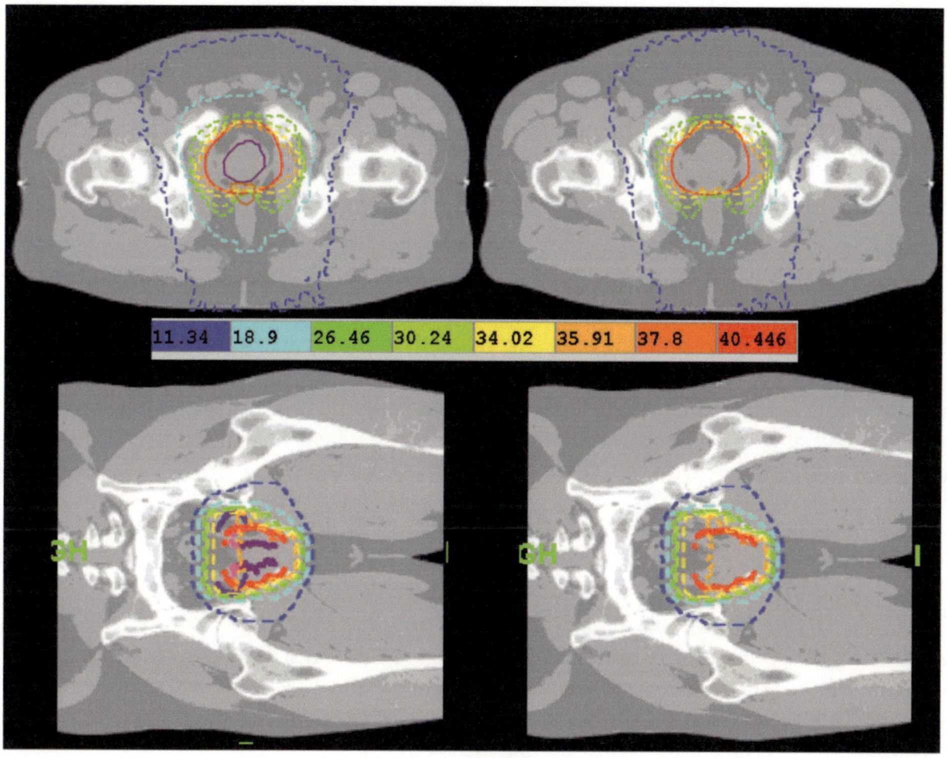

Fig. 4. The reference CT slices of a prostate cancer patient are shown in the transverse and coronal planes for the Helical Tomotherapy dose distributions with (left) and without (right) patient setup correction. In each case, the dose values of the isodose lines are also presented.

In this investigation each patient has a reference kilovoltage CT (kVCT) that was used for the development of the treatment plan. For each fraction, a pre-treatment verification megavoltage CT (MVCT) was obtained in the tomotherapy unit to assess setup accuracy. In order to evaluate the dosimetric effect of setup correction in Helical Tomotherapy, two different cumulative dose distributions were analyzed for the examined clinical cases. One cumulative dose distribution was calculated by adding up the separate delivered fractional dose distributions with setup correction. In this set of merged images, a mutual information based registration (that considered translational and rotational only corrections) was performed between the reference kVCT and the pre-treatment MVCT for each fraction based on anatomical landmarks. The other cumulative dose distribution was computed by adding up the delivered fractional dose distributions as calculated on the daily MVCT, without applying any positional corrections from the daily MVCT-kVCT co-registration. The dose distributions with and without patient repositioning were computed and the final dose volume histograms (DVHs) for both dose calculations were compared (Fig. 5).

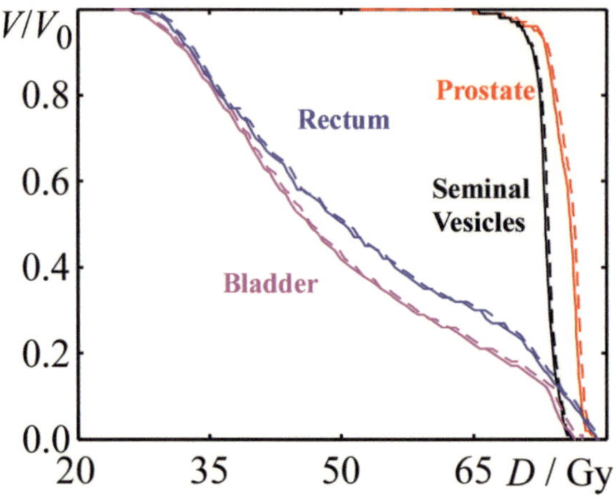

Fig. 5. The dose volume histograms (DVHs) of the targets (Prostate, Seminal Vesicles) and organs at risk (bladder, rectum) are illustrated. The solid lines correspond to the dose distribution with setup correction, whereas the dashed lines correspond to the dose distribution without setup correction (Mavroidis et al. 2011) (published with permission from: Mavroidis et al. Radiobiological and dosimetric analysis of daily megavoltage CT registration techniques on adaptive radiotherapy with Helical Tomotherapy. Technology in Cancer Research and Treatment, Vol.10, pp. 9, 2011, Adenine Press, http://www.tcrt.org).

For this dose prescription of the dose distributions with and without setup correction, the complication-free tumor control probabilities, P_+ are 10.9% and 11.9% for mean doses to the ITV ($\bar{D}_{ITV}$) of 74.7 Gy and 75.2 Gy and biologically effective uniform doses to the ITV ($\bar{\bar{D}}_B$) of 75.2 Gy and 75.4 Gy, respectively. The corresponding total control probabilities, P_B are 14.5% and 15.3%, whereas the total complication probabilities, P_I are 3.6% and 3.4%, which are almost equal to the response probabilities of the rectum (3.6% and 3.4%, respectively). At the dose level of the dose distributions with and without setup correction that maximizes the P_+ index ($\bar{D}_{ITV}$ = 90.0 Gy), the P_+ values are 55.9% and 57.7%, respectively.

Response probability	Clinical Dose Prescription		Optimum Dose Prescription	
	With setup correction	W/o setup correction	With setup correction	W/o setup correction
GTV (%)	15.5	+ 0.8	85.2	- 1.0
Seminal Vesicles (%)	93.6	+ 0.2	99.5	0.0
Bladder (%)	0.1	0.0	5.1	- 0.3
Rectum (%)	3.6	- 0.2	25.0	- 2.6
P_+ (%)	**10.9**	**+ 1.0**	**55.9**	**+ 1.8**
P_B (%)	**14.5**	**+ 0.8**	**84.7**	**- 1.0**
P_I (%)	**3.6**	**- 0.2**	**28.8**	**- 2.8**
$\bar{D}_{ITV}$ (Gy)	**74.7**	**+ 0.5**	**90.0**	**0.0**
$\bar{\bar{D}}_B$ (Gy)	**75.2**	**+ 0.2**	**90.6**	**- 0.4**

Table 1. Summary of the radiobiological comparison.

As it is shown in Fig. 6, the expected complication-free tumor control for the dose distributions with setup correction is equivalent or worse than the delivered dose distributions without setup correction. The reason is that the HT TPS does not have the possibility of performing radiobiological treatment plan optimization, which means that the planned dose distributions could not be produced using the maximum P_+ as objective. By examining the tumor control and normal tissue complication probabilities separately it can be observed that the dose distributions with setup correction have the same or higher response probabilities than the dose distributions without setup correction. However, for normal tissues the classification of the dose distributions with and without setup correction seems to be more sensitive and it varies depending on the case. In all the cases, the ITV is irradiated almost iso-effectively by the delivered dose distributions with and without patient setup correction. This is supported by the tumor control probabilities, P_B that are presented in Table 1 (Mavroidis et al. 2011). On the other hand, the setup uncertainties produce higher normal tissue complications when the OARs move into the high dose region or lower expected responses when the OARs move away from the high dose region.

As far as tissues of parallel internal organizations are concerned, dose inhomogeneity does not affect significantly their response, which is mainly determined by the mean dose. In this case, although the variation of a given dose distribution may be large, the $\bar{\bar{D}}$ value does not deviate much from the corresponding mean dose, $\bar{D}$, due to the low relative seriality value characterizing such a tissue.

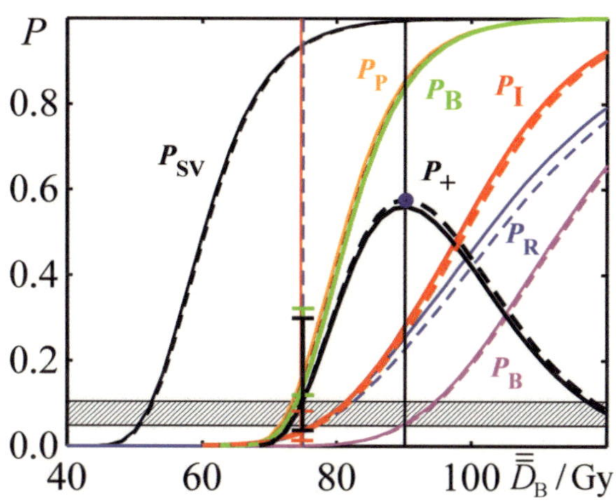

Fig. 6. The dose-response curves that are derived from the radiobiological evaluation of the dose distributions are plotted using $\bar{\bar{D}}$ on the dose axis. The horizontal crossed bar indicates the 5-10% response probability region. The solid and dashed vertical lines indicate the dose levels of the dose distributions with and without setup correction, respectively. The vertical error bars indicate the confidence intervals of the corresponding dose-response curves due to the uncertainties of the radiobiological parameters. The solid lines correspond to the dose distribution with setup correction, whereas the dashed lines correspond to the dose distribution without setup correction.

In Fig. 6, the clinically established dose prescription (solid and dashed vertical lines), deviates from the optimal dose level that is indicated by the radiobiological evaluation. With a small increase in the dose prescription an increase in the complication-free tumor control, P_+ can be achieved because the gain in tumor control is larger than the increment in normal tissue complications until a balance is reached. The dashed vertical line indicates the dose prescription, which intersects with the total complication probability of 10%. Because of these points the clinically prescribed dose level is lower than the optimum level by a $\Delta\bar{\bar{D}}$ of about 15.0 Gy.
In the DVH diagram (Fig. 5) it is observed that a significantly higher dose is delivered to the ITV compared to the OARs, which leads to response curves that are well separated from those of the targets as shown in Fig. 6. The width of the P_+ curve expresses the separation between the response curves of the targets and those of the OARs. At the same time, the most effective dose distribution is indicated, since it generates a higher value of P_+. The more conformal a treatment technique is the more precise and accurate the patient setup process should be. In these techniques the dose distribution is so well matched with the radiosensitivity map of the clinical case that a small misalignment in the setup can rapidly reduce the effectiveness of the delivered therapy. The quality of a treatment does not only depend on the conformity of the applied technique but also on the quality of the supporting services.

4. Radiobiological evaluation of Helical Tomotherapy and MLC-based IMRT treatment plan

Helical Tomotherapy (HT) is a radiation modality that is capable of producing high conformity dose distributions that may be superior than other IMRT techniques (Mackie et al. 1999, Webb 2000). A unique radiation delivery method is employed by HT, which delivers radiation helically through fifty-one projections per rotation. Although HT can produce very conformal dose distributions, it is still unknown how much the effectiveness of the resulted dose distributions differs from that of other radiation therapy modalities such as that of the MLC-based step-and-shoot IMRT. Consequently, the goal of this analysis is to compare IMRT treatment plans generated using MLC-based step-and-shoot IMRT and HT technology based on radiobiological measures, using representative prostate cancer cases. For each case, two sets of treatment plans have been developed (IMRT and HT). A parallel physical and radiobiological evaluation was carried out to assess the different treatment plans. The implemented radiobiological procedure estimates the probability to achieve tumour control without complications based on the knowledge of the dose-response relations of the tumours and organs-at-risk (Emami et al. 1991, Mavroidis et al. 2003, 2005, Ågren 1995).
Fig. 7 illustrates the dose distributions of a conventional, a conformal (CRT), an MLC-based IMRT and a HT treatment plan, of a prostate cancer case, in the form of isodose curves in transverse and coronal views, respectively (Mavroidis et al. 2007). According to the isodose curve distributions, it appears that the HT plan produces slightly lower inhomogeneity inside the ITV as compared to the MLC-based IMRT and very similar dose spread outside the ITV. The MLC-based IMRT radiation modality delivers higher mean doses to the GTV, lymph nodes and bladder and a lower dose to the rectum as compared to the HT (Table 2).

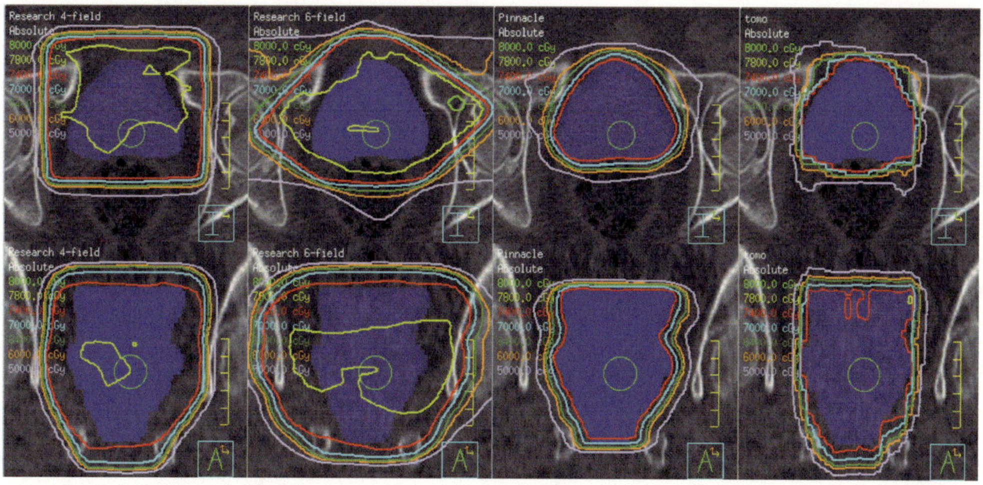

Fig. 7. The reference CT slice of a prostate cancer patient is shown for the treatment plans of four radiation modalities in the transverse and coronal planes. The anatomical structures involved are illustrated together with the dose distributions delivered to the patient.

Tissue	GTV	Lymph nodes	Bladder	Rectum
		Helical Tomotherapy		
P_{Tomo} (%)	39.3	98.0	1.0	2.9
$\bar{\bar{D}}_{Tomo}$ (Gy)	74.8	74.8	61.6	59.6
$\bar{D}_{Tomo}$ (Gy)	74.9	74.8	39.7	34.8
SD_{Tomo}	0.9	0.5	20.6	17.6
$Dmax_{Tomo}$	78.3	77.9	77.9	77.9
$Dmin_{Tomo}$	71.2	73.2	8.3	6.7
		MLC-based IMRT		
P_{IMRT} (%)	44.1	98.4	1.4	1.3
$\bar{\bar{D}}_{IMRT}$ (Gy)	75.6	75.9	62.1	57.7
$\bar{D}_{IMRT}$ (Gy)	75.6	75.9	41.8	34.3
SD_{IMRT}	0.7	0.3	20.2	16.1
$Dmax_{IMRT}$	77.5	77.1	76.7	74.7
$Dmin_{IMRT}$	72.8	74.7	7.9	4.4

Table 2. Summary of the radiobiological evaluation of the Helical Tomotherapy and IMRT treatment plans.

For the applied dose prescription the complication-free tumor control probability (P_+) value is 34.7% for the HT for a mean dose to the ITV ($\bar{D}_{ITV}$) of 74.9 Gy and biologically effective uniform dose to the ITV ($\bar{\bar{D}}_B$) of 74.8 Gy. The total control probability (P_B) is 38.5% and the total complication probability (P_I) is 3.8%. Similarly, of the MLC-based IMRT the P_+ value is 40.8% for $\bar{D}_{ITV}$ = 75.7 Gy and $\bar{\bar{D}}_B$ = 75.6 Gy. The P_B = 43.4% and the P_I = 2.6% (Mavroidis et al 2007). However, if we optimize the dose level of the dose distributions in order to maximize the complication-free tumor control then for the HT, the P_+ value becomes 68.7% for a $\bar{\bar{D}}_B$ of 86.0 Gy stemming from P_B = 87.8% and P_I = 19.1%. Respectively, for the MLC-based IMRT the P_+ value becomes 72.2% for a $\bar{\bar{D}}_B$ of 85.9 Gy having P_B = 87.8% and P_I = 15.5%.

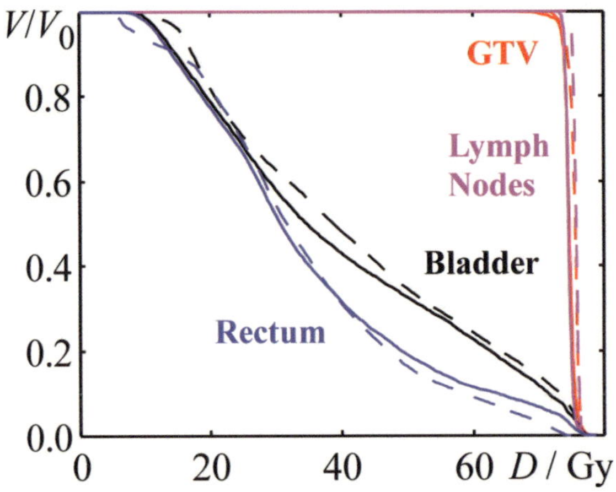

Fig. 8. The DVHs of the GTV and involved lymph nodes as well as those of the organs at risk (bladder and rectum) are illustrated. The solid lines correspond to the dose distribution from Helical Tomotherapy, whereas the dashed lines correspond to the dose distribution from IMRT (Mavroidis et al. 2007) (published with permission from: Mavroidis et al. Treatment plan comparison between Helical Tomotherapy and MLC-based IMRT using radiobiological measures. Physics in Medicine and Biology, Vol.52, pp. 3829, 2007, IOP Publishing Ltd, http://stacks.iop.org/PMB/52/3817).

The dose distribution in the ITV is more homogeneous in the MLC-based IMRT plan as compared to the HT, while achieving a similar sparing of the OARs. As it is shown in Fig. 9, the expected complication-free tumour control for the HT treatment plan is slightly worse than the MLC-based IMRT for the clinical prescribed doses. The reason for this is that the MLC-based IMRT irradiates more effectively the GTV and lymph nodes with better sparing of the rectum as shown in Table 2 and Fig. 9. Although the HT delivers similar mean dose to the rectum with a little larger variation as compared to the MLC-based IMRT, it shows a higher complication probability due to its higher maximum dose and the high relative seriality value of rectum (s = 0.7).

In this analysis, the clinical effectiveness of the Helical Tomotherapy and MLC-based IMRT in prostate cancer radiotherapy was evaluated using both physical and radiobiological criteria. This evaluation shows that the difference between the HT and MLC-based IMRT plans is small with the latter one being more effective over the clinically prescribed dose region. The results of this work indicate that the HT and MLC-based IMRT radiation modalities have almost the same potential of producing treatment plans with small integral doses to the healthy organs and fairly homogeneous doses to the ITV.

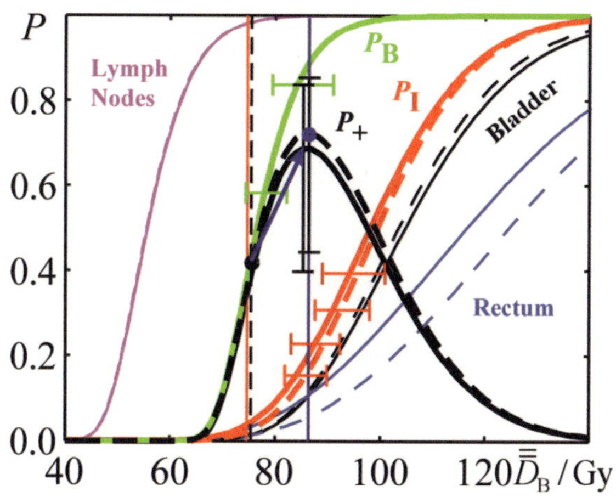

Fig. 9. The dose-response curves of the targets and organs-at-risk are plotted for the HT and MLC-based IMRT radiation modalities using the $\bar{\bar{D}}$ on the dose axis. The vertical lines denote the clinical and optimum dose prescriptions. The solid lines correspond to the dose distribution from Helical Tomotherapy, whereas the dashed lines correspond to the dose distribution from IMRT.

5. Radiobiological evaluation of optimized HDR prostate brachytherapy implants

High Dose Rate (HDR) Brachytherapy is becoming popular for treating localized prostate cancer tumors utilizing 3D ultrasound (U/S) and ^{192}Ir based remote afterloaders. Compared to other 3D imaging modalities (CT, MR) U/S can provide real-time, accurate 3D information on the size and the position of the target volume, on the position of the organs-at-risk and the real time needle tracking and navigation. The use of inverse planning in HDR brachytherapy results in a fast planning process that produces reproducible high quality treatment plans that closely match the clinical protocol constraints (Baltas & Zamboglou 2006, Hsu et al. 2008, Martinez et al. 1989, Milickovic et al. 2002). During the last decade a number of inverse planning algorithms have been proposed (Alterovitz et al. 2006, Karabis et al. 2009, Lahanas et al. 1999, 2003) and many of them have been implemented in modern Treatment Planning Systems (TPS) (Oncentra Prostate™, Nucletron B.V., Veenendaal, The Netherlands, Oncentra Brachy™, Nucletron B.V., Veenendaal, The Netherlands, BrachyVision Treatent Planning™, Varian Medical Systems). It is a common characteristic for HDR implants optimized with such algorithms that there are a few very dominating dwell positions, where the largest part of the total dwell time is spent, which leads to a selective extension of high doses in volumes around such dwell positions. Presently, in HDR brachytherapy, new inverse optimization algorithms enable an adjustment of the source dwell time distribution within the implanted catheters according to user-defined objectives and penalties for the target volume(s) and organs at risk (OARs).

In the present evaluation, the TPS Oncentra Prostate v.3.0 (Nucletron B.V., Veenendaal, The Netherlands) was used, where the Hybrid Inverse treatment Planning and Optimization (HIPO) algorithm has been implemented (Karabis et al. 2005, 2009). HIPO is an inverse planning algorithm that is based on 3D anatomy and it is capable of optimizing the dose distribution for a given needle configuration as well as finding an adequate needle configuration for each application. Furthermore, HIPO has the ability to apply a modulation restriction that limits the free modulation of dwell times eliminating the selective hot spots. It is based on dosimetric objectives, which penalize over/under dosage in target(s) while protecting OARs from overdosage (Karabis et al. 2009). Furthermore, in order to get restriction of the free modulation of dwell times allowing thus more smooth source movements and more smooth distributions of dwell time over dwell positions, HIPO offers the option of a modulation restriction (MR) parameter, which leads to a the dwell time gradient restriction.

The present analysis is based on the treatment plans of 12 prostate cancer patients, which were developed using their 3D ultrasound (U/S) image sets that were obtained intra-operatively right after the needle implantation. The twelve clinical implants for HDR brachytherapy of prostate cancer were selected as monotherapy for low-risk cases and they cover the whole range of prostate volumes with a full range of 26-101 cm^3. In the present clinical protocol, the HDR Monotherapy is delivered in three implants separated by at least 2 weeks interval. In each implant a single fraction with a prescription dose of 11.5 Gy is delivered thus resulting in a total dose of 34.5 Gy. The prostate gland is considered as PTV and urethra, bladder and rectum are used as OARs in the treatment planning. The whole procedure including dose delivery is realized intra-operatively utilizing 3D and 2D Ultrasound imaging.

For the evaluation and report of the quality of the dose distributions, the following DVH-based parameters that have been proposed by GEC/ESTRO-EAU (19-22), have been considered (Baltas & Zamboglou 2006, Kovács et al. 2005, Nag et al. 1999).

D_{100}: The dose that covers 100% of the PTV volume, which is the Minimum Target Dose (MTD).

D_{90}: The dose that covers 90% of the PTV volume, which would be desirable to be equal or greater than the prescription dose.

V_{100}: The percentage of prostate volume (PTV) that has received at least the prescription dose (100% = prescribed dose).

V_{150}: The volume that has received 50% more than the prescribed dose (150% of the prescription dose).

Regarding the OARs, the following dosimetric descriptors for the maximum doses have been considered:

D_{2cm^3}: the dose for the most exposed 2 cm^3 of rectum or bladder,

$D_{0.1cm^3}$: the dose for the most exposed 0.1cm^3 of the urethra as an estimate of the maximum dose

D_{10}: the highest dose covering 10% of the OAR volume (rectum, bladder, urethra)

All the clinical implants have been inversely planned using HIPO with modulation restriction (MR), which was selected based on the maximum values resulting in plans that completely fulfilled the constraints of the dosimetric protocol. In the treatment plan evaluation, the individual tissue DVHs were calculated for each plan (Fig. 10).

The different treatment plans were further evaluated in conjunction with radiobiological dose non-uniformity evaluation measures in order to estimate their expected clinical impact

(Mavroidis et al. 2008). For this evaluation the dose-response parameters of the prostate, urethra, bladder and rectum (Table 3) were used to calculate the corresponding response probabilities as well as the complication-free tumor control probability (P_+) and the biologically effective uniform dose ($\bar{\bar{D}}$).

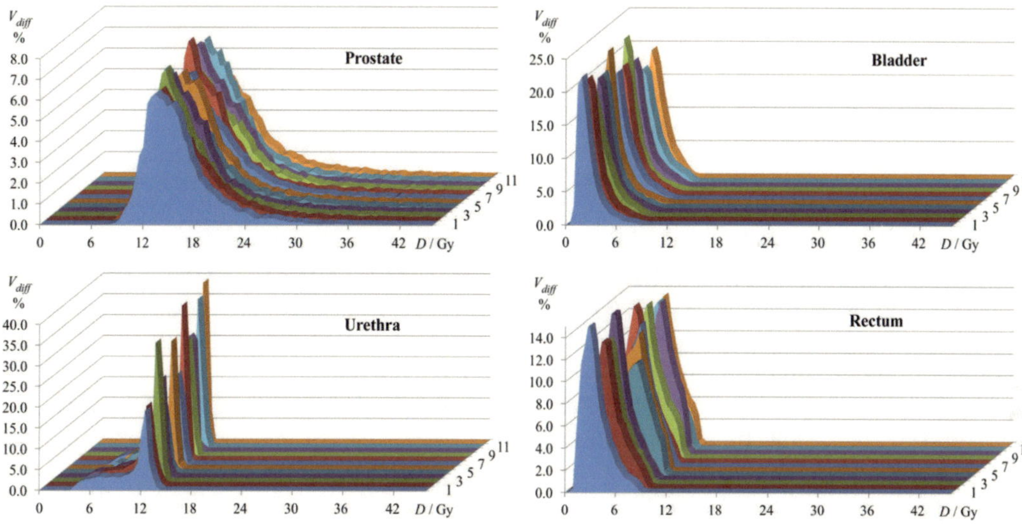

Fig. 10. The differential DVHs of prostate, urethra, bladder and rectum derived from the treatment plans. The prescription dose of the fraction is 11.5 Gy (100%).

Organs	D50 (Gy)	γ	s	α/β
PTV	70.0	4.0	–	3.0
Urethra	120.0	3.0	0.03	3.0
Bladder	80.0	3.0	0.3	3.0
Rectum	80.0	2.2	0.7	3.0

Table 3. Summary of the model parameter values for the prostate cancer cases. D_{50} is the 50% response dose, γ is the maximum normalized value of the dose-response gradient and s is the relative seriality, which characterizes the volume dependence of the organ.

Finally, the conformal index COIN (Baltas et al. 1998), which is a measure of brachytherapy implant quality and dose specification, was applied in evaluation of the examined treatment plans. COIN considers also the conformity of the 3D dose distribution regarding the OARs based on three coefficients. The first coefficient is the fraction of the PTV that is enclosed by the prescription dose. The second coefficient is the fraction of the volume encompassed by the prescription dose that is covered by PTV and it is a measure of how much tissue outside the PTV is covered by the prescription dose. The third coefficient is the fraction of the volume of each OAR that receives doses that exceed their dose limit.

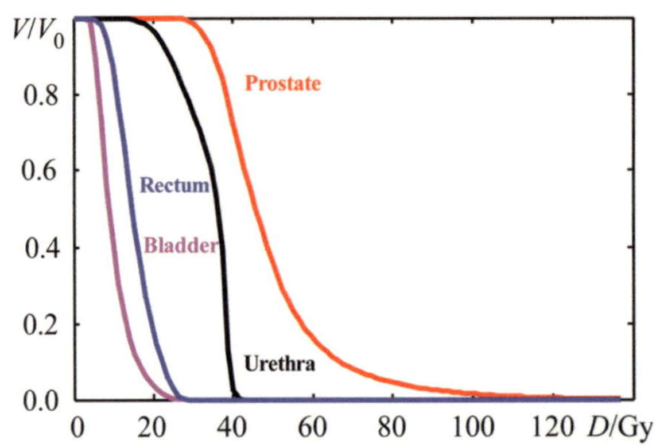

Fig. 11. The average cumulative DVHs of the PTV (prostate gland, red), urethra (black), bladder (pink) and rectum (blue) are presented for the HDR treatment plans, which were optimized with modulation restriction. Here, the total dose of 34.5 Gy delivered by three fractions of 11.5 Gy is considered to be the total prescription dose (100%) (Mavroidis et al. 2010) (published with permission from: Mavroidis et al. Radiobiological evaluation of the influence of dwell time modulation restriction in HIPO optimized HDR prostate brachytherapy implants. Journal of Contemporary Brachytherapy, Vol.2, pp. 126, 2010, Termedia sp.zo.o., DOI: 10.5114/jcb.2010.16923).

Fig. 11 illustrates the average DVHs of the dose distributions examined. Based on the DVHs and the results shown in Table 4, the HIPO optimization with MR has an acceptable variance coefficient, CV, (meaning dose inhomogeneity) inside the PTV. The average mean dose in the PTV in the HIPO with MR plans is 48.4 Gy and the corresponding control probability is 97.8%. Regarding the organs at risk, the HIPO optimization with MR plans deliver fairly low maximum doses in urethra, which results in a clinically acceptable response probability (3.8%) (Mavroidis et al. 2010).

Tissues	CTV	Urethra	Bladder	Rectum
P (%)	97.8	3.8	0.0	0.02
D_{mean} **(Gy)**	48.4	33.0	9.2	14.4
CV **(%)**	30.5	18.2	46.5	33.3
$\bar{\bar{D}}$ **(Gy)**	32.9	34.2	22.3	22.8
D_{max} **(Gy)**	136.6	41.4	27.6	27.6
D_{min} **(Gy)**	23.5	11.0	2.8	2.8

Table 4. Summary of the dosimetric and radiobiological measures averaged over the 12 prostate cancer patients regarding the applied HDR technique.

A quantitative analysis of the dosimetric and radiobiological results of the different dose distributions shows that for the HDR optimization with MR at the clinical dose prescription the P_+ value is 94.0% and the biologically effective uniform dose to the PTV, $\bar{\bar{D}}_B$ is 32.9Gy. The total control probability, P_B is 97.8% and the total complication probability, P_I is 3.8%, which mainly stems from the response probability of urethra (3.8%) (Mavroidis et al. 2010). However, if a different dose level of the dose distributions is selected in order to maximize

the complication-free tumor control then the P_+ value becomes 95.2% for a $\bar{\bar{D}}_B$ of 32.2 Gy having $P_B = 96.3\%$ and $P_I = 1.1\%$.
The average COIN values, which were calculated with and without the inclusion of the organs at risk (OARs) for the 12 implants using HIPO with modulation restriction are 0.867 ± 0.019 and 0.870 ± 0.021, respectively. These values indicate that the examined treatment plans are characterized by high quality.

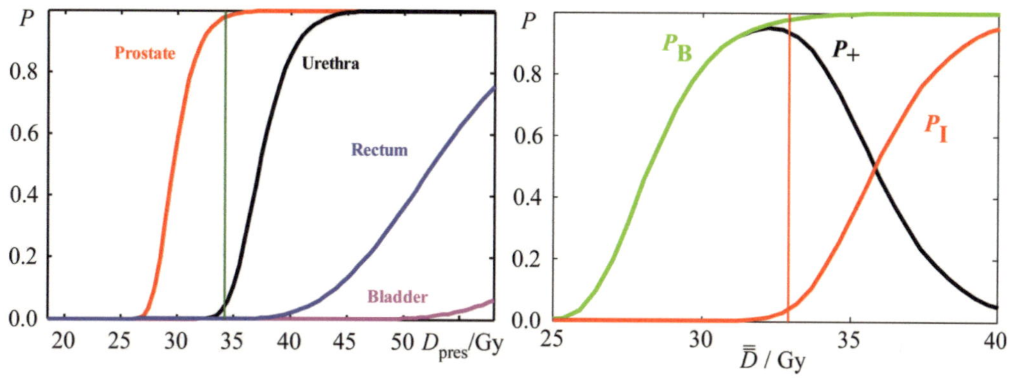

Fig. 12. *Left diagram:* The average dose-response curves of the PTV (red), urethra (black), bladder (pink) and rectum (blue) are presented for the HDR treatment plans, which were optimized with modulation restriction, regarding different prescription doses. *Right diagram:* The average curves of the total tumor control probability, P_B (green), total normal tissue complication probability, P_I (red) and complication-free tumor control probability, P_+ (black) are presented for the HDR treatment plans, regarding different radiobiological prescription doses. The total dose of 34.5 Gy delivered by three fractions of 11.5 Gy is considered to be the total prescription dose (100%) (Mavroidis et al. 2010) (published with permission from: Mavroidis et al. Radiobiological evaluation of the influence of dwell time modulation restriction in HIPO optimized HDR prostate brachytherapy implants. Journal of Contemporary Brachytherapy, Vol.2, pp. 126, 2010, Termedia sp.zo.o., DOI: 10.5114/jcb.2010.16923).

Non-uniform dose distributions, which may be as effective as equivalent uniform dose distributions, which means that a higher number of degrees-of-freedom can be taken advantage of by incorporating radiobiological measures in treatment plan optimization. In this sense, a radiobiologically based optimization algorithm could find dose distributions of smoother non-uniformity that irradiate the target as effectively as the physically optimized dose distributions without modulation restriction and at the same time optimize the dose fall-off towards the organs at risk. This is because the radiobiologically based HDR optimization would take into account the volume effect of all the involved organs at risk in the proximity of the target and optimize the dose fall-off accordingly. It has to be mentioned that radiobiologically based HDR optimization is characterized by more clinically relevant dose constraints for the OARs and normal tissue stroma, which could lead to better results than the HDR optimization without modulation restriction. However, the large hot spots produced in the target volume by this method would increase the risk for secondary cancer (Schneider et al 2006). Consequently, by deteriorating physical dose conformation, the HDR optimization with MR provides slightly better biological conformation.

6. Conclusions

This chapter demonstrates the use of radiobiological measures in prostate cancer treatment plan optimization may have a great impact on the clinical effectiveness of the applied treatment. Taking into account the dose-response relations of the irradiated tumors and normal tissues, a radiobiological dose delivery evaluation can be performed, which combines the information of a given dose distribution with the radiosensitivity map of the patient. The use of $P-\bar{\bar{D}}$ diagrams can complement the traditional tools of evaluation such as DVHs, in order to compare and effectively evaluate different treatment plans.

The findings show that the use of fused CT-MRI images produce dose distributions, which lead on average to better expected treatment outcome compared to the use of CT images alone. The extent of this improvement decreases as we move from conventional to IMRT treatments due to the fact that IMRT delivers already limited doses to OARs. Although 3D conformal radiotherapy techniques are not characterized by very high conformalities, the better knowledge of the CTV extension can considerably improve the effectiveness of their dose distributions. These findings were observed during treatment plan evaluation and comparison based on common dosimetric indices as well as on radiobiological measures.

The clinical effectiveness of delivered Helical Tomotherapy dose distributions with and without patient setup correction, which were evaluated using both physical and biological criteria, showed that the dose distributions with and without patient setup correction are very similar and the expected clinical outcome is not always better in the first case unless a radiobiological treatment plan optimization has been performed first. However, the effectiveness of a HT treatment plan can be considerably deteriorated if an accurate initial patient setup procedure is not available. The application of radiobiological measures on HT prostate cancer treatment plans with and without patient setup correction revealed minor or modest differences in the predicted therapeutic impact of using the MVCT method.

Radiobiological evaluation of treatment plans provides additional information about the fitness of a plan and a closer association of the delivered treatment with the clinical outcome. The simultaneous presentation of the radiobiological evaluation together with the physical data shows their complementary relation in analyzing a dose plan. The use of radiobiological parameters is necessary if a clinically relevant quantification of a plan is needed. The application of the P_+ and $\bar{\bar{D}}$ concepts on representative Helical Tomotherapy and MLC-based IMRT prostate cancer treatment plans revealed differences in the biological impact of the corresponding dose distributions. It can be concluded that for clinical cases, which may look dosimetrically similar, in radiobiological terms they can be quite different. Helical Tomotherapy and MLC-based IMRT can cover the target volume with the clinically prescribed dose while minimizing the volume of the organs at risk receiving high dose. Both radiation modalities have almost the same potential of producing treatment plans of equivalent clinical effectiveness in terms adequate irradiation of the tumor and sparing of the involved OARs.

At the maximum P_+ dose prescription, it was proved that the different modulation restriction approaches do not affect significantly the proper coverage and eradication of the target and the sparing of rectum and bladder but they affect mainly the effective sparing of urethra. In this analysis, which was performed using both physical and radiobiological criteria, it is shown that the HDR optimization with MR can introduce a minor improvement in the effectiveness of the produced dose distribution compared to the HDR optimization without modulation restriction. The likelihood to accomplish a good treatment result can be increased by the use of therapeutic indices such as P_+ and $\bar{\bar{D}}$, which can be used as figures of merit for a treatment.

7. Appendix

Radiobiological treatment plan evaluation

In the present radiobiological treatment plan evaluation method, the Linear-Quadratic-Poisson model is used to describe the dose-response relation of the tumours and normal tissues (Källman et al. 1992b, Ågren et al. 1990). This model takes into account the fractionation effects that are introduced by the clinical protocol:

$$P(D) = \exp\left(-e^{e\gamma - (D/D_{50})\cdot(e\gamma - \ln\ln 2)}\right) \quad (1)$$

where $P(D)$ is the probability to control a tumour or induce a certain injury to a normal tissue that is irradiated uniformly with a dose D. D_{50} is the dose, which gives a 50% response and γ is the maximum normalized dose-response gradient. The parameters D_{50} and γ are specific for every organ and type of clinical endpoint and they are derived directly from clinical data (Emami et al. 1991, Eriksson et al. 2000, Gagliardi et al. 2000, Jackson et al. 1995, Mavroidis et al. 2003, 2005, Roesink et al. 2001, Willner et al. 2002, Ågren 1995). The uncertainties that are associated with these parameters are of the order of 5% for D_{50}, 30% for γ and 90% for s. These uncertainties define the confidence interval of the entire dose-response curve around its best estimate (Deasy 1997). The response of the entire organ to a non-uniform dose distribution is given by an expanded version of Eq. (1) for tumours and the relative seriality model for normal tissues (Lind et al. 1999).
The relative seriality model is a model that account for the volume effect. For a heterogeneous dose distribution, the overall probability of injury (P_I) for a number of OARs is expressed as follows (Källman et al. 1992b, Lind et al. 1999):

$$P_I = 1 - \prod_{j=1}^{N_{organs}} \left(1 - [1 - \prod_{i=1}^{M_j}(1 - P^j(D_i)^{s_j})^{\Delta v_i}]^{1/s_j}\right) \quad (2)$$

where P_I^j is the probability of injuring organ j and N_{organs} is the total number of vital OARs. $P^j(D_i)$ is the probability of response of the organ j having the reference volume and being irradiated to dose D_i as described by Eq. (1). $\Delta v_i = \Delta V_i / V_{ref}$ is the fractional sub-volume of the organ that is irradiated compared to the reference volume for which the values of D_{50} and γ were calculated. M_j is the total number of voxels or sub-volumes in the organ j, and s_j is the relative seriality parameter that characterizes the internal organization of that organ. A relative seriality close to zero ($s \approx 0$) corresponds to a completely parallel structure, which becomes non-functional when all its functional subunits are damaged, whereas $s \approx 1$ corresponds to a completely serial structure which becomes non-functional when at least one functional subunit is damaged. It should be mentioned that other models such as the LKB (Burman et al. 1991, Kutcher et al. 1991, Kwa et al. 1998), parallel (Boersma et al. 1995) etc could also have been used with the appropriate response parameter set.
Tumours are assumed to have a parallel structural organization since the eradication of all of the clonogenic cells is required. Furthermore, in complex multi-target cancer cases, the

eradication of all the clonogenic cells in tumours implies that every individual tumour has to be eradicated. This implication indicates a parallel organization fashion for the tumours. Taking this assumption into account the overall probability of tumour control (P_B), is given by the expression (Lind et al. 1999, Mavroidis et al. 2000):

$$P_{\mathrm{B}} = \prod_{j=1}^{N_{\mathrm{tumours}}} \left(\prod_{i=1}^{M_j} P^j (D_i)^{\Delta v_i} \right) \quad (3)$$

where P_{B}^j is the probability of eradicating tumour j and N_{tumours} is the total number of tumours or targets involved in the clinical case.

To evaluate the effectiveness of the treatment plans, the concept of P_+, which expresses the probability of achieving tumour control without causing severe damage to normal tissues (Källman et al. 1992a), was employed. Using the quantities P_B and P_I, which were defined above, the P_+ can be estimated from the following expression:

$$P_+ = P_{\mathrm{B}} - P_{\mathrm{B} \cap \mathrm{I}} \approx P_{\mathrm{B}} - P_{\mathrm{I}} \quad (4)$$

This concept is based on the accuracy of the models to calculate the probabilities P_B and P_I and the radiobiological parameters, which describe the dose-response relations of the different tumours and normal tissues.

As a measure of the quality of a treatment plan, the mean doses and their standard deviations to the target volumes and organs at risk are usually reported, together with the minimum and maximum doses as well as some DVH-based constraints. In addition to those parameters, the present radiobiological treatment plan evaluation uses the $\bar{\bar{D}}$ concept, which is defined as the dose that causes the same tumour control or normal tissue complication probability as the actual dose distribution given to the patient and it is derived numerically from the following expression (Mavroidis et al. 2000, 2001):

$$P_{\mathrm{B}}(\vec{D}) \equiv P_{\mathrm{B}}(\bar{\bar{D}}_{\mathrm{B}}) \quad (5)$$

where $\vec{D}$ denotes the 3-dimensional dose distribution. This definition is a generalization of the effective uniform dose, D_{eff} introduced by Brahme (Brahme 1984). By normalizing treatment plans to a common prescription point ($\bar{\bar{D}}$) and then plotting out the tissue response probability vs. $\bar{\bar{D}}$ curves, a number of plan trials can be compared based on radiobiological endpoints.

8. References

Alterovitz, R.; Lessard, E.; Pouliot, J.; Hsu, I.; O'Brien, J. & Goldberg, K. (2006). Optimization of HDR Brachytherapy Dose Distributions Using Linear Programming with Penalty Costs. *Medical Physics,* Vol.33, pp. 4012–4019

Baltas, D.; Kolotas, C.; Geramani, K.; Mould, R.F.; Ioannidis, G.; Kekchidi, M. & Zamboglou, N. (1998). A Conformal Index (COIN) to Evaluate Implant Quality and Dose Specification in Brachytherapy. *International Journal of Radiation Oncolology, Biology, Physics*, Vol.40, pp. 515-524

Baltas, D. & Zamboglou, N. (2006). 2D and 3D Planning in Brachytherapy, In: *New Technologies in Radiation Oncology,* of Bortfeld, T.; Grosu, A.-L. & Schlegel, W., pp. 237-254, Springer, Berlin-Heidelberg

Beasley, M.; Driver, D. & Dobbs, H.J. (2005). Complications of Radiotherapy: Improving the Therapeutic Index. *Cancer Imaging,* Vol.5, pp. 78-84

Boswell, S.; Tomé, W.; Jeraj, R.; Jaradat, H. & Mackie, T.R. (2006). Automatic Registration of Megavoltage to Kilovoltage CT Images in Helical Tomotherapy: An Evaluation of the Setup Verification Process for the Special Case of a Rigid Head Phantom. *Medical Physics,* Vol.33, pp. 4395

Brahme, A. (1994). Which parameters of the dose distribution are best related to the radiation response of tumours and normal tissues. *Proceedings of the Interregional Seminars for Europe, the Middle East and Africa Organized by the IAEA,* Leuven, pp. 37-58

Brahme, A. (1997). The Need for Accurate Target and Dose Specifications in Conventional and Conformal Radiation Therapy - An Introduction. *Acta Oncologica,* Vol.36, pp. 789-792

Buffa, F.M.; Davidson, S.E.; Hunter, R.D.; Nahum, A.E. & West, C.M. (2001). Incorporating Biologic Measurements (SF2, CFE) into a Tumor Control Probability Model Increases their Prognostic Significance: A Study in Cervical Carcinoma Treated with Radiation Therapy. *International Journal of Radiation Oncolology, Biology, Physics,* Vol.50, pp. 1113-1122

Chen, L.; Price, R.A. Jr.; Wang, L.; Li, J.; Qin, L.; McNeeley, S.; Ma, C.M.; Freedman, G.M. & Pollack, A. (2004). MRI-Based Treatment Planning for Radiotherapy: Dosimetric Verification for Prostate IMRT. *International Journal of Radiation Oncolology, Biology, Physics,* Vol.60, pp. 636-647

Claus, F.G.; Hricak, H. & Hattery, R.R. (2004). Pretreatment Evaluation of Prostate Cancer: Role of MR Imaging and 1H MR Spectroscopy. *Radiographics,* Vol.24, pp. S167-S180

Creutzberg, C.L.; Althof, V.G.M.; Huizenga, H.; Visser, A.G. & Levendag, P.C. (1993). Quality Assurance Using Portal Imaging: The Accuracy of Patient Positioning in Irradiation of Breast Cancer. *International Journal of Radiation Oncolology, Biology, Physics,* Vol.25, pp. 529-539

Debois, M.; Oyen, R.; Maes, F.; Verswijvel, G.; Gatti, G.; Bosmans, H.; Feron, M.; Bellon, E.; Kutcher, G.; Van Poppel, H. & Vanuytsel, L. (1999). The Contribution of Magnetic Resonance Imaging to the Three-Dimensional Treatment Planning of Localized Prostate Cancer. *International Journal of Radiation Oncolology, Biology, Physics,* Vol.45, pp. 857-865

Emami, B.; Lyman, J.; Brown, A.; Coia, L.; Goitein, M.; Munzenrider, J.E.; Shank, B.; Solin, L.J. & Wesson, A.M. (1991). Tolerance of Normal Tissue to Therapeutic Irradiation. *International Journal of Radiation Oncolology, Biology, Physics,* Vol.21, pp. 109-22

Fenwick, J.D. & Nahum, A.E. (2001). Series Model Volume Effects in a Population of Non-Identical Patients: How Low is Low? *Physics in Medicine and Biology,* Vol.46, pp. 1815-1834

Hou, A.H.; Swanson, D. & Barqawi, A.B. (2009). Modalities for Imaging of Prostate Cancer. *Advances in Urology,* 818065

Hsu, I-C.; Yamada, Y.; Vigneault, E. & Pouliot, J. (2008). *Prostate High-Dose Rate Task Group,* American Brachytherapy Society, Retrieved from www.americanbrachytherapy.org

Jackson, A.; Ten Haken, R.K.; Robertson, J.M.; Kessler, M.L.; Kutcher, G.J. & Lawrence, T.S. (1995). Analysis of Clinical Complication Data for Radiation Hepatitis Using a Parallel Architecture Model. *International Journal of Radiation Oncolology, Biology, Physics*, Vol.31, pp. 883-891

Karabis A, Giannouli S, Baltas D. (2005). HIPO: A Hybrid Inverse Treatment Planning Optimization Algorithm in HDR Brachytherapy. *Radiotherapy and Oncology*, Vol.76, Supplement 2, pp. S29

Karabis, A.; Belotti, P. & Baltas, D. (2009). Optimization of Catheter Position and Dwell Time in Prostate HDR Brachytherapy using HIPO and Linear Programming, *Proceedings of World Congress on Medical Physics and Biomedical Engineering*, Munich, Germany, September 7-12, 2009, pp. 612-615

Kovács, G.; Pötter, R.; Loch, T.; Hammer, J.; Kolkman-Deurloo, I-K.; de la Rosette, J.J.M.C.H. & Bertermann, H. (2005). GEC/ESTRO-EAU Recommendations on Temporary Brachytherapy Using Stepping Sources for Localised Prostate Cancer. *Radiotherapy and Oncology*, Vol.74, pp. 137–148

Källman, P.; Lind, B.K. & Brahme, A. (1992a). An Algorithm for Maximizing the Probability of Complication Free Tumor Control in Radiation Therapy. *Physics in Medicine and Biology*, Vol.37, pp. 871-890

Källman, P.; Ågren, A.K. & Brahme, A. (1992b). Tumor and Normal Tissue Responses to Fractionated Non Uniform Dose Delivery. *International Journal of Radiation Biology*, Vol.62, pp. 249-262

Lahanas, M.; Baltas, D. & Zamboglou, N. (1999). Anatomy-Based Three-Dimensional Dose Optimization in Brachytherapy Using Multiobjective Genetic Algorithms. *Medical Physics*, Vol.26, pp. 1904-1918

Lahanas, M.; Baltas, D. & Giannouli, S. (2003). Global Convergence Analysis of Fast Multiobjective Gradient Based Dose Optimization Algorithms for High-Dose-Rate Brachytherapy. *Physics in Medicine and Biology*, Vol.48, pp. 599-617

Lind, B.K.; Mavroidis, P.; Hyödynmaa, S. & Kappas, C. (1999). Optimization of the Dose Level for a Given Treatment Plan to Maximize the Complication Free Tumor Cure. *Acta Oncologica*, Vol.38, pp. 787-798

Löf, J.; Lind, B.K. & Brahme, A. (1995). Optimal Radiation Beam Profiles Considering the Stochastic Process of Patient Positioning in Fractionated Radiation Therapy. *Inverse Problems*, Vol.11, pp. 1189-1209

Mackie, T.R.; Balog, J.; Ruchala, K.J.; Shepard, D.; Aldridge, J.S.; Fitchard, E.E.; Reckwerdt, P.; Olivera, G.H.; McNutt, T. & Metha, M. (1999). TomoTherapy. *Seminars in Radiation Oncology*, Vol.9, pp. 108-117

Mavroidis, P.; Lind, B.K.; Van Dijk, J.; Koedooder, K.; De Neve, W.; De Wagter, C.; Planskoy, B.; Rosenwald, J.C.; Proimos, B.; Kappas, C.; Danciu, C.; Benassi, M.; Chierego, G. & Brahme, A. (2000). Comparison of Conformal Radiation Therapy Techniques Within the Dynamic Radiotherapy Project 'DYNARAD'. *Physics in Medicine and Biology*, Vol.45, pp. 2459-2481

Mavroidis, P.; Lind, B.K. & Brahme, A. (2001). Biologically Effective Uniform Dose ($\bar{\bar{D}}$) for Specification, Report and Comparison of Dose Response Relations and Treatment Plans. *Physics in Medicine and Biology*, Vol.46, pp. 2607-2630

Mavroidis, P.; Laurell, G.; Kraepelien, T.; Fernberg, J.O.; Lind, B.K. & Brahme, A. (2003). Determination and Clinical Verification of Dose-Response Parameters for

Esophageal Stricture from Head and Neck Radiotherapy. *Acta Oncologica,* Vol.42, pp. 865-881

Mavroidis, P.; al-Abany, M.; Helgason, A.R.; Ågren Cronqvist, A.K.; Wersäll, P.; Theodorou, K.; Kappas, C.; Lind, H.; Lind, B.K.; Steineck, G. & Brahme, A. (2005). Dose-Response Relations for Anal Sphincter Regarding Faecal Leakage and Blood or Phlegm in Stools After Radiotherapy for Prostate Cancer. *Strahlentherapie und Onkologie,* Vol.181, pp. 293-306

Mavroidis, P.; Costa Ferreira, B.; Shi, C.; Lind, B.K. & Papanikolaou, N. (2007). Treatment Plan Comparison Between Helical Tomotherapy and MLC-Based IMRT Using Radiobiological Measures. *Physics in Medicine and Biology,* Vol.52, pp. 3817-3836, © 2007 IOP Publishing Ltd, http://stacks.iop.org/PMB/52/3817

Mavroidis, P.; Komisopoulos, G.; Lind, B.K. & Papanikolaou, N. (2008). Interpretation of the Dosimetric Results of Three Uniformity Regularization Methods in Terms of Expected Treatment Outcome. *Medical Physics,* Vol.35, pp. 5009-5018

Mavroidis, P.; Katsilieri, Z.; Kefala, V.; Milickovic, N.; Papanikolaou, N.; Karabis, A.; Zamboglou, N. & Baltas, D. (2010). Radiobiological Evaluation of the Influence of Dwell Time Modulation Restriction in HIPO Optimized HDR Prostate Brachytherapy Implants. *Journal of Contemporary Brachytherapy,* Vol.2, pp. 117-128

Mavroidis, P.; Su, F.; Giantsoudi, D.; Stathakis, S.; Komisopoulos, G.; Shi, C.; Swanson G. & Papanikolaou, N. (2011). Radiobiological and Dosimetric Analysis of Daily Megavoltage CT Registration Techniques on Adaptive Radiotherapy with Helical Tomotherapy. *Technology in Cancer Research and Treatment,* Vol.10, pp. 1-13

Meeks, S.L.; Harmon Jr., J.F.; Langen, K.M.; Willoughby, T.R.; Wagner, T.H. & Kupelian, P.A. (2005). Performance Characterization of Megavoltage Computed Tomography Imaging on a Helical Tomotherapy Unit. *Medical Physics,* Vol.32, pp. 2673

Milickovic, N.; Lahanas, M.; Papagiannopoulou, M.; Zamboglou, N. & Baltas, D. (2002). Multiobjective Anatomy-Based Dose Optimization for HDR-Brachytherapy with Constraint Free Deterministic Algorithms. *Physics in Medicine and Biology,* Vol.47, pp. 2263-2280

Mitine, C.; Dutreix, A. & Van Der Schueren, E. (1991). Tangential Breast Irradiation: Influence of Technique of Set-Up on Transfer Errors and Reproducibility. *Radiotherapy and Oncology,* Vol.22, pp. 308-310

Martinez, A.A.; Orton, C.G. & Mould, R.F. (Eds.). (1989). *Brachytherapy HDR and LDR.* Nucletron International, B.V, Leersum, The Netherlands

Nag, S.; Beyer, D.; Friedland, J.; Grimm, P. & Nath, R. (1999). American Brachytherapy Society (ABS) Recommendations for Transperineal Permanent Brachytherapy of Prostate Cancer. *International Journal of Radiation Oncolology, Biology, Physics,* Vol.44, pp. 789-799

Parker, C.C.; Damyanovich, A.; Haycocks, T.; Haider, M.; Bayley, A. & Catton, C.N. (2003). Magnetic Resonance Imaging in the Radiation Treatment Planning of Localized Prostate Cancer Using Intra-Prostatic Fiducial Markers for Computed Tomography Co-Registration. *Radiotherapy and Oncology,* Vol.66, pp. 217-224

Rasch, C.; Barillot, I.; Remeijer, P.; Touw, A.; van Herk, M. & Lebesque, J.V. (1999). Definition of the Prostate in CT and MRI: a Multi-Observer Study. *International Journal of Radiation Oncolology, Biology, Physics,* Vol.43, pp. 57-66

Rørvik, J.; Halvorsen, O.J.; Espeland, A. & Haukaas, S. (1993). Inability of CT to Assess Local Extent of Prostate. *Acta Radiologica,* Vol.34, pp. 39–42

Scheidler, J.; Hricak, H.; Vigneron, D.B.; Yu, K.K.; Sokolov, D.L.; Huang, L.R.; Zaloudek, C.J.; Nelson, S.J.; Carroll, P.R. & Kurhanewicz, J. (1999). Prostate Cancer: Localization with Three-Dimensional Proton MR Spectroscopic Imaging Clinicopathologic Study. *Radiology* Vol.213, pp. 473-480

Tzikas, A.; Karaiskos, P.; Papanikolaou, N.; Stathakis, S.; Sandilos, P.; Koutsouveli, E.; Lavdas, E.; Scarleas, C.; Dardoufas, K.; Lind, B.K. & Mavroidis, P. (2011). Investigating the Clinical Aspects of Using CT vs. CT-MRI Images During Organ Delineation and Treatment Planning in Prostate Cancer Radiotherapy. *Technology in Cancer Research and Treatment,* Vol.10, pp. 231-42

Villeirs, G.M.; Van Vaerenbergh, K.; Vakaet, L.; Bral, S.; Claus, F.; De Neve, W.J.; Verstraete, K.L. & De Meerleer, G.O. (2005). Interobserver Delineation Variation Using CT Versus Combined CT+MRI in Intensity-Modulated Radiotherapy for Prostate Cancer. *Strahlentherapie und Onkologie,* Vol.181, pp. 424-430

Villeirs, G.M. & De Meerleer, G.O. (2007). Magnetic Resonance Imaging (MRI) Anatomy of the Prostate and Application of MRI in Radiotherapy Planning. *European Journal of Radiology,* Vol.63, pp. 361-368

Welsh, J.S.; Lock, M.; Harari, P.M.; Tomé, W.; Fowler, J.; Mackie, T.R.; Ritter, M.; Kapatoes, J.; Forrest, L.; Chappell, R.; Paliwal, B. & Mehta, M.P. (2006). Clinical Implementation of Adaptive Helical Tomotherapy: A Unique Approach to Image-Guided Intensity Modulated Radiotherapy. *Technology in Cancer Research and Treatment,* Vol.5, pp. 465-480

Webb S. (2000). *Intensity-Modulated Radiation Therapy,* IOP Publishing, Bristol, UK

Weinreb, J.C.; Blume, J.D.; Coakley, F.V.; Wheeler, T.M.; Cormack, J.B.; Sotto, C.K.; Cho, H.; Kawashima, A.; Tempany-Afdhal, C.M.; Macura, K.J.; Rosen, M.; Gerst, S.R. & Kurhanewicz, J. (2009). Prostate Cancer: Sextant Localization at MR Imaging and MR Spectroscopic Imaging Before Prostatectomy--Results of ACRIN Prospective Multi-Institutional Clinicopathologic Study. *Radiology* Vol.251, pp. 122-133

Ågren, A.-K.; Brahme, A. & Turesson, I. (1990). Optimization of Uncomplicated Control for Head and Neck Tumors. *International Journal of Radiation Oncolology, Biology, Physics,* Vol.19, pp. 1077-1085

Ågren, A.K. (1995). *Quantification of the response of heterogeneous tumors and organized normal tissues to fractionated radiotherapy, PhD Thesis,* Stockholm University, Stockholm, Sweden

Part 4

Medical Management and Its Therapeutic Implications

12

Current Options and Future Directions in Castrate Resistant Prostate (CRPC)

Suzanne Richter and Srikala S. Sridhar
Department of Medical Oncology, Princess Margaret Hospital
University of Toronto
Canada

1. Introduction

Prostate cancer is the most frequently diagnosed malignancy in North America and second leading cause of cancer-related death (Jemal *et al.*, 2010). Despite effective local therapy, prostate cancer often recurs. Standard therapy for recurrent or metastatic prostate cancer remains androgen deprivation therapy (ADT) which is highly effective but not durable (Sharifi *et al.*, 2005). All patients will eventually progress to castrate resistant prostate cancer (CRPC) where there are few treatment options and until recently survival was a dismal 12-18 months (Tannock *et al.*, 1996). In this chapter we will review the current treatment approaches for CRPC, but focus primarily on the newly approved options available in the post-docetaxel setting.

Castrate-resistant prostate cancer (CRPC) is defined as prostate cancer progression despite ADT and may present with either increasing serum prostate-specific antigen (PSA) levels, radiologic progression, and/or the appearance of new metastases (Saad and Hotte, 2010). Over the years, advanced prostate cancer has been referred to as hormone-resistant prostate cancer (HRPC) or androgen-insensitive prostate cancer (AIPC), but the name has changed to CRPC to reflect the fact that intracrine/paracrine androgen production and signaling pathways play an important role in mediating resistance to first line ADT. CRPC presents as a spectrum of diseases ranging from patients with rising PSA alone, without metastases or symptoms to patients with rising PSA, progressive metastatic disease and significant symptoms. In patients who develop CRPC and who are relatively asymptomatic, secondary hormonal treatments may be attempted. To date, no study of secondary hormone treatment has demonstrated survival benefits, but most trials have been small, underpowered and confounded by the use of subsequent treatments. In patients who are progressing on ADT, discontinuation of antiandrogens, introduction of low dose prednisone or ketoconazole to block production of adrenal androgens, can offer transient PSA responses and palliative benefits in 30% to 35% of patients (Storlie *et al.*, 1995; Small *et al.*, 2004; Heng and Chi, 2006).

For CRPC patients with symptoms, rapid PSA progression or visceral disease, docetaxel chemotherapy and prednisone is currently considered standard of care. Docetaxel is a member of the taxane family of drugs which binds to tubulin and causes microtubule stabilization, leading to cell cycle arrest in the G2/M phase and subsequently cell death (Jordan *et al.*, 1993). Docetaxel is adminstered every three weeks intravenously at a dose of 75mg/m2 with oral prednisone 5 mg twice daily. This is based on two pivotal randomized phase III trials, the TAX 327 trial and the SWOG 9916 trial. TAX 327 randomized more than 1000 patients to receive docetaxel plus prednisone (weekly or every 3 weeks) or mitoxantrone plus prednisone (the previous first-line option). The every 3 week docetaxel arm had a median survival of 18.9 months compared with 16.5 months in the mitoxantrone arm. PSA response rates (defined as ≥ 50% drop in serum PSA level) were 48% in the docetaxel group and 32% in the mitoxantrone arm (Tannock *et al.*, 2004). In the SWOG 9916 study, 770 patients were randomized to receive either docetaxel plus estramustine and prednisone or mitoxantrone plus prednisone. Again the median overall survival was longer (17.5 months vs. 15.6 months, P=0.02 by the log-rank test) and PSA response rates were higher (50% vs. 27%, P<0.001) with docetaxel compared with mitoxantrone (Petrylak *et al.*, 2004). Given the efficacy of docetaxel as a single agent and potential thromboembolic toxicity from the addition of estramustine, docetaxel alone with daily prednisone became the standard approach. Although in the trial setting, patients received up to 10 cycles of treatment, in routine practice where patients are less fit, an average of 7 cycles is the length of treatment (Chin *et al.*, 2010). Some patients also appear to respond to retreatment with docetaxel, raising the concept of docetaxel refractory vs. docetaxel resistant disease (Chin *et al.*, 2010). Nonetheless, all patients will eventually develop taxane resistance and progress. In the second line setting, mitoxantrone chemotherapy has palliative benefits, but does not offer a survival advantage, underscoring the need for new strategies in the post-docetaxel setting (Tannock *et al.*, 1996).

Much of the research in the post-docetaxel setting has focused on understanding taxane resistance. Several mechanisms have been proposed including alterations in both docetaxel uptake and retention in cells; changes to tubulin affecting binding sites for docetaxel; and changes in the androgen receptor (AR), which may also contribute in part to the anticancer activity of docetaxel (Gan and Kavallaris, 2008; Seruga *et al.*, 2010). Strategies aimed at overcoming taxane resistance may extend the therapeutic benefit of the taxanes in CRPC.

2. Cabazitaxel

Cabazitaxel is a new semi-synthetic derivative of the taxoid 10-deacetylbaccatin-III, which like docetaxel binds to and stabilizes tubulin. But, unlike docetaxel is a poor substrate for the P-glycoprotein drug efflux pump and may also have enhanced penetration through the blood-brain barrier (Niraula and Tannock, 2011). In a Phase 1 trial of cabazitaxel the dose limiting toxicity at 25 mg/m2 every 3 weeks was grade 4 neutropenia, and the common non-hematologic adverse events included low grade diarrhea (52%), nausea (40%) and vomiting (16%). Two patients with CRPC, including one previously treated with docetaxel showed a partial response (Mita *et al.*, 2009).

A phase III multicenter, multinational trial comparing cabazitaxel with mitoxantrone in the second line setting was conducted with a primary endpoint of overall survival (OS) (de Bono, 2010). Cabazitaxel significantly improved median OS compared with mitoxantrone (15.1 months vs 12.7 months, respectively; HR 0.72; 95% CI 0.61-0.84;

$p<0.0001$). Secondary endpoints including progression free survival (PFS) (2.8 months vs 1.4 months), response rate (14.4% vs 4.4%; $p=0.005$), and median time to progression (TTP) by tumor assessment (8.8 months vs. 5.4 months; $p<0.0001$) also favored cabazitaxel. From a toxicity standpoint febrile neutropenia, neutropenia, leukopenia and diarrhea were more common in the cabazitaxel arm. One major concern with cabazitaxel however was a toxic death rate of 5% compared to only 1.9% for mitoxantrone. As cabazitaxel moves out of the controlled clinical trial setting into general use, early and proactive management of the toxicites will be critical. Cabazitaxel was FDA approved in 2010 for patients progressing on or after docetaxel. In the same year, a second drug, Abiraterone was also approved for use in the post-docetaxel setting.

3. Abiraterone

Over the last decade there has been a paradigm shift in the approach to CRPC, where despite castrate testosterone levels, there appears to be continued androgen receptor expression and signaling, suggesting that the androgen receptor axis is still a rational therapeutic target. In CRPC, androgens are mainly produced by the adrenal glands and by the prostate cancer cells themselves. This occurs by the sequential conversion of cholesterol to dihydrotestosterone and testosterone. This conversion is mediated by the CYP17 enzyme, which when inhibited can block androgen production. Ketoconazole, an antifungal agent, was the first generation CYP17 inhibitor that was tested in prostate cancer, with some benefit, but to date no studies have confirmed a survival benefit. On the other hand, abiraterone acetate (abiraterone), an oral, irreversible and more selective inhibitor of CYP17 has shown very encouraging results in the post-docetaxel setting.

In Phase I/II testing of abiraterone, there were no dose limiting toxicities, the main side effects were hypokalemia and lower-limb edema (due to the mineralocorticoid excess from the upstream inhibition of 17 alpha-hydroxylase), and antitumor activity was seen at all dose levels (Ryan *et al.*, 2010). A Phase III double blind, randomized, placebo-controlled trial of abiraterone 1000 mg daily plus prednisone (to avoid the mineralocorticoid related effects) versus prednisone alone, with the primary endpoint of OS was initiated (de Bono *et al.*, 2011). In total, 1,195 post-docetaxel CRPC patients were accrued, and treated until clinical or radiographic disease progression. Of note, biochemical progression alone (rising PSA) was not considered sufficient for discontinuation of the study drug. Interim analysis demonstrated increased median OS in the abiraterone arm, at 14.8 months compared to 10.9 months (HR 0.65, 95% CI 0.54-0.77) for prednisone leading to early termination of the trial. Other key endpoints including PSA response, time to PSA progression and radiographic progression free survival were all significantly improved in the abiraterone arm. Time to skeletal related events (SRE), defined as pathologic fracture, spinal cord compression, or palliative radiation therapy or surgery also favored the abiraterone arm. Mineralocorticoid related adverse events, consisting of hypertension and hypokalemia were more common in the abiraterone arm, but grade 3+ events were infrequent. A second Phase III trial of abiraterone in the pre-docetaxel setting has closed to accrual and results will likely be available in 2012.

Since both abiraterone and cabazitaxel are now approved in the post-docetaxel setting, a key question will be to determine the optimal sequencing of these agents. At this point it will likely be done on a case by case basis after careful consideration of the rate of disease progression, overall burden of disease, performance status and toxicity profile of either drug.

4. Sipuleucel-T

Aside from cytotoxic therapies and androgen deprivation approaches, immunotherapy has emerged in prostate cancer drug development. Sipuleucel-T (Provenge, Dendreon) is an immunotherapy that can enhance response to the prostate cell tumor antigen, prostatic acid phosphatase. Generation of the immunotherapy involves collection of peripheral blood cells by leukophoresis and subsequent exposure to prostatic acid phosphatase and granulocyte macrophase colony stimulating growth factor. The cells are then reintroduced into the patient. Sipuleucel-T is an autologous dendritic cell vaccine which enhances prostatic acid phosphatase related T cell response.

Encouraging phase I/II trial results led to the pivotal randomized, double-blind, placebo-controlled, multicenter trial (Study 9902B) known as the IMPACT trial (Immunotherapy for Prostate Adenocarcinoma Treatment), with a primary endpoint of overall survival (Kantoff *et al.*, 2010). All patients underwent three leukapheresis procedures (Weeks 0, 2, and 4), followed 3 days later by either sipuleucel-T or the non-activated control. Eligible CRPC patients had metastatic disease in soft tissue and/or bone with evidence of radiologic or biochemical disease progression. Patients with moderate to severe prostate cancer-related pain and/or use of narcotics were excluded. Tumor expression of prostatic acid phosphatase of 25% or more was required. Five hundred twelve patients were randomized (2:1) to sipuleucel-T (n=341) or control (n=171). The sipuleucel-T arm had a 4.1 months improvement in median overall survival (25.8 mos versus 21.7 mo, p= 0.032, HR 0.775, 95% CI 0.61, 0.98). There was no difference in time-to-progression. Common adverse events (AE) for sipuleucel-T were mild or moderate and included chills, fatigue, fever, back pain, nausea, joint ache and headache. Serious adverse reactions (SAE) more common with sipuleucel-T were acute infusion reactions and stroke. Similar survival and tolerability results were seen in two additional trials, which ultimately led to approval by the US Food and Drug Administration in 2010 (Small *et al.*, 2006; Higano *et al.*, 2009). Priced at $31,000 per treatment, Sipuleucel-T is one of the most expensive treatments ever, and as such may not be as widely available as either abiraterone or cabazitaxel.

5. Zoledronic acid

Over the last 10 years, there has also been growing interest in the issue of bone health in prostate cancer as it is known that both androgen deprivation therapy, and bony metastases can promote bone destruction. Zoledronic acid, is a nitrogen-containing bisphosphonate that inhibits osteoclast-mediated bone resorption. In a randomized placebo controlled clinical trial in men with CRPC and bone metastases, zoledronic acid reduced skeletal related events and decreased bone pain leading to its approval by the FDA in 2002 (Saad *et al.*, 2002). Bone resorption is a process that is dependent on RANK Ligand, a protein that acts as the primary mediator of osteoclast formation, function and survival. Preclinical models have demonstrated that inhibiting RANK Ligand significantly improves cortical and trabecular bone density, volume and strength. Studies with a novel bone targeting agent known as Denosumab have been encouraging, and offers another agent to address the bone complications of prostate cancer.

6. Denosumab

Denosumab is a fully humanized monoclonal antibody against the RANK ligand. RANK plays a major role in osteoclast activation. In the phase III trial of 1901 CRPC patients with one or more metastases, compared to zoledronic acid, denosumab delayed time to skeletal related events by approximately 3 months with a 2.3% incidence of osteonecrosis of the jaw compared to 1.3% in the zoledronic acid arm. Notably, there was no difference in overall survival (Fizazi *et al.*, 2011). This phase III study garnered FDA approval for Denosumab for the prevention of skeletal related events (SRE) in CRPC patients with bone metastases. Denosumab is also being evaluated for its ability to delay the development of bone metastases in CRPC patients. A third role for denosumab may be in protecting against ADT related osteoporosis. In this study, 912 patients on ADT received denosumab 60 mg subcutaneously every 6 months. At 24 months followup, denosumab was associated with increased bone mineral density at all sites and a reduction in the incidence of new vertebral fractures (Smith *et al.*, 2009). Denosumab also offers the benefit of being subcutaneously administered, and this might be an advantage for patients who are not otherwise requiring intravenous treatments.

7. Summary

There has been a significant increase in the number of treatment options available to men with CRPC. These advancements have included therapies with new taxane derivatives, drugs targeting the androgen axis, immunotherapy and bone targeting agents. Cabazitaxel, abiraterone and sipuleucel-T all show survival benefits, while Denosumab appears to reduce the risk of new bone metastases and skeletal related events in CRPC patient with bone metastases. But, with these new options comes new questions, such as, what is the optimal sequencing of these agents. As sequencing strategies become increasingly common, comparison of survival against historic data in addition to comparison of outcomes between newer agents and their associated trials will become increasing difficult to analyze. Whether results in the post docetaxel setting will be replicated in the chemonaive prostate cancer population awaits further definition. Also it is unclear if any of these agents will work better in combination with each other or with other molecular targeted therapies, although to date the latter have been disappointing in prostate cancer. What is very exciting however, is the fact that through drug development new information has become available enhancing our understanding of tumor progression in prostate cancer. Future areas of exploration include the use of newer agents in the prechemotherapy and neoadjuvant setting, using objective biologic endpoints such as pathologic response and radiographic response over short treatment intervals. Defining new endpoints may assist in circumventing the eventual difficulty in proceeding with large trials of heterogeneous patients in whom a placebo controlled trial design may not be feasible. Lastly, as the understanding of the molecular drivers of disease progression become increasingly understood, molecular markers that may serve as surrogate clinical trial endpoints may emerge, further enhancing a flourishing field.

8. References

Chin, S.N., Wang, L., Moore, M., and Sridhar, S.S. (2010) A review of the patterns of docetaxel use for hormone-resistant prostate cancer at the princess margaret hospital. *Curr Oncol*, 17, 24-9.

de Bono, J.S., Logothetis, C.J., Molina, A., Fizazi, K., North, S., Chu, L., Chi, K.N., Jones, R.J., Goodman, O.B., Jr., Saad, F., Staffurth, J.N., Mainwaring, P., Harland, S., Flaig, T.W., Hutson, T.E., Cheng, T., Patterson, H., Hainsworth, J.D., Ryan, C.J., Sternberg, C.N., Ellard, S.L., Flechon, A., Saleh, M., Scholz, M., Efstathiou, E., Zivi, A., Bianchini, D., Loriot, Y., Chieffo, N., Kheoh, T., Haqq, C.M., and Scher, H.I. (2011) Abiraterone and increased survival in metastatic prostate cancer. *N Engl J Med*, 364, 1995-2005.

de Bono, J.S., Oudard, S., Ozguroglu, M., Hansen, S., Machiels, J.P., Kocak, I., Gravis, G., Bodrogi, I., Mackenzie, M.J., Shen, L., Roessner, M., Gupta, S., and Sartor, A.O. (2010) Prednisone plus cabazitaxel or mitoxantrone for metastatic castration-resistant prostate cancer progressing after docetaxel treatment: A randomised open-label trial. *Lancet*, 376, 1147-54.

Fizazi, K., Carducci, M., Smith, M., Damiao, R., Brown, J., Karsh, L., Milecki, P., Shore, N., Rader, M., Wang, H., Jiang, Q., Tadros, S., Dansey, R., and Goessl, C. (2011) Denosumab versus zoledronic acid for treatment of bone metastases in men with castration-resistant prostate cancer: A randomised, double-blind study. *Lancet*, 377, 813-22.

Gan, P.P., and Kavallaris, M. (2008) Tubulin-targeted drug action: Functional significance of class ii and class ivb beta-tubulin in vinca alkaloid sensitivity. *Cancer Res*, 68, 9817-24.

Heng, D.Y., and Chi, K.N. (2006) Prednisone monotherapy in asymptomatic hormone refractory prostate cancer. *Can J Urol*, 13, 3335-9.

Higano, C.S., Schellhammer, P.F., Small, E.J., Burch, P.A., Nemunaitis, J., Yuh, L., Provost, N., and Frohlich, M.W. (2009) Integrated data from 2 randomized, double-blind, placebo-controlled, phase 3 trials of active cellular immunotherapy with sipuleucel-t in advanced prostate cancer. *Cancer*, 115, 3670-9.

Jemal, A., Bray, F., Center, M.M., Ferlay, J., Ward, E., and Forman, D. (2010) Global cancer statistics. *CA Cancer J Clin*, 61, 69-90.

Jordan, M.A., Toso, R.J., Thrower, D., and Wilson, L. (1993) Mechanism of mitotic block and inhibition of cell proliferation by taxol at low concentrations. *Proc Natl Acad Sci U S A*, 90, 9552-6.

Kantoff, P.W., Higano, C.S., Shore, N.D., Berger, E.R., Small, E.J., Penson, D.F., Redfern, C.H., Ferrari, A.C., Dreicer, R., Sims, R.B., Xu, Y., Frohlich, M.W., and Schellhammer, P.F. (2010) Sipuleucel-t immunotherapy for castration-resistant prostate cancer. *N Engl J Med*, 363, 411-22.

Mita, A.C., Denis, L.J., Rowinsky, E.K., Debono, J.S., Goetz, A.D., Ochoa, L., Forouzesh, B., Beeram, M., Patnaik, A., Molpus, K., Semiond, D., Besenval, M., and Tolcher, A.W. (2009) Phase i and pharmacokinetic study of xrp6258 (rpr 116258a), a novel taxane, administered as a 1-hour infusion every 3 weeks in patients with advanced solid tumors. *Clin Cancer Res*, 15, 723-30.

Niraula, S., and Tannock, I.F. (2011) Broadening horizons in medical management of prostate cancer. *Acta Oncol*, 50 Suppl 1, 141-7.

Petrylak, D.P., Tangen, C.M., Hussain, M.H., Lara, P.N., Jr., Jones, J.A., Taplin, M.E., Burch, P.A., Berry, D., Moinpour, C., Kohli, M., Benson, M.C., Small, E.J., Raghavan, D., and Crawford, E.D. (2004) Docetaxel and estramustine compared with mitoxantrone and prednisone for advanced refractory prostate cancer. *N Engl J Med*, 351, 1513-20.

Ryan, C.J., Smith, M.R., Fong, L., Rosenberg, J.E., Kantoff, P., Raynaud, F., Martins, V., Lee, G., Kheoh, T., Kim, J., Molina, A., and Small, E.J. (2010) Phase i clinical trial of the cyp17 inhibitor abiraterone acetate demonstrating clinical activity in patients with castration-resistant prostate cancer who received prior ketoconazole therapy. *J Clin Oncol*, 28, 1481-8.

Saad, F., Gleason, D.M., Murray, R., Tchekmedyian, S., Venner, P., Lacombe, L., Chin, J.L., Vinholes, J.J., Goas, J.A., and Chen, B. (2002) A randomized, placebo-controlled trial of zoledronic acid in patients with hormone-refractory metastatic prostate carcinoma. *J Natl Cancer Inst*, 94, 1458-68.

Saad, F., and Hotte, S.J. (2010) Guidelines for the management of castrate-resistant prostate cancer. *Can Urol Assoc J*, 4, 380-4.

Seruga, B., Ocana, A., and Tannock, I.F. (2010) Drug resistance in metastatic castration-resistant prostate cancer. *Nat Rev Clin Oncol*, 8, 12-23.

Sharifi, N., Gulley, J.L., and Dahut, W.L. (2005) Androgen deprivation therapy for prostate cancer. *Jama*, 294, 238-44.

Small, E.J., Halabi, S., Dawson, N.A., Stadler, W.M., Rini, B.I., Picus, J., Gable, P., Torti, F.M., Kaplan, E., and Vogelzang, N.J. (2004) Antiandrogen withdrawal alone or in combination with ketoconazole in androgen-independent prostate cancer patients: A phase iii trial (calgb 9583). *J Clin Oncol*, 22, 1025-33.

Small, E.J., Schellhammer, P.F., Higano, C.S., Redfern, C.H., Nemunaitis, J.J., Valone, F.H., Verjee, S.S., Jones, L.A., and Hershberg, R.M. (2006) Placebo-controlled phase iii trial of immunologic therapy with sipuleucel-t (apc8015) in patients with metastatic, asymptomatic hormone refractory prostate cancer. *J Clin Oncol*, 24, 3089-94.

Smith, M.R., Egerdie, B., Hernandez Toriz, N., Feldman, R., Tammela, T.L., Saad, F., Heracek, J., Szwedowski, M., Ke, C., Kupic, A., Leder, B.Z., and Goessl, C. (2009) Denosumab in men receiving androgen-deprivation therapy for prostate cancer. *N Engl J Med*, 361, 745-55.

Storlie, J.A., Buckner, J.C., Wiseman, G.A., Burch, P.A., Hartmann, L.C., and Richardson, R.L. (1995) Prostate specific antigen levels and clinical response to low dose dexamethasone for hormone-refractory metastatic prostate carcinoma. *Cancer*, 76, 96-100.

Tannock, I.F., de Wit, R., Berry, W.R., Horti, J., Pluzanska, A., Chi, K.N., Oudard, S., Theodore, C., James, N.D., Turesson, I., Rosenthal, M.A., and Eisenberger, M.A. (2004) Docetaxel plus prednisone or mitoxantrone plus prednisone for advanced prostate cancer. *N Engl J Med*, 351, 1502-12.

Tannock, I.F., Osoba, D., Stockler, M.R., Ernst, D.S., Neville, A.J., Moore, M.J., Armitage, G.R., Wilson, J.J., Venner, P.M., Coppin, C.M., and Murphy, K.C. (1996) Chemotherapy with mitoxantrone plus prednisone or prednisone alone for symptomatic hormone-resistant prostate cancer: A canadian randomized trial with palliative end points. *J Clin Oncol*, 14, 1756-64.

13

The Role of PDE-5 Inhibitors in Prostate Cancer

Anindita Das, Fadi N. Salloum and Rakesh C. Kukreja
Division of Cardiology, Pauley Heart Center, Department of Internal Medicine
Virginia Commonwealth University, Richmond
USA

1. Introduction

Prostate cancer currently stands as the most frequently diagnosed solid tumor in men, and remains one of the leading causes of cancer mortality in men in the Western world, accounting for an estimated 32,050 deaths in the United States in 2010 (Jemal *et al.*, 2010). With the well-known use of serum prostate-specific antigen (PSA) as a screening tool, men are being diagnosed with earlier stage disease at younger ages. However, a significant number of men continue to be diagnosed with high-risk localized prostate cancer. Radical prostatectomy, radiotherapy, cryotherapy, high-intensity focused ultrasound, radiation therapy, and androgen deprivation as well as androgen receptor blockade have been the mainstays of treatment for cancer patients with localized and androgen-dependent prostate cancer.

As prostate cancer cell growth is androgen dependent, its deprivation is an important therapeutic strategy. However, long-term androgen-ablation results in androgen-independent cancer cell growth in metastatic patients, leading to hormone refractory prostate cancer (HRPC) (Sonpavde *et al.*, 2006). Prostate cancer tends to invade the pelvic lymph nodes and spread to distant organs, mainly via the blood stream, showing a strong predilection for bones (Koutsilieris, 1993;Sourla *et al.*, 1996). This disease frequently metastasizes to bone and almost invariably progresses from an androgen-sensitive to an androgen-independent status, greatly limiting therapeutic options and significantly reducing life expectancy in patients. Skeletal metastases occur in more than 80% of cases of advanced-stage prostate cancer and they confer a high level of morbidity. Metastasis of prostate cancer, like that of other solid tumors, involves multiple steps, including angiogenesis, local migration, invasion, intravasation, circulation and extravasation of tumor cells and then angiogenesis and colonization in the new site. Treatment-naive metastatic prostate cancer is largely sensitive to androgen-deprivation therapy (ADT), but the effectiveness of ADT is temporary, and tumors in the majority of patients eventually relapse and evolve into castration-resistant prostate cancer (CRPC), from which most patients die (Eisenberger and Walsh, 1999). These tumors eventually become incurable or resistant to antihormonal therapy. Indeed, there is an association between ADT and high risk of cardiovascular disease and mortality, and men with a history of recent or active cardiac disease are particularly at risk (Saigal *et al.*, 2007). In men with a history of coronary artery disease, chronic heart failure, or myocardial infarction, ADT was associated with an increased risk of mortality (Nguyen *et al.*, 2011). Continuous ADT use for at least 6 months in older men is also associated with an increased risk of diabetes and fragility fracture (Alibhai *et al.*, 2009). For this reason, new agents and therapeutic modalities are needed, including non-hormonal systemic chemotherapy, which can provide another option for patients with non-localized HRPC or CRPC.

2.1 Chemotherapeutic agents

Chemotherapy is often used as a main regimen in the overall treatment of most cancers. In the past, clinical trial design has focused on sequential development of chemotherapeutic drugs based on symptoms and number of prior therapies. There are four chemotherapeutic agents that the US Federal Drug Administration (FDA) approved for CRPC: estramustine, mitoxantrone, docetaxel and cabaxitaxel.

2.2 Docetaxel

Chemotherapy, using Taxotere (docetaxel), a member of taxane family, remains the standard option for patients at the advanced stages, in particular, HRPC (Schurko and Oh, 2008). As of April 2010, only one approved chemotherapeutic agent, docetaxel, showed promising results in improving survival in patients with metastatic CRPC (Abdulla and Kapoor, 2011). This drug is a microtubule-polymerizing agent with a well-established antimitotic chemotherapy action. It causes downregulation of anti-apoptotic protein, Bcl-2 (Li *et al.*, 2005;Schiff and Horwitz, 1980;Schurko and Oh, 2008;Stein, 1999;Yoo *et al.*, 2008), enhances the apoptosis induced by "tumor necrosis factor-related apoptosis-inducing ligand" (TRAIL) (Yoo *et al.*, 2008), down regulates genes involved in cell cycle progression (cyclin A, cyclin F, *CDC2*, *CDK2*, *BTG*, etc.), transcription factors (transcription factor A, ATF5, TAF 1 31L, etc.), oncogenes (*GRO*, *BRCA1*, *p120*, etc.) and apoptosis as *GADD45A (Li et al., 2005;Stein, 1999;Yoo et al., 2008)*. A recent study showed that docetaxel upregulates p53 and p21 in a p38-dependent manner to desensitize prostate cancer cells (Gan *et al.*, 2011). The p38/p53/p21 signaling pathway could be important for regulating the susceptibility towards docetaxel in prostate cancer. Docetaxel regimens have been shown to increase survival compared to previous treatment modalities in HRPC, although prognosis remains poor and median survival ranges from 10 to 20 months (Petrylak *et al.*, 2004;Tannock *et al.*, 2004). Cancer cells become resistant to taxanes and other microtubule-binding chemotherapeutic agents and therefore docetaxel therapy is limited. Makarovskiy et al. found that continuity of docetaxel exposure induces the formation of resistant giant multinucleated clones (Makarovskiy *et al.*, 2002). Lack of curative treatments at the advanced prostate cancer, underline the importance of additional trials for the successful development of an effective therapeutic approach. Another study showed that docetaxel and sodium selenite combination plays an antiproliferative synergistic and additive cell death effect (Freitas *et al.*, 2011). That study suggested that docetaxel and sodium selenite combination may be more effective in prostate cancer treatment than docetaxel alone warranting further evaluation of this combination in prostate cancer therapeutic approach.

Docetaxel in combination with prednisone compared with mitoxantrone in combination with prednisone yielded an extension in median survival with HRPC, however, patients eventually developed progressive disease associated with poor outcomes (Berthold *et al.*, 2008). Carbazitaxel, a tubulin-binding semi-synthetic taxane, is the first drug to improve survival in patients with metastatic CRPC whose disease has progressed during or after docetaxel-based therapy, providing a 30% reduction in the risk of death and an improved median overall survival compared with mitoxantrone (de Bono *et al.*, 2010). Carbaxitaxel in combination with prednisone was approved by the FDA in June 2010 for the treatment of patients with metastatic CRPC who had been previously treated with docetaxel (Wu *et al.*, 2011).

Although there are several options after failing hormone therapy to help achieve disease control, HRPC remains incurable, and there continues to be an ongoing need for the development of new therapies that provide significant survival benefits without severely impacting quality of life. Today, not only are hormonal and cytotoxic treatment modalities available to patients with metastatic CRPC, but also more novel treatments in the areas of immune and targeted therapies are being offered. Newer agents currently being investigated for their potential role in metastatic CRPC are sipuleucel T (an autologous dendritic cell-based vaccine), denosumab (antibody), abiraterone (hormonal therapy), TAK-700 (hormonal therapy), MDV3100 (hormonal therapy) and ipilimumab (immune therapy), zibotentan (endothalin-receptor antagonists) and dasatinib (tyrosine kinase inhibitor).

2.3 Doxorubicin

Anthracyclines rank among the most important chemotherapeutic drugs with a large spectrum of antitumor activity, including prostate cancer. The precise mechanisms of action of anthracyclines in tumor cells remain a matter of controversy. The suggested mechanisms include (i) DNA intercalation, leading to inhibition of synthesis of macromolecules; (ii) generation of reactive oxygen species (ROS), leading to DNA damage or lipid peroxidation; (iii) DNA binding and alkylation; (iv) DNA cross-linking; (v) interference with DNA unwinding or DNA strand separation and helicase activity; (vi) direct membrane effects; (vii) initiation of DNA damage via inhibition of topoisomerase II; and (viii) induction of apoptosis in response to topoisomerase II inhibition (Takemura and Fujiwara, 2007). Doxorubicin (DOX, Adriamycin) and its analogue epirubicin, or 4-epidoxorubicin, are the most potent anthracyclines, and have a broad spectrum of activity against solid tumors and hematological malignancies. Monotherapy with DOX or in combination with other agents, have been used extensively for the treatment of HRPC, however, controversial results have been reported (Petrioli *et al.*, 2008). Acquisition of chemoresistance remains one of the major problems of chemotherapy failure in cancer patients. Therefore, there is an urgent need to identify a strategy that can overcome chemoresistance and sensitize tumor cells to chemotherapeutic agents. For this reason, a clinical chemotherapeutic regimen consisting of a combination of drugs can achieve a higher therapeutic efficacy than that provided by a single drug.

2.4 Cardiotoxicity

Despite its clinical efficacy, the use of DOX is associated with their severe toxicity, including a myelosuppression and dose-dependent delayed and progressive irreversible cardiomyopathy often observed several years after cessation of treatment eventually results in refractory cardiac dysfunction (Steinherz *et al.*, 1991;Steinherz *et al.*, 1995). It has been shown that DOX induces cardiomyopathy and heart failure in >30% patients receiving 500 mg/m^2 or higher cumulative doses (Menna *et al.*, 2011;Minotti *et al.*, 2004). The molecular basis for this cardiotoxic effect remains a matter of debate. Several hypotheses have been suggested to explain the acute and chronic cardiotoxicity of DOX; these include the increased level of ROS and lipid peroxidation by DOX-iron cmplexes (Myers, 1998), along with a reduction in the levels of antioxidants and sulfhydryl groups (Takemura and Fujiwara, 2007), alterations in cardiac muscle gene expression, sensitization of Ca^{2+} release from sarcoplasmic reticulum channels, mitochondrial DNA damage and dysfunction and alteration of membrane potentials, and induction of apoptosis (Arola *et al.*, 2000;Burke *et al.*, 2002;Kumar *et al.*, 2001;Olson and Mushlin, 1990). Of these options, the free radical and ROS hypothesis of DOX-induced cardiotoxicity has gained the most support in previous studies.

The target organelles of DOX toxicity in cardiomyocytes are mitochondria wherein DOX accumulates with time (Kalyanaraman *et al.*, 2002;Konorev *et al.*, 1999). DOX-induced cardiomyopathy occurs predominantly via the generation of ROS in the cardiomyocyte mitochondria, a mechanism that is separate from its antineoplastic activity, which occurs primarily through inhibition of topoisomerase II (Myers, 1998). DOX is known to generate free radicals either by redox cycling between a semiquinone form and a quinone form or by forming a DOX-Fe^{3+} complex (Davies and Doroshow, 1986). In both pathways, molecular oxygen is reduced to superoxide anion ($O_2^{-}\cdot$), which is converted to other forms of reactive oxygen species such as hydrogen peroxide (H_2O_2) and hydroxyl radical ($OH\cdot$). Mitochondrial enzymes (e.g. NADH dehydrogenase) activate DOX by converting it to the corresponding semiquinone which generates superoxide in the presence of molecular oxygen. The dismutation of the superoxide, spontaneous or catalyzed by superoxide dismutase (SOD) enzymes, generates hydrogen peroxide in mitochondria (Kalyanaraman *et al.*, 2002). The heart is particularly vulnerable to free radical injury because the drug causes the disappearance of cardiac glutathione peroxidase, leaving the heart with no means of disposing of the hydrogen peroxide (Myers, 1998). These free radicals could then cause membrane and macromolecule damage, both of which lead to injury to the heart, an organ that has a relatively low level of antioxidant enzymes such as SOD and catalase (Doroshow *et al.*, 1980). Several studies demonstrated that DOX-induced cardiotoxicity can be largely reduced by the overexpression of the antioxidant enzymes mitochondrial superoxide dismutase (MnSOD), metallothionein, or catalase (Kang *et al.*, 1996;Kang *et al.*, 1997;Yen *et al.*, 1996). Moreover, free radical scavengers including probucol, amifostine, and dexrazoxane have demonstrated protection from doxorubicin-induced cardiotoxicity, further substantiating the role of ROS in DOX-induced cardiotoxicity (Koning *et al.*, 1991;Kumar *et al.*, 2001;Nazeyrollas *et al.*, 1999). On the other hand, all of these agents have pronounced clinical disadvantages, including a significant decline in high-density lipoprotein (HDL) levels, an inability to prevent DOX-induced mortality and weight loss, and potentiation of myelosuppression (Liu *et al.*, 2002b).
DOX induce cardiotoxicity ultimately results in myocyte apoptosis which plays an important role in the development of heart failure (Hosseinzadeh *et al.*, 2011;Mizutani *et al.*, 2005;Spallarossa *et al.*, 2004;Spallarossa *et al.*, 2009). In fact, apoptosis contributes to cardiomyocyte loss, which eventually leads to structural changes maladaptive to normal cardiac physiological demands (Narula *et al.*, 1996;Singal *et al.*, 2000). Strategies for the prevention of DOX-induced cardiotoxicity during chemotherapy have focused on three main approaches: dose optimization, synthesis of analogues and combination therapy. However, none of the analogues available clinically appear to have any advantage over DOX (Weiss, 1992); a better anthracycline has yet to be found. Today, liposomal formulations of anthracyclines are available; treatments have lower toxicity profiles, especially in terms of cardiac side-effects (Safra, 2003). The activity of anthracyclines is therefore an area worthy of further research in this clinical setting.

3.1 PDE-5 inhibitors

Cyclic nucleotide phosphodiesterases (PDEs) are a family of related phosphohydrolases that selectively catalyze the hydrolysis of the 3′ cyclic phosphate bonds of cAMP and cGMP, second messengers in the cell (Bender and Beavo, 2006). The PDE enzymes, of at least 11 types, are ubiquitous through out the body, and perform a variety of functions (Kukreja *et al.*, 2004). PDE-5 is the primary enzyme in the corpus cavernosum, and plays a crucial role in vascular smooth muscle contraction through controlling the rate of hydrolyzation and subsequent degradation of cGMP (Bender and Beavo, 2006). Three widely prescribed PDE-5 inhibitors, sildenafil (Viagra), vardenafil (Levitra), and tadalafil (Cialis), have proven very effective for the treatment of erectile dysfunction (ED) in men (Boolell *et al.*, 1996;Porst *et al.*, 2001;Porst *et al.*, 2003) and more recently for pulmonary artery hypertension (Galie *et al.*, 2005;Galie *et al.*, 2010). In the lung, inhibition of PDE-5 opposed smooth muscle vasoconstriction and attenuated the rise in pulmonary artery pressure and vascular remodeling (Sebkhi *et al.*, 2003).

Several studies have shown that PDE-5 inhibitors induce a preconditioning-like effect against ischemia/reperfusion (I/R) injury in the intact heart and adult cardiomyocytes (Bremer *et al.*, 2005;Das *et al.*, 2004;Das *et al.*, 2005;Das *et al.*, 2008;Das *et al.*, 2009;Ockaili *et al.*, 2002;Salloum *et al.*, 2003;Salloum *et al.*, 2007;Salloum *et al.*, 2008). The mechanisms of cardioprotection include nitric oxide (NO) generation by activation of eNOS/iNOS (endothelial nitric oxide synthase/inducible nitric oxide synthase), activation of protein kinase C, cGMP-dependent protein kinase (PKG) and ERK, and inactivation of GSK3β and opening of the mitoK_{ATP} channels (Das *et al.*, 2004;Das *et al.*, 2005;Das *et al.*, 2008;Das *et al.*, 2009;Ockaili *et al.*, 2002;Salloum *et al.*, 2003). PDE-5 inhibition attenuated cardiomyocytes cell death resulting from necrosis and apoptosis after SI-RO (simulated ischemia and reoxygenation) by NOS-dependent up-regulation of the Bcl-2/Bax ratio (Das *et al.*, 2005). Sildenafil attenuated ischemic cardiomyopathy in mice by limiting necrosis and apoptosis and by preserving left ventricular (LV) function possibly through a NO-dependent pathway following myocardial infarction by left anterior descending coronary artery ligation (Salloum *et al.*, 2008). Tadalafil also limits myocardial I/R injury and dysfunction through hydrogen sulfide (H_2S) signaling in a PKG-dependent fashion (Salloum *et al.*, 2009).

3.2 PDE-5 inhibitors protect against DOX-induced cardiomyopathy

Sildenafil attenuated cardiomyocyte apoptosis and left ventricular (LV) dysfunction in a chronic model of DOX-induced cardiotoxicity (Fisher *et al.*, 2005). Treatment with clinically relevant doses of sildenafil (0.7 mg/kg IP) prior to DOX treatment inhibited cardiomyocyte apoptosis, preserved mitochondrial membrane potential ($\Delta\psi m$) and myofibrillar integrity, prevented of LV dysfunction as well as ST prolongation. Reduction in fractional shortening and abnormalities in the nonspecific T wave and ST segment of Electrocardiography (ECG) was typically observed in DOX-induced ventricular dysfunction (van Acker *et al.*, 1996). Our ECG study indicated the most marked increase in ST interval occurred between week 4 and week 8 of DOX treatment. Furthermore, ST interval of sildenafil and DOX groups remained unchanged from baseline during the course of the study. This study demonstrated that sildenafil significantly protected against ST-interval prolongation throughout the study period. Exposure of adult mouse ventricular myocytes to DOX resulted in dissipation of $\Delta\psi m$ as illustrated via JC-1 immunofluorescent staining (Figure 1C, G), which leaded to the induction of apoptosis (Figure 1H) compared to control (Figure 1A). In contrast, sildenafil pretreatment with DOX demonstrated preservation of the $\Delta\psi m$ (Figure 1D, G) and reduction of apoptosis (Figure 1H). However, sildenafil-induced protection was abolished by N^G-nitro-L-arginine methyl ester (L-NAME, an inhibitor of NOS) and 5-hydroxydecanoate (5-HD, mitoK_{ATP} channel blocker). These findings implied that sildenafil-mediated protection from DOX-induced cardiomyocyte apoptosis is NOS dependent and established a significant role of mitoK_{ATP} channel opening in sildenafil-induced cardioprotection. Additionally, the anti-apoptotic protein Bcl-2 was significantly declined after treatment in the DOX group compared with the sildenafil + DOX and control groups, suggesting a pivotal role of Bcl-2 in altering the pathological process leading to end-stage heart failure.

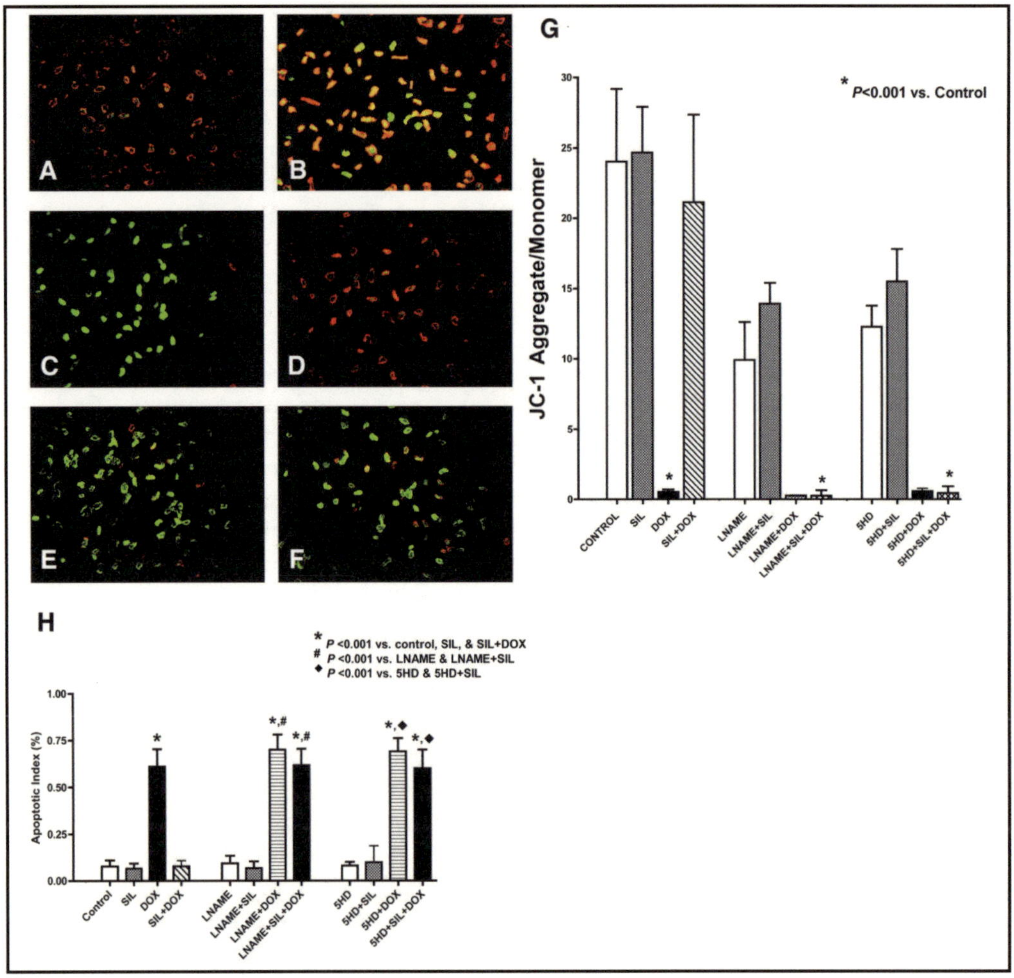

Fig. 1. Effect of sildenafil on Δψm and apoptosis in adult mouse ventricular myocyte. **A to F**, JC-1 staining of cardiomyocytes. Red fluorescence represents the mitochondrial aggregate, indicating intact mitochondrial membrane potential. Green fluorescence represents the monomeric form of JC-1, indicating dissipation of Δψm. **A**, Control; **B**, sildenafil (1 μmol/L); **C**, DOX (1 μmol/L); **D**, sildenafil (1 μmol/L) plus DOX (1 μmol/L); **E**, L-NAME (100 μmol/L)+sildenafil+DOX; **F**, 5-HD (100 μmol/L) +sildenafil+DOX; **G**, ratio of mitochondrial aggregates to monomeric form of JC-1; **H**, Apoptotic Index for TUNEL-positive cardiomyocytes. Data are mean±SEM (n=3; magnification X200). Reprinted from Fisher, P. W. et al. Circulation 2005;111:1601-1610 with permission.

More recently, we showed that tadalafil, the long acting PDE-5 inhibitor, also improved LV function by preserving fractional shortening (LVFS) and ejection fraction (LVEF) compared with DOX-treated mice (Figure 2) (Koka *et al.*, 2010). This study also demonstrated that tadalafil improved survival rates in mice without interfering with the anti-tumor effect of DOX. Tadalafil prevented cardiomyocyte apoptosis in DOX-induced cardiomyopathy through up-regulation of cGMP (Figure 3A) and PKG activity (Figure 3B), by restoring Bcl-2 and GATA-4 in the myocardium, and by reducing the oxidative stress via the up-regulation of mitochondrial superoxide dismutase (MnSOD). Moreover, tadalafil did not interfere with the efficacy of DOX in killing human osteosarcoma cells *in vitro* or its antitumor effect *in vivo* in tumor xenograft model. These studies suggest that prophylactic treatment with the class of PDE-5 inhibitors might become a promising therapeutic intervention for managing the clinical concern of DOX-induced cardiotoxicity in patients.

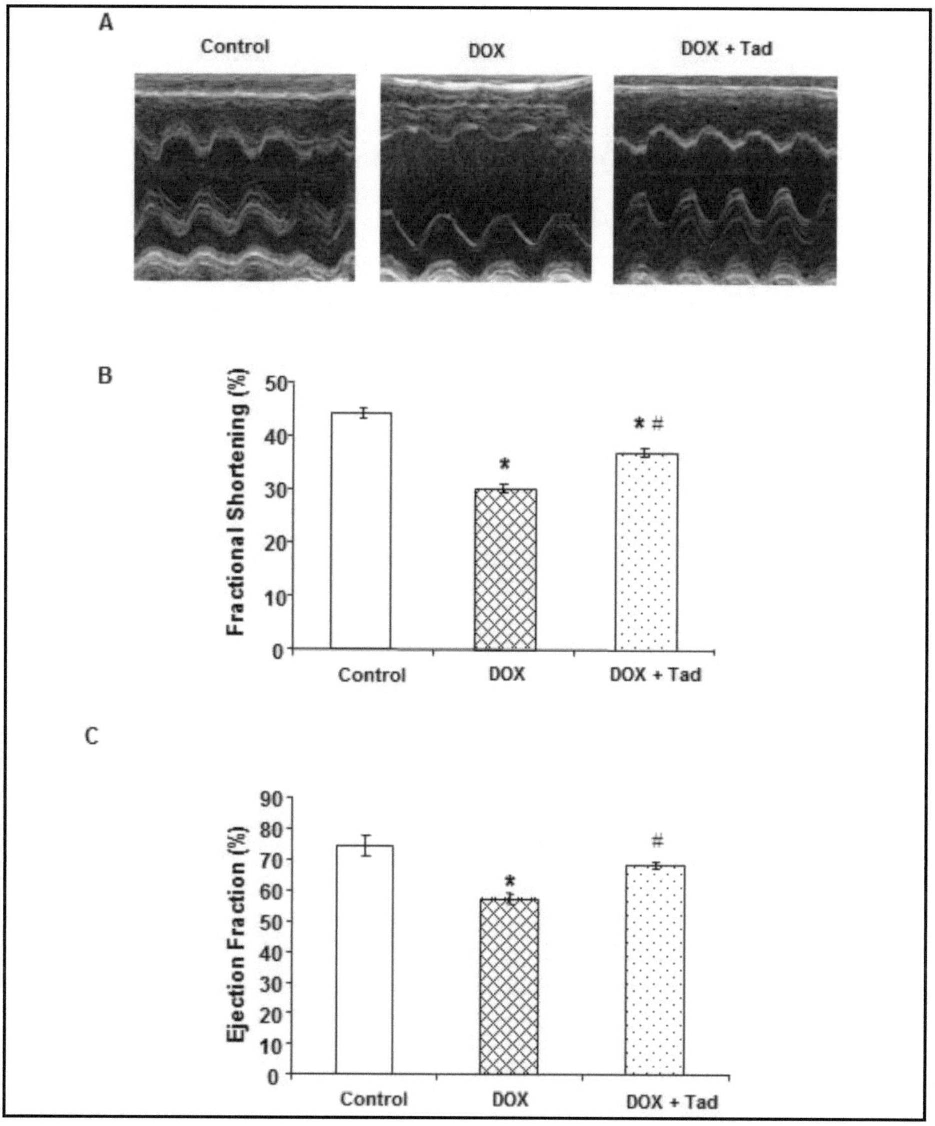

Fig. 2. Transthorasic echocardiography represented the effect of tadalafil on ventricular contractile dysfunction caused by DOX. **A,** representative M-mode images for control, DOX and tadalafil +DOX- treated mice. **B and C,** the averaged data of fractional shortening **(B)** and ejection fraction **(C)** in the mice are presented as mean ± S.E. (n = 6 per group; *, $P < 0.05$ versus control; #, $P < 0.05$ versus DOX). Reprinted from Koka, et al. J Pharmacol Exp Ther. 2010 Sep 1;334(3):1023-1030 with permission.

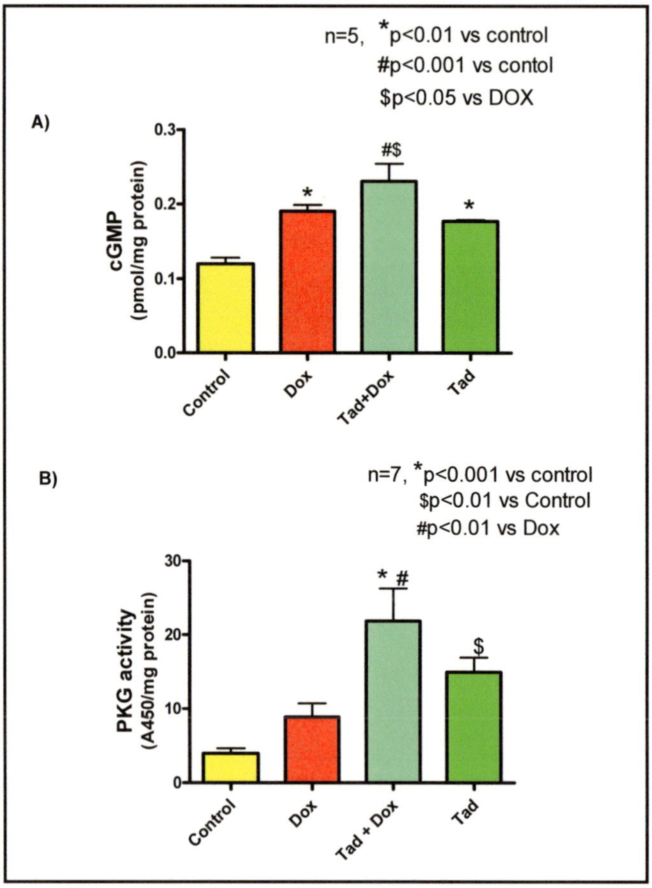

Fig. 3. Tadalafil augments cGMP and protein kinase G after DOX treatment. cGMP level **(A)** and PKG activity **(B)** in the cardiac tissue. Results are presented as mean ± S.E. (n = 5–7/group). *, $P < 0.05$ versus control; #, $P < 0.05$ versus DOX group. Partial data reprinted from Koka, et al. J Pharmacol Exp Ther. 2010 Sep 1;334(3):1023-1030 with permission.

3.3 PDE-5 inhibitors in cancer

Increased PDE-5 expression is reported in multiple human carcinomas including metastatic breast cancers, colon adenocarcinoma, bladder squamous carcinoma, and lung cancers as compared to adjacent normal tissues (Epstein and Hachisu, 1984;Joe *et al.*, 2003;Lim *et al.*, 2003;Piazza *et al.*, 2001;Porst *et al.*, 2001;Singer *et al.*, 1976;Whitehead *et al.*, 2003). PDE-5 was also detected as a predominant isoform of cGMP-PDEs in many carcinoma cells lines in culture, including colonic adenocarcinoma (SW480, HCT116, HT29, T84), breast cancer (HTB-26, MCF-7), lung cancer, bladder and prostate cancer (LNCAP, PC-3), and leukemia (Thompson *et al.*, 2000;Whitehead *et al.*, 2003;Zhu *et al.*, 2005). These studies suggest a functional role of an up-regulated PDE-5 in controlling tumor cell growth and death. PDE-5 selective inhibitors, sildenafil and vardenafil induced caspase dependent apoptosis and antiproliferation in B-cell chronic lymphatic leukemia (Sarfati *et al.*, 2003;Zhu *et al.*, 2005). Vardenafil when given in combination with DOX significantly improved the survival and reduced the tumor size in the brain-tumor-bearing rats (Black *et al.*, 2008). In this study, oral administration of vardenafil and sildenafil increased the rate of transport of compounds across the blood-tumor-brain and improved the efficacy of DOX in treatment of brain tumors. The selective increase in tumor capillary permeability appeared to be mediated by a selective increase in tumor cGMP levels and increased vesicular transport through tumor capillaries, and could be attenuated by iberiotoxin, a selective inhibitor for calcium-dependent potassium (K_{Ca}) channels, that are effectors in cGMP signaling. This study supported the use of PDE5 inhibitors as a novel therapy to selectively increase drug transport to malignant brain tumors. Another PDE-5 inhibitor, exisulind (sulindac sulfone) and its higher affinity analogues also induced apoptosis and inhibited cell proliferation in colon tumor cells lines by activating PKG and increasing phosphorylation of β-catenin (Lim *et al.*, 2003;Liu *et al.*, 2002a).

One of the major causes of chemotherapy failure in cancer treatment is multidrug resistance (MDR). One of the known causes of MDR is overexpression of the ATP-binding cassette (ABC) transporters, such as P-glycoprotein (ABCB1/P-gp/MDR1), multidrug resistance proteins (ABCCs/MRPs) and breast cancer resistant protein (ABCG2/BCRP). Among these transporters, the ABCB1 transporter is the most important mediator of MDR (Ambudkar *et al.*, 2003), and is responsible for chemotherapeutic drug resistance to a variety of drugs, including vinca alkaloids, anthracyclines, epipodophyllotoxins and taxanes (Szakacs *et al.*, 2006). These transporters actively efflux a variety of structurally and functionally diverse chemotherapeutic drugs out of cancer cells, thereby reducing the intracellular drug accumulation, increasing the likelihood of decreased cytotoxic and thus unsuccessful treatment (Dean *et al.*, 2001;Gillet *et al.*, 2007;O'Connor, 2007). Therefore, a promising approach is to inhibit these transporters to restore the sensitivity of drug-resistant cancer cells to chemotherapeutic drugs, which leads to a more efficacious treatment for cancer patients. As a result, a number of compounds have been identified with the ability to inhibit individual or several transporters by blocking drug efflux, increasing drug accumulation and thus sensitizing resistant cancer cells. Several of these agents, including cyclosporine A, VX-710 (biricodar), Verapamil(Germann *et al.*, 1997;Minderman *et al.*, 2004;Qadir *et al.*, 2005), LY475776 (Dantzig *et al.*, 2004), V-104 and GF-120918 (elacridar) (Evers *et al.*, 2000) can inhibit/suppresses the function of multiple transporters including ABCB1, ABCC1, and ABCG2. Unfortunately, most of these inhibitors have not been translated into clinical trials due to unfavorable side effects, toxic pharmacokinetic interactions, or simply because the magnitude of improvement in therapeutic outcome of these inhibitors with conventional chemotherapeutic agents is either nonsignificant or inconclusive (Szakacs *et al.*, 2006). Several tyrosine kinase inhibitors (TKIs), including imatinib (Shen *et al.*, 2009), nilotinib (Tiwari *et al.*, 2009), lapatinib (Dai *et al.*, 2008), and erlotinib (Shi *et al.*, 2007), can also reverse MDR to antineoplastic drugs mediated by ABC-transporters. However, the reversal potential of these TKIs has not been determined in clinical trials. Consequently, there is an urgent need for the discovery of more efficacious, non-toxic and less expensive novel agents to reverse MDR in cancer cells. Recent study showed that the PDE-5 inhibitor, vardenafil, significantly reversed MDR in ABCB1 overexpressing cancer cells, and its efficacy was greater than that of tadalafil (Ding *et al.*, 2011). Sildenafil also inhibited cell surface ABC transporters ABCB1 and ABCG2-midiated drug efflux, resulting in an increase in the intracellular concentrations of anticancer drugs and ensuing drug sensitivity (Shi *et al.*, 2011). However, sildenafil had no effect on efflux mediated by ABCC1. Based on these recent studies, it is reasonable to suggest that sildenafil may have the potential to improve the chemotherapeutic outcome of cancer patients by enhancing the distribution and accumulation of chemotherapeutic drugs and ensuing drug sensitivity.

3.4 PDE-5 inhibitors in prostate cancer

All forms of prostate cancer therapy cause significant risk of erectile dysfunction due to trauma sustained by the cavernosal nerves (Rambhatla *et al.*, 2008). As mentioned earlier, PDE-5 is the predominant enzyme in the corpus cavernosum and plays an essential role in vascular smooth muscle contraction through specific regulation of cGMP. There is an increasing amount of evidence suggesting that PDE-5 inhibitors significantly improve erectile function in men after post-radical prostatectomy (Mydlo *et al.*, 2005;Ohebshalom *et al.*, 2005;Schiff *et al.*, 2006;Teloken *et al.*, 2007). Their efficacy and safety have triggered a number of attempts to determine their potential benefits in non-urological conditions (Vlachopoulos *et al.*, 2009). The rationale behind the use of PDE-5 inhibitors on a prolonged and continuous basis in the post-prostatectomy patient has never been fully and scientifically delineated (Rambhatla *et al.*, 2008). The prolonged and continuous administration of vardenafil, prevented both fibrosis and loss of smooth muscle, subsequently reduced corporal veno-occlusive dysfunction (CVOD) following bilateral cavernosal nerve resection (Ferrini *et al.*, 2006). Similar results were reported both in the unilateral and bilateral nerve resection models using continuous long-term administration of sildenafil (Kovanecz *et al.*, 2008a). A long-term single daily dose of tadalafil also prevented CVOD and the underlying corporal fibrosis in the rat caused by cavernosal nerve damage, as effectively as the previously reported continuous treatment with vardenafil or sildenafil, through a cGMP-related mechanism that appeared to be independent of iNOS induction (Kovanecz *et al.*, 2008b). Sildenafil treatment was also effective for improving erectile function in men with post-radiation, particularly, in the early stages after the completion of radiation (Teloken *et al.*, 2007). Treatment with exisulind, another PDE-5 inhibitor, at 250 mg bid had been evaluated in men with prostate cancer following radical prostectomy (Goluboff *et al.*, 2001). In a randomized, 12 month study; exisulind suppressed the overall rise in prostate specific antigen (PSA) levels compared to placebo group. In addition, PSA doubling time was increased more than two fold for high-risk patients who continued with exisulind. Another study also reported that the early use of PDE-5 inhibitor after prostate brachytherapy maintained erectile function at both 6 and 12 months (Pahlajani *et al.*, 2010). Emerging studies focusing on the molecular mechanisms of apoptosis and fibrosis are beginning to shed some light on the beneficial use of PDE-5 inhibitors.

In recent years, extensive and diverse preclinical and clinical studies indicated that PDE-5 inhibitors also had beneficial effects to enhance the chemotherapeutic efficacy of anticancer drugs in prostate and other cancer. PDE-5 inhibitors, sulindac sulfide and exisulind, inhibited growth and induced apoptosis in both the androgen-sensitive (LNCaP) and androgen-insensitive (PC-3) human prostate cancer cell lines (Lim *et al.*, 1999;Lim *et al.*, 2003). Exisulind also suppressed the growth of human prostate cancer cells in a nude mouse xenograft model (Goluboff *et al.*, 1999). At a low dose, combination of colecoxib, a cyclooxygenase-2 (COX-2) inhibitor, with exisulind prevented prostate carcinogenesis by altering key molecular events (Narayanan *et al.*, 2007). Combination of celecoxib and exisulind not only enhanced apoptosis, but also exerted an anti-inflammatory effect by the reduced levels of COX-2, prostaglandin E_2, and tumor necrosis factor α (TNF-α). Therefore, a combination of potential agents at low doses is considered to be very efficacious in minimizing toxicity compared with the use of individual agents at higher dose levels.

Recently, we demonstrated that co-treatment with the PDE-5 inhibitor, sildenafil, potentiated the antitumor efficacy of DOX in prostate cancer cells, while simultaneously reducing the risk of cardiomyopathy (Das *et al.*, 2010). Cell proliferation of PC-3 and DU145, prostate cancer cells, were reduced in a dose-dependent manner with DOX treatment (Figure 5 A, B). Co-treatment with sildenafil resulted in an additive effect on DOX-induced reduction of cell proliferation (Figure 4 A, B). Co-treatment with sildenafil also enhanced DOX-induced cell killing (Figure 4 C, D). Sildenafil and DOX combination also enhanced the killing of ovarian cancer and sarcoma cells, suggesting a potential efficacy of sildenafil in chemosensitization in multiple malignancies. Co-treatment with sildenafil and DOX enhanced PC-3 and DU145 prostate cancer cell killing through further enhancing ROS generation compared to DOX alone. In contrast, the sildenafil and DOX combination attenuated DOX-induced ROS generation in normal prostate cells. It has been suggested that the basic difference in mitochondrial respiration between normal and cancer cells makes cancer cells more sensitive to oxidative stress (Deberardinis *et al.*, 2008;Vander Heiden *et al.*, 2009). Further investigations need to be warranted to define how sildenafil sensitizes cancer cells to amplify DOX-mediated ROS generation. Interestingly, sulindac, also selectively enhanced killing of cancer cells exposed to oxidizing agents via production of ROS (Resnick *et al.*, 2009). However, low levels of sulindac also induced delayed preconditioning response against I/R injury in the heart through up-regulation of putative effectors of cardioprotection including iNOS and HSP27 (Moench *et al.*, 2009).

We further demonstrated that co-treatment with sildenafil and DOX enhanced DOX-induced apoptosis in PC-3 and DU145 prostate cancer cells (Figure 4 E, F) (Das *et al.*, 2010). The increased apoptosis by sildenafil and DOX was associated with enhanced expression of proapoptotic proteins Bad and Bax and suppression of Bcl-2 and Bcl-xL. Also, sildenafil and DOX combination dephosphorylated Bad, which may enhance Bad heterodimerization with Bcl-xL thereby promoting DOX-induced apoptosis. The ectopic overexpression of Bcl-xL in DU145 cells attenuated the synergistic effect of sildenafil and DOX on cell killing. Caspase-3 and -9 activities were also increased following sildenafil and DOX co-treatment. Overexpression of dominant negative procaspase-9 in DU145 cells blocked the enhanced cell killing by combined treatment with sildenafil and DOX compared with DOX alone.

Treatment with sildenafil and DOX in mice bearing prostate tumor xenografts resulted in significant inhibition of tumor growth (Figure 5A) (Das *et al.*, 2010). The ratio of tumor weight to body weight was also reduced with sildenafil co-treatment with DOX compared to DOX alone (Figure 5B). The reduced tumor size was associated with amplified apoptotic cell death (Figure 6) and increased expression of activated caspase-3. The anti-tumor effect of sildenafil and DOX combination ameliorated DOX-induced cardiac dysfunction, which was consistent with our previous study showing improved left ventricular (LV) function with PDE5 inhibitors (sildenafil and tadalafil) in DOX-treated mice (Fisher *et al.*, 2005;Koka *et al.*, 2010). Fractional shortening (LVFS) and ejection fraction (LVEF) declined in DOX-treated mice. Sildenafil co-treatment with DOX improved LVFS and LVEF compared with the DOX-treated groups.

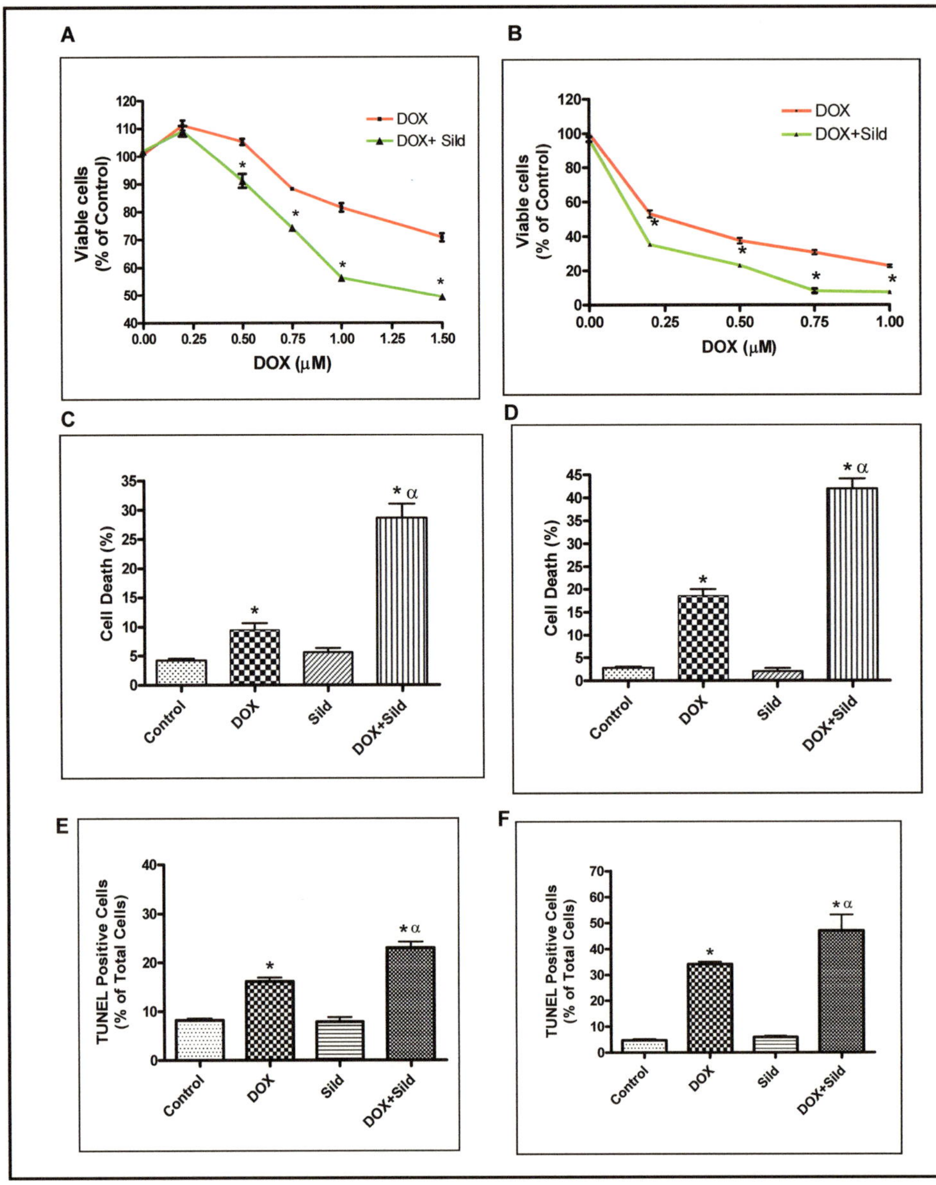

Fig. 4. Sildenafil (Sild) enhances DOX-induced prostate cancer cell death. Cell viability of (A) PC-3 and (B) DU145 cells after 72 h of treatment with different concentrations of DOX and/or sildenafil (10 μM). (*$p<0.001$ vs respective concentration of DOX; n=6). Cell death assessed after 24 h treatment of (C) PC-3 with 1.5 μM DOX and 10 μM sildenafil and (D) DU145 with 0.5 μM DOX and 10 μM sildenafil (*$p<0.001$ vs control and $^{\alpha}p<0.001$ vs DOX; n=6). Apoptosis is assessed by TUNEL staining after 72 hr of treatment. Percentage of TUNEL-positive nuclei in (E) PC-3 cells following treatment with 1.5 μM DOX and 10 μM sildenafil and (F) DU145 with 0.5 μM DOX and 10 μM sildenafil (*$p<0.001$ vs control and $^{\alpha}p<0.001$ vs DOX; n=3). Results are presented as mean ± S.E. Reprinted from Das et al. Proc Natl Acad Sci U S A. 2010 Oct 19;107(42):18202-18207 with permission.

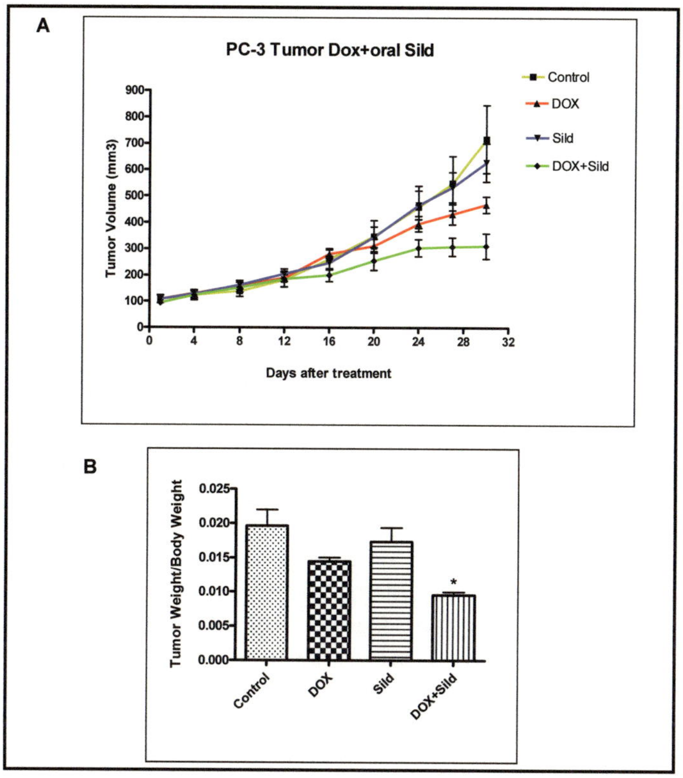

Fig. 5. Oral administration of sildenafil (Sild) potentiates DOX-induced inhibition of prostate tumor xenograft growth. Male nude mice bearing PC-3 human prostate tumors were treated with DOX (3 mg/kg, i.p., twice per week, a total of six times) or sildenafil (10 mg/ kg, orally, everyday) or DOX+sildenfil for 30 days. (A) Tumor growth during 30 d of different treatments (n=8). (B) Bar diagram showing the ratio of tumor weight to body weight after 30 d of treatment (*p<0.05 vs. DOX alone; n=8). Reprinted from Das et al. Proc Natl Acad Sci U S A. 2010 Oct 19;107(42):18202-18207 with permission.

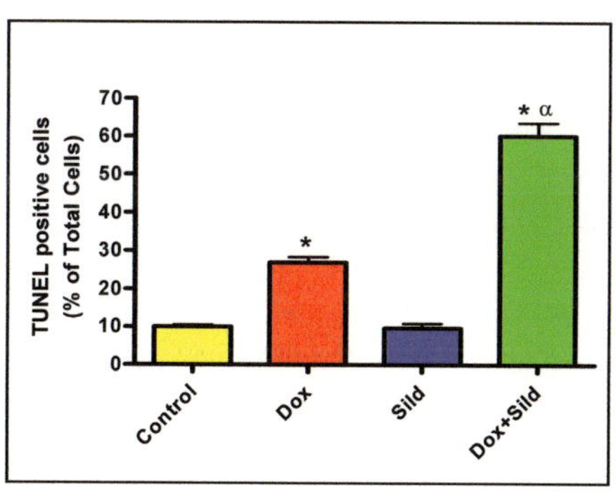

Fig. 6. Sildenafil enhances DOX-induced apoptosis in PC-3 prostate tumors. Bar diagram showing TUNEL-positive cells (*p<0.001 vs. control and $^{\alpha}$p<0.001 vs. DOX; n=3). Results are reported as means ±SE. Reprinted from Das et al. Proc Natl Acad Sci U S A. 2010 Oct 19;107(42):18202-18207 with permission.

4. Concluding comments and future perspective

PDE-5 inhibitors including sildenafil, vardenafil and tadalafil are safe and efficacious first-line on-demand agents for the treatment of erectile dysfunction (Boolell *et al.*, 1996;Porst *et al.*, 2001). Their mechanism of action involves inhibition of the PDE-5 enzyme and resulting increase in cGMP and smooth muscle relaxation in the penis. Their target enzyme, PDE-5 is expressed in several tissues throughout the human body, including the pulmonary and systemic vasculature, hypertrophied myocardium and cancer cells. Preclinical studies have demonstrated that PDE-5 inhibitors have powerful cardioprotective effect in the setting of I/R injury, pressure overload-induced hypertrophy, heart failure and DOX-induced cardiomyopathy. The effects of PDE-5 inhibitors on the pulmonary circulation and hypertrophied right ventricle have made these agents first-line therapy for many patients with pulmonary hypertension. Several reports have indicated that PDE-5 inhibitors improve erectile function following radiation therapy or post-radical prostatectomy in prostate cancer patients. Recent research from our laboratory has reported provocative findings that **sildenafil is both a powerful sensitizer of DOX-induced killing of prostate cancer and provides concurrent cardioprotective benefit (Das *et al.*, 2010).** Moreover, sildenafil and vardenafil have been shown to block or reverse the drug efflux function of the ABC transporters, thereby suggesting that sildenafil can be used as a modulator of ABCB1 and ABCG2 to reverse MDR in cancer cells. Considering the well-established safety profile of PDE-5 inhibitors, clinical studies are needed to fully exploit the beneficial effect of the combination treatment of anti-tumor agents such as DOX with the PDE-5 inhibitors as a therapeutic tool in prostate cancer patients. Also, further studies are needed to gain in depth understanding of the molecular mechanisms by which PDE-5 inhibitors increase the efficacy of chemotherapeutic agents.

5. Acknowledgment

This work was supported in part by National Institutes of Health Grants HL51045, HL59469, and HL79424 (to R.C.K).

6. References

Abdulla A and Kapoor A (2011) Emerging Novel Therapies in the Treatment of Castrate-Resistant Prostate Cancer. *Can Urol Assoc J* 5: pp 120-133.

Alibhai SM, Duong-Hua M, Sutradhar R, Fleshner N E, Warde P, Cheung A M and Paszat L F (2009) Impact of Androgen Deprivation Therapy on Cardiovascular Disease and Diabetes. *J Clin Oncol* 27: pp 3452-3458.

Ambudkar SV, Kimchi-Sarfaty C, Sauna Z E and Gottesman M M (2003) P-Glycoprotein: From Genomics to Mechanism. *Oncogene* 22: pp 7468-7485.

Arola OJ, Saraste A, Pulkki K, Kallajoki M, Parvinen M and Voipio-Pulkki L M (2000) Acute Doxorubicin Cardiotoxicity Involves Cardiomyocyte Apoptosis. *Cancer Res* 60: pp 1789-1792.

Bender AT and Beavo J A (2006) Cyclic Nucleotide Phosphodiesterases: Molecular Regulation to Clinical Use. *Pharmacol Rev* 58: pp 488-520.

Berthold DR, Pond G R, Soban F, de Wit R, Eisenberger M and Tannock I F (2008) Docetaxel Plus Prednisone or Mitoxantrone Plus Prednisone for Advanced Prostate Cancer: Updated Survival in the TAX 327 Study. *J Clin Oncol* 26: pp 242-245.

Black KL, Yin D, Ong J M, Hu J, Konda B M, Wang X, Ko M K, Bayan J A, Sacapano M R, Espinoza A, Irvin D K and Shu Y (2008) PDE5 Inhibitors Enhance Tumor Permeability and Efficacy of Chemotherapy in a Rat Brain Tumor Model. *Brain Res* 1230: pp 290-302.

Boolell M, Allen M J, Ballard S A, Gepi-Attee S, Muirhead G J, Naylor A M, Osterloh I H and Gingell C (1996) Sildenafil: an Orally Active Type 5 Cyclic GMP-Specific Phosphodiesterase Inhibitor for the Treatment of Penile Erectile Dysfunction. *Int J Impot Res* 8: pp 47-52.

Bremer YA, Salloum F, Ockaili R, Chou E, Moskowitz W B and Kukreja R C (2005) Sildenafil Citrate (Viagra) Induces Cardioprotective Effects After Ischemia/Reperfusion Injury in Infant Rabbits. *Pediatr Res* 57: pp 22-27.

Burke BE, Mushlin P S, Cusack B J, Olson S J, Gambliel H A and Olson R D (2002) Decreased Sensitivity of Neonatal Rabbit Sarcoplasmic Reticulum to Anthracycline Cardiotoxicity. *Cardiovasc Toxicol* 2: pp 41-51.

Dai CL, Tiwari A K, Wu C P, Su X D, Wang S R, Liu D G, Ashby C R, Jr., Huang Y, Robey R W, Liang Y J, Chen L M, Shi C J, Ambudkar S V, Chen Z S and Fu L W (2008) Lapatinib (Tykerb, GW572016) Reverses Multidrug Resistance in Cancer Cells by Inhibiting the Activity of ATP-Binding Cassette Subfamily B Member 1 and G Member 2. *Cancer Res* 68: pp 7905-7914.

Dantzig AH, Shepard R L, Pratt S E, Tabas L B, Lander P A, Ma L, Paul D C, Williams D C, Peng S B, Slapak C A, Godinot N and Perry W L, III (2004) Evaluation of the Binding of the Tricyclic Isoxazole Photoaffinity Label LY475776 to Multidrug Resistance Associated Protein 1 (MRP1) Orthologs and Several ATP- Binding Cassette (ABC) Drug Transporters. *Biochem Pharmacol* 67: pp 1111-1121.

Das A, Durrant D, Mitchell C, Mayton E, Hoke N N, Salloum F N, Park M A, Qureshi I, Lee R, Dent P and Kukreja R C (2010) Sildenafil Increases Chemotherapeutic Efficacy of Doxorubicin in Prostate Cancer and Ameliorates Cardiac Dysfunction. *Proc Natl Acad Sci U S A* 107: pp 18202-18207.

Das A, Ockaili R, Salloum F and Kukreja R C (2004) Protein Kinase C Plays an Essential Role in Sildenafil-Induced Cardioprotection in Rabbits. *Am J Physiol Heart Circ Physiol* 286: pp H1455-H1460.

Das A, Salloum F N, Xi L, Rao Y J and Kukreja R C (2009) ERK Phosphorylation Mediates Sildenafil-Induced Myocardial Protection Against Ischemia-Reperfusion Injury in Mice. *Am J Physiol Heart Circ Physiol* 296: pp H1236-H1243.

Das A, Xi L and Kukreja R C (2005) Phosphodiesterase-5 Inhibitor Sildenafil Preconditions Adult Cardiac Myocytes Against Necrosis and Apoptosis. Essential Role of Nitric Oxide Signaling. *J Biol Chem* 280: pp 12944-12955.

Das A, Xi L and Kukreja R C (2008) Protein Kinase G-Dependent Cardioprotective Mechanism of Phosphodiesterase-5 Inhibition Involves Phosphorylation of ERK and GSK3beta. *J Biol Chem* 283: pp 29572-29585.

Davies KJ and Doroshow J H (1986) Redox Cycling of Anthracyclines by Cardiac Mitochondria. I. Anthracycline Radical Formation by NADH Dehydrogenase. *J Biol Chem* 261: pp 3060-3067.

de Bono JS, Oudard S, Ozguroglu M, Hansen S, Machiels J P, Kocak I, Gravis G, Bodrogi I, Mackenzie M J, Shen L, Roessner M, Gupta S and Sartor A O (2010) Prednisone Plus Cabazitaxel or Mitoxantrone for Metastatic Castration-Resistant Prostate Cancer Progressing After Docetaxel Treatment: a Randomised Open-Label Trial. *Lancet* 376: pp 1147-1154.

Dean M, Rzhetsky A and Allikmets R (2001) The Human ATP-Binding Cassette (ABC) Transporter Superfamily. *Genome Res* 11: pp 1156-1166.

Deberardinis RJ, Sayed N, Ditsworth D and Thompson C B (2008) Brick by Brick: Metabolism and Tumor Cell Growth. *Curr Opin Genet Dev* 18: pp 54-61.

Ding PR, Tiwari A K, Ohnuma S, Lee J W, An X, Dai C L, Lu Q S, Singh S, Yang D H, Talele T T, Ambudkar S V and Chen Z S (2011) The Phosphodiesterase-5 Inhibitor Vardenafil Is a Potent Inhibitor of ABCB1/P-Glycoprotein Transporter. *PLoS One* 6: pp e19329.

Doroshow JH, Locker G Y and Myers C E (1980) Enzymatic Defenses of the Mouse Heart Against Reactive Oxygen Metabolites: Alterations Produced by Doxorubicin. *J Clin Invest* 65: pp 128-135.

Eisenberger MA and Walsh P C (1999) Early Androgen Deprivation for Prostate Cancer? *N Engl J Med* 341: pp 1837-1838.

Epstein PM and Hachisu R (1984) Cyclic Nucleotide Phosphodiesterase in Normal and Leukemic Human Lymphocytes and Lymphoblasts. *Adv Cyclic Nucleotide Protein Phosphorylation Res* 16: pp 303-324.

Evers R, Kool M, Smith A J, van Deemter L, de Haas M and Borst P (2000) Inhibitory Effect of the Reversal Agents V-104, GF120918 and Pluronic L61 on MDR1 Pgp-, MRP1- and MRP2-mediated transport. *Br J Cancer* 83: pp 366-374.

Ferrini MG, Davila H H, Kovanecz I, Sanchez S P, Gonzalez-Cadavid N F and Rajfer J (2006) Vardenafil Prevents Fibrosis and Loss of Corporal Smooth Muscle That Occurs After Bilateral Cavernosal Nerve Resection in the Rat. *Urology* 68: pp 429-435.

Fisher PW, Salloum F, Das A, Hyder H and Kukreja R C (2005) Phosphodiesterase-5 Inhibition With Sildenafil Attenuates Cardiomyocyte Apoptosis and Left Ventricular Dysfunction in a Chronic Model of Doxorubicin Cardiotoxicity. *Circulation* 111: pp 1601-1610.

Freitas M, Alves V, Sarmento-Ribeiro A B and Mota-Pinto A (2011) Combined Effect of Sodium Selenite and Docetaxel on PC3 Metastatic Prostate Cancer Cell Line. *Biochem Biophys Res Commun* 408: pp 713-719.

Galie N, Ghofrani H A, Torbicki A, Barst R J, Rubin L J, Badesch D, Fleming T, Parpia T, Burgess G, Branzi A, Grimminger F, Kurzyna M and Simonneau G (2005) Sildenafil Citrate Therapy for Pulmonary Arterial Hypertension. *N Engl J Med* 353: pp 2148-2157.

Galie N, Rubin L J and Simonneau G (2010) Phosphodiesterase Inhibitors for Pulmonary Hypertension. *N Engl J Med* 362: pp 559-560.

Gan L, Wang J, Xu H and Yang X (2011) Resistance to Docetaxel-Induced Apoptosis in Prostate Cancer Cells by P38/P53/P21 Signaling. *Prostate* 71: pp 1158-1166.

Germann UA, Ford P J, Shlyakhter D, Mason V S and Harding M W (1997) Chemosensitization and Drug Accumulation Effects of VX-710, Verapamil, Cyclosporin A, MS-209 and GF120918 in Multidrug Resistant HL60/ADR Cells

Expressing the Multidrug Resistance-Associated Protein MRP. *Anticancer Drugs* 8: pp 141-155.

Gillet JP, Efferth T and Remacle J (2007) Chemotherapy-Induced Resistance by ATP-Binding Cassette Transporter Genes. *Biochim Biophys Acta* 1775: pp 237-262.

Goluboff ET, Prager D, Rukstalis D, Giantonio B, Madorsky M, Barken I, Weinstein I B, Partin A W and Olsson C A (2001) Safety and Efficacy of Exisulind for Treatment of Recurrent Prostate Cancer After Radical Prostatectomy. *J Urol* 166: pp 882-886.

Goluboff ET, Shabsigh A, Saidi J A, Weinstein I B, Mitra N, Heitjan D, Piazza G A, Pamukcu R, Buttyan R and Olsson C A (1999) Exisulind (Sulindac Sulfone) Suppresses Growth of Human Prostate Cancer in a Nude Mouse Xenograft Model by Increasing Apoptosis. *Urology* 53: pp 440-445.

Hosseinzadeh L, Behravan J, Mosaffa F, Bahrami G, Bahrami A and Karimi G (2011) Curcumin Potentiates Doxorubicin-Induced Apoptosis in H9c2 Cardiac Muscle Cells Through Generation of Reactive Oxygen Species. *Food Chem Toxicol* 49: pp 1102-1109.

Jemal A, Siegel R, Xu J and Ward E (2010) Cancer Statistics, 2010. *CA Cancer J Clin* 60: pp 277-300.

Joe AK, Liu H, Xiao D, Soh J W, Pinto J T, Beer D G, Piazza G A, Thompson W J and Weinstein I B (2003) Exisulind and CP248 Induce Growth Inhibition and Apoptosis in Human Esophageal Adenocarcinoma and Squamous Carcinoma Cells. *J Exp Ther Oncol* 3: pp 83-94.

Kalyanaraman B, Joseph J, Kalivendi S, Wang S, Konorev E and Kotamraju S (2002) Doxorubicin-Induced Apoptosis: Implications in Cardiotoxicity. *Mol Cell Biochem* 234-235: pp 119-124.

Kang YJ, Chen Y and Epstein P N (1996) Suppression of Doxorubicin Cardiotoxicity by Overexpression of Catalase in the Heart of Transgenic Mice. *J Biol Chem* 271: pp 12610-12616.

Kang YJ, Chen Y, Yu A, Voss-McCowan M and Epstein P N (1997) Overexpression of Metallothionein in the Heart of Transgenic Mice Suppresses Doxorubicin Cardiotoxicity. *J Clin Invest* 100: pp 1501-1506.

Koka S, Das A, Zhu S G, Durrant D, Xi L and Kukreja R C (2010) Long-Acting Phosphodiesterase-5 Inhibitor Tadalafil Attenuates Doxorubicin-Induced Cardiomyopathy Without Interfering With Chemotherapeutic Effect. *J Pharmacol Exp Ther* 334: pp 1023-1030.

Koning J, Palmer P, Franks C R, Mulder D E, Speyer J L, Green M D and Hellmann K (1991) Cardioxane--ICRF-187 Towards Anticancer Drug Specificity Through Selective Toxicity Reduction. *Cancer Treat Rev* 18: pp 1-19.

Konorev EA, Kennedy M C and Kalyanaraman B (1999) Cell-Permeable Superoxide Dismutase and Glutathione Peroxidase Mimetics Afford Superior Protection Against Doxorubicin Induced Cardiotoxicity: the Role of Reactive Oxygen and Nitrogen Intermediates. *Arch Biochem Biophys* 368: pp 421-428.

Koutsilieris M (1993) Osteoblastic Metastasis in Advanced Prostate Cancer. *Anticancer Res* 13: pp 443-449.

Kovanecz I, Rambhatla A, Ferrini M, Vernet D, Sanchez S, Rajfer J and Gonzalez-Cadavid N (2008a) Long-Term Continuous Sildenafil Treatment Ameliorates Corporal Veno-

Occlusive Dysfunction (CVOD) Induced by Cavernosal Nerve Resection in Rats. *Int J Impot Res* 20: pp 202-212.

Kovanecz I, Rambhatla A, Ferrini M G, Vernet D, Sanchez S, Rajfer J and Gonzalez-Cadavid N (2008b) Chronic Daily Tadalafil Prevents the Corporal Fibrosis and Veno-Occlusive Dysfunction That Occurs After Cavernosal Nerve Resection. *BJU Int* 101: pp 203-210.

Kukreja RC, Ockaili R, Salloum F, Yin C, Hawkins J, Das A and Xi L (2004) Cardioprotection With Phosphodiesterase-5 Inhibition--a Novel Preconditioning Strategy. *J Mol Cell Cardiol* 36: pp 165-173.

Kumar D, Kirshenbaum L A, Li T, Danelisen I and Singal P K (2001) Apoptosis in Adriamycin Cardiomyopathy and Its Modulation by Probucol. *Antioxid Redox Signal* 3: pp 135-145.

Li Y, Hussain M, Sarkar S H, Eliason J, Li R and Sarkar F H (2005) Gene Expression Profiling Revealed Novel Mechanism of Action of Taxotere and Furtulon in Prostate Cancer Cells. *BMC Cancer* 5: pp 7.

Lim JT, Piazza G A, Han E K, Delohery T M, Li H, Finn T S, Buttyan R, Yamamoto H, Sperl G J, Brendel K, Gross P H, Pamukcu R and Weinstein I B (1999) Sulindac Derivatives Inhibit Growth and Induce Apoptosis in Human Prostate Cancer Cell Lines. *Biochem Pharmacol* 58: pp 1097-1107.

Lim JT, Piazza G A, Pamukcu R, Thompson W J and Weinstein I B (2003) Exisulind and Related Compounds Inhibit Expression and Function of the Androgen Receptor in Human Prostate Cancer Cells. *Clin Cancer Res* 9: pp 4972-4982.

Liu L, Underwood T, Li H, Pamukcu R and Thompson W J (2002a) Specific CGMP Binding by the CGMP Binding Domains of CGMP-Binding CGMP Specific Phosphodiesterase. *Cell Signal* 14: pp 45-51.

Liu X, Chen Z, Chua C C, Ma Y S, Youngberg G A, Hamdy R and Chua B H (2002b) Melatonin As an Effective Protector Against Doxorubicin-Induced Cardiotoxicity. *Am J Physiol Heart Circ Physiol* 283: pp H254-H263.

Makarovskiy AN, Siryaporn E, Hixson D C and Akerley W (2002) Survival of Docetaxel-Resistant Prostate Cancer Cells in Vitro Depends on Phenotype Alterations and Continuity of Drug Exposure. *Cell Mol Life Sci* 59: pp 1198-1211.

Menna P, Gonzalez P O, Chello M, Covino E, Salvatorelli E and Minotti G (2011) Anthracycline Cardiotoxicity. *Expert Opin Drug Saf.*

Minderman H, O'Loughlin K L, Pendyala L and Baer M R (2004) VX-710 (Biricodar) Increases Drug Retention and Enhances Chemosensitivity in Resistant Cells Overexpressing P-Glycoprotein, Multidrug Resistance Protein, and Breast Cancer Resistance Protein. *Clin Cancer Res* 10: pp 1826-1834.

Minotti G, Menna P, Salvatorelli E, Cairo G and Gianni L (2004) Anthracyclines: Molecular Advances and Pharmacologic Developments in Antitumor Activity and Cardiotoxicity. *Pharmacol Rev* 56: pp 185-229.

Mizutani H, Tada-Oikawa S, Hiraku Y, Kojima M and Kawanishi S (2005) Mechanism of Apoptosis Induced by Doxorubicin Through the Generation of Hydrogen Peroxide. *Life Sci* 76: pp 1439-1453.

Moench I, Prentice H, Rickaway Z and Weissbach H (2009) Sulindac Confers High Level Ischemic Protection to the Heart Through Late Preconditioning Mechanisms. *Proc Natl Acad Sci U S A* 106: pp 19611-19616.

Mydlo JH, Viterbo R and Crispen P (2005) Use of Combined Intracorporal Injection and a Phosphodiesterase-5 Inhibitor Therapy for Men With a Suboptimal Response to Sildenafil and/or Vardenafil Monotherapy After Radical Retropubic Prostatectomy. *BJU Int* 95: pp 843-846.

Myers C (1998) The Role of Iron in Doxorubicin-Induced Cardiomyopathy. *Semin Oncol* 25: pp 10-14.

Narayanan BA, Reddy B S, Bosland M C, Nargi D, Horton L, Randolph C and Narayanan N K (2007) Exisulind in Combination With Celecoxib Modulates Epidermal Growth Factor Receptor, Cyclooxygenase-2, and Cyclin D1 Against Prostate Carcinogenesis: in Vivo Evidence. *Clin Cancer Res* 13: pp 5965-5973.

Narula J, Haider N, Virmani R, DiSalvo T G, Kolodgie F D, Hajjar R J, Schmidt U, Semigran M J, Dec G W and Khaw B A (1996) Apoptosis in Myocytes in End-Stage Heart Failure. *N Engl J Med* 335: pp 1182-1189.

Nazeyrollas P, Prevost A, Baccard N, Manot L, Devillier P and Millart H (1999) Effects of Amifostine on Perfused Isolated Rat Heart and on Acute Doxorubicin-Induced Cardiotoxicity. *Cancer Chemother Pharmacol* 43: pp 227-232.

Nguyen PL, Chen M H, Goldhaber S Z, Martin N E, Beard C J, Dosoretz D E, Katin M J, Ross R, Salenius S A and D'Amico A V (2011) Coronary Revascularization and Mortality in Men With Congestive Heart Failure or Prior Myocardial Infarction Who Receive Androgen Deprivation. *Cancer* 117: pp 406-413.

O'Connor R (2007) The Pharmacology of Cancer Resistance. *Anticancer Res* 27: pp 1267-1272.

Ockaili R, Salloum F, Hawkins J and Kukreja R C (2002) Sildenafil (Viagra) Induces Powerful Cardioprotective Effect Via Opening of Mitochondrial K(ATP) Channels in Rabbits. *Am J Physiol Heart Circ Physiol* 283: pp H1263-H1269.

Ohebshalom M, Parker M, Guhring P and Mulhall J P (2005) The Efficacy of Sildenafil Citrate Following Radiation Therapy for Prostate Cancer: Temporal Considerations. *J Urol* 174: pp 258-262.

Olson RD and Mushlin P S (1990) Doxorubicin Cardiotoxicity: Analysis of Prevailing Hypotheses. *FASEB J* 4: pp 3076-3086.

Pahlajani G, Raina R, Jones J S, Burdick M, Ali M, Li J, Mahadevan A, Ciezki J and Zippe C (2010) Early Intervention With Phosphodiesterase-5 Inhibitors After Prostate Brachytherapy Improves Subsequent Erectile Function. *BJU Int* 106: pp 1524-1527.

Petrioli R, Fiaschi A I, Francini E, Pascucci A and Francini G (2008) The Role of Doxorubicin and Epirubicin in the Treatment of Patients With Metastatic Hormone-Refractory Prostate Cancer. *Cancer Treat Rev* 34: pp 710-718.

Petrylak DP, Tangen C M, Hussain M H, Lara P N, Jr., Jones J A, Taplin M E, Burch P A, Berry D, Moinpour C, Kohli M, Benson M C, Small E J, Raghavan D and Crawford E D (2004) Docetaxel and Estramustine Compared With Mitoxantrone and Prednisone for Advanced Refractory Prostate Cancer. *N Engl J Med* 351: pp 1513-1520.

Piazza GA, Thompson W J, Pamukcu R, Alila H W, Whitehead C M, Liu L, Fetter J R, Gresh W E, Jr., Klein-Szanto A J, Farnell D R, Eto I and Grubbs C J (2001) Exisulind, a Novel Proapoptotic Drug, Inhibits Rat Urinary Bladder Tumorigenesis. *Cancer Res* 61: pp 3961-3968.

Porst H, Padma-Nathan H, Giuliano F, Anglin G, Varanese L and Rosen R (2003) Efficacy of Tadalafil for the Treatment of Erectile Dysfunction at 24 and 36 Hours After Dosing: a Randomized Controlled Trial. *Urology* 62: pp 121-125.

Porst H, Rosen R, Padma-Nathan H, Goldstein I, Giuliano F, Ulbrich E and Bandel T (2001) The Efficacy and Tolerability of Vardenafil, a New, Oral, Selective Phosphodiesterase Type 5 Inhibitor, in Patients With Erectile Dysfunction: the First at-Home Clinical Trial. *Int J Impot Res* 13: pp 192-199.

Qadir M, O'Loughlin K L, Fricke S M, Williamson N A, Greco W R, Minderman H and Baer M R (2005) Cyclosporin A Is a Broad-Spectrum Multidrug Resistance Modulator. *Clin Cancer Res* 11: pp 2320-2326.

Rambhatla A, Kovanecz I, Ferrini M, Gonzalez-Cadavid N F and Rajfer J (2008) Rationale for Phosphodiesterase 5 Inhibitor Use Post-Radical Prostatectomy: Experimental and Clinical Review. *Int J Impot Res* 20: pp 30-34.

Resnick L, Rabinovitz H, Binninger D, Marchetti M and Weissbach H (2009) Topical Sulindac Combined With Hydrogen Peroxide in the Treatment of Actinic Keratoses. *J Drugs Dermatol* 8: pp 29-32.

Safra T (2003) Cardiac Safety of Liposomal Anthracyclines. *Oncologist* 8 Suppl 2: pp 17-24.

Saigal CS, Gore J L, Krupski T L, Hanley J, Schonlau M and Litwin M S (2007) Androgen Deprivation Therapy Increases Cardiovascular Morbidity in Men With Prostate Cancer. *Cancer* 110: pp 1493-1500.

Salloum F, Yin C, Xi L and Kukreja R C (2003) Sildenafil Induces Delayed Preconditioning Through Inducible Nitric Oxide Synthase-Dependent Pathway in Mouse Heart. *Circ Res* 92: pp 595-597.

Salloum FN, Abbate A, Das A, Houser J E, Mudrick C A, Qureshi I Z, Hoke N N, Roy S K, Brown W R, Prabhakar S and Kukreja R C (2008) Sildenafil (Viagra) Attenuates Ischemic Cardiomyopathy and Improves Left Ventricular Function in Mice. *Am J Physiol Heart Circ Physiol* 294: pp H1398-H1406.

Salloum FN, Chau V Q, Hoke N N, Abbate A, Varma A, Ockaili R A, Toldo S and Kukreja R C (2009) Phosphodiesterase-5 Inhibitor, Tadalafil, Protects Against Myocardial Ischemia/Reperfusion Through Protein-Kinase G-Dependent Generation of Hydrogen Sulfide. *Circulation* 120: pp S31-S36.

Salloum FN, Takenoshita Y, Ockaili R A, Daoud V P, Chou E, Yoshida K and Kukreja R C (2007) Sildenafil and Vardenafil but Not Nitroglycerin Limit Myocardial Infarction Through Opening of Mitochondrial K(ATP) Channels When Administered at Reperfusion Following Ischemia in Rabbits. *J Mol Cell Cardiol* 42: pp 453-458.

Sarfati M, Mateo V, Baudet S, Rubio M, Fernandez C, Davi F, Binet J L, Delic J and Merle-Beral H (2003) Sildenafil and Vardenafil, Types 5 and 6 Phosphodiesterase Inhibitors, Induce Caspase-Dependent Apoptosis of B-Chronic Lymphocytic Leukemia Cells. *Blood* 101: pp 265-269.

Schiff JD, Bar-Chama N, Cesaretti J and Stock R (2006) Early Use of a Phosphodiesterase Inhibitor After Brachytherapy Restores and Preserves Erectile Function. *BJU Int* 98: pp 1255-1258.

Schiff PB and Horwitz S B (1980) Taxol Stabilizes Microtubules in Mouse Fibroblast Cells. *Proc Natl Acad Sci U S A* 77: pp 1561-1565.

Schurko B and Oh W K (2008) Docetaxel Chemotherapy Remains the Standard of Care in Castration-Resistant Prostate Cancer. *Nat Clin Pract Oncol* 5: pp 506-507.

Sebkhi A, Strange J W, Phillips S C, Wharton J and Wilkins M R (2003) Phosphodiesterase Type 5 As a Target for the Treatment of Hypoxia-Induced Pulmonary Hypertension. *Circulation* 107: pp 3230-3235.

Shen T, Kuang Y H, Ashby C R, Lei Y, Chen A, Zhou Y, Chen X, Tiwari A K, Hopper-Borge E, Ouyang J and Chen Z S (2009) Imatinib and Nilotinib Reverse Multidrug Resistance in Cancer Cells by Inhibiting the Efflux Activity of the MRP7 (ABCC10). *PLoS One* 4: pp e7520.

Shi Z, Peng X X, Kim I W, Shukla S, Si Q S, Robey R W, Bates S E, Shen T, Ashby C R, Jr., Fu L W, Ambudkar S V and Chen Z S (2007) Erlotinib (Tarceva, OSI-774) Antagonizes ATP-Binding Cassette Subfamily B Member 1 and ATP-Binding Cassette Subfamily G Member 2-Mediated Drug Resistance. *Cancer Res* 67: pp 11012-11020.

Shi Z, Tiwari A K, Shukla S, Robey R W, Singh S, Kim I W, Bates S E, Peng X, Abraham I, Ambudkar S V, Talele T T, Fu L W and Chen Z S (2011) Sildenafil Reverses A. *Cancer Res* 71: pp 3029-3041.

Singal PK, Li T, Kumar D, Danelisen I and Iliskovic N (2000) Adriamycin-Induced Heart Failure: Mechanism and Modulation. *Mol Cell Biochem* 207: pp 77-86.

Singer AL, Sherwin R P, Dunn A S and Appleman M M (1976) Cyclic Nucleotide Phosphodiesterases in Neoplastic and Nonneoplastic Human Mammary Tissues. *Cancer Res* 36: pp 60-66.

Sonpavde G, Hutson T E and Berry W R (2006) Hormone Refractory Prostate Cancer: Management and Advances. *Cancer Treat Rev* 32: pp 90-100.

Sourla A, Doillon C and Koutsilieris M (1996) Three-Dimensional Type I Collagen Gel System Containing MG-63 Osteoblasts-Like Cells As a Model for Studying Local Bone Reaction Caused by Metastatic Cancer Cells. *Anticancer Res* 16: pp 2773-2780.

Spallarossa P, Altieri P, Aloi C, Garibaldi S, Barisione C, Ghigliotti G, Fugazza G, Barsotti A and Brunelli C (2009) Doxorubicin Induces Senescence or Apoptosis in Rat Neonatal Cardiomyocytes by Regulating the Expression Levels of the Telomere Binding Factors 1 and 2. *Am J Physiol Heart Circ Physiol* 297: pp H2169-H2181.

Spallarossa P, Garibaldi S, Altieri P, Fabbi P, Manca V, Nasti S, Rossettin P, Ghigliotti G, Ballestrero A, Patrone F, Barsotti A and Brunelli C (2004) Carvedilol Prevents Doxorubicin-Induced Free Radical Release and Apoptosis in Cardiomyocytes in Vitro. *J Mol Cell Cardiol* 37: pp 837-846.

Stein CA (1999) Mechanisms of Action of Taxanes in Prostate Cancer. *Semin Oncol* 26: pp 3-7.

Steinherz LJ, Steinherz P G and Tan C (1995) Cardiac Failure and Dysrhythmias 6-19 Years After Anthracycline Therapy: a Series of 15 Patients. *Med Pediatr Oncol* 24: pp 352-361.

Steinherz LJ, Steinherz P G, Tan C T, Heller G and Murphy M L (1991) Cardiac Toxicity 4 to 20 Years After Completing Anthracycline Therapy. *JAMA* 266: pp 1672-1677.

Szakacs G, Paterson J K, Ludwig J A, Booth-Genthe C and Gottesman M M (2006) Targeting Multidrug Resistance in Cancer. *Nat Rev Drug Discov* 5: pp 219-234.

Takemura G and Fujiwara H (2007) Doxorubicin-Induced Cardiomyopathy From the Cardiotoxic Mechanisms to Management. *Prog Cardiovasc Dis* 49: pp 330-352.

Tannock IF, de Wit R, Berry W R, Horti J, Pluzanska A, Chi K N, Oudard S, Theodore C, James N D, Turesson I, Rosenthal M A and Eisenberger M A (2004) Docetaxel Plus Prednisone or Mitoxantrone Plus Prednisone for Advanced Prostate Cancer. *N Engl J Med* 351: pp 1502-1512.

Teloken PE, Ohebshalom M, Mohideen N and Mulhall J P (2007) Analysis of the Impact of Androgen Deprivation Therapy on Sildenafil Citrate Response Following Radiation Therapy for Prostate Cancer. *J Urol* 178: pp 2521-2525.

Thompson WJ, Piazza G A, Li H, Liu L, Fetter J, Zhu B, Sperl G, Ahnen D and Pamukcu R (2000) Exisulind Induction of Apoptosis Involves Guanosine 3',5'-Cyclic Monophosphate Phosphodiesterase Inhibition, Protein Kinase G Activation, and Attenuated Beta-Catenin. *Cancer Res* 60: pp 3338-3342.

Tiwari AK, Sodani K, Wang S R, Kuang Y H, Ashby C R, Jr., Chen X and Chen Z S (2009) Nilotinib (AMN107, Tasigna) Reverses Multidrug Resistance by Inhibiting the Activity of the ABCB1/Pgp and ABCG2/BCRP/MXR Transporters. *Biochem Pharmacol* 78: pp 153-161.

van Acker SA, Kramer K, Voest E E, Grimbergen J A, Zhang J, van der Vijgh W J and Bast A (1996) Doxorubicin-Induced Cardiotoxicity Monitored by ECG in Freely Moving Mice. A New Model to Test Potential Protectors. *Cancer Chemother Pharmacol* 38: pp 95-101.

Vander Heiden MG, Cantley L C and Thompson C B (2009) Understanding the Warburg Effect: the Metabolic Requirements of Cell Proliferation. *Science* 324: pp 1029-1033.

Vlachopoulos C, Terentes-Printzios D, Ioakeimidis N, Rokkas K and Stefanadis C (2009) PDE5 Inhibitors in Non-Urological Conditions. *Curr Pharm Des* 15: pp 3521-3539.

Weiss RB (1992) The Anthracyclines: Will We Ever Find a Better Doxorubicin?. *Semin Oncol* 19: pp 670-686.

Whitehead CM, Earle K A, Fetter J, Xu S, Hartman T, Chan D C, Zhao T L, Piazza G, Klein-Szanto A J, Pamukcu R, Alila H, Bunn P A, Jr. and Thompson W J (2003) Exisulind-Induced Apoptosis in a Non-Small Cell Lung Cancer Orthotopic Lung Tumor Model Augments Docetaxel Treatment and Contributes to Increased Survival. *Mol Cancer Ther* 2: pp 479-488.

Wu Y, Rosenberg J E and Taplin M E (2011) Novel Agents and New Therapeutics in Castration-Resistant Prostate Cancer. *Curr Opin Oncol* 23: pp 290-296.

Yen HC, Oberley T D, Vichitbandha S, Ho Y S and St Clair D K (1996) The Protective Role of Manganese Superoxide Dismutase Against Adriamycin-Induced Acute Cardiac Toxicity in Transgenic Mice. *J Clin Invest* 98: pp 1253-1260.

Yoo J, Park S S and Lee Y J (2008) Pretreatment of Docetaxel Enhances TRAIL-Mediated Apoptosis in Prostate Cancer Cells. *J Cell Biochem* 104: pp 1636-1646.

Zhu B, Vemavarapu L, Thompson W J and Strada S J (2005) Suppression of Cyclic GMP-Specific Phosphodiesterase 5 Promotes Apoptosis and Inhibits Growth in HT29 Cells. *J Cell Biochem* 94: pp 336-350.

14

Entering a New Era – Prostate Cancer Immuno-Therapy After the FDA Approval for Sipuleucel-T

Thomas H. Brill
Technische Universität München (TUM)
Germany

1. Introduction

As cancer is estimated to cause 1,500,000 deaths in Europe and more than 500,000 alone in the US each year (Ferlay et al., 2007; Jemal et al., 2010) newer strategies are needed to improve current treatment success rates. The role of the immune system is designated cancer immunosurveillance as it limits tumor growth (Dunn et al., 2002). This biological principle has been deduced from clinical observations in human as if veterinary cancer patients and has also been proved experimentally in immunodeficient mice characterized by a high incidence of tumors (Shankanan et al., 2001). The evidence on the role of the immune system found in limiting tumor growth and progression is linked to observations showing a positive correlation between the presence of tumor infiltrating lymphocytes (TILs) and improved outcome in most - but not all - tumor entities studied so far; e.g. in colorectal cancer significantly higher levels of memory CD8+T-cell infiltrates are positively correlated with clinical benefit, defined as less advanced pathological stage, absence of metastatic invasion, and increased survival (Pages et al., 2005; Galon et al., 2006). Similarly, the presence of TILs has been associated with decreased tumor cells in the draining lymph nodes of cervical cancer patients limiting the risk of metastatic progression (Piersma et al., 2007). In lung carcinoma patients, increasing numbers of TILs have also been shown to significantly improve disease-specific survival (Al-Shibli et al., 2008). PCa glands are also frequent diffusely infiltrated (CD4+T-cells as if CD8+T-cells) so suggesting that PCa may be immunogenic but the correlation of these findings to clinical data is not that clear as in other tumor entities (McArdle et al., 2004; Zhang et al., 2006). Altogether, these observations support the immunosurveillance hypothesis and form the rationale to use the immune system to control tumor burden by vaccine-based interventions against cancer relying on the stimulation of an effective antitumor immune response in the cancer patient and resulted recently in labelling "avoiding immune destruction" as an emerging hallmark of cancer by the scientific community (Hanahan & Weinberg, 2011). The therapeutic cancer vaccine definition as given by the National Cancer Institute (NCI) is: vaccines, which are intended to treat already existing cancers by strengthening the body´s natural defences against cancer.

But it is of great importance to notice the two paradoxical roles the immune system has in cancer: while at the one hand various components of the immune response - innate as if adaptive - are able to mediate cancer cell destruction, at the other hand specific types of immune cells can also induce an environment that favours tumor growth as also the development of metastasis (DeNardo et al., 2008). Among the latter are, for example, tumor associated macrophages (TAM) (Mantovani et al., 2002; Luo et al., 2006), type 2 helper CD4+(TH2) T-cells (DeNardo et al., 2009; Ziegler et al., 2009), and last not least regulatory T(Treg)-cells (Curiel et al., 2004; Yamaguchi & Sakaguchi, 2006). These various immune cells have been shown to accumulate at tumor sites, negatively impacting the establishment of antitumor T-cell responses, and so creating an immunosuppressive tumor environment. Cancer cells themselves can also evolve mechanisms that allow them to evade immunosurveillance and to negatively affect the functionality of effector T-cells. These so called tumor-escape-mechanisms are: i) down regulation of antigen expression, components of the antigen-processing and presentation machinery, and expression of Major Histocompatibility Complex (MHC) molecules (Marincola et al., 2000), ii) decreased expression of co-stimulatory cytokines which are of crucial importance to T-cell activation (Sica et al., 2003), iii) enhanced surface expression of molecules that negatively regulate T-cell activation, so called "co-inhibitory signals", such as PDL1/B7-H1 and B7-H4 (Dong et al., 2002; Driessens et al., 2009), and iv) secreting a milieu of soluble factors that ultimately inhibit the activation, proliferation, and differentiation of the various components of the immune response; e.g. TGF-β (Thomas & Massague, 2005), IL-10 (Kurte et al., 2004), IL-13 (Terabe et al., 2000), and VEGF (Gabrilovich et al., 1996). And it was shown that the differential genetic and proteomic alterations of cancer cells accumulate in the course of disease from the localised tumor to lymph node positive state to end stage metastatic disease (Taylor et al., 2006). In order to design a successful anti-cancer immunostimulative strategy, it is important not to ignore the discoveries made by scientists working in the areas of immunity, infection and especially autoimmunity. For example, successful immunological clearance of viral as if bacterial infections are naturally accompanied by tremendous expansions of pathogen-reactive cytotoxic T-lymphocytes (CTLs), with up to 50 % of all circulating CD8+T-cells being antigen specific CTLs, which only subside after the infection has been defeated. On the other hand, most cancer vaccines which are in the field today generate poor T-cell responses with antigen-specific CTL rates beneath 1 % that often disappear soon after vaccination. Thus, one should not be surprised that insufficient tumor responses or regressions are observed (Cho & Celis, 2010).

The goal of vaccine-based cancer immunotherapy approaches is to induce a tumor-specific immune response that will reduce tumor burden by tipping the balance from a protumor to an antitumor immune environment - and from a clinicians point of view it is a success if tumor progression is stopped or if the tumor does not even metastasizes. So achieving cure is a high goal, which the so called therapeutic cancer vaccines might never reach, but we would save millions if we could force cancer into a chronic disease patients learn to live with but don't succumb from it. This chapter discusses strategies employed in the field of PCa vaccines aiming to enhance activation of an immune response that has shown impact in clinical trials.

There are many attempts around to describe the different vaccine platforms systematically, but as for most approaches the molecular mode of action is not exactly known attempts to divide into active versus passive, specific versus unspecific vaccines are difficult. It is more practical to categorize each vaccine depending on the vaccine-delivery system used, and whether specific or multiple antigens are targeted (Palena & Schlom, 2010). In the multi-antigen vaccine formulations often known and unknown antigens are included. A list of the various types of vaccine-delivery systems under investigation in the field of PCa in clinical stages is presented in Table 1.

1. Immunisation against multiple (not specified) antigens	Ref. (e.g.)	2. Immunisation against specified antigen(s)	Ref. (e.g.)
1.1 Cell-based		2.1 Cell-based	
1.1.1 DCs pulsed ex vivo with allogeneic whole-tumor cell mRNA	(Mu et al., 2005)	2.1.1 DCs pulsed ex vivo with a single peptide	
1.1.2 DCs pulsed ex vivo with autologous whole-tumor cell lysates	(Pandha et al., 2004)	human PAP as target (e.g. sipuleucel-T) xenogeneic PAP as target	(Higano et al., 2009a; Kantoff et al., 2010a) (Fong et al., 2001)
1.1.3 Allogeneic whole-tumor cells (modified ex vivo)		PSMA as target	(Tjoa et al., 1999; Fishman, 2009)
e.g. GVAX	(Simons et al., 2006; Small et al., 2007; Higano et al., 2008; Higano et al., 2009b)	PSA as target	(Barrou et al., 2004) (Hildenbrand et al., 2007)
e.g. OnyP	(Michael et al., 2005)	PSCA as target	(Thomas-Kaskel et al., 2006)
e.g. LNCaP/IL2/IFNγ	(Brill et al., 2007, 2009)	Telomerase as target	(Vonderheide et al., 2004; Su et al., 2005)
1.1.4 whole tumor cells (modified in situ - "in situ vaccination")		2.1.2 DCs pulsed ex vivo with multiple peptides	
Cell modification via viral vectors e.g. AdV-IL2	(Simons et al., 1999)	DCs pulsed "peptide cocktail" diff. epitopes from prostate TAAs	(Fuessel et al., 2006; Waeckerle-Men et al., 2006)
		2.2 Viral vector-based	
		PSA in VV and FV (e.g. Prostvac-VF)	(Kaufman et al., 2004; Kantoff et al., 2010b; Gulley et al., 2010)
		PSA in AdV	(Lubaroff et al., 2009)
		MUC1 in MVA	(Dreicer et al., 2009)
		2.3 DNA based	
		PSMA	(Low et al., 2009)
		human PAP	(McNeel et al., 2009)

1. Immunisation against multiple (not specified) antigens	Ref. (e.g.)	2. Immunisation against specified antigen(s)	Ref. (e.g.)
		2.4 Peptide based	
		2.4.1 Multiple peptides used: "peptide cocktail" diff. epitopes from prostate TAAs	(Feyerabend et al., 2009)
		2.4.2 Single peptide used: e.g. HER2/neu epitope (776-790)	(Perez et al., 2010)

AdV = Adenovirus; DCs = dendritic cells; diff. = different; FV = Fowl pox virus; mRNA = messenger RNA; PAP = prostatic acid phosphatase; PSMA = prostate-specific membrane antigen; PSCA = prostate stem cell antigen; TAA = tumor associated antigen; VV = Vaccinia virus

Table 1. Systematic list of vaccine-delivering systems in PCa vaccine approaches

Novel therapeutic options for patients of this stage of disease have been stated as an urgent medical need. Thus besides vaccine therapies a number of agents (e. g. endothelin receptor antagonists, receptor activator of nuclear factor κB ligand inhibitors, anti-angiogenic drugs, cytochrome P17 enzyme inhibitors, vitamin D analogues) are now tested in phase III registration trials either alone or in combination with docetaxel for first- or second-line use in mCRPC patients (Antonarakis & Drake, 2010; Antonarakis & Eisenberger, 2011).
Clinical trails that have engrossed most interest include i) Dendritic Cell (DC)-based vaccines (with clinically meaningful outcome for sipuleucel-T), ii) DNA vaccines (e.g. viral vector-based Prostvac-VF) together with recombinant peptide vaccines, and iii) whole-tumor cell vaccines (e.g. GVAX).

2. DC-based vaccines

Since cancer in fact develops and evolves in the presence of an intact immune system TAAs are by definition inadequately immunogenic. This results in a suboptimal T-cell activation, induction of immune tolerance and thus an ineffective immune reaction. Cancer vaccines are intended to break this immune tolerance. Strong presentation of antigen by antigen-presenting cells (APCs) is essential. Dendritic cells (DCs), which are the most powerful APCs, are known to be deficient in number and function in cancer patients. Activating APCs that are able to appropriately process and present the TAA is pivotal to activating an adaptive immune response and breaking peripheral tolerance.

2.1 The sipuleucel-T (PROVENGE®) approach

The history of this new treatment option began with phase I and phase II clinical trials in the academic field back in the 1990th. In the early 2000th the first phase III accrual of patients started and first data published in 2006 and FDA approval was asked for. But the FDA concluded that further confirmation would be obligatory prior to approval. This judgment sparked protests from patients and advocates who urged the FDA to repeal its decision. In 2009 preliminary results of that phase III pivotal trial, named Imunotherapy for Prostate

Adenocarcinoma Treatment (IMPACT) study, were presented to the community at an AUA national conference and to the FDA (Schellhammer et al., 2009). After re-analysis of these facts the FDA finally permitted sipuleucel-T end of April 2010, so it is worth to have a closer look into the prescription information (FDA, 2010a) and the approval letter (FDA, 2010b) as this product is not just another in a row of existing PCa vaccines but - as the first active immune therapy granted with approval for use in human subjects - opens an entire new entity for curative intervention. Finally in July 2010 the IMPACT trial data were presented in a peer reviewed journal (Kanthoff et al., 2010b) and as a result the prostate panel of the National Comprehensive Cancer Network (NCCN) has changed its guidelines how to treat mCRPC patients by adding sipuleucel-T as a category 1 treatment recommendation (NCCN, 2010).

Sipuleucel-T is an antigen specific cellular immunotherapy based on autologoues DCs (see Tab. 1) and indicated in metastatic but asymptomatic or minimally symptomatic patients who are in a hormone refractory and disease progressive stage. Sipuleucel-T consists of APCs and other cells of the peripheral blood mononuclear cells (PBMC) compartment, that have been activated during a defined ex vivo period with a recombinant human fusion protein combining PAP and GM-CSF. To obtain patient's PBMCs a standard leukapheresis procedure approximately 72 hours prior to the infusion date has to be performed. During ex vivo culture period the PAP protein can bind to and be processed by APCs into smaller TAA fragments, so the recombinant antigen should target the DCs, and is thought to direct the immune response to PAP (Kanthoff et al., 2010a).

Due to the autologoues nature of sipuleucel-T and the individuality of this approach its final cellular composition (T-, B-, NK-, and other cells) depends on the cells obtained from the patient's leukapheresis and will vary from patient to patient and from dose to dose, but the ex vivo procedure is regulated in that a minimum of 50 million PAP-GM-CSF activated CD54+ cells are included, suspended in 250 mL of Lactated Ringer's solution, and reinfused intravenously to the patient (FDA, 2010a; Kanthoff et al., 2010a).

The IMPACT trial was randomized, placebo-controlled, double-blind, multicentered. A total of 512 patients were randomized (2:1 ratio) to receive sipuleucel-T ($n = 341$) or control ($n = 171$). The placebo material used in control subjects was peripheral blood mononuclear cells that had not been PAP-activated, but given back to the patients under equal clinical conditions. In case of disease progression control subjects were allowed to cross over to an open-label use of the vaccine. The effectiveness of sipuleucel-T showed an increase in OS of 4.1 months in the pivotal phase III trial (25.8 vs 21.7 months) and OS benefit (3-year OS of 31.7 % vs 23.0 %). Sipuleucel-T successfully reached the prespecified level of statistical significance and reduced the overall risk of death by 22 % compared to control ($p < 0.05$) (Kanthoff et al., 2010b). Analyses of time to disease progression did not differ between verum and placebo patients and thus not meet statistical significance.

As sipuleucel-T is intended and produced solely for personalized use in a central laboratory there is no routine testing for transmissible infectious diseases so general precautions for handling blood products has to be employed. Due to the expiration time being as short as 18 h the product safety testing is challenging and sipuleucel-T has to be released for use based on the sterility and microbial results from a number of tests. If the sterility results show positive for microbial contamination after the use of sipuleucel-T, the manufacturer will inform the treating doctor. As, due to the character of the product, no cell filter can be used during the i.v. re-infusion of the ex vivo stimulated blood compounds, acute infusion reactions are the most common solely adverse event (AE) in patients receiving sipuleucel-T but also in control subjects receiving the non-activated peripheral blood mononuclear cells. Such events included, but were not limited to, vomiting, fatigue, fever, chills, respiratory events (dyspnea, hypoxia, and bronchospasm), nausea, hypertension, and tachycardia. To minimize potential acute infusion reactions e.g. chills and/or fever, it is recommended to premedicate patients orally with an antihistamine prior to infusion of sipuleucel-T (Kanthoff et al., 2010b).

The safety evaluation of sipuleucel-T, released by the FDA, is based on 601 PCa patients who received at least one dose of sipuleucel-T reported in four different clinical trials (Small et al., 2006; Harzstark et al., 2009; Higano et al., 2009a; Kanthoff et al., 2010a). Almost all (98.3 %) indivduals in the sipuleucel-T group and 96.0 % in the control group reported an adverse event. In 67.4 % of patients in the sipuleucel-T group, these adverse events were mild or moderate. Severe (grade 3) and life-threatening (grade 4) adverse events were reported in 23.6 % and 4.0 % of patients in the sipuleucel-T group compared with 25.1 % and 3.3 % of control group patients. Fatal (grade 5) adverse events were reported in 3.3 % of patients in the sipuleucel-T group compared with 3.6 % of patients in the control group. The FDA recommended the manufacturer to run a post-marketing study to assess the risk of cerebrovascular events in 1,500 PCa patients who receive sipuleucel-T and awaits completion of this study till December 31, 2015 (FDA, 2010b).

Each dose of sipuleucel-T requires a leukapheresis approximately three days prior to the infusion. AE´s that were reported within one day following the leukapheresis procedure included citrate toxicity (14.2 %), oral paresthesia (12.6 %), general paresthesia (11.4 %), and fatigue (8.3 %) (FDA, 2010a).

Due to its novelty in the market as if the pricey production process and due to the high research and development costs sipuleucel-T as a pharmaceutical product is quite expensive - more than 90.000 USD. So there is a discussion whether or not these costs should be covered by the public. In comparison to other recently introduced drugs in other tumor entities (e.g. lung cancer or breast cancer) and based on the calculation of the achievable duration in life time the costs of sipuleucel-T has been calculate as about 10 times higher (Longo, 2010).

2.2 Other DC based vaccines

A wide variety of other approaches using DCs have been studied, including evaluation of DCs pulsed with defined proteins like PSMA (Tjoa et al., 1999; Fishman, 2009), PSA (Barrou et al., 2004; Hildenbrand et al., 2007), xenogeneic PAP (Fong et al., 2001), PSCA (Thomas-Kaskel et al., 2006), and telomerase (Vonderheide et al., 2004; Su et al., 2005). Strategies based on peptides included pulsing DCs with multiple but defined peptides (prostate stem cell antigen (PSCA14–22), prostatic acid phosphatase (PAP299–307), prostate-specific membrane antigen (PSMA4–12), Prostein (31-39), Survivin (95–104), Trp-p8 (187–195), and prostate-specific antigen (PSA154–163)) (Fuessel et al., 2006; Waeckerle-Men et al., 2006). To expand antitumor reactivity and prevent tumor escape from the immune system, researchers have used DCs genetically engineered to express an enlarged range of antigens by the use of tumor cell lysates (Pandha et al., 2004), and allogeneic PCa cell lines (DU145, LNCaP and PC-3) messenger RNA (Mu et al., 2005).

3. DNA vaccines

DNA vaccines are focused to the TAA which is used in a specific approach to switch the patient's immune system. Most DNA vaccines have focused on tissue-specific (PAP, PSMA,

PSCA and PSA) rather than tumor-specific antigens. The major advantages of DNA vaccines is, at least compared with DC-based vaccines, that they are easy and inexpensive to produce and that with some viral vectors used in this attempt there is a huge body of experience as they have been used in millions of persons for preventive vaccinations against infective disease (Fioretti et al., 2010).

3.1 Prostvac-VF approach

This approach has been tested clinically in a number of phase I studies demonstrating safety of the vectors (Sanda et al., 1999; DiPaola et al., 2006; Arlen et al., 2007), and three phase II studies. Prostvac-VF consists of two genetically engineered viruses (recombinant Vaccinia (V) virus and Fowl pox (F) virus) administered in a sequential regimen. The virus strain used in Prostvac-V is a to some extent attenuated version of the virus used for smallpox immunization. Fowl pox viruses are unable to replicate in human cells but have been shown to be an effective way of boosting cellular immune responses primarily initiated using Vaccinia virus. The viral vectors are engineered to contain a gene encoding human PSA which contains an alteration in the HLA-A2 specific epitope that is planned to enhance the immunogenicity of the expressed antigen. In addition, these viruses both contain the genes encoding three co-stimulatory molecules, B7.1, ICAM-1 and LFA-3 (together named TRICOM). The academic work to establish this vaccine platform was done in cooperation with industrial sponsorship initially with Therion Biologics Cambridge, MA and subsequently with BN ImmunoTherapeutics, Garcia Ave, CA (Madan et al., 2009). The first phase II trial conducted by the Eastern Cooperative Oncology group enrolled 64 eligible patients and assigned them randomly to receive i) four vaccinations with fowl pox-PSA (rF-PSA), ii) three rF-PSA vaccines followed by one vaccinia-PSA (rV-PSA) vaccine, or iii) one rV-PSA vaccine followed by three rF-PSA vaccines. In this trial the TRICOM-component was not included. The prime/boost schedule was well tolerated with a small amount of adverse events. Of the eligible patients, 45.3% of men remained free of PSA progression at 19.1 months and 78.1 % demonstrated clinical progression free survival. There was a trend favouring the treatment group that received a priming dose of rV-PSA (Kaufman et al., 2004).

So in further trials using this approach rV-PSA priming was always followed by rF-PSA boostering. In the second phase II trial (n = 125 patients) it could be shown that at 3 years post study analysis, Prostvac-VF patients (n = 82) had a better OS with 25 (30 %) of 82 alive versus 7 (17 %) of 40 controls, longer median survival by 8.5 months (25.1 vs 16.6 months for controls), an estimated hazard ratio of 0.56 (95% CI, 0.37-0.85), and stratified log-rank $p < 0.01$. There was a minor imbalance in favour of the Prostvac-VF arm in mean and median of some laboratory values. But integration of these factors plus performance status in the Halabi nomogram revealed a 1-month mean and 2-month median difference in predicted survival (mean and median of 20.4 months for controls vs mean of 21.4 months and median of 22.5 months for Prostvac-VF). The observed survival difference of 8.5 months far exceeds that predicted by the Halabi nomogram. So these data are - despite of OS being not the primary end point - considered clinically meaningful and strongly suggests that Prostvac-VF immunotherapy may produce an OS benefit, but still regarded as hypothesis generating data as the authors state in the discussion of there recently published work (Kantoff et al., 2010b). The National Cancer Institute (NCI) has also recently completed a third phase II study in 32 PCa bearing men in whom immune and regulatory T-cell responses were evaluated. In that study, 13 of 28 evaluable patients had more than two-fold increases in PSA epitope specific immune responses, and four of five high responders (more than a six-fold increase) survived >40 months, while low or non-responders had a median OS of 20 months. The Halabi predicted survival of these metastatic CRPC patients was 17 months. Of interest is the Treg-cell course reported: Treg-cell suppressive function was shown to decrease following vaccine in patients surviving longer than predicted, and increase in patients surviving less than predicted (Gulley et al., 2010). Prostvac-VF immunotherapy is a promising approach, and a larger pivotal phase III trial is planned. If the data gained to date (OS benefit of 8.5 months) could be approved in a pivotal phase III trial - this platform is considered to be the next immunotherapy candidate for FDA approval.

Main components of this approach (rV-PSA, rF-PSA and rV-B7.1) have also been tested in a two armed phase II trial with or without combining the vaccine and docetaxel (plus dexamethasone) showing that docetaxel can be administered safely with immunotherapy without inhibiting vaccine specific T-cell responses. The authors state that patients previously vaccinated with an anti-cancer vaccine respond longer to docetaxel compared with a historical control of patients receiving docetaxel alone (Arlen et al., 2006).

3.2 Other viral vector-based vaccines

A group at the University of Iowa, USA, used an adenovirus genetically engineered to carry the genetic information for PSA and injected one single amount of recombinant virus. They included 32 patients with measurable mCRPC in a phase I trial. Patients were treated with a single s.c. vaccine injection at one of three dose levels, either suspended in a Gelfoam matrix or as an aqueous solution. The vaccine was judged safe in both administration forms at all doses. Anti-PSA antibodies and anti-PSA T-cell responses were detected in the majority of individuals. As PSA doubling time (PSA-DT) was increased and half of the patients survived longer than predicted by the Halabi nomogram this vaccine could be stated safe and potentially clinical effective and should proceed to phase II (Lubaroff et al., 2009).

A multicenter phase II trial in 40 patients with PSA progression used TG4010, a recombinant MVA vector expressing the tumor-associated antigen mucin 1 (MUC1) and Interleukin-2 (IL-2) as an adjuvant. Despite the primary endpoint of a 50 % decrease in PSA values from baseline was not observed, in 13 of 40 patients a more than two fold improvement in PSA-DT could be observed ($p < 0.01$ for all 40 patients) and ten patients had a PSA plateau for over 8 months demonstrating evidence of biologic activity (Dreicer et al., 2009).

3.3 Other DNA-vaccines

A phase I/II, dose escalation, DNA vaccination trial with plasmid DNA, coding for PSMA, fused to a domain (DOM1) of the C fragment of tetanus toxin was performed in patients with recurrent PCa. The DNA, was delivered either by i.m. injection without further manipulation or i.m. followed by electroporation. The PSMA epitope used in this study is a short stretch of 9 amino acids. Preliminary analysis of CD8+ T-cell reactivity against the PSMA target peptide indicated significant responses in three out of three patients and CD4+ T-cell responses against the DOM1. These data suggest electroporation as an effective method for stimulating the humoral system induced by DNA vaccination in humans (Low et al., 2009).

Results of a phase I/II trial, conducted with DNA vaccine encoding human PAP co-administered intradermally with GM-CSF, in PCa patients (stage D0) showed an increased PSA-DT, 6.5 months pretreatment versus 9.3 months in the 1 year post treatment (McNeel et al., 2009).

In a phase I/II trial a composition of 13 prostate-associated synthetic peptides (e.g. PSA, PSCA, PSMA, Survivin and Prostein) was used to counteract tumor escape mechanisms by genetic mutations or antigen loss. The TAA-epitopes were presented on HLA-A2 and on HLA-DR molecules, with the aim to activate a broad spectrum of CD8+ and CD4+ specific T-cells. The peptides were applied s.c. with or without immune stimulants (imiquimod, GM-CSF, MUC1-protamin complex). Four out of 19 men had a fivefold elevation of PSA-DT. Four individuals had minor PSA changes during vaccination and 11 patients showed progressive disease. In four men the vaccination was discontinued due to adverse events graded moderate. Although underpowered to draw definitive results imiquimod as an adjuvant seems beneficial (Feyerabend et al., 2009).

In contrast to the later approach using a peptide cocktail it is also possible to induce immune responses (elevated DTH-reaction, increased IFNγ ELISPOT activity and decreased Treg-cell frequency) by only using a short active sequence existing of fourteen amino acids of the TAA HER2/neu. Such synthetic fragments (500 μg) were administered together with GM-CSF in a phase I trial using a schedule of six intradermal vaccinations (Perez et al., 2010).

A slightly different but unique approach is used by a group at the university of Kurume, Japan. They tested an individualized method of peptide vaccination based on preexisting cytotoxic T-cell and immunoglobulin (IgG) reactivity. Each patient was tested for reactivity among 16 immunogenic peptides known to bind to HLA-A24. Peptides were derived from a number of targets, including PAP, PSMA, multidrug resistance protein, PSA, and a variety of other epithelial tumor antigens. Each patient was immunized with four peptides on the basis of his reactivity panel. This personalized medicine approach was tested as monotherapy and in combination with chemotherapy. As the peptides were injected s.c. vaccines were well tolerated and showed reactivity (DTH-reactions, CTL and IgG responses) and clinical activity (PSA declines up to 30 % in four out of 17 patients (Uemura et al., 2010). In a second trial the combination with estramustine showed a better PFS as estramustine alone ($p < 0.05$) (Noguchi et al., 2010).

4. Whole-tumor-cell vaccines

While autologous whole-tumor-cell vaccines are derived from the patient's own tumor cells in an often lengthy and pricey process, allogeneic whole-tumor-cell vaccines originate from various tumor cell lines and are easier to set up (Risk & Corman, 2009).

4.1 Prostate GVAX®

The GM-CSF-secreting cancer cell immunotherapy platform (GVAX®) (managed by Cell Genesys, South San Francisco, CA) was set up to be used in diverse types of carcinomas. The prostate GVAX® form uses two different PCa cell lines (PC3 and LNCaP) which have been modified through adenoviral transfer to secrete GM-CSF (Ward & McNeel, 2007). Analyses of these two cell lines showed up many genes well-known in human PCa metastases, including previously described prostate TAAs. The PC-3 cell line was derived from a PCa bone metastasis, and LNCaP was derived from a PCa metastasis to a lymph node. LNCaP was shown to express PAP, PSMA, PSA, urokinase-type plasminogen activator and prostate stem cell antigen (PSCA) (Simons et al., 1999; Kiessling et al., 2002; Lu & Celis, 2002). PC-3

was shown to express glutathione S-transferase, mutant p53, CEA, and urokinase-type plasminogen activator (Warren & Weiner, 2000). GM-CSF - the cytokine the GVAX inventors have chosen as to further augment their vaccine - has shown some impact in PCa patients (PSA modulations) if administered as a solely therapeutic agent (Small et al., 1999; Dreicer et al., 2001; Schwaab et al., 2006). However, the use of GM-CSF might be challenged by counterregulatory immune responses that aim to reduce the expansion of cytotoxic T cells, thereby limiting antitumor activity. The use of GM-CSF for anti-cancer immunostimulation has caused some concerns as GM-CSF is associated with the presence of CD34+myeloid suppressor cells. Besides that it has been shown that GM-CSF is secreted by some carcinomas (Bronte et al., 1999) with a clinically relevant worse outcome (e. g. higher rate of recurrence) as in tumors with lesser CD34+cells which release Transforming Growth Factor (TGF) β inhibiting T-cell functions (Young, et al., 1997). This knowledge is important to determine the best use of GM-CSF and generally, low doses of GM-CSF are associated with greater stimulation of the immune response than higher doses which might create a counterproductive immune response via inducible nitric oxide synthase (iNOS) in well designed mouse data. This immunosupression could be abandoned by the specific iNOS inhibitor, L-NMMA, resulting in restored antigenspecific T-cell responsiveness in vitro (Serafini et al., 2004). Therefore, it is critical to optimize the use of GM-CSF, in order to improve, rather than hamper, the immune response (Harzstark et al., 2009).
In a first phase I/II trial (coded G9802) a fixed total cell dose of 1.2×10^8 cells (6×10^7 per cell line) was used in hormone therapy-naïve patients with PSA recurrence following radical prostatectomy and absence of radiologic metastases. GM-CSF secretion from the clinical lots used in this trial was 150 ng/10^6 cells/24 h (LNCaP) and 450 ng/10^6 cells/24 h (PC-3). Patients were vaccinated weekly via intradermal injections for 8 weeks and resulted in one patient having a partial PSA response of 7 month duration. The injection sites were found to have invasion of inflammatory cells and APCs on histopathology. At 20 weeks after the first treatment, 16 of 21 treated patients showed a statistically significant decrease in PSA velocity (slope) compared with prevaccination PSA course (Simons et al., 2006) (Urba et al., 2008). Two further uncontrolled single-arm phase II studies included asymptomatic CRPC patients with (n = 34) or without (n = 21) metastases (G9803 trial) and only men with metastases (n = 80) (G0010 trial). The two trials have shown anti-tumor effects of prostate GVAX®, the first one (G9803 trial) demonstrating an overall survival benefit of 34.9 versus 26.2 months in the mCRPC subgroup (n = 34) (Small et al., 2007) and the other (G0010 trial), a study in which the vaccine was re-engineered to secrete a higher dose of GM-CSF, showing an OS ranging from 20.0 to 29.1 months (n = 80) depending on dosing regimen. Dose levels ranged from 1×10^8 cells q28d × 6 to as many as 5×10^8 cells prime/3×10^8 cells boost q14d × 11. Besides the differences in OS also the proportion of men who generated an antibody response to one or both cell lines increased with dose and included 10 of 23 in the low-dose up to 16 of 18 in the highest dose group ($p < 0.01$; Cochran-Armitage trend test) (Higano et al., 2008). A combined expanded retrospectively analyses of antibody response using the data from the three above mentioned trials indicated a significant ($p < 0.05$) association of alternative reading frame protein (TARP) antibody induction and median survival time (Nguyen et al., 2010). No dose-limiting or autoimmune toxicities were seen. The most common adverse events in both studies were injection-site erythema, myalgias, fatigue, malaise, and arthralgias. Based on these promising findings, two powerful sized randomized phase III studies of GVAX immunotherapy (VITAL-1 and VITAL-2) were set

up. VITAL-1 involved 626 men with asymptomatic chemotherapy-naïve CRPC, and randomized them to GVAX or docetaxel/prednisone, with OS as the primary endpoint. The trial was terminated in October 2008 based on the results of a previously unplanned futility analysis conducted by the study´s Independent Data Monitoring Committee (IDMC), which indicated that the trial had a less than 30 % chance of showing OS (predefined primary endpoint) (Higano et al., 2009b). VITAL-2 was designed initially to enrol 600 men with symptomatic mCRPC, randomizing them to docetaxel/prednisone or docetaxel/GVAX. It was haltered after having enrolled patients for two years (n = 408) in August 2008 as mortality appeared to be higher in men on the investigational arm receiving docetaxel/GVAX (67 vs. 47 respectively). Preliminary analysis revealed no significant difference in the patients baseline characteristics of toxic effect that could explain the unexpected discrepancy in death rate. A survival advantage (14.1 vs 12.2 moths; HR 1.7, 95 % CI 1.15-2.53) was seen in the control arm (doxetacel-prednisone) over the experimental (GVAX-doxetacel) arm (Small et al., 2009). Further evaluation has not yet been released and due to this contradictory data the future of GVAX is unclear.
Two other whole-tumor-cell vaccines (ONY-P1 and LNCaP-IL2-IFNγ) have finished phase I/II trials and released results.

4.2 ONY-P1

ONY-P1 (managed by Onyvax, Ltd, London, UK) consists of three irradiated PCa cell lines given to 26 patients with nonmetastatic CRPC intradermally (2.4×10^7 cells per injection), once a month for up to 12 month. In total 11 of the 26 patients demonstrated a prolonged decrease in their PSA-velocity (PSAV). None of the treated patients experienced any significant toxicity. Median time to disease progression was 58 weeks. PSAV-responding patients showed a titratable TH1 cytokine release profile in reply to restimulation with a vaccine lysate, while non-responders showed a mixed TH1 and TH2 response. Furthermore, immunologic profile correlated with PSAV response by artificial neural network analysis (Michael et al., 2005).

4.3 LNCaP-IL2-IFNγ

This approach uses only LNCaP cells retrovirally transduced with a N2/huIL2/huIFNγ-vector, resulting in IL-2 and IFNγ secretion. The two cytokines chosen for this approach have been used for immunostimulation solely and in combination in a variety of tumors (Brill et al., 2007; Dieli et al., 2007) and both substances are FDA approved single agents. Expression of tumor-associated antigens is upregulated after treatment with IFNγ via IFNγ-inducible genes, thereby increasing the susceptibility of tumors to MHC restricted CD8+CTL-mediated killing (Gansbacher et al., 1990a; Shankanan et al., 2001; Propper et al., 2003; Dunn et al., 2005). IL-2 is a well-known T cell growth factor, which is traditionally implicated in the agonistic stimulation of immune responses (Gansbacher et al., 1990b; Rosenthal et al., 1994) and FDA approved for systemic application against metastatic renal cell cancer. IL-2 is the only cytokine to date not been detected to be produced by any cancer. LNCaP cells, as mentioned above (see GVAX) express some relevant TAAs but in contrast to other PCa cell lines used as cancer vaccines, do not express transforming growth factor (TGF)-β. After detailed investigation of the safety profile with special attention to induction of autoimmunity (n = 3 patients at a dose level of $7{,}5 \times 10^6$ cells) (Brill et al., 2007), further patients (n = 27) were scheduled to receive four intradermal vaccine injections (dose level of

1.5×10^7 cells) on days 1, 15, 29, and 92. In the absence of disease progression, patients received further vaccinations every three months - resulting in a total amount of more or less 100 million cells/year - as compared to 4,600 million used in other trials (see GVAX). The primary study criteria were safety and the difference in PSA-DT, determined in the pretreatment phase (before the start of vaccination) and in the trial treatment phase (during vaccination). During vaccination there was a significant prolongation of the PSA-DT compared with the prevaccination period (from 63 to 114 days ($p < 0.01$; intention to treat analyses)). The median overall survival time from first vaccination was 32 months - the median Halabi-predicted survival in these thirty heavily pretreated mCRPC-patients was calculated as low as 15 months. Despite such comparisons of assessed and Halabi-predicted survival are widely accepted to compare patients groups and even different approaches (Lubaroff et al., 2009; Gulley et al., 2010; Kantoff et al., 2010b) these data are to be categorized somehow as speculative. ELISPOT based immune monitoring revealed T-cell stimulation in the majority of patients and artificial network analysis showed best predictive value for a response to the vaccination for survirvin-reactivity at day 36 (Brill et al., 2009).

5. Approaches to overcome tumor induced immunosuppression

Three strategies have reached clinical phases in this respect: i) Inhibition of CTLA-4, ii) depletion of Treg-cells, and blocking programmed death-1 (PD-1) checkpoint.

CTLA-4 is a T-cell surface glycoprotein that is up regulated following T-cell activation to restrain the immune response. Its main task is to prevent autoimmunity by regulating the body's immune response to self antigens. Two fully human mAbs focussed to block CTLA-4 are at this time in clinical development: ipilimumab (MDX-010; Medarex/Bristol-Myers Squibb, Princeton, NJ) and tremelimumab (CP-675,206; Pfizer, New York, NY). The later is an immunoglobulin G2 antibody and ipilimumab is an immunoglobulin G1κ antibody; both bind to CTLA-4 with affinities less than 1 nmol/L. T-cells express two counteracting receptors on their cell surface - CD28 and CTLA-4. Both bind to the same ligands or co-stimulatory molecules on the outside of APCs (B7.1 and B7.2). Binding to CD28 results in activating T-cells, while interacting with CTLA-4 inhibits T-cell stimulation. In the first human phase I trial the use of an anti–CTLA-4 antibody alone in men with PCa, 14 patients with progressive mCRPC, seven of whom had received prior chemotherapy, were given one single dose of ipilimumab. Two patients demonstrated PSA declines of > 50 % and two patients established prolongation of their PSA-DT (Small et al., 2007b). These data suggest - as these end stage patients got no other therapy besides anti-CTLA-4 mAb - that some degree of immune "autopriming" exists even in a difficult stage of disease, with an ongoing low-level presentation of antigen, perhaps from basal apoptotic rates, which can then be enhanced with CTLA-4 blockade (Harzstark et al., 2009). Blocking CTLA-4 has been shown to prolong and potentiate immune responses to vaccine in two phase I trials (one as combination with GVAX; the other as combination with Prostvac-VF) (Arlen et al., 2009). Combinations of ipilimumab with chemotherapy as if vaccine has been successful in malignant melanoma and ipilimumab was recently approved for this purpose by the FDA (Hodi et al., 2010; Robert et al., 2011).

Treg-cells are induced during vaccination and the expansion of Treg-cells already present in the patient are possible factors causative to impaired vaccine efficacy by suppressing CD4+ and CD8+ effector T-cells through IL-2 consumption, the secretion of suppressive cytokines, and cytolysis. Therefore, combining the elimination of Treg-cells - achieved in specific (via mAb) or unspecific (via low dose chemotherapy) manor - with therapeutic immunotherapy approaches seems promising. When comparing DC vaccination in patients with renal cell carcinoma (RCC) with/without previous elimination of Treg-cells by an IL-2 diphtheria toxin conjugate (Denileukin diftitox; ONTAK®), a higher immune response rate was achieved in the Denileukin diftitox group (Dannull et al, 2005). Low, i.e. not tumoricidal doses of chemotherapy can also synergize with vaccination: It could be shown that low dose cyclophosphamide selectively diminishes quantity and function of Treg-cells with little effect on other lymphocyte subpopulations (Ghiringhelli et al., 2007). Besides low dose chemotherapy it has been noticed in individuals with RCC that the multi-kinase inhibitor sunitinib shows depletion of Treg-cells (Finke et al, 2008; Kusmartsev & Vieweg, 2009). Besides Treg-cells (CD4+CD25highFoxP3+T-cell) other subsets of immune cells with suppressive function are focused in preclinical studies (e.g. CD4+NKT-cells, MDSCs, tumor associated Macrophages, and CD4+TH2-cells) (Palena & Schlom, 2010).

PD-1 is another co-inhibitory receptor molecule expressed on activated T-lymphocytes and functioning as an immune checkpoint. When PD-1 is bound by its ligand, T-cell proliferation and activation are inhibited, resulting in inhibition of anti-tumor immune responses (Blank & Mackensen, 2007). Expression of the PD-1 ligand has been described on a variety of human tumor cells including PCa, leading to decreased tumor-specific immunogenicity (Ebelt et al., 2009). In addition, expression of the PD-1 ligand correlates with a poorer prognosis in some human malignancies. MDX-1106, a fully human anti-PD-1 blocking antibody, is the first agent in its class to reach human clinic. Results of a phase I trial using MDX-1106 in patients with refractory metastatic solid tumors (including metastatic CRPC) were recently published and shows signs of immunological impact and clinical response - but not jet in the included PCa patients (Brahmer et al., 2010). Common side effects of this agent - but also seen in trials blocking CTLA-4 and after depleting Treg-cells - include subclinical hypothyroidism, colitis and autoimmune arthritis.

Other targets but to date only in preclinical research are TH17 cells and B7-inhibitors. For TH17cells it is known that TGF-β together with IL-6 in addition to IL-1-β, IL-21 or IL-23 promotes development of TH17 cells (OConnor et al., 2010). The role of that TH-subtype in cancer vaccine settings is not clear yet. They have a well defined function in autoimmune or autoinflammatory-associate pathology as they at least in some aspects (e.g. production of IL-10) act like Treg-cells. The frequency of IL-17 producing T-cells might correlate with clinical response to therapeutic vaccination in CRPC patients (Derhovanessian et al., 2009). B7 is a co-signal important in T-cell development (see Prostvac-VF) and B7-inhibitors are constitutively expressed in numerous types of human tumors and had been shown to support evasion of tumor immunity by promoting apoptosis of activated effector T-cells, inhibiting IL-2 production and tumor resistance to T-cell mediated lysis. B7-inhibtors can be blocked by new drugs tested in preclinical models resulting in enhanced cytotoxic T-cell responses against TAAs (Palena & Schlom, 2010).

6. Points to consider: Safety, regulatory and ethical issues

Immunostimulatory trials in various cancer entities has often been judged as limited in the impact but have always been seen as at least non toxic and so not harming the patients. AEs seen in vaccine trials have in most cases be limited to local injection side reactions. Vaccines which use a cytokine in addition reported flu-like symptoms but not above grade 2. If

CTLA4-antibodies are used or Tregs-cells depleted some aspects of autoimmunity and other immunological break through events has been seen up to grade 3. In a combination of chemotherapy with vaccine (see GVAX) there were more deaths and diminished OS noticed in the combination arm.

AEs seen in the sipuleucel-T trials could be explained by the i.v. re-infusion of cells which had been manipulated outside the body as the AEs were as common in the verum group (stimulated T-cell re-infusion) as in the control group (unstimulated T-cell re-infusion). Also in other clinical trials severe up to fatal acute infusion reactions had caused concerns after re-infusion of immune cells. While for sipuleucel-T the total amount of cells is unknown - only the total amount of CD54+ cells is adjusted to a minimum of 5×10^8 APCs - patients with fatal AE received 2×10^9 and 10×10^{10} gene modified T-cells respectively (Brentjens et al., 2010; Morgan et al., 2010). So one could state that for vaccines based on DCs the i.v. application route seems not to be ideal and even more doubtful as other routes of application with a better safety profile are well established (e. g. intranodal (inguinal lyph node) (Mu et al., 2005), subcutaneous (Vonderheide et al., 2004; Hildenbrand et al., 2007) or intradermal re-infusion of DCs (Mu et al., 2005; Su et al., 2005; Waeckerle-Men et al., 2006; Hildenbrand et al., 2007; Sampson et al., 2009; Toh et al., 2009)) in urological and other tumor entities.

Cancer vaccines are a diverse array of therapeutics with several mechanisms of action - and some times the mode of action is not well known even for products having succeeded in late-stage trials. So cancer vaccines are a challenge for the regulators, researchers and sponsors in several aspects: i) preclinical testing and the need for relevant animal models, ii) finding the proper dose, iii) trial design especially assessment of the right end point, and iv) attempts to conduct cancer vaccine trials in early state patients.

Besides some basic ethical questions - e.g. is it ethical to do a placebo treatment in a cancer patient at all - an other challenge in cancer vaccine research is to investigate what healthcare strategies and interventions offer the greatest benefits to individual patients and the population as a whole, that means to do comparative effectiveness research (CER) which to date has not been performed in the cancer vaccine field at all (Stewart et al., 2010). Undertaking any type of CER in oncology, calls for an outcomes measurement that can capture quality-of-life (QOL) measures. Most treatment decisions in cancer care are made with palliative intent or with probabilities of cure that must be weighed against the toxicity side-effects of the treatment. Although great strides have been made in the use of targeted therapies with more favourable side-effect profiles, oncologists remain extremely aware of the clinical tradeoffs between length of life and quality of life. Last points to mention are attempts to use earlier patients or even to test cancer vaccines in the preventive setting (Gray et al., 2008) and to define special vaccine adjuvants tailored to be used in the new therapeutic area of therapeutic cancer vaccines (Dubensky & Reed, 2010; Young, 2010).

7. References

Al-Shibli, K.I.; Donnem, T.; Al-Saad, S. et al. (2008). Prognostic effect of epithelial and stromal lymphocyte infiltration in non-small cell lung cancer. *Clin Cancer Res,* 14:5220-5227

Antonarakis, E.S. & Drake, C.G. (2010). Current status of immunological therapies for prostate cancer. *Curr Opin Urol,* 20:241-246

Antonarakis, E.S. & Eisenberger, M.A. (2011). Expanding treatment options for metastatic prostate cancer. *New Engl J Med,* 364:2055-2058

Arlen, P.M.; Gulley, J.L.; Parker, C. et al (2006). A randomized phase II study of concurrent Docetaxel plus vaccine versus vaccine alone in metastatic Androgen-independent prostate cancer. *Clin Cancer Res,* 12:1260-1269

Arlen, P.M.; Skarupa, L.; Pazdur, M. et al. (2007). Clinical safety of a viral vector based prostate cancer vaccine strategy. *J Urol,* 178:1515-1520

Arlen, P.M.; Mohebtash, M.; Madan, R.V. et al. (2009). Promising novel immunotherapies and combinations for prostate cancer. *Future Oncol,* 5:187-196

Barrou, B.; Benoit, G.; Ouldkaci, M. et al. (2004). Vaccination of prostatectomized prostate cancer patients in biochemical relapse, with dendritic cells pulsed with recombinant human PSA. *Cancer Immunol Immunother,* 53:453-460

Blank, C. & Mackensen, A. (2007). Contribution of the PD-L1/PD-1 pathway to T-cell exhaustion: an update on implications for chronic infections and tumor evasion. *Cancer Immunol Immunother,* 56:739-745

Brahmer, J.R.; Drake, C.G.; Wollner, I. et al. (2010). Phase I study of single-agent anti-programmed death-1 (MDX-1106) in refractory solid tumors: safety, clinical activity, pharmacodynamics, and immunologic correlates. *J Clin Oncol,* 28: 3167-3175

Brentjens, R.; Yeh, R.; Beral, Y. et al. (2010). Treatment of chronic lymphocytic leucemia with genetically targeted T cells: Case report of an unforeseen adverse event in a phase I clinical trial. *Mol Therapy,* 18:666-668

Brill, T.H.; Kübler, H.R.; v. Randenborgh, H. et al. (2007). Allogeneic retrovirally transduced, IL-2- and IFN- -secreting cancer cell vaccine in patients with hormone refractory prostate cancer - a phase I clinical trial. *J Gene Med,* 9: 457-560

Brill, T.H.; Kübler, H.R.; Pohla, H. et al. (2009). Therapeutic Vaccination with an Interleukin-2–Interferon-γ-Secreting Allogeneic Tumor Vaccine in Patients with Progressive Castration-Resistant Prostate Cancer: A Phase I/II Trial. *Hum Gene Therapy,* 20:1641-1651

Bronte, V.; Chapell, D.B.; Apolloni, E. et al. (1999). Unopposed production of granulocyte-macrophage colony-stimulating factor by tumors inhibits CD8+ T cell responses by dysregulating antigen-presenting cell maturation. *J Immunol,* 162:5728-5737

Cho, H.-I. & Celis, E. (2010). Overcoming doubts and other obstacles in the development of effective peptide-based therapeutic vaccines against cancer. *Expert Rev Vaccines,* 9:343-345

Curiel, T.J.; Coukos, G.; Zou, L. et al. (2004). Specific recruitment of regulatory T cells in ovarian carcinoma fosters immune privilege and predicts reduced survival. *Nat Med,* 10:942-949

Danull, J.; Su, Z.; Rizzieri, D. et al. (2005). Enhancement of vaccine-mediated antitumor immunity in cancer patients after depletion of regulatory T cells. *J Clin Invest,* 115:3623-3633

DeNardo, D.G.; Johansson, M.; Coussens, L.M. (2008). Immune cells as mediators of solid tumor metastasis. *Cancer Metastasis Rev,* 27:11-18

DeNardo, D.G.; Barreto, J.B.; Andreu, P. et al. (2009). CD4+ T cells regulate pulmonary metastasis of mammary carcinomas by enhancing protumor properties of macrophages. *Cancer Cell,* 16:91-102

Dendreon Inc.; Dendreon's second randomized phase 3 D9902A trial of Provenge extends survival in patients with advanced prostate cancer (press release 10/31/2005). <http://investor.dendreon.com/releasedetail.cfm>?ReleaseID=178106, (accessed 08.05.09)

Derhovanessian, E.; Adams, V.; Hähnel, K. et al. (2009). Pretreatment frequency of circulating IL-17+CD4+T-cells, but not Tregs; correlates with response to whole-cell vaccination in prostate cancer patients. *Int J Cancer,* 15:1372-1379

Dieli, F.; Vermijlen, D.; Fulfaro, F. et al. (2007). Targeting human gamma delta T cells with zoledronate and interleukin-2 for immunotherapy of hormone refractory prostate cancer. *Cancer Res,* 67:7450-7457

DiPaola, R.S.; Plante, M.; Kaufman, H. et al. (2006). A phase I trial of pox PSA vaccines (PROSTVAC-VF) with B7-1, ICAM-1, and LFA-3 co-stimulatory molecules (TRICOM) in patients with prostate cancer. *J Transl Med,* 4:1-5

Dreicer, R.; See, W.A.; Klein, E.A. (2001). Phase II trial of GM-CSF in advanced prostate cancer. *Invest New Drugs,* 19:261-265

Dong, H.; Strome, S.E.; Salomao, D.R. et al. (2002). Tumorassociated B7-H1 promotes T-cell apoptosis: a potential mechanism of immune evasion: *Nat Med,* 8:793-800

Drake, C.G. & Antonarakis, E.S. (2010). Update: immunological strategies for prostate cancer. *Curr Urol Rep,* 11:202-207

Dreicer. R.; Stadler, W.M.; Ahmann, F.R. et al. (2009). MVA-MUC1-IL2 vaccine immunotherapy (TG4010) improves PSA doubling time in patients with prostate cancer with biochemical failure. *Invest New Drugs,* 27:379-386

Driessens, G.; Kline, J. & Gajewski, T.F. (2009). Costimulatory and coinhibitory receptors in anti-tumor immunity. *Immunol Rev,* 229:126-144

Dubensky, T.W. & Reed, S.G. (2010). Adjuvants for cancer vaccines. *Seminars Immunol,* 22:155-161

Dunn, G.P.; Bruce, A.T.; Ikeda, H. et al. (2002). Cancer immunoediting: from immunosurveillance to tumor escape. *Nat Immunol,* 3:991-998

Dunn, G.P.; Ikeda, H.; Bruce, A.T. et al. (2005). Interferon-g and cancer immunoediting. *Immunol Res,* 32:231-245

Ebelt, K.; Babaryka, G.; Frankenberger, B. et al. (2009). Prostate cancer lesions are surrounded by FOXP3(+), PD-1(+) and B7-H1(+) lymphocyte clusters. *Eur J Cancer,* 45:1664-1672

Ferlay, J.; Autier, P.; Boniol, M. et al. (2007). Estimates of the cancer incidence and mortality in Europe in 2006. *Annals Oncol,* 18:581-592

Feyerabend, S.; Stevanovic, S.; Gouttefanggeas, C. et al. (2009). Novel multi-peptide vaccination in HLA-A2+ hormone sensitive patients with biochemical relapse of prostate cancer. *Prostate,* 69-917-927

FDA; 29th April 2010: Prescription Information for PROVENGE®

FDA; 29th April 2010: Approval Letter for PROVENGE®

Finke, J.H.; Rini, B.; Ireland, J. et al. (2008). Sunitinib reverses type-1 immune suppression and decreases T-regulatory cells in renal cell carcinoma patients. *Clin Cancer Res,* 14:6674-6682

Fioretti, D.; Iurescia, S.; Fazio, V.M. et al. (2010). DNA vaccines: developing new strategies against cancer. *J Biomed Biotech,* Published online 2010 March 28. doi: 10.1155/2010/174378

Fishman, M. (2009). A changing world for DCvax: a PSMA loaded dendritic cell vaccine for prostate cancer. *Expert Opin Biol Ther,* 9:1565-75

Fong, L.; Brockstedt, D.; Benike, C. et al. (2001). Dendritic cell-based xenoantigen vaccination for prostate cancer immunotherapy. *J Immunol,* 167:7150-7156

Fuessel, S.; Meye, A.; Schmitz, M. et al. (2006). Vaccination of hormone-refractory prostate cancer patients with peptide cocktail-loaded dendritic cells: results of a phase I clinical trial. *Prostate,* 66:811-821

Gabrilovich, D.I.; Chen, H.L.; Girgis, K.R. et al. (1996). Production of vascular endothelial growth factor by human tumors inhibits the functional maturation of dendritic cells. *Nat Med,* 2:1096-1103

Galon, J.; Costes, A.; Sanchez-Cabo, F. et al. (2006). Type, density, and location of immune cells within human colorectal tumors predict clinical outcome. *Science,* 313:1960-1964

Gansbacher, B.; Bannerji, R.; Daniels, B. et al. (1990a). Retroviral vector-mediated γ interferon gene transfer into tumor cells generates potent and long lasting antitumor immunity. *Cancer Res,* 50:7820-7825

Gansbacher, B.; Zier, K.; Daniels, B. et al. (1990b). Interleukin-2 gene transfer into tumor cells abrogates tumorigenicity and induces protective immunity. *J Exp Med,* 172:1217-1724

Ghiringhelli, F.; Menard, C.; Puig, P.E. et al. (2007). Metronomic cyclophosphamide regimen selectively depletes CD4(+)CD25(+) regulatory T cells and restores T and NK effector functions in end stage cancer patients. *Cancer Immunol Immunother,* 56:641-648

Gulley, J.L.; Arlen, P.M.; Madan, R.A. et al. (2010). Immunologic and prognostic factors associated with overall survival employing a poxviral-based PSA vaccine in metastatic castrate-resistant prostate cancer. *Cancer Immunol Immunother,* in press

Gray, A.; Raff, A.B.; Chiriva-Internati, M. et al. (2008). A paradigm shift in therapeutic vaccination of cancer patients: the need to apply therapeutic vaccination strategies in the preventive setting. *Immunol Rev,* 222:316-327

Harzstark, A.L. & Small, E.J. (2009). Immunotherapeutics in development for prostate cancer. *Oncologist,* 14:391-398

Hanahan, D. & Weinberg, R.A. (2011). Hallmarks of cancer : the next generation. *Cell,* 144: 646-674

Higano, C.S.; Corman, J.M.; Smith, D.C. et al. (2008). Phase 1/2 dose escalation study of a GM-CSF-secreting, allogeneic, cellular immunotherapy for metastatic hormone-refractory prostate cancer. *Cancer,* 113:975-984

Higano, C.S.; Schellhammer, P.F.; Small, E.J. et al. (2009). Integrated data from 2 randomized double-blind, placebo-controlled, phase 3 trials of active cellular immunotherapy with sipuleucel-T in advanced prostate cancer. *Cancer,* 115:3670-3679

Higano, C.S.; Saad, F.; Somer, B. et al. (2009). A phase III trial of GVAX immunotherapy for prostate cancer versus docetaxel plus prednisone in asymptomatic, castration-resistant prostate cancer, in: Genitourinary Cancer Symposium 2009, Abstract 150

Hildenbrand, B.; Sauer, B.; Kalis, O. et al. (2007). Immunotherapy of patients with hormone-refractory prostate carcinoma pre-treated with interferon-g and vaccinated with PSA-peptide loaded dendritic cells - A pilot study. *Prostate,* 67:500–508

Hodi, S.F.; O´Day, S.J.; McDermont, D.F. et al. (2010). Improved survival with ipilimumab in patients with metastatic melanoma. *New Engl J Med,* 636: 711-723

Jemal, A.; Siegel, R.; Xu, J. et al. (2010). Cancer statistics, 2010, CA Cancer J Clin 60:277-300

Kantoff, W.P.; Higano, C.S.; Shore, N.D. et al.. (2010). Sipuleucel T immunotherapy for castration resistant prostate cancer. *New Engl J Med,* 363:411-422

Kantoff, W.P.; Schuetz, T.J.; Blumenstein, B.A. et al. (2010). Overall survival analysis of a phase II randomized controlled trial of a poxviral-based PSA-targeted immunotherapy in metastatic castration-resistant prostate cancer. *J Clin Oncol,* 28:1099-1105

Kaufman, H.L.; Wang, W.; Manola, J. et al. (2004). Phase II randomized study of vaccine treatment of advanced prostate cancer (E7897): A trial of the Eastern Cooperative Oncology Group. *J Clin Oncol,* 22:2122-2132

Kiessling, A.; Schmitz, M.; Stevanovic, S. et al. (2002). Prostate stem cell antigen: Identification of immunogenic peptides and assessment of reactive CD8+ T cells in prostate cancer patients. *Int J Cancer,* 102:390-397

Kurte, M.; Lopez, M.; Aguirre, A. et al. (2004). A synthetic peptide homologous to functional domain of human IL-10 down-regulates expression of MHC class I and transporter associated with antigen processing 1/2 in human melanoma cells. *J Immunol,* 173:1731-1737

Kusmatsev. S. & Vieweg, J. (2009). Enhancing the efficacy of cancer vaccines in urologic onconlogy: new directions. *Nat Rev Urol,* 6:540-549

Longo, D.L. (2010). Sipuleucel-T immunotherapy for castrate-resistant prostate cancer. *New Engl J Med,* 363:1968

Low, L.; Mander, A.; McCann, K. et al. (2009). DNA vaccination with electroporation induces increased antibody responses in patients with prostate cancer. *Human Gene Therapy,* 20:1269-1278

Lu, J. & Celis, E. (2002). Recognition of prostate tumor cells by cytotoxic T lymphocytes specific for prostate-specific membrane antigen. *Cancer Res,* 62:5807-5812

Lubaroff, D.M.; Konety, B.R.; Link, B. et al. (2009). Phase I Clinical Trial of an adenovirus/Prostate-Specific Antigen vaccine for prostate cancer: safety and immunologic results. *Clin Cancer Res,* 15:7375-7380

Luo, Y.; Zhou, H.; Krueger, J. et al. (2006). Targeting tumorassociated macrophages as a novel strategy against breast cancer. *J Clin Investig,* 116:2132-2141

Madan, R.A.; Arlen, P.M.; Mohebtash, M. et al. (2009). ProstVac-VF: a vector-based vaccine targeting PSA in prostate cancer. *Expert Opin Investig Drugs,* 18:1001-1011

Mantovani, A.; Sozzani, S.; Locati, M. et al. (2002). Macrophage polarization: tumor-associated macrophages as a paradigm for polarized M2 mononuclear phagocytes. *Trends Immunol,* 23:549-555

Marincola, F.M.; Jaffee, E.M.; Hickljn, D.J. et al. (2000). Escape of human solid tumors from t-cell recognition: molecular mechanisms and functional significance. *Advances Immunol,* 74:181-273

McArdle, P.A.; Canna, K.; McMillan, D.C. et al. (2004). The relationship between T-lymphocyte subset infiltration and survival in patients with prostate cancer. *Br J Cancer,* 91: 541-543

McNeel, D.G.; Dunphy, E.J.; Davies, J.G. et al. (2009). Safety and immunological efficacy of a DNA vaccine encoding prostatic acid phosphatase in patients with stage D0 prostate cancer. *J Clin Oncology,* 27:4047-4054

Michael, A.; Ball, G.; Quatan, N. et al. (2005). Delayed disease progression after allogeneic cell vaccination in hormone-resistant prostate cancer and correlation with immunologic variables. *Clin Cancer Res,* 11:4469–4478

Morgan, R.A.; Yang, J.C.; Kitano, M. et al. (2010). Case report of a serious adverse event following the administration of T cells transduced with a chimeric antigen receptor recognizing ERBB2. *Mol Therapy,* 18:1-9

Mu, L.J.; Kyte, J.A.; Kvalheim, G. et al. (2005). Immunotherapy with allotumour mRNA-transfected dendritic cells in androgen-resistant prostate cancer patients. *Br J Cancer,* 93:749-756

Nguyen, M.C.; Tu, G.H.; Koprivnikar, K.E. et al. (2010). Antibody responses to galectin-8, TARP and TRAP1 in prostate cancer patients treated with a GM-CSF-secreting cellular immunotherapy. *Cancer Immunol Immunother,* (May2010; Epub - ahead of print)

Noguchi, M.; Kakuma, T.; Uemura, H. et al. (2010). A randomized phase II trial of personalized peptide vaccine plus low dose estramustine phosphate (EMP) versus standard dose EMP in patients with castration resistant prostate cancer. *Cancer Immunol Immunother,* 59:1001-1009

OConnor, W.Jr.; Zenewicz, L.A. & Flavell, R.A (2010). The dual nature of TH17 cells: shifting the focus to function. *Nat Immunol,* 6:471-476

Pages, F.; Berger, A.; Camus, M. et al. (2005). Effector memory T cells, early metastasis, and survival in colorectal cancer. *New Eng J Med,* 353:2654-2666

Palena, C. & Schlom, J. (2010). Vaccines against human carcinomas: strategies to improve antitumor immune responses. *J Biomed Biotech,* Published online 2010 March 16. doi: 10.1155/2010/380697

Pandha, H.S.; John, R.J.; Hutchinson, J. et al. (2004). Dendritic cell immunotherapy for urological cancers using cryopreserved allogeneic tumour lysate pulsed cells: a phase I/II study. *BJU Int,* 94:412-418

Perez, S.A.; Kallinteris, N.L.; Bisias, S. et al. (2010). Results from a phase I clinical study of a novel li-Key/HER2/neu(776-790) hybrid peptide vaccine in patients with prostate cancer. *Clin Cancer Res,* 16:3495-3506

Piersma, S.J.; Jordanova, E.S.; van Poelgeest, M.I.E. et al. (2007). High number of intraepithelial CD8+ tumor-infiltrating lymphocytes is associated with the absence of lymph node metastases in patients with large early-stage cervical cancer. *Cancer Res,* 67:354-361

Propper, D.J.; Chao, D.; Braybrooke, J.P. et al. (2003). Low-dose IFNγ induces tumor MHC expression in metastatic malignant melanoma. *Clin Cancer Res,* 9:84-92

Risk, M. & Corman, J.M. (2009). The role of immunotherapy in prostate cancer: an overview of current approaches in development. *Rev Urol,* 11:16-27

Robert, C.; Thomas, L.; Bondarenko, I. et al. (2011). Ipilimumab plus dacarbazine in previously untreated melanoma patients. *New Engl J Med* : e-pub 5th June 2011

Rosenthal, F.; Cronin, K.; Bannerji, R. et al. (1994). Synergistic induction of cytotoxic effector cells by tumor cells transduced with a retroviral vector carrying both the IL-2 and IFNγ cDNAs. *Blood,* 83:1289-1298

Sampson, J.H.; Archer, G.E.; Mitchell, D.A. et al. (2009). An epidermal growth factor receptor variant III-targeted vaccine is safe and immunogenic in patients with glioblastoma multiforme. *Mol Cancer Therapy,* 8:2773-2779

Sanda, M.G.; Smith, D.C.; Linda, G.C. et al. (1999). Recombinant vaccinia-PSA (PROSTVAC) can induce a prostatespecific immune response in androgen-modulated human prostate cancer. *Urology,* 53:260-266

Schellhammer, P.F.; Higano, C.; Berger, E.R. et al. (2009). A randomized, double-blind, placebo-controlled, multi-center, phase III trial of sipuleucel-T in men with metastatic, androgen independent prostatic adenocarcinoma (AIPC). Presented at the Annual Meeting of the American Urological Association, Chicago, IL, April 25-30

Schwaab, T.; Tretter, C.P.G.; Gibson, J.J. et al. (2006). Tumor-related immunity in prostate cancer patients treated with human recombinant Granulocyte Monocyte-Colony Stimulating Factor (GM-CSF). *Prostate,* 66:667-674

Serafini, P.; Carbley, R.; Noonan, K.A. et al. (2004). High-dose Granulocyte-Macrophage Colony-Stimulating Factor-producing vaccines impair the immune response through the recruitment of myeloid suppressor cells. *Cancer Res,* 64: 6337–6343

Shankaran, V.; Ikeda, H.; Bruce, A.T. et al. (2001). IFNγ, and lymphocytes prevent primary tumour development and shape tumour immunogenicity. *Nat,* 410:1107-1111

Sica, G.L.; Choi, I.-H.; Zhu, G. et al. (2003). B7-H4, a molecule of the B7 family, negatively regulates T cell immunity. *Immunity,* 18:849-861

Simons, J.W.; Mikhak, B.; Chang, J.F. et al. (1999). Induction of immunity to prostate cancer antigens: results of a clinical trial of vaccination with irradiated prostate tumor cells engineered to secrete granulocyte-macrophage colony-stimulating factor using ex vivo gene transfer. *Cancer Res,* 59:5160-5168

Simons, J.W.; Carducci, M.A.; Mikhak, B. et al. (2006). Phase I/II trial of an allogeneic cellular immunotherapy in hormone-naive prostate cancer *Clin Cancer Res,* 12:3394-3401

Small, E.J.; Reese, D.M.; Um, B. et al. (1999). Therapy of advanced prostate cancer with granulocyte macrophage colony-stimulating factor. *Clin Cancer Res,* 5:1738–1744

Small, E.J.; Schellhammer, P.F.; Higano, C.S. et al. (2006). Placebo-controlled phase III trial of immunologic therapy with sipuleucel-T (APC8015) in patients with metastatic, asymptomatic hormone refractory prostate cancer. *J Clin Oncol,* 24:3089-3094

Small, E.J.; Sacks, N.; Nemunaitis, J. et al. (2007). Granulocyte macrophage colony stimulating factor - secreting allogeneic cellular immunotherapy for hormone-refractory prostate cancer. *Clin Cancer Res,* 13:3883-3891

Small, E.J.; Tchekmedyian, N.S.; Rini, B.I. et al. (2007). A pilot trial of CTLA-4 blockade with human anti-CTLA-4 in patients with hormone-refractory prostate cancer. *Clin Cancer Res,* 13:1810-1815

Small, E.J.; Demkow, T.; Gerritsen, W.R. et al. (2009). A phase III trial of GVAX immunotherapy for prostate cancer in combination with docetaxel versus docetaxel plus prednisone in symptomatic, castration resistant prostate cancer, in: Genitourinary Cancer Symposium 2009, Abstract 7

Stewart, D.J.; Whitney, S.N.; Kurzrock, R. (2010). Equipoise Lost: ethics, cost, and the regulation of cancer clinical research. *J Clin Oncol,* 28:1-11

Su, Z.; Dannull, J.; Yang, B.K. et al. (2005). Telomerase mRNA-transfected dendritic cells stimulate antigen-specific CD8+ and CD4+ T cell responses in patients with metastatic prostate cancer. *J Immunol,* 174:3798-3807

Taylor, B.S.; Varambally, S. & Chinnaiyan, A.M. (2006). Differential proteomic alterations between localised and metastatic prostate cancer. *Br J Cancer,* 95:425-430

Terabe, M.; Matsui, S.; Noben-Trauth, N. et al. (2000). NKT cell mediated repression of tumor immunosurveillance by IL-13 and the IL-4R-STAT6 pathway. *Nat Immunol,* 1:515-520

Thomas, D.A. & Massague, J. (2005). TGF-β directly targets cytotoxic T cell functions during tumor evasion of immune surveillance. *Cancer Cell,* 8:369-380

Thomas-Kaskel, A.K.; Zeiser, R.; Jochim, R. et al. (2006). Vaccination of advanced prostate cancer patients with PSCA and PSA peptide-loaded dendritic cells induces DTH responses that correlate with superior overall survival. *Int J Cancer,* 119:2428-2434

Toh, H.C.; Wang, W.W.; Chia, W.K. et al. (2009). Clinical benefit of allogeneic melanoma cell lysate-pulsed dendritic cell vaccine in MAGE-positive colorectal cancer patients. *Clin Cancer Res,* 15:7726-7736

Tjoa, B.A.; Simmons, S.J.; Elgamal, A. et al. (1999). Follow-up evaluation of a phase II prostate cancer vaccine trial. *Prostate,* 40:125-129

Uemura, H.; Fujimoto, K.; Mine, T. et al. (2010). Immunological evaluation of personalized peptide vaccination monotherapy in patients with castration-resistant prostate cancer. *Cancer Sci,* 101:601-608

Urba, W.J.; Small, E.J.; Higano, C.S. et al. (2008). Treatment of biochemical recurrence of prostate cancer with granulocyte-macrophage colony-stimulating factor secreting, allogeneic. *Cellular Immunotherapy J Urol,* 180:2011-2017

Waeckerle-Men, Y.; Uetz-von Allmen, E.; Fopp, M. et al. (2006). Dendritic cell-based multi-epitope immunotherapy of hormone-refractory prostate carcinoma. *Cancer Immunol Immunother,* 55:1524-1533

Ward, J.E. & McNeel, D.G. (2007). GVAX: an allogeneic, whole-cell, GM-CSF secreting cellular immunotherapy for the treatment of prostate cancer. *Expert Opin Biol Ther,* 7:1893-1902

Warren, T.L. & Weiner, G.J. (2000). Uses of granulocyte-macrophage colony-stimulating factor in vaccine development. *Curr Opin Hematol,* 7:168–173

Yamaguchi, T. & Sakaguchi, S. (2006). Regulatory T cells in immune surveillance and treatment of cancer. *Semin Cancer Biol,* 16:115-123

Young, R.C. (2010). Cancer clinical trials - a chronic but curable crisis. *New Engl J Med,* 3634:306-309

Young, M.R.; Wright, M.A.; Lozano, Y. et al. (1997). Increased recurrence and metastasis in patients whose primary head and neck squamous cell carcinomas secreted granulocyte-macrophage colony-stimulating factor and contained CD34+ natural suppressor cells. *Int J Cancer,* 74:69 -74

Zhang, Q.; Jang, T.L. & Yang, X. (2006). Infiltration of tumor-reactive transforming growth factor-beta insensitive CD8+ T cells into the tumor parenchyma is associated with apoptosis and rejection of tumor cells. *Prostate,* 66: 235-247

Ziegler, A.; Heidenreich, R.; Braumuller, H. et al. (2009). EpCAM, a human tumor-associated antigen promotes Th2 development and tumor immune evasion. *Blood,* 113:3494-3502

15

Skeletal Related Events in Prostate Cancer: Important Therapeutic Considerations

Miguel Álvarez Múgica[1], Jesús Mª Fernández Gómez[2,3], Antonio Jalón Monzón[2], Verónica Bulnes Vázquez[4], Erasmo Miguelez[1] and Francisco Valle González[1]

[1]*Urology Department, Hospital Valle del Nalón*
[2]*Urology Department. HUCA*
[3]*University of Oviedo*
[4]*Radiology Department, Hospital Álvarez Buylla*
Spain

1. Introduction

In western countries, prostate cancer is the most common non-dermatological malignant disease in men. An estimated 217730 new cases will have been diagnosed in 2010 in the USA (Jemal A et al., 2010) and 382250 cases were diagnosed in 2008 in Europe (Ferlay J et al., 2010), accounting for 28% and 22% of new non-cutaneous cancer diagnoses, respectively.

Bone is one of the most common sites of metastatic disease in patients with cancer, affecting approximately 400,000 patients each year. Nearly 70% of patients with advanced breast or prostate cancer will experience bone lesions; 50% of these patients will develop a secondary skeletal complications which represents a substantial disease and economic burden (Schulman KL & Kohles J, 2007).

The pathologic penetration of bone by tumour tissue can lead to numerous skeletal-related events, such as hypercalcemia, fracture, spinal cord compression, and potentially debilitating bone pain (Berruti A et al., 2002). Often these consequences result in the need for radiological and surgical intervention. Along with these therapies, pharmacological management is required to help reduce symptoms, prevent recurrence and further improve patients' quality of life.

Prostate carcinoma is the most common visceral malignancy and the second leading cause of death from cancer in men (Diamond T et al., 2004). Androgen-deprivation therapy (ADT), either alone (as depot gonadotrophin releasing hormone agonist) or in combination with antiandrogens (such as flutamide, bicalutamide, or cyproterone acetate), is recommended treatment for men with metastatic or locally advanced, non-metastatic prostate carcinoma (Fowler JE et al., 2002). Although it has been demonstrated that this form of therapy significantly reduces tumour growth and improves survival beyond 3 years after completion (Bolla M et al., 1997), there is growing concern regarding the negative effects of ADT on the skeleton. Accelerated bone loss, osteoporosis, and a potential for increased. Fracture rates have been reported in men with prostate carcinoma who are receiving ADT. Because many patients who present with prostate carcinoma are elderly and may have preexisting osteoporosis, subclinical vitamin D deficiency, or any of a multitude of medical problems, the risk of skeletal deterioration is increased (Elliot ME et al., 2002).

2. Diagnosis of osteoporosis in men

Bone mineral density (BMD) is considered to be the gold standard for diagnosing and assessing the severity of osteoporosis and fracture risk in women. The role of BMD in men is less clear. BMD is measured most commonly by dual-energy X-ray absorptiometry (DXA), but quantitative computed tomography (QCT) of the lumbar spine also is used, particularly in research studies (Faulkner KG et al., 1998).

BMD of the wrist and hip, after adjusting for age, is a strong predictor of fracture risk (Melton L et al., 1998). Although the BMD criteria for diagnosing osteoporosis in men remain controversial (Binkley NC et al., 2002), a definition based on World Health Organization recommendations is accepted currently.

According to definition, osteoporosis exists when the BMD value is > 2.5 standard deviations (SD) below the peak young normal mean reference range (T-score < 2.5). Accurate T-score calculations in individual men can be obtained from bone densitometers using standardized software derived from reference databases for 'healthy' Caucasian men ages 20–40 years. In elderly men, it has been reported that advanced spondyloarthropathy, facet joint disease, and aortic calcification elevate spinal BMD falsely, as assessed by DXA (Zmuda JM et al., 2000)). Spinal BMD of the second through fourth lumbar vertebrae should be measured routinely to diagnose osteoporosis. Interpretation of the results often requires the addition of spinal radiographs to improve diagnostic accuracy. QCT of the lumbar spine, using the new three-dimensional multislice scanners, may overcome this problem, but it is not available at many centers; this technique has the ability to accurately define a region of interest unconfounded by extravertebral calcification (Faulkner KG et al., 1998; Weigert JM & Cann CE, 1988). Femoral neck DXA in elderly men, for practical purposes, is used routinely for the diagnosis of osteoporosis, especially if spinal BMD is pseudoelevated. Both spinal BMD and total hip BMD are the preferred sites for monitoring changes in BMD in response to therapies (Kaufman JM et al., 2000; Lenchik L et al., 2002). In a recent study, the relative risk of hip fracture in men was 3.0 (range, 1.7–5.4) for each SD decrease in femoral neck BMD (Delaet C et al., 1998). Longitudinal studies suggest that the rate of lumbar spine bone loss in elderly men is approximately 5–10% per decade, with acceleration after age 75 years. Femoral neck bone loss in normal elderly men is estimated at approximately 0.7% per year (Jones G et al., 2004). A number of factors may increase the bone loss normally associated with aging. These include physical immobility, poor nutrition, reduced calcium dietary intake and intestinal absorption, vitamin D deficiency, increased cytokines, reduced growth factors and osteoblastic activity, and a gradual decline in gonadal androgen production (Kaufman JM et al., 2000). Accelerated bone loss similar to that seen in women undergoing bilateral oophorectomy has been demonstrated in men with hypogonadism who undergo gonadectomy (Daniell HW, 1997) or who receive ADT (Bruder JM & Welch MD, 2002; Yaturu S et al., 2002). In male sex offenders who underwent surgical castration, spinal bone loss occurred at a rate of 4% per year (Stepan JJ et al., 1999). Because these rates of loss are higher compared with the rates of loss observed in otherwise healthy elderly men, the abrupt loss of sex steroids appears to initiate a period of rapid bone loss.

3. Bone health in prostate cancer

In advanced prostate cancer, 65–75% of patients may eventually develop bone metastases. It is also important to note that approximately 10% of men with prostate cancer have bone metastases at initial presentation. Almost all patients who die of prostate cancer have bone involvement (Greenspan SL, 2008).

Men with prostate carcinoma who are treated with ADT are elderly and are at risk for a wide variety of metabolic bone problems. In a recent retrospective study of 125 men with a mean age of 77 years who were treated with ADT, Bruder and Welch reported a 27% prevalence of osteoporosis and a 51% prevalence of osteopenia (lumbar spine or femoral neck BMD T-score, -2.5 to -1.0) (Bruder JM & Welch MD, 2002); furthermore, 44% of the cohort had biochemical evidence of vitamin D insufficiency and secondary hyperparathyroidism.

Osteoporosis has become an increasingly important problem in men's health, accounting for significant morbidity in the aging male population. Patients with prostate cancer treated with ADT are at a high risk of osteoporosis. These patients may have additional morbidity from decreased bone mineralization, such as skeletal fractures. Moreover, a direct association has been noted between fractures and a decreased quality of life and increased mortality (Gilbert SM & Mckiernan JM, 2005).

The prevalence of osteoporosis is lower in men than in women for several physiologic reasons, including a greater accumulation of skeletal mass during growth, greater bone size, absence of midlife menopause, a slower rate of bone loss, and a shorter male life expectancy (Amin S & Felson DT, 2001). The rates of annual bone mass loss in aging men range from 0.5% to 1% compared with 1% to 2% in women (Gilbert SM & Mckiernan JM, 2005; Smith MR, et al., 2001). The prevalence of osteoporosis increases progressively during ADT, reaching almost 50% after 4 years of ADT and more than 80% after 10 years. In contrast, it affects 35.4% of hormone-naive patients with prostate cancer (Morote J, et al., 2007).

4. Mechanism of metastatic development

In healthy adults, bone physiology is a dynamic, coordinated process controlled by 2 types of cells: osteoclasts and osteoblasts. Through a balanced remodeling process, osteoclasts resorb bone, and osteoblasts build bone at the same site (Coleman RE, 2001; Rosen LS, et al., 2003). This bone remodeling sequence consists of 4 distinct phases: activation, resorption, reversal, and formation.

Bone metastases are often characterized by their radiographic appearance as either osteolytic, osteoblastic, or mixed or mixed. Most patients with breast cancer have predominantly mixed or osteolytic lesions (Coleman RE, 2001; Rosen LS, et al., 2003). In contrast, patients with prostate cancer are often found to have predominantly osteoblastic lesions. However, regardless of appearance, there is significant osteolytic activity. In fact, osteolytic activity in these lesions often is comparable with, if not higher than, that typically seen in breast cancer and multiple myeloma. Such activity has been demonstrated by markedly elevated biochemical markers of bone resorption in the serum and urine of such patients. Only in multiple myeloma do purely lytic bone lesions develop (Coleman RE, 2001; Rosen LS, et al., 2003).

Several mechanisms have been proposed for metastatic spread to the bone. Early animal and human evaluations demonstrated that breast and pelvis tissue drain directly into the veins of the spine, increasing the deposition of metastatic cells into the bone marrow (Coleman

RE, 2006). More recent studies have demonstrated how metastatic lesions develop once cancer cells reside in the marrow. Cellular modulators such as Receptor Activator for Nuclear Factor κ B Ligand (RANKL), parathyroid hormone-related protein (PTHrP), and serine protease urokinase (uPA) disrupt the balance of osteoblast and osteoclast activity that are involved in the formation of metastatic lesions (Mundy GR, 2002). Most bone lesions are classified as osteolytic or osteoblastic, depending on the direction of the bone breakdown/rebuilding imbalance. In osteoblastic lesions (prostate cancer metastases), the production of endothelin-1, transforming growth factor β (TGF-β) and uPA directly increase osteoblast activity and the formation of space-occupying bone lesions. In osteolytic lesions (primarily breast and lung cancer metastases), osteoclast activity is increased through the production of PTHrP, which stimulates nuclear factor κB (NF-κB) from stromal cells of bone, leading to increased osteoclast differentiation and activity (Mundy GR, 2002; Saad F, 2008).
Newer studies have also shown that RANKL activity in both osteolytic and osteoblastic lesions also may lead to increased tumour proliferation (Uehara H, et al., 2003; Yin JJ, et al., 1999). As osteoclasts break down bone, growth factors are released to stimulate the production of osteoblasts, allowing for bone repair and remodeling. These factors, including TGF-β and platelet derived growth factor have been shown to perpetuate bone metastases in both breast and prostate cancer models (Uehara H, et al., 2003; Yin JJ, et al., 1999).

In metastatic bone disease, RANK Ligand has been implicated in a "vicious cycle" of bone destruction and tumour growth. Some tumours that have metastasized to the bone produce growth factors that can increase expression of RANK Ligand by osteoblasts. This stimulates osteoclast activity and leads to excess bone loss (Coleman RE, 2001; Rosen LS, et al., 2003). Osteoclast-mediated bone resorption leads to the release of growth factors and calcium from the bone matrix, that can in turn stimulate the tumour cell, further contributing to this cycle of bone destruction (Rosen LS, et al., 2003).

5. Bone tissue and effects of hormonal therapy

In life, bone is a rigid yet dynamic organ that is continuously moulded, shaped and repaired. Bone microstructure is patterned to provide maximal strength with minimal mass, as determined by the physiological needs of the organism. How are bone structure and function maintained, and how are changes in bone metabolism induced? Once formed, bone undergoes a process termed remodelling that involves break down (resorption) and build-up (synthesis) of bone; this occurs in micro scale throughout the skeleton. This remodeling cycle is a coupled process; in a normal young adult after completion of normal linear growth, bone resorption and formation are roughly equivalent, resulting in a net bone balance. Bones are composed of 2 main types of tissues: cortical bone and trabecular bone. Cortical bone is 80% to 90% calcified and has mainly mechanical and protective functions. Trabecular bone is only 15% to 25% calcified and constitutes only 20% of the total bone mass, but carries out most of the bone's metabolic function. Bone strength is a function of bone mass and of other parameters including geometry (the diameter of the cortical bone), material properties (the quality of the bone matrix and inorganic crystals) and microstructure (the diameter and interconnectivity of the trabeculae) (Gruber R, et al., 2008). The bone mass of a normal adult is the outcome of a dynamic equilibrium between bone formation (mediated by osteoblasts) and bone resorption (mediated by osteoclasts).
Most adult skeletal diseases are due to excess osteoclastic activity, leading to an imbalance in bone remodelling which favours resorption. Such diseases would include osteoporosis, periodontal disease, rheumatoid arthritis, multiple myeloma and metastatic cancers. For

individuals with osteoporosis, bone fractures represent life-threatening events, and today there are in excess of 70 million people worldwide at risk (Brown JP & Jasse RG, 2002).

Recent breakthroughs in our understanding of osteoclast differentiation and activation have come from the analysis of a family of biologically related tumour necrosis factor (TNF) receptor (TNFR)/TNF-like proteins: osteoprotegerin (OPG), receptor activator of nuclear factor (NF)-kB (RANK) and RANK ligand (RANKL), which together regulate osteoclast function. Binding of RANKL to RANK on the surfaces of osteoclast precursors will trigger maturation, activation, and prolonged survival of these cells. Thus, RANKL promotes bone resorption. In contrast, OPG is a "decoy receptor" that binds and neutralizes RANKL, thus inhibiting bone resorption (Bayle WJ, et al., 2003). There is interplay between RANKL and OPG.

The ratio of RANKL to OPG is a critical factor determining the balance between bone resorption and bone formation. Vitamin D3, parathyroid hormone, tumour necrosis factor-α (TNF-α), activated T-cells, and glucocorticoid therapy all increase this ratio, promoting bone resorption. Estrogen deficiency states (including menopause) also produce osteoporosis because normal levels of 17β-estradiol inhibit RANKL production and stimulate OPG. (Bayle WJ, et al., 2003; Hofbauer LC & Schoppet M, 2004). Testosterone stimulates osteoblasts, inhibits the apoptosis of both osteoblasts and osteoclasts, and is a precursor of estrogen via aromatization; its net effect is to stimulate bone formation. Estrogens are essential in bone formation and resorption in men, and low levels are associated with loss of BMD and fracture risk. (Boonen S, et al., 2008).

In osteoporosis, resorption usually exceeds formation with the net effect of bone loss, decreased strength, and an increased risk of fracture. The hypogonadal state resulting from cancer therapy enhances osteoclastic bone resorption, promoting bone loss, which along with other important clinical factors such as age, prior fragility fracture, and family history lead to increasing fracture risk (Gleason D, et al., 2003; Major PP & Cook R, 2002). In males with hypogonadism (whether induced by orchiectomy, ADT, hyperparathyroidism, or other causes), both testosterone and estrogen levels fall, shifting the balance of bone turnover toward resorption (Higano CS, 2008; Perez et al., 2006). It has been hypothesized that several malignancies including prostate and breast cancer and multiple myeloma also promote bone resorption by expressing or stimulating RANKL (Boyle WJ, 2003).

The use of androgen deprivation therapy (ADT) in prostate cancer patients induces hypogonadism causing significant bone loss often leading to osteoporosis and an increased risk of fracture that may be compounded by the presence of bone metastases. Bone metastases disrupt the normal bone remodeling process by increasing bone resorption, which weakens the bone matrix and increases the risk of other bone complications, such as spinal cord compression, impaired mobility and bone pain (Berruti A, et al., 2001). Bone mineral density (BMD) is reduced by 0.6–5.3% annually in patients with locally advanced disease and 2.3–6.6% in patients with metastatic disease receiving ADT, exceeding by 5 to 10 fold the normal bone loss rates of similarly aged otherwise healthy men and prostate cancer patients not receiving ADT (Casey R, et al., 2006; Michaelson MD, et al., 2007; Smith MR, et al., 2008). Consequently, patients receiving ADT are 7–45% more likely to experience a fracture than patients not receiving ADT (Shahinian VB, et al., 2005; Smith MR, et al., 2006). Bisphosphonates have been shown to prevent bone loss and related complications in patients with locally advanced and metastatic prostate cancer and should be considered as part of cancer treatment when ADT is initiated in these patients. Androgen deprivation therapy is increasingly being prescribed both for men with locally advanced or high-risk non-metastatic prostate cancer and for those with recurrent disease (Meng MW, et al., 2002; Sharifi N, et al., 2005). With this increased exposure to ADT, clinicians have seen the emergence of longer-term treatment complications, including osteoporosis and osteopenia. Although osteoporosis is generally less frequent in men, it is increasingly recognized as a source of substantial morbidity and even mortality in the aging male. Men suffer one third of all hip fractures. Osteoporotic vertebral fractures have a radiological prevalence of up to 50% in both sexes; they often cause chronic pain, and even clinically silent fractures are associated with increased risks of future fracture (both vertebral and hip), kyphosis, restricted lung function, impaired activities of daily living and even increased mortality (Mavrokokki A, et al., 2007). A study of Canadian prostate cancer patients who were orchiectomized found that their 5-year risks of vertebral and hip fractures were 2.2 fold higher than those of patients who had not been orchiectomized ($p < 0.001$ for both) (Body JJ, 2003).

Fractures also independently predict diminished survival in prostate cancer patients on ADT. In one retrospective study, a history of fracture since the diagnosis of prostate cancer decreased median overall survival from 160 months to 121 months ($p = 0.04$) (Oefelein MG, 2002).

6. Non-invasive markers of bone turnover in normal men and in men with prostate carcinoma treated with androgen deprivation therapy

The slow dynamics of bone turnover and the infrequency with which bone density is monitored following castration in prostate cancer cases justify the recent increasing interest in studying the effects of ADT and the pathophysiology of bone metastasis.

Bone loss in elderly men occurs predominantly as a result of increased bone turnover. On bone histomorphometry, trabecular plate thinning and endocortical bone resorption is evident (Clarke BL, 1996). Non-invasive serologic and urinary markers of bone turnover now can be quantitated accurately. Markers of bone formation, such as bone-specific serum alkaline phosphatase, osteocalcin, procollagen type I propeptides and bone glaprotein, are usually normal in elderly men; whereas markers of bone resorption, such as urinary deoxypyridinoline excretion rates and the NTx and CTx telopeptides of Type I collagen and pyridinolines, often are found to be elevated (Khosla S, 1998).

7. Patients at high risk of bone disease. Who should be screened?

Gold-standard therapeutic care for relapsed hormone-sensitive prostate cancer (HSPC) patients demands chemical or surgical hormonal blockade over the course of the therapeutic strategy. With the advent of prostate-specific antigen (PSA), early detection of HSPC recurrence and early hormonal blockade has become possible. In turn, this may lead to osteoporosis and bone fragility (Smith MR, 2003). Pathological fractures related to osteoporosis are very expensive (Groot MT, et al., 2003) and highly correlated with decreased survival with mortality in the first year as high as 70% (Berruti A, et al., 2000).

There are 4 robust, independent risk factors for osteoporotic fracture described: low bone mineral density (BMD), a prior fragility fracture, age ≥65 and a family history of osteoporosis (Brown JP, & Josse RG, 2002). There are also other risk factors for osteoporosis, including lifestyle and dietary factors, such as smoking, excessive intake of alcohol or caffeine, inadequeate dietary calcium intake, weight < 57 kg or loss of > 10% of weight at age 25 and diseases and treatments associated with bone loss (Brown JP, & Josse RG, 2002; Greenspan SL, 2008).

Prostate cancer itself is associated with osteoporosis, even among ADT-naïve patients without metastatic disease. In a cross-sectional study, 45.2% of such patients had osteopenia and 35.4% had osteoporosis even before starting ADT. Systematic retrospective reviews have also shown the association between ADT and increased fracture risk (Saad F, et al., 2008; Brufsky AM, 2008).

Because age and hypogonadism are both considered major risk factors for osteoporosis, all prostate cancer patients beginning ADT should be screened with DXA scans at baseline; anyone aged ≥ 65 and anyone with kyphosis, back pain, substantial height loss, or other symptoms suggesting vertebral fractures should also be screened with thoracic and lumbar spine x-rays.

8. Incidence and presentation of skeletal-related events

The progression of metastatic bone disease in patients with prostate cancer can lead to debilitating skeletal-related events (SREs) (Oofelein MG, et al., 2002). About 70–80% of patients with metastatic prostate cancer present with or develop bone metastasis (Polascik TJ, 2008), and are at increased risk for skeletal-related events (SREs), which include pathological fractures, spinal cord compression (figure 4), and severe pain requiring radiotherapy or surgery for bone lesions. These SREs result in significant complications that reduce quality of life (Botteman MF, et al., 2010).

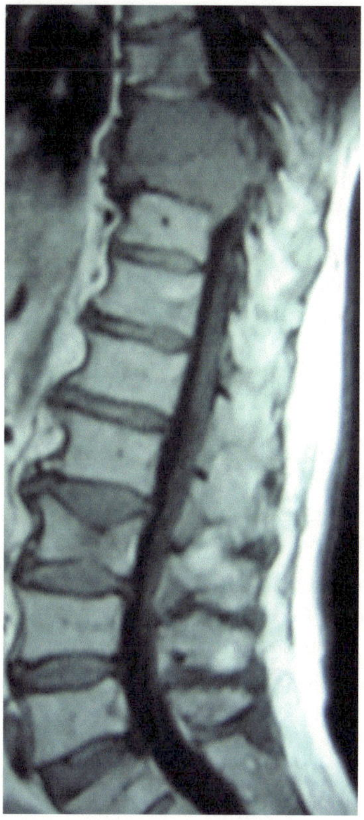

Fig. 4. Total disruption of the 9th dorsal vertebral body due to a metastatic prostate carcinoma, with spinal cord compression.

Skeletal-related events (SRE) include any secondary complication from the presence of bone metastases and can occur in both osteolytic and osteoblastic lesions. Pain is the most common symptom of bone disease and is thought to be due to increased sensitization of nociceptors, tumor infiltration of nerve channels, and local tissue acidification during the bone resorption process. Often the pain is described as dull, aching, or constant, with increasing intensity with weight-bearing activities. In many patients, this is localized to the area of infiltration (most often the thoracic spine), but may be referred or radicular if there is compression of the nerve channels. In nearly one-third of patients with bone metastasis, pain is caused by pathologic fracture. Similar to osteoporosis, this is often caused by the lytic breakdown of bone, often in the ribs, spine, and long bones. Pain is the most common symptom of fracture, although some patients may develop kyphosis from compression of the spine. In approximately 6% of patients, fracture may lead to the development of neurologic symptoms (Boyle WJ, et al., 2003).

Another cause of neurologic symptoms in patients with metastatic bone disease is malignant spinal cord compression. This medical emergency often is caused by direct compression of the spinal canal by osteoblastic tumor formation and edema or necrosis of the spinal cord from alteration of arterial and venous blood flow. Patients often present with severe back pain, weakness, paralysis, paresthesias and decrease in bowel or bladder control (Sathiakumar N, et al., 2011). At presentation, up to 68% of patients are unable to walk. Prompt management of this complication is necessary to decrease the progression of irreversible neurologic damage. Prevention and early treatment is paramount because the ability to regain ambulation after treatment is a strong predictor of overall survival (Sathiakumar N, et al., 2011; Aljumaily R, & Mathew P, 2011).

Hypercalcemia, defined as serum calcium >10.5 mg/dl, is another common presentation of skeletal metastasis. While the release of calcium into the blood from bone breakdown is the most common mechanism in patients with bone metastasis, hypercalcemia may also occur due to parathryroid hormone imbalances in patients without skeletal lesions. Hypercalcemia is a multifactorial complication of malignancy. Radiation therapy, surgical stabilization, and/or decompression often are necessary in patients with bone metastasis, particularly when the spinal column is involved. Pharmacotherapy is the mainstay of hypercalcemia treatment and is almost always used adjunctively with surgery or radiation to manage fractures, malignant spinal cord compression, and the pain of skeletal-related events (Shahinia V, et al., 2005).

Bone pain is the most common type of cancer-related pain, and was deemed to be severe and debilitating in two-thirds of patients. Treating bone pain therefore remains a consideration when managing metastatic bone disease (Coleman RE, 2006).

SRE is a pathology of high cost. A study in 342 patients with prostate cancer and bone metastases revealed that the annual economic effect of medically treating SREs for these patients was $12,469. Patients most frequently had radiation therapy (89%), followed by pathologic fracture (23%) and bone surgery (12%). Among patients diagnosed as having at least 1 SRE, 78% experienced 1 type of SRE, 17% had 2 types of SREs, and 5% had 3 or more distinct types of SREs. The mean costs associated with SREs in the year after the initial diagnosis of an SRE, adjusted for the censoring of the data, was $12,469, with the highest costs associated with radiation therapy ($5930), followed by pathologic fracture ($3179) and bone surgery ($2218) (Lage MJ, et al., 2008).)

In advanced prostate cancer, 65–75% of patients may eventually develop bone metastases. It is also important to note that approximately 10% of men with prostate cancer have bone

metastases at initial presentation. Almost all patients who die of prostate cancer have bone involvement (Egerdie B et al., 2010).
Men with prostate cancer that develops SRE have a poor prognosis. In a cohort study of 23,087 incident patients with prostate cancer, 569 (almost 3%) presented with bone metastasis at prostate cancer diagnosis, of whom 248 (43.6%) experienced a skeletal related event during follow-up. Of the 22,404 men (97% overall) without bone metastasis at diagnosis 2,578 (11.5%) were diagnosed with bone metastasis and 1,329 (5.9%) also experienced a skeletal related event during follow-up. One and 5-year survival was 87% and 56% in patients with prostate cancer without bone metastasis, 47% and 3% in those with bone metastasis, and 40% and less than 1% in those with bone metastasis and skeletal related events, respectively. Compared with men with prostate cancer without bone metastasis the adjusted 1-year mortality rate ratio was 4.7 (95% CI 4.3-5.2) in those with bone metastasis and no skeletal related events, and 6.6 (95% CI 5.9-7.5) in those with bone metastasis and a skeletal related event. The result of this study brings the conclusion, that bone metastasis and skeletal related events predict poor prognosis in men with prostate cancer (Norgaard M, et al., 2010).

9. Treatment for prostate cancer induced bone loss: Current options and new horizons

Prostate cancer is the most frequently diagnosed non-cutaneous cancer and the second leading cause of cancer deaths among men in the United States. The 5-year relative survival among men aged 65 years or older is 99.8% for all tumour stage groups combined but is considerably lower (5%) among men with distant metastatic disease at diagnosis (Aapro M, et al., 2008).
Advances in cancer therapies have extended patients' lives and improved patients' outcomes. Because cancer patients are living longer, they may be at an increased risk of metastatic bone pain and untreated bone metastases. As anticancer therapies have extended overall survival, the likelihood that a patient with advanced cancer will live long enough to experience an SRE increases.
Approximately 70% of patients with advanced prostate cancer develop skeletal metastases, which are often associated with significant morbidity and mortality (Coleman RE, 2001). In addition to the skeletal effects of cancer itself, bone loss resulting from treatment is an emerging problem. The causes of cancer treatment-induced bone loss (CTIBL) include the hypogonadal state induced by cancer therapies (testosterone deficiency secondary to androgen deprivation from gonadotrophin-releasing hormone [GnRH] agonists and surgical castration in prostate cancer). This hormone depletion promotes osteoporosis and increases the risk of fracture. This type of patients with malignant bone disease are at risk for skeletal-related events, including pathological fracture, metastases requiring surgery or radiation therapy to bone, and spinal cord compromise. They may experience fragility fractures either because of co-morbid conditions or because of toxicities of their cancer therapy, thus the prevalence of osteoporosis increases during ADT, preventive measures are recommended.
Fracture remains the most significant clinical end point related to CTIBL resulting from ADT. Moreover, fractures are an independent adverse predictor of survival in patients with prostate cancer (Oefelein MG, et al., 2002). No prospective data are yet available regarding the impact of ADT on fracture rates; nevertheless, several retrospective analyses provide

significant evidence for increased fracture risk. An analysis of 15,716 men with fractures and 47,149 matched controls in a nationwide, population-based, case-control study found that prostate cancer is associated with increased risk of fracture (odds ratio [OR] 1.8; 95% CI, 1.6 to 2.1), with an even higher increased risk of hip fracture (OR 3.7; 95% CI, 3.1 to 4.4). However, there was no increased risk of vertebral fractures, which are frequently underreported in the absence of sequential spine x-rays. When adjusted for prostate cancer, age, and previous fracture, an increased fracture risk was seen for both GnRH agonists, with or without non-steroidal anti-androgens (OR 1.7; 95% CI, 1.2 to 2.5; *P* .01), and orchiectomy (OR 1.7; 95% CI, 1.2 to 2.4; *P* .01).

Because survival in men with non-metastatic prostate cancer treated with hormone therapy is long (median survival time is 7 years), (Antonarakis ES, et al., 2007) long-term issues of bone health are of particular significance. Moreover, men with untreated disease tend to have lower BMD than their peers and, therefore, are at higher risk for fracture before beginning ADT (Smith MR, et al., 2001).

The identification of the incidence of CTIBL among patients with prostate cancer raises issues for clinicians, including the identification of those at increased fracture risk and appropriate preventative strategies. These questions are of concern not only for the specialist, but also for general practitioners who will frequently encounter these patients. Pharmacotherapy is key to the prevention and treatment of skeletal-related events. Successful treatment of the tumour is the best method of preventing skeletal-related events. Current measures in the treatment of CTIBL and others are cited below.

9.1 Lifestyle measures, calcium and vitamin D supplementation

Lifestyle modifications to address osteoporosis include exercise, smoking cessation and moderating alcohol and caffeine intake. In addition, men over 50 should have a total of 1500 mg daily of calcium and 800 IU daily of vitamin D (D3 being preferable to D2) (Brown JP, et al., 2002). However, the Osteoporotic Society of Canada guidelines state that while adequate calcium and vitamin D (whether dietary or supplemented) are essential adjuncts to prevent and treat osteoporosis, they are insufficient by themselves as treatments.

9.2 Bisphosphonates

Bisphosphonates (BPs) are often used for patients with bone metastases to prevent pathologic fractures, reduce bone pain or control hypercalcemia, but they are not specifically indicated for the prevention and treatment of cancer treatment induced bone loss. Numerous randomized controlled trials have explored the effects of BPs on BMD in the setting of ADT for non-metastatic prostate cancer (Greenspan SL, et al., 2007; Greenspan SL, et al., 2008), but to date none have had sufficient power to demonstrate a reduction in fractures. These trials demonstrate clearly that BPs are effective in reducing BMD loss associated with ADT for at least 1 year (Saad F, et al., 2008).

Since the mid-1990s, bisphosphonates have become a mainstay of the management of metastatic bone disease from breast, lung, and prostate cancer. They are the primary treatment of hypercalcemia, widely recommended to reduce the pain associated with metastatic disease and are the only class of agents approved to prevent the development of skeletal-related events.

Several placebo-controlled trials have demonstrated the (Coleman RE, 2004) benefit of using these agents to prevent skeletal-related events in patients with known bone metastasis.

Bisphosphonates have some limitations. First, long-term efficacy data are sparse. Oral BPs are poorly absorbed, must be taken on an empty stomach and often produce gastrointestinal side effects. Thus, long-term adherence to oral BPs tends to be poor; studies of 1-year adherence to BPs in postmenopausal women have found adherence rates under 60% even with once monthly treatments (Boonen S, et al., 2008). Due to lack of compliance, intravenous BPs are preferred to oral BPs; influenza-like acute phase reactions on initial administration are common but mild, while acute tubular necrosis is rare but serious.

9.2.1 Effect of bisphosphonates on preventing or treating bone complications

The use of bisphosphonates is an emerging therapy for preventing and treating osteoporosis and fractures in the management of recurrent and advanced prostate cancer disease. Moreover, these substances can act as pain relief agents (Verreuther R, 1993; Rodrigues P, et al., 2004). Bisphosphonates, synthetic analogs of the endogenous pyrophosphate molecule, inhibit osteoclast-mediated bone destruction by a decrease bone resorption in patients receiving ADT and/or with metastatic disease (Smith MR, 2003; Ryan CW, et al., 2006; Lipton A, 2004). These drugs selectively adsorb to mineral surfaces on bone that are surrounded by osteoclasts. The bisphosphonates are then released from the bone surface, where they are internalized by and disrupt the bone-resorbing action of osteoclasts (Lipton A, 2004). At least two types of bisphosphonates exist: non-nitro-gen-containing bisphosphonates (clodronate, etidronate) and the more potent nitrogen-containing bisphosphonates (alendronate, ibandronate, pamidronate, risedronate, zoledronic acid) (Lipton A, 2004). Both types of bisphosphonates have been evaluated in prostate cancer patients at risk of bone complications. Pamidronate has been shown to maintain BMD during ADT, whereas alendronate and zoledronic acid have been shown to increase BMD during ADT (Casey R, et al., 2006; Greenspan SL, et al., 2007). Zoledronic acid has also been shown to prevent metastatic disease induced bone complications (for example, fractures, spinal cord compression) in patients with hormone-refractory disease (Saad F, et al., 2002; Saad F, et al., 2004). At this time, no bisphosphonate is indicated for the prevention or treatment of ADT-induced bone loss; however, alendronate is indicated for treatment of men with osteoporosis (Higano CS, 2004). A randomized controlled trial demonstrated that a single infusion of zoledronic acid suppressed bone turnover for at least 12 months and increased BMD of the hip and spine in men receiving a GnRH agonist for non-metastatic prostate cancer. Compared with placebo, zoledronic acid increased BMD of the lumbar spine and hip by 7.1% and 2.6%, respectively (Berenson JR, 2005).

Bisphosphonates have been shown to decrease the risk of skeletal complications by approximately one third (Body JJ, 2003). In addition, bisphosphonates are clinically important for the treatment of hypercalcemia of malignancy and can reduce cancer induced bone pain. The two bisphosphonates approved by the FDA for use in patients with cancer involving bone are pamidronate and zoledronic acid. Clodronate and ibandronate have been licensed for use in malignant bone disease in other countries. Because of the high frequency of skeletal involvement in advanced cancers, bisphosphonates are routinely prescribed in the practice of medical oncology (Ramaswamy B & Shapiro CL, 2003).

A head-to-head non-inferiority trial of zoledronic acid vs pamidronate demonstrated no significant difference between the treatments. One thousand six hundred forty eight patients with osteolytic multiple myeloma or bone metastasis (osteoblastic or osteolytic) from breast cancer were randomized to receive monthly treatments with zoledronic acid (4 mg) or pamidronate (90 mg). The development of skeletal-related events was equivalent in the zoledronic acid and pamidronate groups (47% vs 51%, respectively), although fewer patients on zoledronic acid required radiotherapy (19% vs 24%; p = 0.037). Likewise, the time to skeletal-related events was similar at 376 days in the zoledronic acid group vs 356 days in patients treated with pamidronate (p = 0.151), although in a subgroup analysis of breast cancer patients on hormonal therapy, zoledronic acid appeared slightly more efficacious (p = 0.047). From this trial it was determined that there was equal benefit for patients using pamidronate or zoledronic acid (Rosen LS, 2003). When treating patients with skeletal lesions from cancer, current oncology practice in the United States typically uses either pamidronate, 90 mg, infused over at least 2 h every 3–4 wk, or zoledronic acid, 4 mg, infused over at least 15 min every 3–4 wk (Hillner BE, et al., 2003; Coleman RE, 2004). With the FDA approval of zoledronic acid in 2001, this agent has gained popularity in clinical practice because of its efficacy in reducing skeletal-related events and the shorter infusion time. Because of the lifelong risk of skeletal-related events in patients with metastatic bone disease, the clinical practice in the palliative setting has been to continue bisphosphonate therapy indefinitely.

9.2.2 Adverses effects of biphosphonates

Bisphosphonate-associated osteonecrosis of de jaw (ONJ) in patients with malignancy has come to the attention of the medical and dental communities primarily through case reporting, and the number of reported cases has been increasing over the past 3 yr. All bisphosphonates have been associated with cases of ONJ; however, this must be tempered with the acknowledgment of the lack of a consensus definition for ONJ and the unknown incidence of ONJ in the general population. The published literature reviewed by the task force identified <1000 cases (Khosla S, et al., 2007)). There are established guidelines for oral health care before initiating chemotherapy (Bamia A, et al., 2005).

A confirmed case of bisphosphonate-associated ONJ was defined as an area of exposed bone in the maxillofacial region that did not heal within 8 wk after identification by a health care provider, in a patient who was receiving or had been exposed to a bisphosphonate and had not had radiation therapy to the craniofacial region (Khosla S, et al., 2007).

A suspected case of bisphosphonate-associated ONJ was defined as an area of exposed bone in the maxillofacial region that had been identified by a health care provider and had been present for <8 wk in a patient who was receiving or had been exposed to a bisphosphonate and had not had radiation therapy to the craniofacial region (Khosla S, et al., 2007).

The risk factors for bisphosphonate-associated ONJ are:

Oral bone manipulating surgery, poor fitting dental appliances, intraoral trauma, duration of exposure to bisphosphonate treatment, co-administration of glucocorticoids, comorbid conditions (such as alcohol, tabacco, and malignancies), and pre-existing dental or periodontal disease.

Suggest recommendations for clinical management before initiating bisphosphonate therapy and when the diagnosis of ONJ has been made are as follows.

General recommendations:

- There should be free and complete communication between health care professionals (physicians and dentists) involved in treatment and between health care professionals and patients (Ruggerio SL, et al., 2004). Physicians should encourage patients to inform their dentist that they are taking a bisphosphonate.
- All patients starting or taking bisphosphonates should be informed of the benefits of bisphosphonate treatment. They should also be informed of the risks of

bisphosphonates, including the risk of ONJ, the signs and symptoms of ONJ, and the risk factors for developing ONJ (Ruggerio SL, et al., 2004).

- Patients taking bisphosphonates should be encouraged to maintain good oral hygiene and to have regular dental visits during which they can be instructed in proper dental hygiene and can receive proper dental care. They should be urged to report any oral problems to their dentist and physician.
- Education of physicians and patients about bisphosphonate-associated ONJ is vitally important in all circumstances and particularly in circumstances or locations where the resources to provide dental examinations and treatment are limited.

9.3 Raloxifene

Raloxifene is a selective estrogen receptor modulator (SERM) often used to treat osteoporosis in women. In a 12-month open-label study enrolling 48 men with nonmetastatic prostate cancer receiving Antiandrogen theraphy, the addition of raloxifene 60 mg daily significantly improved bone mass density at the total hip and spine (Smith MR, et al., 2004).

9.4 Bicalutamide

Bicalutamide is a non-steroidal anti-androgen, which increases estradiol levels when given as monotherapy. A 12-month, openlabel comparison of leuprolide versus bicalutamide (150 mg daily) in 52 men with non-metastatic prostate cancer showed that bicalutamide increased bone mass density (BMD) at several sites (e.g., lumbar spine BMD +2.5% vs. −2.5%; $p < 0.001$), as well as decreasing fat mass, fatigue, loss of libido and hot flushes compared with leuprolide. Breast tenderness and enlargement were seen more frequently in the bicalutamide group (Smith MR, et al., 2004). Finally, a recent prospective study whose population included 253 prostate cancer patients with osteoporosis found that bicalutamide treatment maintained BMD over 6 years (Wadhwa VK, et al., 2009).

9.5 Corticosteroids

Corticosteroids are used most commonly in patients that develop spinal cord compression, but may also be used in those with diffuse pain unresolved with bisphosphonate and analgesic use. As potent anti-inflammatory agents, they improve neurologic symptoms and pain through the reduction of vasogenic edema around the spinal cord. Dexamethasone is often the preferred agent due to its increased potency and central nervous system penetration (Kilmo P, et al., 2004).

Often a loading dose of 10 to 100 mg is administered, followed by a 16- to 96-mg/day maintenance dose, although controversy exists over which dose is more efficacious. High doses have been recommended (100 mg loading dose followed by 24 mg every 6 hours × 3 days) to quickly restore ambulation, although may increase the incidence of serious adverse effects (Kilmo P, et al., 2004; Cole J, et al., 2008; Heimdal K, et al., 1992). Systematic reviews of the literature found a shortage of quality data, but came to the following conclusions: "There is good evidence to support the use of high-dose dexamethasone (96 mg/d)" in non-ambulatory patients, "but inconclusive evidence for the use of moderate-dose steroids (16 mg/d) in conjunction with radiotherapy for the treatment of MSCC (Loblaw D, et al., 1998). They also state that there is fair evidence for not using steroids in non-paretic patients, although this is not common practice (Loblaw D, et al., 1998; Coleman RE, 2004).

Adverse effects of steroids include insomnia, increased appetite, edema, hyperglycemia, leukocytosis, increased risk of infection, and gastrointestinal bleeding. Patients receiving high doses are at increased risk of these effects and should receive close monitoring; ulcer prophylaxis should be considered. Since adrenal suppression is likely when doses are continued beyond 5 to 7 days, doses should be tapered when discontinuing therapy with these agents (Loblaw D, et al., 1998; Coleman RE, 2004).

9.6 Analgesics

Both opioid and non-opioid analgesics are recommended for the symptomatic treatment of pain. Clinical trials show that bisphosphonate therapy improves pain control and allows most patients to use lower opioid doses; however, bisphosphonates should be viewed as adjunctive for pain control because nearly all patients will require analgesics.
In patients with mild pain, non-steroidal anti-inflammatory drugs (NSAIDs) and acetaminophen are acceptable agents to use. Acetaminophen is preferred in patients with thrombocytopenia, renal dysfunction, those receiving nephrotoxic agents, or at risk for gastrointestinal bleeds. In patients with liver dysfunction, NSAIDs are preferred for mild pain (Wadhwa VK, et al., 2008).
Since most patients experience moderate to severe pain, opioid analgesics often are used. Patients naïve to opioid therapy should begin with low doses of immediate release agents (typically 5-15 mg orally morphine or 2-4 mg intravenous morphine) and reassessed every 1 to 2 hours for effect. After 24 hours of pain control on a short-acting regimen, patients should be converted to a long-acting agent such as sustained release morphine, oxycodone, fentanyl, or methadone for basal control. Patients who are opioid tolerant should begin with higher doses of short-acting agents; if they are on a long-acting product, this should be continued, increasing the dose as needed to account for short-acting opioid use. A similar approach should be taken in patients initiating opioid therapy as an outpatient, with a short-acting opioid available every 3 to 4 hours and close follow-up. A bowel regimen with a stimulant plus stool softener should be initiated to prevent constipation from opioid use. The National Comprehensive Cancer Network (NCCN) provides a useful guideline for pain management in cancer patients (Coleman RE, 2004).
Adjunct agents such as anticonvulsants (gabapentin, lamotrigine, topiramate), tricyclic antidepressants (amitriptyline, imipramine, desipramine, nortriptyline), venlafaxine, duloxetine, or topical analgesics (lidocaine or capsaicin) may also help to reduce neuropathic pain caused by nerve compression (Cole J, et al., 2008).

9.7 Upcoming agents: Toremifene citrate and denosumab

The effects on BMD of toremifene citrate, a new SERM, were tested in a 6-month, placebo-controlled dose-finding study with 46 men with prostate cancer receiving ADT. An oral dose of 60 mg daily significantly improved BMD and decreased hot flushes (Steiner MS, et al., 2004). A 2-year, double blind, placebo- controlled phase-III multicentre study of oral toremifene 80 mg has been completed in 1389 ADT patients with advanced prostate cancer; this compound reduced new morphometric vertebral fractures (the primary endpoint) by 53% ($p = 0.034$). Bone mineral density at lumbar spine, hip, and femur was also increased significantly ($p < 0.0001$), and lipid profiles were improved compared with placebo (Smith MR, et al., 2004; Schwarz EM & Ritchlin CT, 2006).
In advanced prostate cancer, metastasis is sadly inevitable. Although bone metastases from prostate cancer have a predominantly osteoblastic appearance, histological findings

(Roudier MP, et al., 2008) and analysis of bone turnover markers (Brown JE, et al., 2005; Demers LM, 2003), support the view that excess osteoclastic activity induces bone destruction in these metastases. The Receptor Activator of NF-B Ligand (RANKL) is the main driver of osteoclast formation, function, and survival (Boyle WJ, et al., 2003). Lymphocytes infiltrate the tumour, causing upregulation of nuclear factor-Kappa B (RANK) ligand (RANKL) and lymphotoxin (Luo et al., 2007). Denosumab is a fully human monoclonal antibody that specifically targets RANKL and is delivered by subcutaneous injection twice a year (Schwarz EM & Ritchlin CT, 2006). This therapy was found to be very effective in reducing fractures and was well-tolerated in the clinical settings of osteoporotic postmenopausal women (McClung MR, et al., 2006; Cummings SR, et al., 2009) and protecting BMD in osteopenic postmenopausal women receiving adjuvant aromatase inhibitors for breast cancer (Ellis GK, et al., 2008). More recently, denosumab (60 mg subcutaneously, every 6 months) was evaluated in a 36-month, phase-III, placebo-controlled randomized clinical trial involving 1468 men with non-metastatic prostate cancer who were receiving ADT.48 Compared with placebo, denosumab significantly improved BMD at all sites measured, including lumbar spine (the primary endpoint) by 6.7% ($p < 0.001$), total hip by 4.8% ($p < 0.001$), femoral neck by 3.9% ($p < 0.001$), and distal radius by 5.5% ($p < 0.001$) at 24 months; by the end of the trial (36 months), denosumab dramatically reduced the risk of new vertebral fractures (a secondary endpoint) by 62% ($p = 0.006$), but not overall survival in prostate cancer (Fizzazi et al., 2011).
A recent phase-III study comparing denosumab versus zoledronic acid (Fizazi K, et al., 2011) showed that denosumab was better than the established therapy, zoledronic acid, for the delay or prevention of skeletal-related events in patients with advanced prostate cancer, while there was no difference in overall survival or disease progression.

10. Conclusions

Disease-related skeletal complications are common in men with metastatic prostate cancer. Such events, including fracture, hypercalcemia, spinal cord compression, and severe pain are serious complications of several malignancies. Agents such as bisphosphonates should be used to prevent skeletal-related events; they and other agents such as corticosteroids and analgesics are effective in symptom management of skeletal-related events. Through the use of these agents, along with radiation and surgical therapy, outcomes and quality of life can be improved in patients with metastatic disease. Bone metastasis and skeletal related events predict poor prognosis in men with prostate cancer.

11. References

Jemal, A. Siegel, R. Xu, J. & Ward, E. Cancer statistics, 2010. (2010). CA *Cancer Journal Clinics* 60: 277-300.

Ferlay, J. Parkin, DM. & Steliarova-Foucher, E. (2010). Estimates of cancer incidence and mortality in Europe in 2008. *European Journal of Cancer* 46: 765-81.

Schulman, KL. & Kohles, J. (2007). Economic burden of metastatic bone disease in the US. *Cancer* 109: 2334-42.

Berruti, A. Dogliotti, L. & Terrone, C. (2002). Changes in bone mineral density, lean body mass and fat content as measured by dual energy X-ray absorptiometry in patients with prostate cancer without apparent bone metastases given androgen deprivation therapy. *Journal of Urology* 167: 2361-2367.

Diamond, TH. Higano, CS. Smith, MR. Guise, T. & Singer, F. (2004). Osteoporosis in men with prostate carcinoma receiving androgen-deprivation therapy. *Cancer* 100 (5): 892-9.

Fowler, JE. Bigler, SA. White, PC. & Duncan, W. (2002). Hormone therapy for locally advanced prostate cancer. *Journal of Urology* 168: 546-9.

Bolla, M. Gonzalez, D. & Warde, P. (1997). Improved survival in patients with locally advanced prostate cancer treated with radiotherapy and gosarelin. *New England Journal of Medicine* 337: 295-300.

Elliot, ME. Wilcox, AJ. & Carnes, ML. (2002). Androgen deprivation in veterans with prostate cancer: implications for skeletal health. *Journal of Bone Mineral Research* 17: 366-71.

Melton, LJ. Atkinson, EJ. O´Connor, MK. O´Fallon, WM. & Riggs, BL. (1998). Bone density and fracture risk in men. *Journal of Bone Mineral Research* 13: 1915-23.

Binkley, NC. Schmeer, P. Wasnich, RD. & Lenchik, L. (2002). What are the criteria by which a densitometric diagnosis of osteoporosis ca be made in males and non-Caucasians?. *Journal of Clinical Densitometry* 5: 19-27.

Zmuda, JM. Cauley, JA. Glynn, NY. & Finkelstein, JS. (2000). Posterior-anterior and lateral dual-energy X-ray absorptometry for the assessment of vertebral osteoporosis and bone loss among older men. *Journal of Bone Mineral Research* 15: 1417-24.

Faulkner, KG. (1998). Bone densitometry: choosing the proper skeletal site to measure. *Journal of Clinical Densitometry* 1: 279-85.

Weigert, JM. & Cann, CE. (1998). 3D QCT: a useful tool in following therapy. In: International Society of Clinical Densitometry. *Proceedings of the 4th annual Scientific Meeting of the International Society of Densitometry.* West Hartford: ISCD, 1-4.

Kaufman, JM. Johnell, O. & Abadie, E. (2000). Background for the studies on the treatment of male osteoporosis: state of the art. *Annals of Rheumathology Diseases* 59: 765-772.

Lenchik, L. Kiebzak, GM. & Blunt, BA. (2002). What is the role of serial bone mineral density measurements in patient management?. *Journal of Clinical Densitometry* 5: 29-38.

Delaet, C. van Hout, BA. Burger, H. Weel, AE. Hofman, A. & Pols, HA. Hip fracture prediction in elderly men and women: validation in the Rotterdam study. J Bone Miner Res 1998; 13: 1587-93.

Jones, G. Nguyen, T. Sambrook, P. Kelly, P. & Eisman, JA. (2004). Progressive loss of bone in the femoral neck in elderly people: longitudinal findings from the Dubbo Osteoporosis Epidemiology Study. *British Medicine Journal* 309: 691-95.

Stepan, JJ. Lachman, MA. Svereina, J. Pacovsky, V. & Baylink, D. (1989). Castrated men exhibit bone loss: effect of calcitonin treatment on biochemical indices of bone remodelling. *Journal of Clinical Endocrinology and Metabolism* 69: 523-27.

Daniell, HW. (1997). Osteoporosis after orchiectomy for prostate cancer. *Journal of Urology* 157: 439-44.

Bruder, JM. & Welch, MD. (2002). Prevalence of osteopenia and osteoporosis by central and peripheral bone mineral density in men with prostate cancer during androgen deprivation. *Journal of Bone Mineral Research* 17: 411-21.

Yaturu, S. DePrisco, C. & DjoDjo, S. (2002). Effect of bisphosphonates in osteoporosis secondary to LHRH analogs for prostate cancer. *Journal of Bone Mineral Research* 17: 474-79.

Greenspan, SL. (2008). Approach to the prostate cancer patient with bone disease. *Journal of Clinical Endocrinology and Metabolism* 93: 2-7.

Gilbert, SM. & McKiernan, JM. (2005). Epidemiology of male osteoporosis and prostate cancer. *Current Opinion in Urology* 15: 23-27.

Amin, S. & Felson, DT. (2001). Osteoporosis in men. *Rheumathology Diseases Clinics of North America* 27: 19-47.

Smith, MR. McGovern, FJ. & Zietmna, AL. (2001). Pamidronate to prevent bone loss during androgen-deprivation therapy for prostate cancer. *New England Journal of Medicine* 341: 948-55.

Morote, J. Planas, J. Orsola, A. Abascal, JM. Salvador, C. Trilla, E. Raventos, C. Cecchini, L. Encabo, G. Reventos J. (2007). Prevalence of osteoporosis during long-term androgen deprivation therapy in patients with prostate cancer. *Urology* 69 (3): 500-4.

Casey, R. Love, W. Mendoza, C. Reymond, D. & Zarenda, M. (2006). Zoledronic acid reduces bone loss in men with prostate cancer undergoing androgen deprivation therapy. *The 2006 Multidisciplinary Prostate Cancer Symposium*, 2006.

Michaelson, MD. Kaufman, DS. Lee, H. McGovern, FJ. Kantoff, PW. & Fallon, MA. (2007). Randomized controlled trial of annual zoledronic acid to prevent gonadotrophin-releasing hormone agonist-induced bone loss in men with prostate cancer. *Journal of Clinical Oncology* 25: 1038-42.

Smith, MR. Eastham, J. Gleason, DM. Shasha, D. Tchekmedyian, S. & Zinner, N. (2003). Randomized controlled trial of zoledronic acid to prevent bone loss in men receiving androgen deprivation therapy for non-metastatic prostate cancer. Journal of Urology 169: 2008-12.

Shahinian, VB. Kuo, YF. Freeman, JL. & Goodwin, JS. (2005). Risk of fracture after androgen deprivation for prostate cancer. *New England Journal of Medicine* 352: 154-64.

Smith, MR. Boyce, Sp. Moyneur, E. Duh, MS. Raut, MK. & Brandman, J. (2006). Risk of clinical fractures after gonadotrophin-releasing hormone agonist therapy for prostate cancer. *Journal of Urology* 175: 136-9.

Meng, MW. Grossfeld, GD. & Sadetsky, N. (2002). Contemporary patterns of androgen deprivation therapy use for newly diagnosed prostate cancer. *Urology* 60 (3): 7-11.

Sharifi, N. Gulley, JL. & Dahut, WL. (2005). Androgen deprivation therapy for prostate cancer. *Journal of the American Medical Association* 294: 238-44.

Mavrokokki, A. Cheng, A. Stein, B. & Goss, AN. (2007). Nature and frequency of bisphosphonate-associated osteonecrosis of the jaws in Australia. *Journal of Oral Maxillofacial Surgery* 65: 415 23.

Body, JJ. (2003). Effectiveness and cost of bisphosphonate therapy in tumour bone disease. *Cancer* 97 (3): 859-65.

Oefelein, MG. Ricchiuti, V & Conrad, W. (2002). Skeletal fractures negatively correlate with overall survival in men with prostate cancer. *Journal of Urology* 168: 1005-7.

Coleman, RE. (2001). Metastatic bone disease: clinical features, pathophysiology and treatment strategies. *Cancer Treatment Reviews* 27: 165-76.

Rosen, LS. Gordon, D. & Tchekmedyian, NS. (2003). Zoledronic Acid Versus Placebo in the Treatment of Skeletal Metastases in Patients With Lung Cancer and Other Solid Tumours: A Phase III, Double-Blind, Randomized Trial-The Zoledronic Acid Lung Cancer and Other Solid Tumours Study Group. *Journal of Clinical Oncology* 21: 3150-57.

Coleman, RE. (2006). Clinical features of metastatic bone disease and risk of skeletal morbidity. *Clinical Cancer Research* 12 (20): 6243-49.

Mundy GR. (2002). Metastasis: metastasis to bone: causes, consequences and therapeutic opportunities. *Nature Reviews of Cancer* 2 (8): 584.

Saad F. (2008). Targeting the receptor activator of nuclear factor-B (RANK) ligand in prostate cancer bone metastases. *British Journal of Urology Internationalis* 101(9): 1071-5.

Uehara, H. Kim, SJ. & Karashima, T. (2003). Effects of blocking platelet-derived growth factor-receptor signaling in a mouse model of experimental prostate cancer bone metastases. *Journal of the National Cancer Institute* 95 (6): 458-70.

Yin, JJ. Selander, K. & Chirgwin, JM. (1999). TGF-B signaling blockade inhibits PTHrP secretion by breast cancer cells and bone metastases development. *Journal of Clinical Investigation* 103 (2): 197-206.

Gruber, R. Pietshcmann, P. & Peterlik, M. (2008). Introduction to bone development remodelling and repair. In: Grampp S, ed. *Radiology of Osteoporosis.* 2nd Ed. Springer, 2008.

Brown, JP. & Josse, RG. (2002). Scientific advisory council of the osteoporosis society of Canada. 2002 Clinical practice guidelines for the diagnosis and management of osteoporosis in Canada. *Canadian Medical Association Journal* 167 (10): 1-34.

Boyle, WJ. Simone, WS. Lacey, DL. (2003). Osteoclast differentiation and activation. *Nature* 423: 337-42.

Hofbauer, LC. & Schoppet, M. (2004). Clinical implications of the osteoprotegerin/RANKL/RANK system for bone and vascular diseases. *Journal of the American Medical Association* 292: 490-95.

Boonen, S. Vanderschueren, D. & Venkek, K. (2008). Recent developments in the management of postmenopausal osteoporosis with bisphosphonates: enhanced efficacy by enhanced compliance. *Journal of Internal Medicine* 264: 315-32.

Oefelein, MG. Ricchiuti, V. & Conrad, W. (2002). Skeletal fractures negatively correlate with overall survival in men with prostate cancer. Journal of Urology 168: 1005-7.

Gleason, D. Saad, F. Goas, A. & Zheng, M. (2003). Continuing benefit of zoledronic acid in preventing skeletal complications after the first occurrence in patients with prostate cancer and bone metastases. *American Society of Clinical Oncology* 22: 379-83.

Major, PP. & Cook, R. (2002). Efficacy of bisphosphonates in the management of skeletal complications of bone metastases and selection of clinical endpoints. *American Journal of Clinical Oncology* 25 (6): 10-18.

Egerdie, B. & Saad, F. (2010). Bone health in the prostate cancer patient receiving androgen deprivation therapy: a review of present and future management options. *Can Urol Assoc J* 4 (2): 129–35.

Higano, CS. (2008). Androgen-deprivation therapy-induced fractures in men with non-metastatic prostate cancer: what do we really know?. *Nature Clinical of Practice Urology* 5: 24-34.

Perez, EA. Serene, M. & Durling, FC. (2006). Aromatase inhibitors and bone loss. *Oncology* 20: 1029-48.

Clarke, BL. Ebeling, PR. & Jones, JD. (1996). Changes in qualitative bone histomorphometry in aging healthy men. *Journal of Clinical Endocrinology and Metabolism* 81: 2264-70.

Singer, FE. Eyre, DR. (2008). *Cleveland Clinic Journal of Medicine.* 75: 739-50.

Khosla, S. Melton, LJ. Atkinson, EJ. O'Fallon, WM. Klee, GG. & Riggs, BL. (1998). Relationship of serum sex steroid levels and bone turnover markers with bone mineral density in men and women: a key role for bioavailable estrogen. *Journal of Clinical Endocrinology and Metabolism* 83: 2266-74.

Smith, MR. (2003). Diagnosis and management of treatment-related osteoporosis in men with prostate carcinoma. *Cancer* 97 (3): 789-92.

Groot, MT. Kruger, CG. Pelger, RC. & Uyl-de Groot, CA. (2003). Financial cost of patients with prostate cancer osseous metastasis in the Netherlands. *European Urology* 43: 226-30.

Berruti, A. Dogliotti, R. Bitossi, R. Fasolis, G. Gorzegno, G. & Bellina, M. (2000). Incidence of skeletal complications in patients with bone metastatic prostate cancer and hormone refractory disease. Predictive role of bone resorption and formation markers evaluated at baseline. *Journal of Urology* 164: 1248-51.

Saad, F. Adachi, JD. & Brown, JP. (2008). Cancer treatment-induced bone loss in breast and prostate cancer. *Journal of Clinical Oncology* 26: 5465-76.

Brufsky, AM. (2008). Cancer treatment-induced bone loss: pathophysiology and clinical perspectives. *Oncology* 13: 187-95.

Polascik, TK. (2008). Bone health in prostate cancer patients receiving androgen-deprivation therapy: the role of bisphosphonates. *Prostate Cancer* 11: 13-9.

Botteman, MF. Meijboom, M. Foley, I. Stephens, JM. Chen, YM. & Kaura, S. (2010). Cost-effectiveness of zoledronic acid in the prevention of skeletal-related events in patients with bone metastases secondary to advanced renal cell carcinoma: application to France, Germany and the United Kingdom. *European Journal of Health Economy* 31: 1117-23.

Sathiakumar, N. Delzell, E. Morrisey, MA. Falkson, C. Yong, M. Chia, V. Blackburn, J. Arora, T. & Kilgore, ML. (2011). Mortality following bone metastasis and skeletal-related events among men with prostate cancer: a population-based analysis of US Medicare beneficiaries. 1999-2006. *Prostate Cancer Prostatic Disease* 14 (2): 177-83.

Aljumaily, R. & Mathew, P. (2011). Optimal management of bone metastases in prostate cancer. *Current Oncology Reports* 13 (3): 222-30.

Shahinian, V. Yong-Fang, K. Freeman, JL. & Goodwin, JS. (2005). Risk of fracture after androgen deprivation for prostate cancer. *New England Journal of Medicine* 352 (2): 154-64.

Lage, MJ. Barber, BL. Harrison, DJ. & Jun, S. (2008). The cost of treating skeletal-related events in patients with prostate cancer. *American Journal of Management Care* 14 (5): 317-22.

Norgaard, M. Jensen, A. Jacobsen, JB. Cetin, K. Fryzek, JP. & Sorensen, HT. (2010). Skeletal related events, bone metastasis and survival of prostate cancer: a population based cohort study in Denmark (1999 to 2007). *Journal of Urology* 184 (1): 162-7.

Aapro, M. Abrahamsson, PA. Body, JJ. Coleman, RE. Colomer, R. Costa, L. Crino, L. Dirix, L. Gnant, M. Gralow, J. Hadji, P. Hortobagyi, GN. Jonat, W. Lipton, A. Monnier, A. Paterson, AH. Rizzoli, R. Saad, F. & Thürlimn, B. (2008). Guidance on the use of bisphosphonates in solid tumours: recommendations of an international expert panel. *Annals of Oncology* 19: 420-32.

Antonarakis, ES. Blackford, AL. & Garrett-Mayer, E. Survival in men with non-metastatic prostate cancer treated with hormone therapy: A quantitative systematic review. *Journal of Clinical Oncology* 25: 4998-5008.

Greenspan, SL. Nelson, JB. & Trump, DL. (2007). Effect of once-weekly oral alendronate on bone loss in men receiving androgen deprivation therapy for prostate cancer: a randomised trial. *Annals of Internal Medicine* 146: 416-24.

Coleman, RE. (2004). Bisphosphonates: clinical experience. *Oncologist* 9 (4): 14-27.

Verreuther, R. (1993). Bisphosphonates as an adjunct to palliative therapy of bone metastases from prostatic carcinoma. A pilot study on Clodronate. *British Journal of Urology* 72: 792-5.

Rodrigues, P. Hering, F. & Campagnari, JC. (2004). Use of bisphosphonates can dramatically improve pain in advanced hormone refractary prostate cancer patients. *Prostate Cancer Prostatic Diseases* 7: 350-54.

Ryan, CW. Huo, D. Demers, LM. Beer, TM. & Lacerna, LV. (2006). Zoledronic acid initiated during the first year of androgen deprivation therapy increases bone mineral density in patients with prostate cancer. *Journal of Urology* 176: 972-78.

Lipton, A. (2004). Pathophysiology of bone metastases: how this knowledge may lead to therapeutic intervention. *Journal of Support Oncology* 2: 205-13.

Saad, F. Gleason, DM. Murray, R. Tchekmedyian, S. Venner, P. & Lacombe, L. (2002). A randomized, placebo-controlled trial of zoledronic acid in patients with hormone-refractory metastatic prostate carcinoma. *Journal of the National Cancer Institute* 94: 1458-68.

Saad, F. Gleason, DM. Murray, R. Tchekmedyian, S. Venner, P. & Lacombe, L. (2004). Long-term efficacy of zoledronic acid for the prevention of skeletal complications in patients with metastatic hormone-refractory prostate cancer. *Journal National Cancer Institute* 96: 879-82.

Berenson, JR. (2005). Recommendations for zoledronic acid treatment of patients with bone metastases. *Oncologist* 10: 52-62.

Ramaswamy, B. & Shapiro, CL. (2003). Bisphosphonates in the prevention and treatment of bone metastases. *Oncology* 17: 1261-70.

Rosen, LS. Gordon, D. & Kaminski, M. (2003). Long-term efficacy and safety of zoledronic acid compared with pamidronate disodium in the treatment of skeletal complications in patients with advanced multiple myeloma or breast carcinoma. *Cancer* 98 (8): 1735-44.

Hillner, BE. Ingle, JN. Chlebowski, RT. Gralow, J. Yee, GC. Janjan, NA. Cauley, JA. Blumenstein, BA. Albain, KS. Lipton, A. & Brown, S. (2003). American Society of

Clinical Oncology update on the role of bisphosphonates and bone health issues in women with breast cancer. *Journal of Clinical Oncology* 21: 4042-57.

Khosla, S. Burr, D. Cauley, J. Dempster, D. Eheling, PR. Felsenberg, D. Gagci, RF. & Gilsanz V. (2007). Bisphosphonate-associated osteonecrosis of the jaw: report of a task force of the American Society for bone and mineral research *Oncology* 22: 1479-91.

Bamias, A. Kastritis, E. Bamia, C. Moulopoulos, LA. Melakopoulos, I. Bozas, G. Koutsoukou, V. Gika, D. Anagnostopoulos, A. Papadimitriou, C. & Terpos, E. (2005). Osteonecrosis of the jaw in cancer after treatment with bisphosphonates: incidence and risk factors. *Journal of Clinical Oncology* 23: 8580-87.

Ruggiero, SL. Mehrotra, B. Rosenberg, TJ. & Engroff, SL. (2004). Osteonecrosis of the jaws associated with the use of bisphosphonates: a review of 63 cases. *Journal of Oral Maxillofacial Surgery* 62: 527-34.

Wadhwa, VK. Weston, R. & Mistry, R. (2009). Long-term changes in bone mineral density and predicted fracture risk in patients receiving androgen-deprivation therapy for prostate cancer, with stratification of treatment based on presenting values. *British Journal of Urology Internationalis* 104: 800-5.

Kilmo, P. Kestle, JR. & Schmidt, MH. (2004). Clinical trials and evidence-based medicine for metastatic spine disease. *Neurosurgery Clinics of North America* 15 (4): 549-64.

Cole, J. & Patchell, R. (2008). Metastatic epidural spinal cord compression. *Lancet Neurology* 7 (5): 459-66.

Heimdal, K. Hirschberg, H. Slettebo, H, Watne, K. & Nome, O. (1992). High incidence of serious side effects of high-dose desamethasone treatment in patients with epidural spinal cord compression. *Journal of Neurooncology* 12 (2): 141-4.

Loblaw, D. & Laperriere, N. (1998). Emergency treatment of malignant extradural spinal cord compression: An evidence-based guideline. *Journal of Clinical Oncology* 16 (4): 1613-24.

Steiner, MS. Patterson, A. & Israeli, R. (2004). Toremifene citrate versus placebo for treatment of bone loss and other complications of androgen deprivation therapy in patients with prostate cancer. ASCO Annual Meeting Proceedings. *Journal of Clinical Oncology* 22: 4597-99.

Schwarz, EM. & Ritchlin, CT. (2007). Clinical development of anti-RANKL therapy. *Arthritis Research Therapy* 2007; 9: 57-63.

Roudier, MP. Morrissey, C. True, LD. Higano, CS. Vessella, RL. & Ott, SM. (2008). Histopathological assessment of prostate cancer bone osteoblastic metastases. *Journal of Urology* 180: 1154-60.

Demers, LM. (2003). Bone markers in the management of patients with skeletal metastases. *Cancer* 97: 874-9.

Luo, JL. Tan, W. Ricono, JM, Korchynskyi, O. Zhang, M. Gonias, SL. Cheresh, DA. Karin, M. (2007). Nuclear cytokine-activated IKKalpha controls prostate cancer metastasis by repressing Maspin. *Nature* 446: 690-94.

McClung, MR. Lewiecki, EM. & Cohen, SB. (2006). Denosumab in postmenopausal women with low bone mineral density. *New England Journal of Medicine* 354: 821-31.

Cummings, SR. San Martin, J. & McClung, MR. (2009). Denosumab for prevention of fractures in postmenopausal women with osteoporosis. *New England Journal of Medicine* 2009; 361: 756-65

Ellis, GK. Bone, HG. & Chlebowski, R. (2008). Randomized trial of denosumab in patints receiving adjuvant aromatase inhibitors for non-metastatic breast cancer. *Journal of Clinical Oncology* 26: 4875-82.

Fizazi, K. Carducci, M. Smith, M. Damiao, R. Brown, J. Karsh, L. Milecki, P. Shore, N. Rader, M. Wang, H. Jiang, Q. Tadros, S. Dansey, R. & Goessl, C. (2011). Denosumab versus zoledronic acid for treatment of bone metastases in men with castration-resistant prostate cancer: a randomised, double-blind study. *Lancet* 377 (68): 813-22.

16

Androgen Deprivation Therapy for Prostate Cancer

Stanislav Ziaran
University Hospital in Bratislava, Urology Clinic, Comennius University
Slovakia

1. Introduction

Since 1941, when Huggins and Hodges proved the favourable effect of surgical castration and oestrogen administration on the progression of metastatic prostate cancer (PCa) (1,2), androgen deprivation therapy (ADT) became the mainstay of management of advanced PCa till now. They demonstrated for the first time the responsiveness of PCa to androgen deprivation.

ADT effectively palliates the symptoms of advanced disease, significantly reduces tumor growth, but there is no conclusive evidence at present that it prolongs survival. Moreover, significant amount of data report that ADT is associated with several adverse effects. The most prominent include: loss of bone mineral density (BMD), which leads into increased fracture risk (3), induction of insulin resistance (4), unfavorable changes in serum lipid profile (5), changes in body composition (6) which can lead into increased cardiovascular morbidity (7) and changes in cognitive functions (8).

The aim of ADT is to cause severe hypogonadism, and adverse effects of ADT clearly demonstrate the essential and pluripotent role of male´s most important androgen - testosterone (TST).

2. Testosterone: A basal overview of biosynthesis, metabolism and its action

In the human male, the main circulating androgen is testosterone (TST). More than 95% of circulating TST is secreted by the testis (Leydig cells) which produce aproximately 6-7 mg of TST daily (9). The rest is secreted by the adrenal cortex, and very small quantities (especially pregnan derivatives) are formed by the cells of the brain (10).

Physiologic TST level in a male is 3-8 ng / ml. The source for the synthesis of steroids is cholesterol. This substrate may be synthetized *de novo* from acetate but it may be also taken up from plasma lipoproteins. Cleavage of the side chain of cholesterol in the mitochondria and the formation of pregnenolone (biologically inactive) is the start of steroidogenic cascade. Pregnenolone is further converted into various steroids by enzymes (cytochromes P450) in the endoplasmatic reticulum.

TST secretion is regulated by the hypothalamic-pituitary-gonadal axis. The hypothalamic luteinising hormone-releasing hormone (LHRH) stimulates the anterior pituitary gland to release luteinising hormone (LH) and follicle-stimulating hormone (FSH). The main regulator of Leydig cell function is LH, acting through the LH receptor (LHr) in Leydig cells.

LH and FSH are required for the development and maintance of testicular functions.The natural ligand for the LHr is LH, but also human choriogonatropin (hCG) can equally well activate the LHr. Activated LHr stimulate adenylyl cyclase via GTP binding proteins and this results in increased production of cyclic AMP (cAMP). cAMP increases steroid production (11).

The total concentration of steroids in target tissues (central and peripheral nervous system, bone, muscle, adipose tissue, haematopoetic system and myocardium) and body fluids is dependent on the presence of binding proteins (sex hormone binding globulin, SHBG, albumin). Binding proteins represent a storage form of circulating steroids, which bind 98% of circulating TST. The rest-2% is "free testosterone" (fTST), which is biologically active. Homeostasis is achieved by "closed" steroid feedback inhibition mechanism, where the plasmatic level of steroids affects the secretion of LH from adenohypophysis.

The effect of TST on target tissues is modulated by metabolic pathways.

1. *Aromatisation* of TST gives rise to 17b- estradiol. When the target cell is estrogen-dependent, the aromatase activity in target cells and supply of androgen substrate (TST) are of major importance for determining the rate of synthesis of estrogens. Aromatase cytochrome P450 enzyme is expressed in many tissues including placenta, ovary, testis, fat tissue, liver, brain, hair follicles.
2. *Reduction* of TST into 5-alfa-dihydrotestosterone (DHT) is achieved by 5a-reductase. This active form of TST (5 to 10 times more biologically effective) can fully activate the androgen receptor (AR) (12). There are 3 isoforms of 5a-reductase. Isoform 2 is clinically more important because its deficiency is associated with distinct clinical manifestations (13). Isoform 2 predominates in cells of the prostate and external genitalia, while isoform 1 predominates in the cells of the skin (except genitals), and in liver cells in small amounts. However, in prostate cancer cells, overexpression of isoform 1 is a common finding, thus increasing its clinical significance (14). In the total deficiency of isoform 2 (autosomal recessive) there is a serious alteration of the development of sex organs in utero (male pseudohermafroditism). Many mutations of the gene encoding isoform 2 are known and can result into a number of different clinical manifestations. Signs of its deficiency are small phallus, severe hypospadias, scrotum bifidum, residual prostate utriculus (15). The newly discovered isoform 3 may play an important role in the development of hormone-refractory prostate cancer (HRCaP) as its overexpression is found in the HRCaP cells (16).

In addition to these metabolic pathways, the level of DHT in target tissues is affected by other enzymes (hydroxysteroid dehydrogenases), which "fine-tune" the effect of androgens in the target tissues (17). Owing to these local conversions the peripheral plasma concentration of androgens are only a rough indicator for their biological activities (12).

The mechanism of action of androgens can be divided into genomic and non-genomic effect (12). Non - genomic effects of androgens include mechanisms affecting the flow of calcium in the cells and the effect on phosphorylation cascade of Map-kinase (18, 19), or membrane effects (20). Genomic effects are mediated by activation of androgen receptor (AR). AR acts as a transcription factor activated by its ligand (TST). By androgen binding, AR is translocated from the cytoplasm to the nucleus where it binds to its DNA domain and interacts as a homodimer with specific DNA sequences that are referred as androgen responsive elements (ARES) (21). Its binding to DNA leads into interactions with transcription factors (22) and other co-factor proteins (21). This results into the "up" or "down" regulation of transcription of target genes (23).

Androgen metabolites are excreted as free steroids or bound (conjugated). Conjugated steroids are bound to glucuronide or sulfate group. Androgens are mostly degraded in the liver (glucuronate, sulphates), but the prostate the skin also contribute significantly to the metabolism of androgens. All the steroid - metabolising enzymes constitute a network for transforming androgens into secretion products (conjugated, unconjugated) that finally leave the body via the urine or the skin. The flux though this network is great, because the half-life of TST in men is only 12 minutes (12).

3. Androgens and bone metabolism

Growth and resorption of bone tissue are mediated by *osteoblasts* and *osteoclasts*. Both types of cells exert mutual influence on each other and equilibrium between the activity of both cell lines maintains net bone mass during constant renewal and turnover. Decreased osteoblast activity and increased activity of osteoclasts leads into loss of bone mass. AR have been located on normal human osteoblasts (24) and both aromatizable and non-aromatizable androgens can stimulate of human osteoblasts proliferation in vitro (25).

Bone deformation strain represents a stimulus for osteoblastic activity. Androgens modify the effects induced by the mechanoreception of human osteoblastic cells by affecting adhesion molecule expression, i.e. fibronectin and the fibronectin receptor. These substances facilitate the adhesion of bone cells to the extracellular matrix, which represents a crucial requirement for osteoblastic development and function (26). In addition, the secretion of osteoprotegerin (OPG), which is unaffected by mechanical strain alone, is doubled when this stimulus occurs in the presence of androgens. OPG is a decoy receptor for RANKL (receptor activator of nuclear factor-kappaB ligand). RANKL is secreted by osteoblasts, it induces osteoclastogenesis stimulates osteoclast differentiation (27). Thus, OPG inhibits bone resoptive effect induced by RANKL (26). Accordingly, TST levels directly correlate with OPG concentrations in healthy men (28).

Parathyroid hormone (PTH) induces osteoclast formation a differentiation. Androgens have direct inhibiting effect on this process via osteoclasts, which express AR and these cells are also blocked form PTH effects by androgens when no conversion to estrogens occurs (29).

Androgens decrease the number of bone remodeling cycles by modifying the genesis of osteoclasts and osteoblasts from their respective progenitor cells. In addition, androgens also exert effects on the lifespan of mature bone cells: they exert pro apoptotic effects on osteoclasts and anti-apoptotic effects on osteoblasts and osteocytes. TST also modulates effects induced by other hormones and cytokines involved in bone metabolism (30).

Osteoblast activity is reflected by concentration of procollagen type 1 (carboxy-terminal: P1CP or amino-terminal: P1NP) and other non collagenous proteins secreted by osteoblasts, eg. osteocalcin and bone specific alkaline phosphatase (BSAP). Also OPG as a decoy receptor for RANKL, can serve as marker of osteoblast activity. Bone resorption, hence osteoclast activity, therefore, can be estimated by urinary excretion of degradation products of type I collagen, such as deoxypyridinoline (DPD) and collagen type I cross- linked N-telopeptide (NTX) (31).

An independent role of androgens in protecting bone mass, both by promoting bone formation and attenuating bone resorption has been demonstrated in humans. Nevertheless, the role of its metabolite estradiol is pivotal in bone metabolism (30).

Aromatization of TST to estradiol is a pivotal event concerning effects of sex steroids on bone metabolism. Estrogen receptors (ER) have been localized in human osteoblasts (32), osteoclasts (33), and osteocytes (34). Human males with mutations of ER or aromatase genes do not achieve normal bone density, despite normal or increased levels of serum TST (35).

4. Androgen deprivation therapy (ADT) and its side effects

ADT is increasingly attained through the use of luteinizing hormone-releasing hormone (LHRH) agonists, which down-regulate anterior pituitary receptors and lead to therapeutic hypogonadism, or directly by inhibiting pituary receptors by LHRH antagonists. The standard castration level is < 50 ng/dL. Prostate cells are physiologically dependent on androgens which stimulate its growth, function and proferation. TST, although not tumorigenic, is essential for the growth and perpetuation of tumor cells (36).
Prostate cancer (PCa) displays a range of clinical behavior, from slow-growing tumors of no clinical significance to aggressively metastatic and lethal disease. Most PCa cases diagnosed with present diagnostic techniques fall into the moderately differentiated group (grade 2, Gleason 6), of which the cancer-specific 10–15-year mortality is 18–30%. This is even lower in the group of PCa diagnosed with grade 1 and 2 or Gleason 4–6, and there are subgroups of patients who are not at risk of dying from PCa even within 15years. Overall mortality is then determined by comorbidity (37). While both short- and long-term ADT are effective for treating PCa, it can often have significant side-effects. It is important that these complications are recognized and managed appropriately so that adverse effects on the patient's quality of life (QoL) are minimized. There has been an increase in the use of ADT at all stages of PCa in recent years. The extensive use of ADT is raising concerns about adverse effects - loss of BMD being the most prominent.

5. Bone loss and osteoporosis

As shown above, androgens are important for maintenance of bone tissue. Although ADT is used in medical practice for more than 60 years, it's only few years that the clinicians became aware of serious and potentially catastrophic consequences resulting form long-term ADT.
Bone density is determined both by peak bone mass achieved during skeletal development and the subsequent amount of maintenance and resorption of bone tissue. Androgens affect both processes and thus are a pivotal determinant of bone mass in men.

5.1 Osteoporosis

Osteoporosis is defined as a systemic metabolic bone disease characterized by low bone mass density (BMD) and microarchitectural deterioration of bone tissue, with a consequent increase in bone fragility and susceptibility to fracture (38). Diagnosis of osteoporosis based on WHO definitions is developed for women originally (39). When based on male cutoffs, 1-2 million (3 - 6%) of men have osteoporosis and 8 -13 million (28 - 47%) have osteopenia; when based on female cutoffs, 280,000 - 1 million (1 - 4%) have osteoporosis and 4 - 9 million (15 - 33%) have osteopenia (40, 41). While this numbers may seem disturbing, it is believed that osteoporosis in men is substantially underdiagnosed and undertreated in the United States (42).
Female osteoporosis has been studied extensively and characterized due to its high prevalence (43) whereas male osteoporosis, especially that associated with ADT has gained focus only recently.

In men, osteoporosis occurs later than in women (44), but the prevalence of osteopenia does not differ significantly between men and women aged more than 50 years. Conversely, the prevalence of osteoporosis in men is lower than in women (40). Even though it may be underestimated when standard female BMD parameters are considered suitable for normal mineralization in men (45). Men generally have a higher BMD than women at the same age (46). Accordingly, the prevalence of male osteoporosis is greater when male-specific ranges are used in men above fifties: ranging from 1% to 4% of elderly men when the diagnosis is based on female cut-off points vs. 3% to 6% when based on male cut-off points (40).
Men are estimated to lose bone mineral density (BMD) at a rate of up to 1% per year with advancing age (47, 48), and one in eight men over age 50 years will experience an osteoporosis-related fracture in their lifetime (49). Of all osteoporotic fractures, hip fractures contribute to the greatest morbidity as well as mortality, both of which are much greater in men than in women (50-52).

5.2 Diagnosis of osteoporosis

Current guidelines recommend assessment of bone mineral density (BMD) previous to ADT and yearly thereafter (53) with dual-energy x-ray absorptiometry (DXA) which is considered the standard method to measure BMD (54). International Society for Clinical Densitometry (ISCD) recommends that central skeleton sites (lumbar spine, total hip and femoral neck) are the most appropriate locations to asses BMD (55).
Diagnosis of osteoporosis can than be made according to WHO classification: if T- score is less than 2,5 of standard deviation. Values between (-) 1 and (-) 2.5 SD (standard deviation) is defined as osteopenia. T - score stands for the number of standard deviations (SD) from the density of young healthy individuals of the same sex (39).(Table 1)
To improve the identification of patients at highest risk of fracture, WHO has developed an algorithm to predict fractures - FRAX ™ http://www.shef.ac.uk/FRAX/
According to European Association of Urology (EAU) guidelines, a precise evaluation of BMD should be performed by dual X-ray absorptiometry before starting long-term ADT. An initial low BMD (T-score below 2.5, or below 1 if other risk factors are present) indicates a high risk of subsequent non-metastatic fracture, suggesting the need for early use of preventive bisphosphonate therapy (56).

Clasiffication	T-score
Normal	>-1
Osteopenia	-1 - -2,5
Osteoporosis	<-2,5

Table 1.

5.3 ADT, prostate cancer (PCa) and clinical aspects of bone disease

At presence, significant amount of data report that ADT is associated with the loss of BMD in a time-dependent manner (57-59) which leads into increased fracture risk (60). Skeletal fractures negatively correlate with overall survival in men with PCa (61) and maintaining skeletal health is crucial for QoL and survival (62).
Treatment of complications of pathological fractures is complicated and expensive (63). Moreover, the typical feature of PCa is the ability to metastasize into bone in more than 80 % of cases (64). Most bone lesions in PCa are osteoblastic in nature (65). However, studies

show that osteoblastic lesions in PCa have excessive bone growth, but on the other hand also simultaneously increased osteolysis (66). The new bone formed by tumor stimulated osteoblast is weak and poorly mineralized and subsequent osteopenia leads into increased osteolysis - result to the creation of bone matrix with seriously compromised integrity. The risk of developing bone complications is therefore increased.

Treatment of PCa does not focus on skeletal complications that may arise from bone metastases. The main symptom of bone metastases is severe bone pain, which often requires strong narcotic therapy or palliative radiation therapy. Other complications include spinal cord compression and pathological fractures, which may require surgery. These skeletal complications have a negative effect on QoL (65).

Data from a double-blind, placebo-controlled studies show that approximately half of patients treated with ADT had one or more events associated with the skeleton. Most of these events required palliative radiotherapy, or were pathological fractures (67). Skeletal complications are also associated with significant financial expenditure. A recent analysis of the costs of health insurance in the U.S. since 1994 until 2002 revealed that the total cost to treat patient with PCa who had skeletal event were 20 000 dollars higher than in patient who did not experience skeletal event (68).

Interestingly, it has been reported that hormone naive patients with advanced PCa have lower baseline BMD than healthy control, and relatively high prevalence of osteopenia and osteoporosis (69, 70). The largest study that investigated the association of BMD measures with PCa risk in older men enrolled was the Osteoporotic Fractures in Men Study (MrOS) (71).

MrOS was prospective study conducted on 4597 men with mean follow up 5.2 years, which evaluated the association of BMD and incidental PCa in a cohort of older men with no history of PCa. Unexpectedly, the authors found that higher total body BMD was significantly related to reduced risk for PCa. This result was „unexpected" because authors presumed that the higher levels of androgens lead into higher prevalence of PCa, which positively correlates with BMD. Additionally, total body BMD was inversely associated with the development of high-grade, but not low-grade disease. A similar but weaker association was observed for total hip BMD with high-grade PCa. This study confirms the association, although still not elucidated, between low BMD and PCa.

5.4 Treatment of ADT induced osteoporosis

Lifestyle changes: Immobilization is an important cause of bone loss. Immobile patients lose bone mass more rapidly than mobile patients. Regular daily activities, overcoming gravity, walking, and exercise have a positive impact on bone density: it stimulates osteoblasts to produce new bone and inhibits osteoclasts, thereby decreasing resorption of bone. It also improves physical coordination (prevention of falls). Cessation of smoking, decreased alcohol consumption and normalization of body mass index (BMI) helps to maintain BMD (72).

Ca supplementation: The ideal is to ensure that the amount of calcium is taken in the normal diet. If the patient is unable to take the recommended amount of calcium in the diet (lactose intolerance, hyperlipoproteinemia, etc) it is recommended for calcium supplementation (1000mg - 1500 mg daily) (72).

Vitamin D: Supplementation of vitamin D is recommended when its deficiency can be assumed or proven. The recommended daily dose is 400-800 IU (10-20 mg).

Bisphosphonates are one of the most potent inhibitors of bone resorption. The effect on the reduction of osteoporotic fractures has been demonstrated for treatment with alendronate, risedronate, ibandronate, etidronate and zoledronic acid. The effectiveness in reducing vertebral and nonvertebral fractures were confirmed by many studies (73, 74, 75). The optimal regimen for zoledronic acid is unclear, because one study recommends treatment every 3 weeks (76), while another trial has produced similar results with an annual injection (77), and finally, another study reports that single infusion of zoledronic acid in patients receiving ADT reduces bone mineral loss and maintains BMD at least for 12 months during ADT (78).
One of the most important and serious adverse effect of bisphoshonate administration is jaw necrosis (79) The initial BMD could be used to guide the choice of regimen (80).Thus, a 3-month injection might be given in osteoporotic patients, for whom a yearly injection is likely to provide insufficient protection (56).
Denosumab is a fully human monoclonal antibody against RANKL (see above). In the largest, well conducted study to date, denosumab was associated with 5.6% increase in the lumbar BMD versus 1% decrease in the placebo arm. There were also significant BMD increases at the total hip, femoral neck and distal third of the radius. 60 mg was delivered subcutaneously every 6 months, was not associated with any significant toxicity, or delayed healing in vertebral fractures (81).

6. Androgens and cognitive functions

It is known that during certain developmental stages- especially during the first years of life, during adolescence, girls surpass in boys several verbal skills. Males excel after about the tenth year of life in non-verbal skills in adulthood, especially in spatial orientation and manipulation (82).
Evidence of a link between sex hormones and spatial abilities came from studies of individuals with Turner syndrome (XO karyotype, no gonadal hormones) or testicular feminization syndrome- (XY karyotype, the tissues are refractory to normal levels of TST). These patients have female external genitalia, they are raised as girls. In these patients verbal skills surpass their spatial abilities, which is a typical pattern of cognitive abilities of women (83).
Studies on men with idiopathic or acquired hypogonadotrophic hypogonadism confirm the importance of TST for spatial abilities. Short-term androgen supplementation did not restore spatial function, suggesting that low levels of sex hormones during the intrauterine and neonatal period have a lifelong impact (84).
Direct sex hormones manipulation supports the conclusion that androgens play an important role in cognition. The first experiments with direct hormonal manipulation can be traced back to 1941 when Simonson et al. (85) published their experiment using methyl TST that was administered to eunuchoids, castrated males, and elderly men. The result was an improved ability to perceive the flicker (critical flicker frequency), a measure of attention and alertness, as long as the androgen treatment lasted (86).
Androgen therapy was also administered to female to male transsexuals in high doses as a preparation before gender reassignment. Their spatial skills have significantly improved, while verbal skills declined considerably (87).
For ethical reasons, nowadays the manipulation of gonadal hormones is restricted to patients in clinical studies. Thus, the last such study was conducted in 1971. Klaiber et al. (88) studied the effect of infused TST on mental abilities in healthy male students. After a 4-

hour infusion of TST or saline in the control group, performance of the control group (saline infusion) showed a significant decline in mental performance when compared to TST infused group.

6.1 Potential mechanisms of action

TST may impact cognition through several mechanisms. For example, activation of calcium channels in the brain occurs through rapid, nongenomic methods of action on G-protein-coupled, agonist sequestrable testosterone membrane receptors that initiate a transcription-independent signal pathway (89). TST also may impact cognitive performance directly through modulating neurotransmitters and stimulating neuronal connectivity, decreasing β-amyloid peptide production, and preventing N-methyl-D-aspartate excitotoxicity (90) mechanisms implicated in cognitive disorders such as Alzheimer disease or dementia. Furthermore, some estrogen studies have highlighted several possible mechanisms through which this hormone can impact cognitive functioning (91). These include increasing cholinergic activity through its action of choline acetyltransferase, maintenance of dendritic spine density on CA1 pyramidal cells of the hippocampus and facilitating induction of long-term potentiation in the hippocampus, increasing serotonergic and cholinergic activity to maintain neural circuitry, altering lipoprotein, and decreasing risk of cerebral ischemia (92, 93).

6.2 Cognitive functions and ADT

Green et al were the first to systematically research the impact of androgen-ablation therapy on the cognitive functioning of men with PCa. Sixty-five men (mean age, 73 years) with advanced PCa were assigned randomly to 1 of 4 groups: leuprolide (N = 19), goserelin (N = 20), cyproterone acetate (N = 11), and monitoring without hormone treatment (N = 15). All men participated in a battery of neuropsychological assessments at baseline (ie, 1 week before treatment) and then 6 months later. PSA and TST levels decreased significantly from baseline to 6 months for the 3 hormonally treated groups. Conflicting results emerged in the memory domain; men in the goserelin group surprisingly improved on 2 measures of memory (verbal [Wechsler Memory Scale-Revised] and visual [Rey-Osterrieth Complex Figure test]) but declined in another measure of verbal memory (Auditory Verbal Learning Test). The goserelin group also declined in a measure of executive functioning (Trails B). Of the 50 men on active treatments, 24 men showed a reliable decline (ie, >1 standard deviation) on at least 1 cognitive task, and 7 men showed a reliable change on 2 tasks, whereas the monitoring-only group showed no decline on any of the tasks (94).

Salminen et al researched the cognitive effects of ADT on 26 men who were diagnosed recently with PCa and who began ADT 2 months before radiotherapy. From baseline to 12 months, tests of visuomotor speed and of reaction time saw significant decreases. The decline in TST coincided with a decline in visuomotor processing (digit symbol), reaction time (10-choice reaction time), working memory speed (subtraction), sustained attention (vigilance), and recognition speed (recognition of letters) (95).

Jenkins et al assessed 32 men with standard neuropsychological assessments at 3 time intervals: at baseline, 3 months, and 9 months. The average age of these men was 67.5 years, and they used ADT for 3 to 5 months. Twenty-five healthy men, similar in age, served as the control group. Although there was no overall group effect, a greater percent of men in the ablation group reported a significant cognitive decline in 1 task (47%)

compared with the control group (17%; odds ratio, 4.412; $P < .05$) at the 3-month time point. There were no significant differences between the groups at the 9-month time point. On specific domain analysis, the tasks most impacted at the 3 month time point were spatial memory and ability (96).

Joly et al compared physical and cognitive function in a cross-sectional study of 57 patients who were receiving ADT for nonmetastatic PCa and 51 healthy, age-matched controls. Thirty patients received ADT as adjuvant treatment after prostatectomy or radiotherapy, and 27 patients received ADT for increasing levels of PSA. The median duration on ablation therapy was 1.8 years (range, 0.4-7.4 years). To assess cognitive functioning, the researcher administered the Sensitivity Cognitive Screen and a self-reported assessment on cognitive deficits (the Functional Assessment of Cancer Treatment-Cognitive Scale [FACT-COG]). In contrast to other studies cited above, Joly and colleagues observed that, although men with nonmetastatic PCa who received ADT experienced more treatment-related symptoms, no differences in cognitive function on either the High Sensitivity Cognitive Screen or the FACT-COG. The authors suggested that the High Sensitivity Cognitive Screen may not be sensitive enough to detect the subtle cognitive changes that occur after ADT. In addition, self-report of cognitive function has not been correlated consistently with actual neuropsychological testing (97).

In conclusion, the data show that androgen ablation does have cosequences for cognitive functioning. Larger longitudinal studies are warranted.

6.3 ADT and changes in body composition

Male hypogonadism (of any etiology) results in a decline in lean body mass (LBM) and an increase in fat mass, which is reversed with TST replacement (98). A cross-sectional study showed that men undergoing long-term ADT (12–101 months) have increased fat mass in the trunk and all extremities- measured by dual-energy x-ray absorptiometry (DXA), compared with eugonadal men with PCa not undergoing ADT (treated with prostatectomy and/or radiation therapy) and age-matched eugonadal controls (99).

Another case control study examined the prevalence and magnitude of obesity and fat mass in a group of 62 men with PCa receiving ADT for 1–5 yr (100). Healthy men ($n = 47$) with a PSA of less than 4.0 ng/ml were recruited as controls. The study showed that men with PCa had significantly higher body weight (86.5 vs. 80.6 kg) and percent body fat (30 vs. 26%) than controls.

Meta-analysis of sixteen studies showed that ADT increased percentage of body fat by on average 7.7% (95% CI 4.3, 11.2, from seven studies, $P < 0.0001$) and decreased % LBM by on average -2.8% (95% CI -3.6, -2.0, from six studies, $P < 0.0001$) but for both there was marked heterogeneity between studies ($I2 = 99\%$ $I2 = 73\%$, respectively). Similarly, body weight (2.1%, $P < 0.0001$ from nine studies) and BMI (2.2%, $P < 0.0001$, from eight studies) increased significantly. More extensive changes were seen with longer duration of treatment (101).

These studies prove that ADT results in an unfavorable body composition. The increase of fat mass in patients on ADT correlates positively with rising insulin levels (102). Hence, this increasing adiposity may be the primary event leading to these metabolic complications (possibly via elaboration of adipokines and inflammatory cytokines). Similarly, it is possible that a decrease in muscle mass may result in decreased glucose uptake by the muscle. These changes may ultimately lead to insulin resistance and diabetes in this population, hence predisposing them to cardiovascular disease. Lifestyle changes or suitable interventions to minimize the effect of ADT on body composition need to be investigated.

7. ADT and insulin resistance

Epidemiological studies have shown that low TST levels predict the development of insulin resistance and type 2 diabetes (103, 104, 105). Studies have also confirmed a direct relationship between serum TST and insulin sensitivity (106). These findings are further supported by interventional studies showing an improvement in insulin sensitivity with TST replacement in hypogonadal obese men (107).

7.1 Early metabolic changes

There is some evidence, that the onset of insulin resistance can be detectable after 3 months of ADT (108, 109). 3-month prospective study using combined androgen blockade with leuprolide and bicalutamide showed a 43% increase in fat mass and a 26% increase in insulin levels from baseline, again indicating development of insulin resistance with increasing adiposity (110). Although there was no significant change in fasting glucose levels, a statistically significant increase in glycosylated hemoglobin was seen (though this increase was within the normal range from 5.46–5.62%). These observations suggest that insulin resistance develops within a few months of initiating ADT; however, this compensatory hyperinsulinemia prevents the development of diabetes.

7.2 Late metabolic changes

Observational study of a population-based cohort found that men undergoing ADT with GnRH agonists had a higher risk of incident diabetes (11%), coronary artery disease (25%), myocardial infarction, and sudden death (111). Interestingly, orchiectomy was associated only with a higher risk of diabetes. In some men, this risk was evident within 4 months of starting ADT. These findings suggest that although both medical and surgical modalities of ADT result in increased metabolic burden, GnRH analogs are also associated with cardiovascular events.

After 12 months of ADT, serum fasting glucose increased significantly (112), suggesting that men with PCa who are receiving long-term ADT are at risk for developing insulin resistance and hyperglycemia, thus leading to their increased risk of cardiovascular disease (113).

A retrospective study which enrolled 396 patients with a median follow-up of 60.1 months, 36 (11.3%) patients developed new- onset diabetes mellitus (NODM). In 77 patients with pre-existing diabetes, there was an increase of >/=10% in serum HbA1c or fasting glucose levels in 15 (19.5%) and 22 (28.6%), respectively. On multivariate analysis, a BMI of >/=30 kg/m(2) was associated with an increased risk of developing NODM (odds ratio 4.65, $P = 0.031$) (114).

In conclusion, patients receiving ADT for PCa with or with no history of diabetes should have routine surveillance of glycaemic control, with appropriate preventive and treatment measures.

8. ADT and lipid alterations

Hyperlipidemia is a known risk factor for cardiovascular disease. Recent epidemiological research suggests that low serum TST levels in men are associated with an adverse lipid profile, especially elevated total cholesterol, LDL cholesterol, and triglycerides (115). Furthermore, interventional studies have shown that TST replacement in hypogonadal men results in an improvement in lipid profile (116).

During long-term ADT, triglycerides rise by approximately 26% and total cholesterol approximately 10%. (117, 118, 119) In addition, high-density lipoprotein (HDL) rises approximately 8% to 11%. The net effect of these changes on cardiovascular risks is unknown. Significant changes can be observed within the first 3 months of treatment, with more modest subsequent change (110).

9. ADT, metabolic syndrome and cardiovascular disease

Metabolic syndrome (MS) is a known risk factor for cardiovascular disease (CVD) (120). According to the Adult Treatment Panel III guidelines (121), a man is considered to have MS if he meets 3 of the following 5 criteria: fasting plasma glucose level >110 mg/dL, serum triglyceride level 150 mg/dL, serum high-density lipoprotein level <40 mg/dL, waist circumference >102 cm, and blood pressure ≥ 130/85 mmHg. Subjects on antihypertensive and antilipid medications are also considered positive for the respective criteria. Recently, male hypogonadism has surfaced as an independent risk factor for MS. Cross-sectional studies have shown that men with hypotestosteronemia have a higher prevalence of MS (122). Longitudinal studies also show that lower androgen levels in men independently predict the development of MS (105).

These observations suggest that profound hypogonadism due to ADT imparts increased metabolic burden. Long-term prospective studies are needed to determine the time of onset of various metabolic alterations in these men.

Since MS is associated with CVD, large studies were conducted to assed the CV risk and ADT. A large SEER-Medicare–based analysis of 73,196 men aged 66 years and older with PCa identified significant GnRH agonist-associated elevations in risk for myocardial infarction (HR, 1.11; p= .03), sudden cardiac death (HR, 1.16; p = .004), and new diagnosis of coronary heart disease (HR, 1.16; p< .001) (123). Similarly, a second SEER-Medicare–based study of 23,000 men with PCa found a 20% ADT-attributable rise in CV morbidity at 1 year (124).

In contrast, a recently reported matched cohort analysis of approximately 20,000 men in an On-tario database found no association between ADT and acute myocardial infarction (HR, 0.91; 95% CI, 0.84–1.00) (125).

A smaller population-based observational study of 3262 men who had undergone prostatectomy for PCa found that ADT was significantly associated with CV mortality, although only in the subset of men aged 65 years and older (126). This analysis failed to validate baseline coronary artery disease and diabetes as risk factors for CV mortality. Finally, combined analysis of 3 randomized trials involving men with localized PCa found that in the subset of men aged 65 years and older, 6 months of treatment with a GnRH agonist led to earlier onset of fatal myocardial infarction (127).

Three large randomized, controlled trials by the Radiation Therapy Oncology Group (RTOG) have been retrospectively analyzed for an association between neoadjuvant/ concomitant/adjuvant ADT and CV mortality. These analyses have not found convincing evidence of an association (128-130). Secondary analyses of a randomized controlled trial from the EORTC found no association between ADT and CV mortality. The RTOG and EORTC trials were randomized, featured large enrollments, and had long-term follow-up.

Bone metabolism	Loss of BMD, skeletal events (fractures), increased morbidity&mortality
Bone marrow	Anaemia
Lipid profile alterations	Increased: overall cholesterol, TAG, LDL, HDL
Impaired insuline sensitivity	Hyperinsulinemia, new onset diabetes, worsening existing DM
Body composition	Increase in fat mass, decrease in muscle mass, increased BMI
Cardiovascular disease	Increased risk of CV morbidity and mortality (?)
Metabolic syndrome	See above
Cognitive functions	Impaired spatial cognition, reaction time, other (?)
Other	Mood changes, loss of libido

Table 2. Summary of main organ systems affected by severe hypogonadism (by ADT)

10. References

[1] Huggins C, Hodges CV. Studies on prostatic cancer. I. The effect of castration, of estrogen and of androgen injection on serum phosphatase in metastatic carcinoma of the prostate. J Urol 2002 Feb;167(2P 2):948-51, discussion 952.

[2] Huggins C, Stevens RE Jr, Hodges CV. Studies on prostate cancer. II. The effect of castration on advanced carcinoma of the prostate gland. Arch Surg 1941;43:209-23.

[3] Shahinian V, Kuo Y, JLFreeman, Goodwin J. Risk of fracture after androgen deprivation for prostate cancer. N Engl J Med 2005; 352:154-164.

[4] Smith MR, Lee H, Nathan DM. Insulin sensitivity during combined androgen blockade for prostate cancer. J Clin Endocrinol Metab. 2006;91(4):1305-8.

[5] Hakimian P, Blute M, Jr, Kashanian J, et al. Metabolic and cardiovascular effects of androgen deprivation therapy. BJU Int. 2008;102:1509–1514

[6] Smith MR, Finkelstein JS, McGovern FJ, et al. Changes in body composition during androgen deprivation therapy for prostate cancer. J Clin Endocrinol Metab. 2002;87:599–603

[7] Saigal CS, Gore JL, Krupski TL, et al. Androgen deprivation therapy increases cardiovascular morbidity in men with prostate cancer. Cancer. 2007;110:1493–1500

[8] Nelson CJ, Lee JS, Gamboa MC, Roth AJ. Cognitive effects of hormone therapy in men with prostate cancer: a review. Cancer. 2008;113(5):1097-106.

[9] Coffey DS (1988) Androgen action and the sex accesory tissues. In: Knobil E, Neill (eds): The physiology of reproduction. J. Raven Press, New York,pp 1081-1119

[10] Baulieu EE (1997) Neurosteroids: of the nervous system, by the nervous system, of the nervous system. In: Rec Prog Horm Res 52: pp 1-32

[11] Saez JM (1994) Leydig cells: endocrine, paracrine and autocrine regulation. Endocr Rev 16: 574-626

[12] Rommerts FFG (2004), Testosterone: Action, Deficiency, Subsitution. Third Edition In:Nieschlag E, Behre HM (Eds): Testosterone: an overview of biosynthesis, transport, metabolism and non genomic functions. Cambrigde University Press, pp 1-39

[13] Wilson JD, Griffin JE, Russel DW (1993) Steroid 5a-reductuase 2 deficiency. Endocr. Rev. 14:577-593

[14] Tindall DJ, Rittmaster RS (2008) : The rationale for inhibiting 5alpha-reductase isoenzymes in the prevention and treatment of prostate cancer. J Urol. 2008 Apr;179(4):1235-42.
[15] Baskin LS (2004) Abnormalities of sexual determination &differentation In:Tanagho EA, McAninch WJ (Eds) Smith´s general urology, 16th Edition, Lange Medical Books, p660 (2004)
[16] Uemura M, Tamura K, Chung S, Honma S, Okuyama A, Nakamura Y, Nakagawa H. (2008): Novel 5 alpha-steroid reductase (SRD5A3, type-3) is overexpressed in hormone-refractory prostate cancer., Cancer Sci. 2008 Jan;99(1):81-6.
[17] Ziaran S, Goncalves FM, Štefančík J, Breza J Sn. The effect of androgens on cognitive function and bone. Lek Obzor. 2009; 3:116-20
[18] Guo Z, Benten WP, Krucken J, Wunderlich F (2002), Nogenomic testosterone calcium signaling. Genotropic actions in androgen receptor-free macrophages J Biol Chem 277:29600-29607
[19] Castoria G, Lombardi M, Barone MV, Bilancio A, Di Domenico M, Bottero D, Vitale F, Migliaccio A, Auricchio F.: Androgen-stimulated DNA synthesis and cytoskeletal changes in fibroblasts by a nontranscriptional receptor action., J Cell Biol. 2003 May 12;161(3):547-56.
[20] Papakonstanti E.A, Kampa M, Castanas E, and Stournaras C. A rapid, nongenomic, signaling pathway regulates the actin reorganization and PSA secretion induced by membrane testosterone receptors' activation. Mol. Endocrinol. 17(5), 870-881 (2003).
[21] Klocker H, Gromoll J, Cato ACB, (2004) The androgen receptor: molecular biology, Third Edition In:Nieschlag E, Behre HM (Eds) Testosterone: Action, Deficiency, Subsitution. Cambrigde University Press,pp 39-92
[22] Lee DK, Duan HO, Chang C.: From androgen receptor to the general transcription factor TFIIH. Identification of cdk activating kinase (CAK) as an androgen receptor NH(2)-terminal associated coactivator.,: J Biol Chem. 2000 Mar 31;275(13):9308-13
[23] Quingley CA, DeBellis A, Marschke KB, El-Awady MK, Wilson EM, French FS (1995). Androgen receptor defects: historical, clinical and molecular perspectives., Endocr Rev 16:271-321
[24] Colvard DS., Erikse EF., Keeting PE., Wilson EM., Lubahn DB., French FS., Riggs BL., Spelsberg TC., (1989) Identification of androgen receptors in normal human osteobast-like cells. Proc Natl Acad Sci USA 86: 854-857
[25] Kasperk CH., Wakley GK., Hierl T., Ziegler R., (1997) Gonadal and adrenal androgens are potent regulators of human bone cell metabolism in vitro. J Bone Miner Res 12: 464-471
[26] Liegibel UM., Sommer U., Tomakidi P., Hilscher U., Van den Heuvel L., Pirzer R., Hillmeier J., Nawroth P., Kasperk C., (2002) Concerted action of androgens and mechanical strain shifts bone metabolism from high turnover into an osteoanabolic mode. J Exp Med 196: 1387- 1392
[27] Khosla S., (2001) Minireview: the OPG/RANKL/RANK system. Endocrinology 142: 5050-5055
[28] Szulz P., Hofbauer LC., Heufelder AE., Roth S., Delmas PD., (2001) Osteoprotegerin serum levels in men: correlation with age, estrogen, and testosterone status. J Clin Endocrinol Metab 86: 3162- 3165

[29] Chen Q, Kaji H, Sugimoto T, Chihara K (2001). Testosterone inhibits osteoclast formation formation stimulated by parathyroid hormone through androgen receptor. FEBS Lett 491:91-93

[30] Zitzmann M, Nieschlag E (2004), Androgens and bone metabolism. In: Nieschlag E, Behre HM (Eds): Testosterone: Action, Deficiency, Subsitution. Third Edition Cambrigde University Press, pp 233-254

[31] Riggs BL., Khosla S., Melton JR., 3 rd (2002) Sex steroid and the construction and conservation of the adult skeleton. Endocr Rev 23: 279-302

[32] Eriksen EF, Colvard DS, Berg NJ, Graham ML, Mann KG, Spelsberg TC, Riggs BL (1988). Evidence of estrogen receptors in normal human osteoblast-like cells. Science 241:84-86

[33] Ourlsler MJ, Pederson L, Fitzpatrick L, Riggs BL (1994). Human giant cell tumors of the bone (osteoclastomas) are estrogen target cells. Proc Natl Acad Sci USA 96:505-510

[34] Braidman I, Baris C, Wood L, Selby P, Adams J, Feemont A, Hoyland J (2000). Preliminary evidence for impaired estrogen receptor protein expression in ostetoblast and osteocytes from men with idiopatic osteoporosis. Bone 26:423-427

[35] Grumbach MM (2000) Estrogen, bone, growth and sex: a sea change in conventional wisdom. J Pediatr Endocrinol Metab 13:1439-1455

[36] Walsh PC. Physiologic basis for hormonal therapy in carcinoma of the prostate. Urol Clin North Am 1975 Feb;2(1):125-40

[37] Bangma CH, Roemeling S, Schröder FH. Overdiagnosis and overtreatment of early detected prostate cancer.World J Urol. 2007 Mar;25(1):3-9.

[38] WHO Assessment od fracture risk and its application to screening for postmenopausal osteoporosis. WHO Technical report series. Geneva, WHO, 1994.

[39] Kanis JA, Melton LJ, Christiansen C, Johnston CC, Khaltaev N. The diagnosis of osteoporosis. J Bone Miner Res 1994; 9: 1137-1141.

[40] Looker AC, Orwoll ES, Johnston Jr CC, Lindsay RL, Wahner HW, Dunn WL, Calvo MS, Harris TB, Heyse SP. Prevalence of low femoral bone density in older US adults from NHANES III. J Bone Miner Res 1997; 12: 1761-1768.

[41] Bilezikian JP. Osteoporosis in men. J Clin Endocrinol Metab 1999; 84: 3431-3434.

[42] Kiebzak GM, Beinart GA, Perser K, Ambrose CG, Siff SJ, Heggeness MH. Undertreatment of osteoporosis in men with hip fracture. Arch Intern Med 2002; 162: 2217-2222

[43] Krane SM, Holik MF. Metabolic bone disease. In: Fauci AS, Braunwald E, Isselbacher KJ, et al., editors. Harrison's principles of internal medicine. 14th edition. Volume 2. New York: McGraw-Hill, 1998:2247–2253.

[44] Orwoll ES, Klein RF. Osteoporosis in men. Endocrine Reviews 1995; 16: 87–116.

[45] Seeman E. Pathogenesis of bone fragility in women and men. Lancet 2002; 359: 1841-1850.

[46] Smith MR. Diagnosis and management of treatment-related osteoporosis in men with prostate carcinoma. Cancer 2003; 97: 789-795.

[47] Hannan MT, Felson DT, Dawson-Hughes B, Tucker KL, Cupples LA, Wilson PWF, Kiel DP. Risk factors for longitudinal bone loss in elderly men and women: the Framingham osteoporosis study. J Bone Miner Res 2000; 15: 710-720.

[48] Jones G, Nguyen T, Sambrook P, Kelly PJ, Eisman JA. Progressive loss of bone in the femoral neck in elderly people: longitudinal findings from the Dubbo osteoporosis epidemiology study. BMJ 1994; 309: 691–695.
[49] Melton LJ, Chrischilles EA, Cooper C, Lane AW, Riggs BL. How many women have osteoporosis. J Bone Miner Res 1992; 7: 1005-1010.
[50] Forsen L, Sogaard AJ, Meyer HE, Edna T, Kopjar B. Survival after hip fracture: short- and long-term excess mortality according to age and gender. Osteoporos Int 1999; 10: 73-78.
[51] Center JR, Nguyen TV, Schneider D, Sambrook PN, Eisman JA. Mortality after all major types of osteoporotic fracture in men and women: an observational study. Lancet 1999; 353: 878-882.
[52] Abrahamsen B, van Staa T, Ariely R, Olson M, Cooper C. Excess mortality following hip fracture: a systematic epidemiological review. Osteoporos Int 2009; 20(10): 1633-1650.
[53] Diamond T, Higano C, Smith M, Guise T, Singer F. Osteoporosis in men with prostate cancinoma receiving androgen deprivation therapy: recommendatios for diagnosis and therapies. Cancer 2004; 100: 892-899.
[54] WHO: Assessment of fracture risk and its application to screening for postmenopausal osteoporosis repot of WHO Study Group. Geneva, 1994: World Health Organization
[55] Kanis J, Seeman E, Johnell O, Rizzoli R, Delmas P. The perspective of the International Osteoporosis Foundation on the official positions of the International Society for Clinical Densitometry. Osteoporosis Int 2005; 16: 456-459.
[56] http://www.uroweb.org/guidelines/online-guidelines/
[57] Daniell HW, Dunn SR, Fergusson DW, Lomas G, Niazi Z, Srtatte PT. Progressive osteoporosis during andorgen deprivation therapy for prostate cancer. J Urol 2000; 163: 181-186.
[58] Greenspan SL, Coates P, Sereika SM, Nelson JB, Trump DL, Resnick NM. Bone loss after initiation of androgen deprivation therapy in patients with prostate cancer. J Clin Endocrinol Metab 2005; 12: 6410-6417.
[59] Ahlborg HG, Nguyen ND, Center JR, Eisman JA, Nguyen TV. Incidence and risk factors for low trauma fractures in men with prostate cancer. Bone 2008; 43: 556-660.
[60] Oefelein MG, Ricchiuti V, Conrad W, Resnick MI. Skeletal fractures negatively correlate with overall survival in men with prostate cancer. J Urol 2002; 168 (3): 1005-1007.
[61] Inoue T, Segawa T, Kamba T, Yoshimura K, Nakamura E, Nishiyama H, Ito N, Kamoto T, Habuchi T, Ogawa O. Prevalence of skeletal complications and their impact on survival of hormone refractory prostate cancer patients in Japan. Urology 2009; 73 (5): 1104-1109.
[62] Saad F, Olsson C, Schulman CC. Skeletal morbidity in men with prostate cancer: quality-of-life considerations throughout the continuum of care. Eur Urol 2004; 46 (6): 731-739.
[63] McKiernan JM, Delea TE, Liss M. et al. Impact of skeletal complications on total medical care costs in prostate cancer patients with bone metastases. Proc Am Soc Clin Oncol 2004; 23: 531 (abstract no. 6057)

[64] Bubendorf L, Schopfer A, Wagner U, Sauter G, Moch H, Willi N, Gasser TC, Mihatsch MJ. Metastatic patterns of prostate cancer: an autopsy study of 1,589 patients. Hum Pathol 2000; 31:578–583.
[65] Liotta LA, Kohn E. Cancer invasion and metastases. JAMA 1990; 263: 1123–6
[66] Garnero P, Buchs N, Zekri J, Rizzoli R, Coleman RE, Delmas PD. Markers of bone turnover for the management of patients with bone metastases from prostate cancer. Br J Cancer 2000; 82: 858–64
[67] Saad F., Gleason DM., Murray R. Long-term efficacy of zoledronic acid for the prevention of skeletal complications in patients with metastatic hormone-refractory prostate cancer. J Natl Cancer Inst 2004; 96: 879–82
[68] McKiernan JM, Delea TE, Liss M. et al. Impact of skeletal complications on total medical care costs in prostate cancer patients with bone metastases. Proc Am Soc Clin Oncol 2004; 23: 531
[69] Ziaran S, Goncalves FM, Wendl J, Trebaticky B, Breza J Sn. Evaluation of bone mass density on patients with prostate cancer prior to the start of androgen deprivation therapy. Bratisl Med J 2009; 110(9):559-562.
[70] Ziaran S, Goncalves FM, Breza J Sn. Hormone naive patients with advanced prostate cancer have lower baseline bone mass density than healthy control. Bratisl Med J 2011; 131 (article in press)
[71] Farhat GN, Taioli E, Cauley JA, Zmuda JM, Orwoll E, Bauer DC, Wilt TJ, Hoffman AR, Beer TM, Shikany JM, Daniels N, Chan J, Fink HA, Barrett-Connor E, Parsons JK, Bunker CH. Osteoporotic Fractures in Men (MrOS) Study Group. The association of bone mineral density with prostate cancer risk in the Osteoporotic Fractures in Men (MrOS) Study. Cancer Epidemiol Biomarkers Prev 2009; 18: 148-154.
[72] Murphy et al. Management of Postmenopausal Osteoporosis. JAOA 2003; 103: 6-11
[73] Smith MR, McGovern FJ, Zietman AL, Fallon MA, Hayden DL et al. Pamidronate to prevent bone loss during androgen-deprivation therapy for prostate cancer. N Engl J Med 2001; 13:948-955.
[74] Ishizaka K, Machida T, Kobayashi S, Kanbe N, Kitahara S et al. Preventive effect of risedronate on bone loss in men receiving androgen-deprivation therapy for prostate cancer. Int J Urol 2007; 12:1071-1075.
[75] Planas J, Trilla E, Raventós C, Cecchini L, Orsola A, Salvador C, Placer J, Encabo G, Morote J. Alendronate decreases the fracture risk in patients with prostate cancer on androgen-deprivation therapy and with severe osteopenia or osteoporosis. BJU Int. 2009;104(11):1637-40.
[76] Smith MR, Eastham J, Gleason DM, et al. Randomized controlled trial of zoledronic acid to prevent bone loss in men receiving androgen deprivation therapy for nonmetastatic prostate cancer. J Urol 2003;169(6):2008-12.
[77] Michaelson MD, Kaufman DS, Lee H, et al. Randomized controlled trial of annual zoledronic acid to prevent gonadotropin-releasing hormone agonist-induced bone loss in men with prostate cancer. J Clin Oncol 2007;25(9):1038-42.
[78] Satoh T, Kimura M, Matsumoto K, Tabata K, Okusa H, Bessho H, Iwamura M, Ishiyama H, Hayakawa K, Baba S. Single infusion of zoledronic acid to prevent androgen deprivation therapy-induced bone loss in men with hormone-naive prostate carcinoma. Cancer. 2009;115(15):3468-74.

[79] Migliorati CA, Siegel MA, Elting LS. Bisphosphonate-associated osteonecrosis: a long-term complication of bisphosphonate treatment. Lancet Oncol 2006;7(6):508-1
[80] Wadhwa VK, Weston R, Parr NJ. Frequency of zoledronic acid to prevent further bone loss in osteoporotic patients undergoing androgen deprivation therapy for prostate cancer. BJU Int 2009, 13. [Epub ahead of print]
[81] Smith MR, Egerdie B, Hernández Toriz N, et al; Denosumab HALT Prostate Cancer Study Group. Denosumab in men receiving androgen-deprivation therapy for prostate cancer. N Engl J Med 2009;361(8):745-55.
[82] Halpern DF (2000), Sex differences in cognitive abilities (3rd Ed) Lawrence Erlbaum, Hillsdale (NJ)
[83] Collaer ML, Hines M (1995) Human behavioral sex differences: A role for gonadal hormones during early development? Psycholl Bull 118:55-107
[84] O´Connor DB, Archer J, Hair WM, Wu FCW (2001) Activational effects of TST on cognitive function in men. Neuropsychologia 39:1385-1394
[85] Simonson E, Kearnes Wm, Enzer N (1941) Effect of oral administration of methyltestosterone on fatigue in eunuchoids and castrates. Endocrinilogy 28:506-512
[86] Duker H (1957) Leistungfahigkeit und Keimdrusenhormone. Barth, Munchen
[87] Slabbekoorn D, van Goozen SHM, Megens J, Gooren LJG (1999) Activating effects of cross-sex hormones on cognitive functioning: A study of short term and long term hormone effects in transsexuals. Psychoneuroendocrinology 24:423-447
[88] Klaiber EL, Broverman DM, Vogel W, Abraham GE, Cone FL (1971) Effects of infused TST on mental performances and serum LH. J Clin Endrocrinol Metab 32:341-349
[89] Cherrier MMM. Androgens and cognitive function. J Endocrinologic Invest. 2005; 28 (3 suppl): 65–75.
[90] Yaffe K. Testosterone and the brain: uncharted territory [letter]. Lancet Neurol. 2004; 3: 270.
[91] Yaffe K,Grady D,Pressman A,Cummings S. Serum estrogen levels, cognitive performance, and risk of cognitive decline in older community women. J Am Geriatr Soc. 1998; 46: 816–821.
[92] Wefel JS,Kayl AE,Meyers CA. Neuropsychological dysfunction associated with cancer and cancer therapies: a conceptual review of an emerging target. Br J Cancer. 2004; 90: 1691–1696.
[93] Yaffe K,Lui LY,Zmuda J,Cauley J. Sex hormones and cognitive function in older men. J Am Geriatr Soc. 2002; 50: 707–712.
[94] Green HJ,Pakenham KI,Headley BC, et al. Altered cognitive function in men treated for prostate cancer with luteinizing hormone-releasing hormone analogues and cyproterone acetate: a randomized controlled trial. BJU Int. 2002; 90: 427–432
[95] Salminen EK,Portin RI,Koskinen A,Helenius H,Nurmi M. Associations between serum testosterone fall and cognitive function in prostate cancer patients. Clin Care Res. 2004; 10: 7575–7582.
[96] Jenkins VA,Bloomfield DJ,Shilling VM,Edginton TL. Does neoadjuvant hormone therapy for early prostate cancer affect cognition? Results from a pilot study. BJU Int. 2005; 96: 48–53.

[97] Joly F,Alibhai SM,Galica J, et al. Impact of androgen deprivation therapy on physical and cognitive function, as well as quality of life of patients with nonmetastatic prostate cancer. J Urol. 2006; 176 (6 pt 1): 2443–2447

[98] Basaria S, Wahlstrom JT, Dobs AS 2001 Anabolic-androgenic steroid therapy in the treatment of chronic diseases. J Clin Endocrinol Metab 86:5108–5117

[99] Basaria S, Lieb 2nd J, Tang A, DeWeese T, Carducci M, Eisenberger M, Dobs AS 2002 Long-term effects of androgen deprivation therapy in prostate cancer patients. Clin Endocrinol (Oxf) 56:779–786

[100] Chen Z, Maricic M, Nguyen P, Ahmann FR, Bruhn R, Dalkin BL 2002 Low bone density and high percentage of body fat among men who were treated with androgen deprivation therapy for prostate carcinoma. Cancer 95:2136–2144

[101] Haseen F, Murray LJ, Cardwell CR, O'Sullivan JM, Cantwell MM. The effect of androgen deprivation therapy on body composition in men with prostate cancer: systematic review and meta-analysis. J Cancer Surviv. 2010;4(2):128-39

[102] Smith JC, Bennett S, Evans LM, Kynaston HG, Parmar M, Mason MD, Cockcroft JR, Scanlon MF, Davies JS2001 The effects of induced hypogonadism on arterial stiffness, body composition, and metabolic parameters in males with prostate cancer. J Clin Endocrinol Metab

[103] Haffner SM, Shaten J, Stern MP, Smith GD, Kuller L 1996 Low levels of sex hormone-binding globulin and testosterone predict the development of non-insulin-dependent diabetes mellitus in men. MRFIT Research Group. Multiple Risk Factor Intervention Trial. Am J Epidemiol 143:889–897

[104] Haffner SM, Valdez RA, Mykkanen L, Stern MP, Katz MS 1994 Decreased testosterone and dehydroepiandrosterone sulfate concentrations are associated with increased insulin and glucose concentrations in nondiabetic men. Metabolism 43:599–603

[105] Laaksonen DE, Niskanen L, Punnonen K, Nyyssönen K, Tuomainen TP, Valkonen VP, Salonen R, Salonen JT2004 Testosterone and sex hormone-binding globulin predict the metabolic syndrome and diabetes in middle-aged men. Diabetes Care 27:1036–1041

[106] Pitteloud N, Hardin M, Dwyer AA, Valassi E, Yialamas M, Elahi D, Hayes FJ 2005 Increasing insulin resistance is associated with a decrease in Leydig cell testosterone secretion in men. J Clin Endocrinol Metab 90:2636–2641

[107] Marin P, Holmang S, Jonsson L, Sjöström L, Kvist H, Holm G, Lindstedt G, Björntorp P 1992 The effects of testosterone treatment on body composition and metabolism in middle-aged obese men. Int J Obes Relat Metab Disord 16:991–997

[108] Smith JC, Bennett S, Evans LM, Kynaston HG, Parmar M, Mason MD, Cockcroft JR, Scanlon MF, Davies JS2001 The effects of induced hypogonadism on arterial stiffness, body composition, and metabolic parameters in males with prostate cancer. J Clin Endocrinol Metab 86:4261–4267

[109] Dockery F, Bulpitt CJ, Agarwal S, Donaldson M, Rajkumar C 2003 Testosterone suppression in men with prostate cancer leads to an increase in arterial stiffness and hyperinsulinaemia. Clin Sci (Lond) 104:195–201

[110] Smith MR, Lee H, Nathan DM 2006 Insulin sensitivity during combined androgen blockade for prostate cancer. J Clin Endocrinol Metab 91:1305–1308

[111] Keating NL, O'Malley AJ, Smith MR 2006 Diabetes and cardiovascular disease during androgen deprivation therapy for prostate cancer. J Clin Oncol 24:4448–4456

[112] Mohamedali HZ, Breunis H, Timilshina N, Alibhai SM. Changes in blood glucose and cholesterol levels due to androgen deprivation therapy in men with non-metastatic prostate cancer. Can Urol Assoc J. 201;5(1):28-32.

[113] Basaria S, Muller DC, Carducci MA, Egan J, Dobs AS. Hyperglycemia and insulin resistance in men with prostate carcinoma who receive androgen-deprivation therapy. Cancer. 2006;106(3):581-8.

[114] Derweesh IH, Diblasio CJ, Kincade MC, Malcolm JB, Lamar KD, Patterson AL, Kitabchi AE, Wake RW. Risk of new-onset diabetes mellitus and worsening glycaemic variables for established diabetes in men undergoing androgen-deprivation therapy for prostate cancer. BJU Int. 2007;100(5):1060-5.

[115] Haffner SM, Mykkanen L, Valdez RA, Katz MS 1993 Relationship of sex hormones to lipids and lipoproteins in nondiabetic men. J Clin Endocrinol Metab 77:1610–1615

[116] Malkin CJ, Pugh PJ, Jones RD, Kapoor D, Channer KS, Jones TH 2004 The effect of testosterone replacement on endogenous inflammatory cytokines and lipid profiles in hypogonadal men. J Clin Endocrinol Metab 89:3313–3318

[117] Smith MR, Finkelstein JS, McGovern FJ, et al. Changes in body composition during androgen deprivation therapy for prostate cancer. J Clin Endocrinol Metab. 2002;87:599–603.

[118] Dockery F, Bulpitt CJ, Agarwal S, et al. Testosterone suppression in men with prostate cancer leads to an increase in arterial stiffness and hyperinsulinaemia. Clin Sci (Lond) 2003;104:195–201

[119] Eri LM, Urdal P, Bechensteen AG. Effects of the luteinizing hormone-releasing hormone agonist leuprolide on lipoproteins, fibrinogen and plasminogen activator inhibitor in patients with benign prostatic hyperplasia. J Urol. 1995;154:100–104

[120] Eckel RH, Grundy SM, Zimmet PZ. The metabolic syndrome. Lancet. 2005;365: 1415 - 1428

[121] Expert Panel on Detection, Evaluation and Treatment of High Blood Cholesterol in Adults. Executive summary of the third report of the National Cholesterol Education Program (NCEP) Expert Panel on Detection, Evaluation, and Treatment of High Blood Cholesterol in Adults (Adult Treatment Panel III). JAMA. 2001;285: 2486 -2497

[122] Muller M, Grobbee DE, den Tonkelaar I, Lamberts SW, van der Schouw YT. Endogenous sex hormones and metabolic syndrome in aging men. J Clin Endocrinol Metab. 2005; 90: 2618 -2623

[123] Keating NL, O'Malley AJ, Smith MR. Diabetes and cardiovascular disease during androgen deprivation therapy for prostate cancer. J Clin Oncol. 2006;24:4448–4456.

[124] Saigal CS, Gore JL, Krupski TL, et al. Androgen deprivation therapy increases cardiovascular morbidity in men with prostate cancer. Cancer. 2007;110:1493–1500.

[125] Alibhai SM, Duong-Hua M, Sutradhar R, et al. Impact of androgen deprivation therapy on cardiovascular disease and diabetes. J Clin Oncol. 2009;27:3452–3458

[126] Tsai HK, D'Amico AV, Sadetsky N, et al. Androgen deprivation therapy for localized prostate cancer and the risk of cardiovascular mortality. J Natl Cancer Inst. 2007;99:1516–1524

[127] D'Amico AV, Denham JW, Crook J, et al. Influence of androgen suppression therapy for prostate cancer on the frequency and timing of fatal myocardial infarctions. J Clin Oncol. 2007;25:2420–2425

[128] Efstathiou JA, Bae K, Shipley WU, et al. Cardiovascular mortality and duration of androgen deprivation for locally advanced prostate cancer: analysis of RTOG 92-02. Eur Urol. 2008;54:816–823.

[129] Roach M, III, Bae K, Speight J, et al. Short-term neoadjuvant androgen deprivation therapy and external-beam radiotherapy for locally advanced prostate cancer: long-term results of RTOG 8610. J Clin Oncol. 2008;26:585–591

[130] Efstathiou JA, Bae K, Shipley WU, et al. Cardiovascular mortality after androgen deprivation therapy for locally advanced prostate cancer: RTOG 85-31. J Clin Oncol. 2009;27:92–99

17

A Review of Quality of Life Following Treatments for Localized Prostate Cancer

Sunao Shoji
Department of Urology, Tokai University Hachioji Hospital
Japan

1. Introduction

Recently, a number of alternative, less invasive treatments have been developed for patients with localized prostate cancer, who are not indicated for surgery, or who do not want to experience the potential side effects of surgery. Laparoscopic radical prostatectomy, robotic assisted laparoscopic radical prostatectomy (RALP), 3-dimensional conformal radiotherapy (3D-CRT), brachytherapy, intensity-modulated external beam radiotherapy (IMRT), high-intensity focused ultrasound (HIFU) and cryoablation of the prostate have all been applied to treat this group of patients.

QOL measurements for prostate cancer therapy have become an essential component of clinical trial evaluations, and should be integrated into comprehensive cancer care. Health-related QOL (HRQOL) concerns, urinary function, and potency rate after treatment are important to patients when selecting treatment options for clinically localized prostate cancer, and they also play a critical role in evaluating outcome following intervention.

Many studies have been carried out with the aim of improving QOL, urinary function, and potency rate after treatment for localized prostate cancer with many modalities. Clinicians have an obligation to assess the impacts these treatments have on QOL, and use this knowledge in an overall evaluation of efficacy.

2. QOL changes after treatment for localized prostate cancer

There are few changes in general HRQOL after a retropubic radical prostatectomy (RRP) or interstitial brachytherapy.[1-3] However, disease-specific QOL, especially bowel function and urinary irritative symptoms, is worse in the interstitial brachytherapygroup, and urinary incontinence and sexual function are worse in the RRP group.[1] Hamada *et al.* evaluated QOL immediately before surgery and at several points during the 6-month period after retropubic radical prostatectomy (RRP). They reported that a radical prostatectomy aggravates the Social/Family well-being score and the FACT-P score.[4] Other studies have also showed that prostatectomy and interstitial brachytherapy continuously decreased health-related QOL.[5-8] Hanlon *et al.* showed that external beam radiotherapy for localized prostate cancer aggravates bowel function.[9] Hubosky *et al.* reported that HRQOL showed patients undergoing cryoablation on average achieved urinary and bowel domain scores

comparable to baseline, but sexual domains remained well below baseline at 12 months follow-up and compared to brachytherapy, cryotherapy results in less irritative and obstructive voiding systems in the early post-treatment period, and may improve the urinary function for up to 24 months after treatment.[10]
We reported QOL after HIFU for localized prostate cancer.[11] In our report the total FACT score significantly improved at 24 months, and Physical well-being factor(at 6 and 12 months after HIFU therapy) and Functionalwell-being factor (at 24 months after HIFU therapy) in FACT-G showed significant improvements. Further analysis of the elements of FACT-G showed such responses as "I am bothered by the side-effects of treatment" (at 12 months after HIFU therapy), "I am able to enjoy life" (at 24 months afterHIFU therapy) and "I have accepted my illness" (at 24 months after HIFU therapy) to have all statistically improved.

3. Urinary function after treatment for localized prostate cancer

3.1 Urinary incontinence after radical prostatectomy

Urinary incontinence is the most prominent side effect of radical prostatectomy. Urinary incontinence after treatment for localized prostate cancer is caused by sphincter malfunction. So, several technical modifications of open, laparoscopic and robot-assisted laparoscopic radical prostatectomy have been advocated to improve early and late urinary incontinence.
Pardo *et al.* reported that urinary incontinence rates of patients treated with non-nerve sparing RRP and nerve sparing RRP were 69% and 54%.[12] It has recently been demonstrated that reconstruction of the posterior aspects of the rhabdoshincter allows a rapid recovery of continence after retropubic radical prostatectomy and laparoscopic radical prostatectomy.[13] But, Joshi *et al.*reported that there was no significant difference in early urinary incontinence between the group for which the posterior aspects of the rhabdoshincter were reconstructed and the group for which they were not reconstructed in cases of RALP.[14] They suggested the reason why there was no significant difference was a magnified stereoscopic view and/or the finer, more maneuverable instruments in robot system may allow better preservation of sphincter supporting musculature, hence improving continence, and may obviate the advantages of posterior reinforcing sutures.
Di Pierro *et al.* compared continence rate between groups of patients treated with RRP and RALP, and reported that the continence rate of the RALP group was significantly higher than the RRP group at 3 and 12 months after RALP.[15] Wang *et al.* reported that continence was achieved in 82%, 87%, and 91% of men at 3, 6, and 12 months after RALP.[16] They also reported that the mean IPSS scores of these patients preoperatively and 3, 6, and 12 months after surgery were 14.1, 5.2, 3.0, and 2.9 and corresponding mean QOL scores were 3.4, 2.1, 1.6, and 1.6.[13]

3.2 Urinary function after radiation therapy, cryotherapy, and HIFU

Sanda *et al.*reported that 18% of patients in the brachytherapy group, 11% of those in the radiotherapy group, and 7% of those in the prostatectomy group had moderate or worse distress from overall urinary symptoms at 1 year.[17] Pardo *et al.* reported that compared to the brachytherapy group, the prostatectomy group showed a greater deterioration of urinary incontinence but better urinary irrigative-obstructive results.[12]

Hubosky *et al.* reported that the urinary function was similar for the groups of patients treated with cryoablation and brachytherapy until 18 months, at which time cryoablation patients fared better and this was sustained up to 24 months.[10]
We reported that the QOL index improved significantly at 6 months after HIFU therapy. Our data on uroflowmetry showed that maximum flow rate and residual urine volume were significantly impaired at 6 months after HIFU. However, the data on maximum flow rate and residual urine volume recovered to baseline at 12, 24 months after HIFU.[11]

4. Erectile function

It is important to preserve erectile function during treatment of prostate cancer. Postoperative potency depends on the preservation of neurovascular bundles (NVB), which are some times affected by tumor invasion.
Hanlon *et al.* reported a normal potency rate at 1 year after treatment of 50% for patients in the RRP group, 65% for patients in the brachytherapy group, and 69% for patients in the radiotherapy group.[17]

4.1 Erectile function after radical prostatectomy

Generally, the potency rate is aggravated by injury to NVB after radical prostatectomy. Poel *et al.* reported a potency rate 53.3 %at 6 months after RALP, and 42% of patients had potency without using a PDE5 inhibitor. They concluded that prostatic fascia preservation resulted to good potency rates after RALP.[18] Consequently, preservation of NVB and prostatic fascia is important to preserve erectile function. Di Pierro *et al.* compared potency rates between groups of patients treated with RRP and RALP. They performed RALP with a procedure using a transperitoneal approach and preserved the NVB through a tension- and energy-free technique[19] as far as cancer localization allowed, and reported that the potency rate without PDE-5 inhibitors of the RALP group (68% and 55%) was significantly higher than that of the RRP group (25% and 26%) at 3 and 12 months after RALP.[15]

4.2 Erectile function after radiation therapy, cryotherapy, and HIFU

Pardo *et al.* reported that among patients with no relevant sexual problems at baseline, approximately 40% in the external and interstitial brachytherapy groups had preserved their pretreatment sexual status.[12]
Merrick *et al.* reported that 39% of patients maintained potency after prostate brachytherapy with a plateau on the potency preservation curve at 6-year follow-up, and preservation of potency after brachytherapy correlated with preimplant erectile function, patients age, use of supplemental external beam radiation therapy, and diabetes, and was statistically significant.[20]
Asterling *et al.* reported that 3.7% and 14.3% of patients had partial erections at 6 weeks and 9 months after cryosurgical ablation. Besides, 21% and 24% of the patients had regained full potency at 18 and 24 months after cryosurgical ablation.[21]
Hubosky *et al.* reported that cryotherapy patients experienced more negative impacts on sexual function steadily up to 12 months compared to brachytherapy patients.[10]
We reported that potency rates were 52%, 63% and 78% for patients who did not undergo NADT at 6, 12and 24 months after HIFU therapy. Furthermore, potency rates were 39%, 62% and 67% at 6, 12, and 24 months, respectively, after HIFUtherapy without the use of

PDE5 inhibitors.[11] HIFU therapy can, therefore, preserve erectile function better than RRP and cryotherapy, and is similar to RALP.

5. Conclusion

5.1 QOL

RRP and interstitial brachytherapy continuously decreased health-related QOL. External beam radiotherapy for localized prostate cancer aggravates the bowel function. Health-related QOL was significantly improved in patients treated with HIFU therapy at 24 months after HIFU.

5.2 Urinary function

Urinary incontinence is the most prominent side effect of radical prostatectomy. But, RALP might improve incontinence rates of patients. The urinary function of patients after brachytherapy and cryotherapy were similar. In HIFU, however maximum flow rate and residual urine volume were significantly impaired at 6 months after treatment, and data on maximum flow rate and residual urine volume recovered to baseline at 12, 24 months after HIFU.

5.3 Erectile function

Generally, potency rate was aggravated by injury to NVB after radical prostatectomy. Consequently, using RALP to preserve the NVB and prostatic fascia is important for preserving erectile function. Approximately 40% of patients in the external and interstitial brachytherapy groups preserved their pretreatment sexual status. In cryoablation, 3.7% and 14.3% of patients had partial erections at 6 weeks and 9 months after treatment. And, 21% and 24% of the patients had regained full potency at 18 and 24 months after cryosurgical ablation. After HIFU, 52%, 63% and 78% of patients who did not undergo NADT had regained full potency at 6, 12, and 24 months after treatment therapy. Furthermore, the potency rates were 39%, 62%, and 67% at 6, 12, and 24 months, respectively, without the use of PDE5 inhibitors. HIFU therapy can, therefore, preserve erectile function better than RRP, radiotherapy, or cryotherapy.

6. References

[1] Litwin MS, Gore JL, Kwan L, et al. Quality of life after surgery, external beam irradiation, or brachytherapy for early-stage prostate cancer. *Cancer* 2007; 109: 2239-47.

[2] Davis JW, Kuban DA, Lynch DF, et al. Quality of life after treatment for localized prostate cancer: differences based on treatment modality. *J Urol* 2001; 166: 947-52.

[3] Brandeis JM, Litwin MS, Burnison CM, et al. Quality of life outcomes after brachytherapy for early stage prostate cancer. *J Urol* 2000; 163: 851-7.

[4] Hamada Y, Kitani K, Kawano T, et al. Assessment of Quality of life in men treated for localized prostate cancer: before and after radical prostatectomy. *Nishinihon J Urol* 2004; 66: 241-8.

[5] Clark JA, Inui TS, Silliman RA *et al.* Patients' perceptions of quality of life after treatment for early prostatic cancer. *J. Clin. Oncol.* 2003; 21: 3777–84.

[6] Litwin MS, Lubeck DP, Spitalny GM, Henning JM, Carroll PR. Mental health in men treated for early stage prostate carcinoma: A posttreatment, longitudinal quality of life analysis from the cancer of the prostate strategic urologic research endeavor. *Cancer* 2002; 95: 54–60.

[7] Clark JA, Bokhour BG, Inui TS, Silliman RA, Talcott JA. Measuring patients' perceptions of the outcomes of treatment for early prostate cancer. *Med. Care* 2003; 41: 923–36.

[8] Bradley E, Bissonette E, Theodorescu D. Determinants of long-term quality of life and voiding function of patients treated with radical prostatectomy or permanent brachytherapy for prostate cancer. *BJU Int.* 2004; 94: 1003–9.

[9] Hanlon L, Watkins D, Peter R, Hanks E. A prospective quality-of-life study in men with clinically localized prostate carcinoma treated with radical prostatectomy, external beam radiotherapy, or interstitial brachytherapy. *Int. J. Radiat. Oncol. Biol. Phys.* 2001; 51: 614–23.

[10] Hubosky SG, Fabrizio MD, Schellhammer PF, et al. Single center experience with third-generation cryosurgery for management of organ-confined prostate cancer: critical evaluation of short-term outcome, complications, and patient quality of life. J Endourol 2007; 21: 1521-31.

[11] Shoji S, Nakano M, Nagata Y, et al. Quality of life following high-intensity focused ultrasound for the treatment of localized prostate cancer: a prospective study. Int J Urol 2010; 17: 715-9.

[12] Pardo Y, Guedea F, Aguilo F, et al. Quality of life impact of primary treatment for localized prostate cancer in patients without hormonal treatment. *J Clin Oncol* 2010; 28: 4687-96.

[13] Rocco B, Gregori A, Stener S, et al. Posterior reconstruction of the rhabdoshincter allows a rapid recovery of continence after transperitoneal videolaparoscopic radical prostatectomy. *Eur Urol* 2007; 51: 996-1003.

[14] Joshi N, Blok W, Muilekom E, et al. Impact of posterior musculofascial reconstruction on early continence after robot-assisted laparoscopic radical prostatectomy: results of a prospective parallel Group Trial. *Eur Urol* 2010; 58: 85-9.

[15] Di Pierro GB, Baumeister P, Stucki P, et al. A prospective trial comparing consecutive series of open retropubic and robot-assisted laparoscopic radical prostatectomy in a centre with a limited caseload. *Eur Urol* 2011; 59: 1-6.

[16] Wang L, Chung SFCM, Yip SKH, et al. The natural history of voiding function after robot-assisted laparoscopic radical prostatectomy. *Urol Oncol* 2009; 29: 177-82.

[17] Sanda MG, Dunn RL, Michalski J *et al.* Quality of life and satisfaction with outcome among prostate-cancer survivors. *N. Engl. J. Med.* 2008; 358: 1250–61.

[18] Wang L, Chung SFCM, Yip SKH, et al. The natural history of voiding function after robot-assisted laparoscopic radical prostatectomy. *Urol Oncol* 2009; 29: 177-82.

[19] Poel HG, Blok W. Role of extent of fascia preservation and erectile function after robot-assisted laparoscopic prostatectomy. *Urology* 2009; 73: 816-21.

[20] Mattei A, Naspro R, Annino F, et al. Tension and energy-free robotic-assisted laparoscopic radical prostatectomy with interfacial dissection of the neurovascular bundles. *Eur Urol* 2007; 52: 687-95.

[21] Merrick GS, Butler WM, Galbreath RW, et al. Erectile function after permanent prostate brachy therapy. *Int J Radiat Oncol Biol Phys* 2002; 52: 893-902.
[22] Asterling A and Greene DR. Prospective evaluation of sexual function in patients receiving cryotherapy as a primary radical treatment for localized prostate cancer. *BJU int* 2008; 103: 788-92.

18

Intermittent Androgen Suppression Therapy for Prostate Cancer Patients: A Choice for Improved Quality of Life?

Gerhard Hamilton[1], Ulrike Olszewski-Hamilton[1] and Gerhard Theyer[2]
[1]*Ludwig Boltzmann Cluster of Translational Oncology, Vienna*
[2]*LKH Kittsee, Burgenland*
Austria

1. Introduction

Prostate cancer is among the most common types of malignancies and causes of cancer-related deaths in men worldwide (Fitzpatrick, *et al.*, 2009). Primary tumor involvement outside the prostatic capsule or relapse following radical prostatectomy results generally in incurability (Lassi & Dawson, 2009). Androgen deprivation therapy has progressed since attempts in 1941, when surgical castration had been shown to improve outcomes for the first time. Palliative treatment consists of hormonal manipulation to deprive the cancer cells of androgenic stimulation by orchidectomy or use of LHRH analogs and steroidal or nonsteroidal antiandrogens (Kollmeier & Zelefsky, 2008). Although continuous androgen suppression therapy (CAS) has been a cornerstone of the management of prostate cancer for more than 50 years, controversy remains regarding its optimum application. Generally, androgen suppression (AS) is performed as continuous treatment, resulting in apoptotic regression of the tumor cells in a high percentage of cases. However, surgical or medical castration results in median progression-free survival of only 2–3 years, with no other effective treatment left (Mellado, *et al.*, 2009). Responses to cytotoxic therapy are low and only recently several studies revealed a possible benefit of incorporating chemotherapeutic agents in treatment regimen for prostate cancer (Chang & Kibel, 2009). Taxanes like docetaxel and cabazitaxel, therapeutic cancer vaccines and newly developed agents targeting androgen receptor signaling are expected to improve therapy (Madan *et al.*, 2011).

Following experimental research using animal models, intermittent androgen suppression (IAS) was introduced as new clinical concept, assuming that during limited regrowth in the treatment cessation periods tumorigenic cells are residing in an androgen-responsive state (Goldenberg, *et al.*, 1995). Since induction of androgen independence may occur early after treatment initiation, cessation of antiandrogen therapy prior to this switch is expected to maintain the apoptotic potential of the tumor cells and keep them sensitive to retreatment. Providing an easy method for selection of the type of treatment and early assessment of tumor growth during the off-periods serial serum PSA determinations made IAS feasible. In detail, IAS consists of an initial androgen suppression period of up to nine months combining LHRH antagonists and antiandrogens, which is followed by treatment cessation until a certain PSA threshold is reached; then, androgen suppression is reinitiated until a maximal effect is observed again. In initial pilot trials regrowing tumors of patients undergoing IAS were consistently reported to be sensitive over several cycles of androgen withdrawal (figure 1).

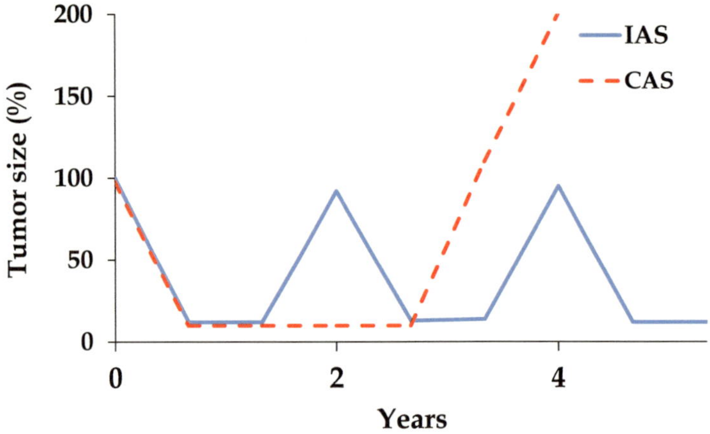

Fig. 1. Schematic model of CAS and IAS. CAS treatment of prostate cancer rapidly results in appearance of androgen-insensitive cells and tumor progression within 2–3 years in advanced stages. On the contrary, IAS preserves the hormone sensitivity of the cells through cycling between androgen suppression and treatment cessation phases in order to prolong the time to hormone refractoriness and possibly survival.

Therefore, the primary goal of IAS has been the prolongation of the hormone-sensitivity of the tumors, which in turn has been expected to result in increased survival eventually. Based on the available evidence, IAS nowadays represents a valid treatment option for patients with nonmetastatic prostate cancer, including those with locally advanced disease, either with or without lymph node involvement, and those who relapsed following apparently curative treatment. IAS has been researched since the mid-1980s in a number of clinical phase II and III trials in an effort to prolong hormone-dependency and reduce adverse effects and costs of CAS (Goldenberg, et al., 1995; Bales, et al., 1996; Buchan & Goldenberg, 2010, da Silva, 2011). With preclinical evidence suggesting a potential benefit of IAS in terms of time to androgen independence, with phase II and phase III studies producing optimistic results and with the potential for decreased costs and complications, IAS has now become a popular modality of therapy worldwide.

2. Experimental development of intermittent androgen suppression

The concept of IAS was experimentally developed using the androgen-dependent Shionogi mouse mammary tumor, investigating regular phases of growth, regression and recurrence of xenograft tumors during serial transplantation (Bruchovsky, *et al.*, 1985). Since postcastrational progression of tumors towards an androgen-independent state appears to be linked to the cessation of androgen-induced differentiation of tumorigenic stem cells, it was hypothesized that the replacement of androgens at the end of apoptotic regression might result in the reappearance of differentiated tumor cells that maintain their apoptotic potential. To determine the effect of intermittent application of androgens on the androgen-dependent Shionogi carcinoma, the tumor was transplanted into a succession of male mice, each of which was castrated when the estimated tumor weight became about 3g. After the tumor had regressed to 30% of the original weight, it was transplanted into the next noncastrated male (Akakura, *et al.*, 1993). This cycle of transplantation and castration-induced regression was successfully repeated four times before tumor growth became androgen-independent during the fifth cycle (figure 2).

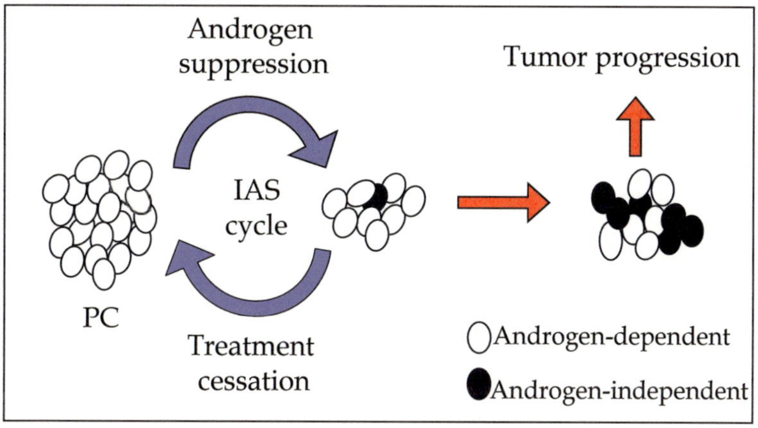

Fig. 2. Experimental animal model of IAS using androgen-dependent Shionogi tumor cells. Tumor cells are androgen-depleted by castration and, following tumor shrinkage to a defined degree, treatment cessation re-establishes a hormone-sensitive tumor. This cycle can be repeated four times until androgen-insensitive cells constitute a population of approximately 50% of all tumor cells in the fifth cycle and progression to a hormone-refractory tumor occurs.

The average duration of one cycle was 30 days and progression to androgen-insensitivity was observed after 150 days. After castration, the concentration of testosterone in the tumor was demonstrated to decline more rapidly than the dihydrotestosterone levels and spontaneous recurrent growth was not accompanied by significant elevation of the whole-tissue concentration of either androgen. These results suggested that a recurrent tumor may contain hormone-sensitive cells, which are capable of resuming growth in an androgen-depleted environment. The data also imply that progression from the androgen-dependent to the androgen-autonomous condition involves the selection and outgrowth of heterogeneous hormone-insensitive cells.

The effects of castration on gene expression were measured in the androgen-dependent Shionogi mouse tumor model (Rennie, *et al.*, 1988). During the first 48-72 h after castration, the tumor continued to increase its mass, but began to regress at 72-144 h. In the surviving cells there were no major decreases in RNA synthesis. Under these conditions, selected genes become overexpressed and, in particular, the concentration of the transcripts encoding testosterone-repressed prostate message-2 (TRPM-2/clusterin) was enhanced only when tumor regression was most evident, i.e. 72-144 h after castration. The TRPM-2 (clusterin) gene also became expressed constitutively in non-regressing tumors after the first and subsequent cycles of androgen withdrawal. TRPM-2 is a membrane-stabilizing protein that appears to be involved in limiting the autophagic lysis of epithelial cells during apoptosis and is possibly preserving the nuclear environment, suppressing the lethal effect of anti-androgenic treatment (Akakura, *et al.*, 1993). Therefore, tumor progression, characterized by the loss of the apoptotic potential, appears to be linked in part to the inappropriate activation of the TRPM-2 gene.

Since postcastrational progression of tumors to an androgen-independent state appears to be linked to the cessation of androgen-induced differentiation of tumorigenic stem cells, the replacement of androgens at the end of a period of apoptotic regression might result in the regeneration of differentiated tumor cells with maintained apoptotic potential. (Akakura, *et al.*, 1993). The frequency of androgen-dependent and -independent tumorigenic stem cells in parent and recurrent Shionogi tumors was determined with help of an *in vivo* limiting dilution test (Rennie, *et al.*, 1990). When assayed in male hosts a marked enrichment of stem cells in the recurrent tumors (1/200 tumor cells) relative to the parent tumors (1/4000 tumor cells) was detectable. By measuring tumor takes in female mice, a 500-fold increase in androgen-independent stem cells was found in the recurrent carcinoma. No enrichment of androgen-independent stem cells was evident in regressing parent tumors. This finding implies that the androgen-independent cells that survived androgen-withdrawal may result from the ability of a small number of initially androgen-independent stem cells to adapt to an altered hormonal environment. These results again indicated that the tumor mass mainly consisted of differentiated cells and that stem cells are initially androgen-dependent, but the apoptosis-inducing effect of androgen withdrawal will be limited to a factor of 100–1000, before compensatory adaptive mechanisms lead to progression of stem cells to an androgen-independent state. In recurrent tumors the amount of dihydrotestosterone was reduced by approximately 85% in comparison to the parent tumor and expression of nuclear androgen receptor was completely abolished within 24 h after castration (Bruchovsky, *et al.*, 1990). However, later on the amount of androgen receptor mRNA in androgen-dependent and -independent cells derived from the Shionogi carcinoma was similar, showing no relationship to progression (Akakura, *et al.*, 1996). The uncoupling of TRPM-2 expression and apoptosis observed in androgen-independent tumor cells implicates that the function of androgen receptor becomes more restricted with tumor progression. There is evidence that the androgen receptor still plays an important role in progression to the castration-resistant incurable state in prostate cancer. While castration proved to be ineffective in castration-resistant prostate tumors in an animal model, knockdown of androgen receptor was demonstrated to decrease serum PSA, inhibit cancer growth and frequently resulted in tumor regression (Snoek, *et al.*, 2009). This study provided evidence that elimination of the androgen receptor might constitute a promising therapeutic strategy for treatment of prostate tumors that had progressed to the castration-resistant state.

Serial determinations of the proportion of stem cells in the Shionogi tumor revealed a constant part during the first three cycles but a 15-fold increase between the third and fourth cycles (Rennie, *et al.*, 1994). In the parent androgen-dependent tumor before androgen ablation they formed 0.8% of the total stem cell compartment. After the fourth cycle the androgen-independent stem cell population increased to 47% and a population of similar size was found in the androgen-independent recurrent of the tumor, which was induced by one-time castration. Therefore, it was concluded that independent of intermittent or continuous androgen withdrawal, conversion to hormone-insensitivity occurs as soon as the tumor has accumulated one-third to one-half of the total stem cell compartment with androgen-independent cells.

The next step included the switch to a human prostate cancer xenograft model using the LNCaP androgen-dependent prostate cell line, where serum PSA levels correlated well with tumor volume and decreased rapidly after castration, followed by appearance of androgen-independency after 3-4 weeks (Gleave, *et al.*, 1996). IAS-treated mice were implanted with testosterone pellets two weeks after castration and were subjected to cycles of testosterone replacement for 1 week and withdrawal for 2 weeks until serum PSA levels returned to baseline no longer. IAS therapy prolonged time to androgen-independent PSA production 3-fold, from an average of 26 days in the CAS group to 77 days in the IAS group. It was concluded that IAS in the LNCaP model delayed the onset of androgen-independent PSA gene regulation markedly most likely due to androgen-induced differentiation and/or downregulation of androgen-suppressed gene expression. In summary, the animal experimental data indicated that androgen-dependent tumor xenografts can be subjected to several cycles of androgen withdrawal/replacement and revealed prolonged hormone-dependency compared to continuous androgen suppression.

3. Clinical development of intermittent androgen suppression

Since the introduction of PSA screening in the late 1980s, more prostate cancers have been detected, and at an earlier stage (Gjertson & Albertsen, 2011). Consequently, the majority of prostate cancers are now detected years before the emergence of clinically evident disease, which usually represents locally advanced or metastatic cancer. PSA screening has remained controversial, because many of the prostate cancers detected are low grade and slow growing and will not need aggressive therapy. Prostate cancer is biologically and clinically a heterogeneous malignancy and its imaging evaluation will need to be tailored to the specific phases of the disease in a patient-specific, risk-adapted manner (Jadvar, 2011). With this long natural history and a median survival without treatment that often approaches at least 15-20 years, many patients will die rather with than of prostate cancer. Approximately one-third of patients who undergo radical prostatectomy will develop a detectable PSA level within 10 years (Tzou, *et al.*, 2011). Biochemical relapse is defined as a rising PSA level in the absence of clinical or radiographic evidence of tumor. Management of PSA recurrence is controversial, as prostate cancer may take an indolent course, or it may develop aggressively into metastatic disease. The only potentially curative treatment for biochemical failure after prostatectomy is radiotherapy and the other treatment options include hormone therapy or clinical trials of new agents.

Research on hormonal treatment of prostate cancer over the past 20 years has focused on maximizing androgen ablation through combination therapy. This increases treatment-related side-effects and expenses and fails to prolong time to progression to androgen-independence (Gleave, *et al.*, 1998, Kollmeier & Zelefsky, 2008). Preliminary evidence indicates that a low androgen milieu is associated with tumor aggressiveness. Transition to androgen-independence is a complex process and involves both selection and outgrowth of preexisting androgen-resistant clones as well as adaptative upregulation of genes that enable cancer cells to survive and grow after CAS (Corona, et al., 2011). CAS in men with prostate cancer increases the risk of osteoporotic fractures, type 2 diabetes and, possibly, cardiovascular events (Grossmann, *et al.*, 2011). The benefits of CAS in treating non-metastatic prostate cancer need to be carefully weighed against the risks of CAS-induced adverse events. Management of the metabolic sequelae of CAS includes optimal reduction of cardiovascular risk factors, with particular attention to weight, blood pressure, lipid profile, smoking cessation and glycemic control.

The rationale behind IAS is based on the hypothesis that, if tumor cells, which survive androgen withdrawal, are forced into a normal differentiation pathway by androgen replacement, their apoptotic potential might be restored and progression to androgen independence may be delayed. Furthermore, immediate androgen ablation can be accomplished with less side effects and quality of live can be improved in a palliative setting. Observations from animal model studies suggest that progression to androgen-independence involves adaptive responses to androgen deprivation, which seem to be delayed by intermittent androgen replacement. Supported by these results, several centers tested the feasibility of IAS in non-randomized groups of prostate cancer patients with serum PSA as trigger point (Buchan & Goldenberg, 2010).

For example, in a small pilot trial in four stage C and three stage D patients with prostate cancer androgen withdrawal was initiated with cyproterone acetate and diethylstilbestrol and then maintained with cyproterone acetate in combination with the LHRH agonist goserelin acetate (Akakura, *et al.*, 1993). After 6 or more months of suppression, treatment was interrupted for 2-11 months. After recovery of testicular function, androgen-withdrawal was resumed when serum PSA increased to a level of about 20 ng/ml. This cycle was sequentially repeated to a total of 2-4 times over treatment periods of 21-47 months with no loss of androgen-dependence. These early results demonstrate that IAS can be used to induce multiple apoptotic regressions of a tumor.

Overall, these trials suggest that IAS is neither inferior nor superior to CAS, with respect to time to castration resistance and cancer-specific survival, but has significant advantages in terms of adverse effects, quality of life and costs (Buchan & Goldenberg, 2010). A number of unresolved questions remain regarding patient selection for therapy, optimum duration of treatment, optimal time point of reinitiation oftherapy after the off-phase and definition of progression to castration-resistant disease. In future, the use of second-line drugs during off-treatment phases holds potential for delaying disease progression in men undergoing IAS. In a review data from 19 phase II studies were discussed with respect to PSA values for treatment suspension/reinitiation, treatment regimen, cycle lengths, testosterone normalization and tolerability. Most trials reported an improvement in quality of life during the off-therapy periods. Interim data from 8 phase III trials comparing IAS and CAS were found to corroborate the phase II results (Abrahamsson, 2009). Phase II/III data suggested that IAS was as effective as CAS but was characterized by better tolerability and quality-of-life advantages; however, more data are required to determine the effect of IAS on the long-term complications of androgen deprivation. Disease progression in 96 patients with biochemically relapsed prostate cancer under IAS was associated with pretreatment PSA doubling time (PSADT) ≥6 vs. <6 months, first off-treatment interval PSADT of ≥3 vs. <3 months and PSA nadir during the first treatment interval of <0.1 vs. ≥0.1 ng/ml. During IAS PSADT became shorter and was associated with testosterone recovery (Keizman, *et al.*, 2011). The duration of the first off-treatment interval (< or > 40 weeks) was correlated with shorter time to hormone-insensitivity and death after adjusting for age, stage, grade and PSA at diagnosis (Yu *et al.*, 2010, Sciarra, *et al.*, 2011).

Few randomized studies compared IAS with CAS for the treatment of advanced prostate cancer. Early survival results from phase III trials were limited and inconsistent. Mottet and colleagues reported no significant difference between patients receiving IAS and CAS with respect to median overall survival and median progression-free survival (Mottet, *et al.*, 2006).

In another IAS study, 127 patients from the intermittent arm and 107 patients from the continuous arm progressed, with a hazard ratio (HR) of 0.81 (da Silva, *et al.*, 2009). There was no difference in survival, with a HR of 0.99. The greater number of cancer deaths in the IAS arm (106 vs 84) was balanced by a greater number of cardiovascular deaths in the continuous arm (52 vs 41). Side effects were more pronounced in the continuous arm and patients treated with IAS reported better sexual function. Median time off therapy for the IAS-treated patients was 52 weeks. However, significant differences were reported in one study: de Leval and colleagues published that the estimated risk of 3-year progression in CAS patients was significantly higher than in the IAS group. This difference was highlighted in patients with a Gleason score >6, where the 3-year progression rates were significantly higher in CAS rather than in IAS patients (de Leval, *et al.*, 2002). Large phase III clinical trials of intermittent vs continuous androgen deprivation in men with metastatic disease or recurrent disease after localized therapy were requested for more than 2 decades in order to obtain reliable data for the comparative impact of these therapies on quality of life and survival.
Finally, the Intergroup randomized phase III trial, which compared IAS vs CAS to test for non-inferiority of IAS with respect to overall survival was presented in February 2011 (Klotz, *et al.*, 2011). Eligible men had rising PSA > 3.0 ng/ml >1 year post irradiation that was either initial or salvage for treatment of localized prostate cancer. IAS was delivered for 8 months in each cycle with restart when PSA reached >10 ng/ml in the off-treatment phase. Primary endpoint was overall survival (OS); secondary endpoints included time to hormone refractory state, quality of live, duration of treatment/non-treatment intervals and time to recovery of testosterone and potency. 1,386 patients were randomized to IAS (690) or CAS (696) arms and median follow-up was 6.9 years. IAS patients completed a median of 2 x 8 months cycles (range: 1-9). Median OS was 8.8 vs 9.1 years in IAS and CAS arms, respectively, with more disease-related (122 vs 97) in the IAS and fewer disease-unrelated (134 vs. 146) deaths in the CAS arm. Time to hormone resistance was statistically significantly improved in the IAS arm (HR 0.80, p = 0.024). Time to development of castration resistance was close to 10 years and in favour of IAS, but the trial design was biased towards IAS. In order to achieve castration resistance status, patients had to be being on treatment. Therefore, some patients who had a rising PSA off-treatment may in fact have had castration-resistant disease, but treatment had to be restarted and the PSA seen to continue to rise before this status could be defined. IAS patients had reduced occurrences of hot flashes, but there was no evidence of differences in adverse events, including myocardial problems or osteoporotic fractures. Thus, in men with PSA recurrence after irradiation IAS is non-inferior to CAS with respect to OS. IAS was suggested to be considered as the new standard of care for most patients with PSA recurrence after radical surgery. High-risk patients seem to be poor candidates for any type of androgen suppression. In summary, it can be concluded from the clinical trials that IAS is neither inferior nor superior to CAS, with respect to the end points, namely the time period until hormone-resistance as well as cancer-specific survival, but offers significant advantages in terms of adverse effects, quality of life and costs. Still, a number of important questions are remaining, regarding appropriate patient selection for therapy, optimum duration of therapy and exact scheduling of treatment reinstallation after the off-cycle. The off-treatment periods particularly hold the possibility to apply drugs such as finasteride or chemotherapeutics, in order to delay disease progression (Locke & Bruchovsky, 2010). Moreover, the study has economic implications: patients in the IAS arm were on therapy only 27% of the time, reducing the cost of therapy significantly.

4. Side effects of androgen suppression therapy

The well-known side effects of CAS like sexual dysfunction, hot flushes, fatigue, cardiovascular complications, osteoporosis, weight gain and anemia have significant implications for quality of life (Malone, *et al.*, 2005; Freedland, *et al.*, 2009; Galvão, *et al.* 2009). Since androgens are essential for the regulation of fat distribution, insulin sensitivity and lipid and bone metabolism, recent publications focussed on the concept that CAS may also be associated with an increase in overall and in particular cardiovascular morbidity and mortality (Corona, *et al.*, 2011). A multivariate analysis by Saigal and colleagues evaluating over 22,000 men concluded that patients receiving CAS had a 20% higher risk of cardiovascular morbidity (Saigal, *et al.*, 2007). CAS leads to increased incidence of osteoporosis and concomitant bone fractures (Kiratli, *et al.*, 2001). Therefore, it was expected that off-treatment periods during IAS would allow for recovery of testosterone levels and cessation of bone material degradation. With regards to bone loss, a large, retrospective study evaluated more than 50,000 men with prostate cancer, showing increased occurrence of bone fracture in the CAS group (19.4% vs 12.6%). There was a significant relationship between the number of CAS doses and fracture risk (Shahinian, *et al.* 2005). In the elderly population of prostate cancer patients increased incidence of osteoporosis and resulting bone fractures are of major concern. Higano and colleagues observed loss of bone mineral density during 9 months of androgen suppression significantly greater than the expected 0.5%-1% annual loss in IAS; however, interruption of androgen suppression attenuated the rate of bone loss without full recovery (Higano, *et al.*, 2004).

In the study by Malone and colleagues, general loss of potency occurred during the treatment period, but was regained by half of the evaluable patients when therapy was withdrawn (Malone, *et al.*, 2005). There was no significant overall change in body mass index at the end of the treatment periods. Osteoporosis was documented for at least one site evaluated in one third of the patients. Quality of life and sexual function seem to follow testosterone normalization (Mearini, *et al.*, 2011). Phase II clinical trials demonstrated improved sexual function and quality of life in men undergoing IAS (Dawson, 2000). The average percentage of time spent off androgen deprivation ranges from 37%-58% and most men were responsive to retreatment with hormonal therapy. While IAS seems feasible and holds the potential to improve quality of life of the patients, the degree of reversal of the long-term side effects of androgen suppression still remains to be confirmed.

4.1 Bone matrix turnover and androgen suppression therapy

Our group examined the effect of IAS on bone metabolism by determinations of CrossLaps levels, a biochemical marker of collagen degradation in blood samples of prostate cancer patients. These measurements revealed that increased bone degradation, which was associated with the androgen suppression phases, was rapidly reversed during treatment cessation periods, in good agreement with the clinical observations of reduced loss of bone mineral density (BMD) in IAS (Theyer, *et al.*, 2010). 140 patients have been recruited since 1993, with first patients reaching their seventh treatment cycle (Theyer & Hamilton, 1998). All patients with disseminated adenocarcinoma of the prostate fulfilling the inclusion criteria of a histologically confirmed tumor, stage ≥T2, not having received pretreatment by hormone ablation or chemotherapy and PSA >6 ng/ml were recruited for a nonrandomized open IAS trial consisting of an initial 8 months course of androgen suppression (goserelin acetate/Zoladex® and cyproterone acetate/ Androcur®), followed by treatment cessation and resuming of the therapy upon increases of PSA >4 and >20 ng/ml, respectively. Serum testosterone was measured using an ELISA assay (Biomar Diagnostics, Marburg, Germany) according to the manufacturer´s instructions. PSA was determined by the microparticulate enzyme immunoassay (MEIA, AxSYM PSA assay, Abbott, USA). CrossLaps ELISA was obtained from Nordic Bioscience Diagnostics, Herlev, Denmark, and used according to the manufacturer´s instructions (Rosenquist, *et al.*, 1998). This assay is used for follow-up of anti-resorptive treatment of patients with metabolic bone diseases (Okabe, *et al.*, 2004).

Amino-terminal propeptide of type I procollagen (PINP) and PSA were determined using the Elecsys 2010 Chemistry Analyzer (Roche Diagnostics, Vienna, Austria). All patients (n=75; mean age ±SD: 68±7 years, range: 53-84 years) exhibited progression of disease without metastases following radical prostatectomy and/or irradiation therapy. The lengths of the treatment cessation periods (mean ±SEM) for the respective off-treatment cycles (I–VI) in months were: 16±2 (n=75), 10±1 (n=31), 8±2 (n=18), 8±1 (n=12), 10±2 (n=8), 7±6 (n=2), respectively. The first treatment cessation period (PI) was significantly longer compared to the following breaks, which were not significantly different among each other. Individual time courses of testosterone and CrossLaps for a representative patient and four IAS cycles is depicted in figure 3A.

CrossLaps are elevated during androgen suppression phases indicating bone matrix degradation and normalize during treatment cessation periods on a regular basis (Theyer, *et al.*, 2010). After a prolonged time without androgen suppression, CrossLaps values exhibited a gradual increase, most likely due to regrowth of the tumor (data not shown; Nguyen-Pamart, *et al.*, 1997). Time courses of PINP and PTH were compared with PSA during the same IAS cycles in further measurements (figure 3B). The results show that PINP is a suitable alternative parameter for the assessment of bone matrix turnover during androgen suppression phases that are accompanied by low PSA levels. The parallel course of blood PTH indicates a participation of this hormone in androgen suppression-induced bone loss. This finding corroborates reports of decreased loss of BMD in bone scans in prostate cancer patients under IAS therapy. Since pretreatment concentrations of CrossLaps were restored within several months of therapy cessation and mean duration of the off-treatment periods ranged from 8–16 months in our patients, this protective effect of IAS is expected to be effective for several treatment cycles (Theyer, *et al.*, 2010). The bone matrix synthesis product PINP was used to assess bone turnover in metastatic prostate and breast cancer among other malignancies (Jung, *et al.*, 2011; Koopmans, *et al.*, 2007; Pollmann, *et al.*, 2007). Studies in metastatic prostate cancer patients showed that both PINP and ICTP (carboxy-terminal telopeptide of type I collagen) were most indicative of predicting metastatic progression and skeletal complications, respectively. Although androgen deprivation has been associated with bone loss in patients with prostate cancer, its mechanism remains unclear. The growth hormone (GH)/insulin-like growth factor-1 (IGF-1)/parathyroid hormone (PTH) axis that plays a critical role in bone synthesis was investigated during CAS (Isahaya, *et al.*, 2010). PTH is secreted by the chief cells of the parathyroid glands as a polypeptide containing 84 amino acids and effects to increase the concentration of calcium in blood (Poole & Reeve, 2005). The serum PTH level was reduced after CAS by approximately 25% compared with baseline levels, concomitant with increases of bone resorption markers like blood and urinary N-telopeptides (NTx), in good agreement with our measurements during androgen suppression in IAS cycles.

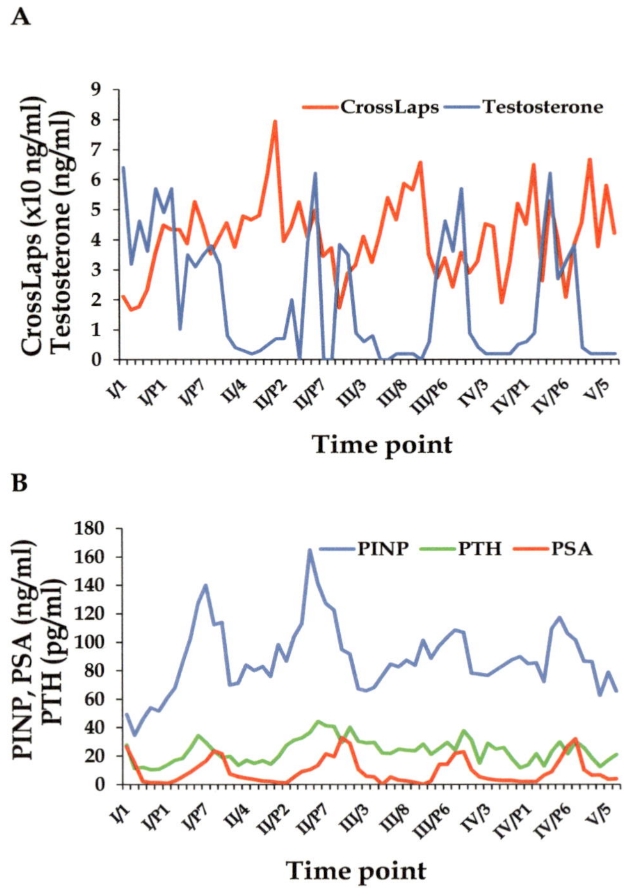

Fig. 3. (A) Individual time courses of testosterone and CrossLaps levels for a representative patient under IAS. Values cover androgen suppression phases (I–IV) and treatment cessation periods (I/P-IV/P). (B) Time courses of PSA, PINP and PTH are shown for the same patient.

4.2 Anemia and intermittent androgen suppression

Anemia was previously reported as a common side-effect of CAS. In an IAS study involving 95 patients receiving 245 cycles the median duration of resting periods was 8 months and median time to treatment failure 47 months (Malone *et al.*, 2005). Testosterone recovery during treatment cessation was observed in 60% of cycles with mild anemia, which was more frequently detected in successive cycles (33%, 44% and 67%). Thus, the observed anemia (hemoglobin level of < 30 g/l) was normochromic, normocytic, temporally related to the initiation of CAS and usually resolved after discontinuation of therapy in half of the cases. The improvement in hemoglobin during the off-treatment intervals probably contributes to improvements in the sense of well-being and vitality in these patients.

We collected data regarding anemia in our prostate cancer patients and a typical course of erythrocyte count, hemoglobin content and hematocrit is shown in figure 4. The data show that small decreases and increases in erythrocyte parameters coincide with IAS phases and levels of PSA. Such determinations can be used to assess the extent of anemia and the impact of treatment cessations on erythropoiesis.

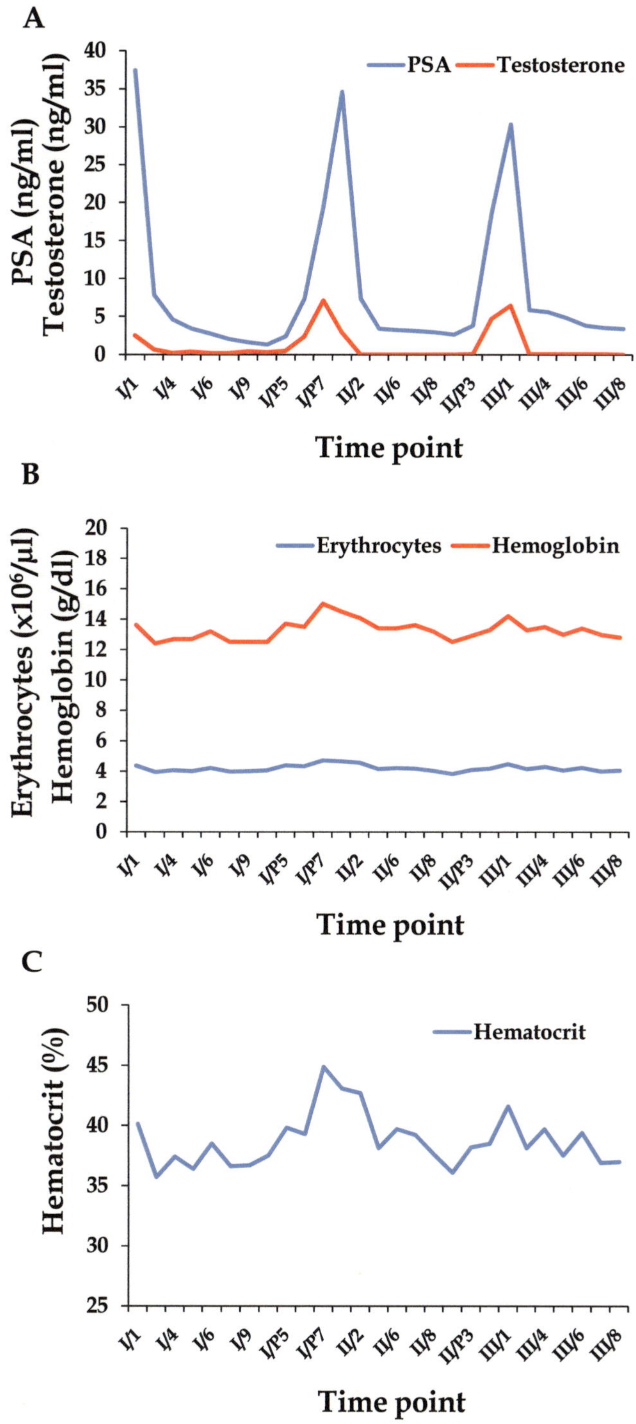

Fig. 4. (A) Time courses of testosterone and PSA, (B), hemoglobin and erythrocyte count and (C) and hematocrit are shown for 3 cycles of IAS for a typical prostate cancer patient.

5. Conclusions

In the past 25 years, IAS has developed from an unproven theoretical framework to a promising therapeutic option for subgroups of prostate cancer patients equal to CAS in respect to overall survival. Many questions in regard to the most suitable patient population and the optimal application of IAS remain to be investigated. With the exception of the frequency of hot flashes the improvement of other side effects of androgen suppression by intermittent therapy needs further careful assessment. This can be supported by determination of laboratory parameters of bone matrix turnover, blood chemistry and lipid profiles and correlation with the clinical characteristics. Last but not least, the reduced costs of intermittent therapy are expected to promote a more general application.

6. References

Abrahamsson, P.A. (2010) Potential Benefits of Intermittent Androgen Suppression Therapy in the Treatment of Prostate Cancer. *Eur Urol* 57(1), 49-59.

Akakura, K., Bruchovsky, N., Goldenberg, S.L., Rennie, P.S., Buckley, A.R. & Sullivan L.D.(1993) Effects of intermittent androgen suppression on androgen-dependent tumors. Apoptosis and serum prostate-specific antigen. *Cancer* 71(9), 2782-2790.

Akakura, K., Bruchovsky, N., Rennie, P.S., Coldman, A.J., Goldenberg, S.L., Tenniswood, M. & Fox, K. Effects of intermittent androgen suppression on the stem cell composition and the expression of the TRPM-2 (clusterin) gene in the Shionogi carcinoma. *J Steroid Biochem Mol Biol* 59(5-6), 501-511.

Bales, G.T., Sinner, M.D., Kim, J.H. & Chodak, G.W. (1996) Impact of intermittent androgen deprivation on quality of live (QOL). *J Urol* 155, 578A.

Brawer, M.K. (2006) Hormonal therapy for prostate cancer. *Rev Urol* 8, S35-47.

Bruchovsky, N., Rennie, P.S., Coldman, A.J., Goldenberg, S.L., To, M. & Lawson, D. (1990) Effects of androgen withdrawal on the stem cell composition of the Shionogi carcinoma. *Cancer Res* 50(8), 2275-2282.

Bruchovsky, N., Rennie, P.S., Otal, N., Vanson, A., Giles, M. & Pontifex, H. (1985) Variability of androgen-related phenotypes in the Shionogi mammary carcinoma during growth, involution, recurrence, and progression to hormonal independence. *Cancer Res* 45(2), 682-689.

Bruchovsky, N., Snoek, R., Rennie, P.S. Akakura, K., Goldenberg, L.S. & Gleaves, M. (1996) Control of tumor progression by maintenance of apoptosis. *Prostate* 6S, 13-21.

Bruchovsky, N., Rennie, P.S., Van Doom, E. & Noble, R.L. (1978) Pathological growth of androgen-sensitive tissues resulting from the latent actions of steroid hormones. *J Toxicol Environ Health* 4, 391-408.

Buchan, N. C. & Goldenberg, S.L. (2010) Intermittent androgen suppression for prostate cancer. *Nature Rev Urol* 7, 552-560.

Bruchovsky, N., Goldenberg, S.L., Rennie, P.S. & Gleaves, M. (1995) Theoretical considerations and initial clinical results of intermittent hormone treatment of patients with advanced prostatic carcinoma. *Urologe-A* 34, 389-392.

Calais da Silva, F.E., Bono, A.V., Whelan, P., Brausi, M., Marques Queimadelos, A., Martin, J.A., Kirkali, Z., Calais da Silva, F.M. & Robertson, C. (2009) Intermittent androgen deprivation for locally advanced and metastatic prostate cancer: results from a randomised phase 3 study of the South European Uroncological Group. *Eur Urol* 55(6), 1269-1277.

Chang, S.S., & Kibel, A.S. (2009) The role of systemic cytotoxic therapy for prostate cancer. *BJU Int* 103, 8-17.

Corona, G., Baldi, E. & Maggi, M. (2011) Androgen regulation of prostate cancer: Where are we now? *J Endocrinol Invest* 34(3), 232-243.

Dawson, N.A. (2000) Intermittent androgen deprivation. *Curr Oncol Rep* 2(5), 409-416.

Fitzpatrick, J.M., Schulman, C., Zlotta, A.R. & Schroeder, F.H. (2009) Prostate cancer: a serious disease suitable for prevention. *BJU Int* 103, 864-870.

Freedland, S.J., Eastham, J. & Shore, N. (2009) Androgen deprivation therapy and estrogen deficiency induced adverse effects in the treatment of prostate cancer. *Prostate Cancer Prostatic Dis* 12(4), 333-338.

Galvão, D.A., Taaffe, D.R., Spry, N., Joseph, D. & Newton, R.U. (2009) Cardiovascular and metabolic complications during androgen deprivation: exercise as a potential countermeasure. *Prostate Cancer Prostatic Dis* 12(3), 233-240.

Gjertson, C.K. & Albertsen, P.C. (2011) Use and assessment of PSA in prostate cancer. *Med Clin North Am* 95(1), 191-200.

Gleave, M.E, Goldenberg, S.L., Jones, E.C., Bruchovsky N. & Sullivan L.D. (1996) Maximal biochemical and pathological downstaging requires eight months of neoadjuvant hormonal therapy prior to radical prostatectomy. *J Urol* 155, 213-219.

Gleave, M., Bruchovsky, N., Goldenberg, S.L. & Rennie, P. (1998) Intermittent androgen suppression for prostate cancer: rationale and clinical experience. *Eur Urol* 34, Suppl 3, 37-41.

Gleave, M., Santo, N., Rennie, P.S., Goldenberg, S.L., Bruchovsky, N. & Sullivan, L.D. (1996) Hormone release and intermittent hormonal therapy in the LNCaP model of human prostate cancer. *Prog Urol* 6(3), 375-385.

Goldenberg, S.L., Bruchovsky, N., Gleave, M.E., Sullivan, L.D. & Akakura, K. (1995) Intermittent androgen suppression in the treatment of prostate cancer: A preliminary report. *Urology* 47, 956-961.

Grossmann, M., Hamilton, E.J., Gilfillan, C., Bolton, D., Joon, D.L. & Zajac, J.D. (2011) Bone and metabolic health in patients with non-metastatic prostate cancer who are receiving androgen deprivation therapy. *Med J Aust* 194(6), 301-306.

Higano, C., Shields, A., Wood, N., Brown, J. & Tangen, C. (2004) Bone mineral density in patients with prostate cancer without bone metastases treated with intermittent androgen suppression. *Urology* 64, 1182-1186.

Higano, C.S., Ellis, W., Russell, K. & Lange, P.H. (1996) Intermittent androgen suppression with leuprolide and flutamide for prostate cancer. *Urology* 48: 800.

Huggins, D. & Hodges, C.V. (1941) Studies on prostatic cancer. I. The effect of castration, of estrogen and of androgen injection on serum phosphatases in metastatic carcinoma of the prostate. *Cancer Res* 1:293-297.

Isahaya, E., Hara, N., Nishiyama, T., Hoshii, T., Takizawa, I. & Takahashi, K. (2010) Bone metabolic disorder in patients with prostate cancer receiving androgen deprivation therapy (ADT): impact of ADT on the growth hormone/insulin-like growth factor-1/parathyroid hormone axis. *Prostate* 70(2), 155-161.

Jadvar, H. (2011) Prostate cancer. *Methods Mol Biol* 727, 265-290.

Jung, K., Miller, K., Wirth, M., Albrecht, M. & Lein, M. (2011) Bone turnover markers as predictors of mortality risk in prostate cancer patients with bone metastases following treatment with zoledronic acid. *Eur Urol* 59(4), 604-612.

Kiratli, B.J., Srinivas, S., Perkash, I. & Terris, M.K. (2001) Progressive decrease in bone density over 10 years of androgen deprivation therapy in patients with prostate cancer. *Urology* 57, 127-132.

Klotz, L.H., Herr, H.W., Morse, M.J. & Whitmore, W.F. (1986) Intermittent endocrine therapy for advanced prostate cancer. *Cancer* 58, 2546-2550.

Klotz, L., O'Callaghan, C.J., Ding, K., Dearnaley, D.P., Higano, C.S., Horwitz, E.M., Malone, S., Goldenberg, S.L., Gospodarowicz, M.K. & Crook, J.M. (2011) A phase III randomized trial comparing intermittent versus continuous androgen suppression for patients with PSA progression after radical therapy: NCIC CTG PR.7/SWOG JPR.7/CTSU JPR.7/UK Intercontinental Trial CRUKE/01/013. *J Clin Oncol* 29, S7; Abstract # 3.

Kollmeier, M.A. & Zelefsky, M.J. (2008) What is the role of androgen deprivation therapy in the treatment of locally advanced prostate cancer? *Nat Clin Pract Urol* 5, 584-585.

Koopmans, N., de Jong, I.J., Breeuwsma, A.J. & E. van der Veer, E. (2007) Serum bone turnover markers (PINP and ICTP) for the early detection of bone metastases in patients with prostate cancer: a longitudinal approach. *J Urol* 178, 849-853.

Lassi, K. & Dawson, N.A. (2009) Emerging therapies in castrate-resistant prostate cancer. *Curr Opin Oncol* 21, 260-265.

de Leval, J., Boca, P., Yousef, E., Nicolas, H., Jeukenne, M., Seidel, L., Bouffioux, C., Coppens, L., Bonnet, P., Andrianne, R. & Wlatregny, D. (2002) Intermittent versus continuous total androgen blockade in the treatment of patients with advanced hormone-naive prostate cancer: results of a prospective randomized multicenter trial. *Clin Prostate Cancer* 1(3), 163-171.

Locke, J.A. & Bruchovsky, N. (2010) Prostate cancer: finasteride extends PSA doubling time during intermittent hormone therapy. *Can J Urol* 7(3), 5162-5169.

Madan, R.A., Pal, S.K., Sartor, O. & Dahut, W.L. (2011) Overcoming chemotherapy resistance in prostate cancer. *Clin Cancer Res* 17(12), 3892-3902.

Malone, S., Perry, G., Segal, R., Dahrouge, S. & Crook, J. (2005) Long-term side-effects of intermittent androgen suppression therapy in prostate cancer: results of a phase II study. *BJU Int* 96, 514-520.

Mearini, L., Zucchi, A., Costantini, E., Bini, V. & Porena, M. (2011) Intermittent androgen suppression in prostate cancer: testosterone levels and its implication. *J Sex Med* 8(4), 1218-1227.

Mellado, B., Codony, J., Ribal, M.J., Visa, L. & Gascon, P. (2009) Molecular biology of androgen-independent prostate cancer: the role of the androgen receptor pathway. *Clin Transl Oncol* 11, 5-10.

Mottet, N., Prayer-Galetti, T., Hammerer, P., Kattan, M.W. & Tunn, U. (2006) Optimizing outcomes and quality of life in the hormonal treatment of prostate cancer. *BJU Int* 98, 20-27.

Nguyen-Pamart, M., Caty, A., Feutrie, M.L., Fournier, E., Gosselin, P. & Mazeman, E. (1997) The diagnostic value of urinary CrossLaps and serum alkaline phosphatase in patients with prostate cancer. *BJU* 80, 452-455.

Okabe, R., Inaba, M., Nakatsuka, K., Miki, T., Naka, H., Moriguchi, A. & Nishizawa, Y. (2004) Significance of serum CrossLaps as a predictor of changes in bone mineral density during estrogen replacement therapy; comparison with serum carboxyterminal telopeptide of type I collagen and urinary deoxypyridinoline. *J Bone Miner Metab* 22, 127-131.

Pollmann, D., Siepmann, S., Geppert, R., Wernecke, K.D., Possinger, K. & Lüftner, D. (2007) The amino-terminal propeptide (PINP) of type I collagen is a clinically valid indicator of bone turnover and extent of metastatic spread in osseous metastatic breast cancer. *Anticancer Res* 27(4A), 1853-1862.

Poole, K. & Reeve, J. (2005). Parathyroid hormone - a bone anabolic and catabolic agent. *Curr Opin Pharmacol* 5(6): 612–617.

Raghavan, D., Koczwara, B. & Javle, M. (1997) Evolving strategies of cytotoxic chemotherapy for advanced prostate cancer. *Eur J Cancer* 33, 566-574.

Rennie, P.S., Bruchovsky, N., Buttyan, R., Benson, M. & Cheng, H. (1988) Gene expression during the early phases of regression of the androgen-dependent Shionogi mouse mammary carcinoma. *Cancer Res* 48(22), 6309-6312.

Rennie, P.S., Bruchovsky, N. & Coldman, A.J. (1990) Loss of androgen dependence is associated with an increase in tumorigenic stem cells and resistance to cell-death genes. *J Steroid Biochem Mol Biol 37(6)*, 843-847.

Rennie, P.S, Bruchovsky, N., Akakura, K., Goldenberg, S.L., Otal, N., Akakura, S., Wong, P. & Tenniswood, M. (1994) Effect of tumour progression on the androgenic regulation of the androgen receptor, TRPM-2 and YPT1 genes in the Shionogi carcinoma. *J Steroid Biochem Mol Biol* 50(1-2), 31-40.

Rosenquist, C., Fledelius, C., Christgau, S., Pedersen, B.J., Bonde, M., Qvist, P. & Christiansen, C. (1998) SerumCrossLaps® ELISA. First application of monoclonal antibodies for measurement in serum of bone-related degradation products from C-terminal telopeptides of type I collagen. *Clin Chem* 44, 2281-2289.

Saigal, C.S., Gore, J.L., Krupski, T.L, Hanley, J., Schonlau, M. & Litwin, M.S. (2007) Androgen deprivation therapy increases cardiovascular morbidity in men with prostate cancer. *Cancer* 110(7), 1493-1500.

Sciarra, A., Cattarino, S., Gentilucci, A., Alfarone, A., Innocenzi, M., Gentile, V. & Salciccia, S. (2011) Predictors for response to intermittent androgen deprivation (IAD) in prostate cancer cases with biochemical progression after surgery. *Urol Oncol*, in press.

Seruga, B. & Tannock, I.F. (2008) Intermittent androgen blockade should be regarded as standard therapy in prostate cancer. *Nat Clin Pract Oncol* 5, 574-576.

Shahinian, V.B., Kuo, Y.F., Freeman, J.L. & Goodwin, J.S. (2005) Risk of fracture after androgen deprivation for prostate cancer. *N Engl J Med* 352(2), 154-164.

da Silva, F.C. (2011) Intermittent hormonal therapy for prostate cancer. *Curr Opin Urol* 21(3), 248-251.

Snoek, R., Cheng, H., Margiotti, K., Wafa, L.A., Wong, C.A., Wong, E.C., Fazli, L., Nelson, C.C., Gleave, M.E. & Rennie, P.S. (2011) In vivo knockdown of the androgen receptor results in growth inhibition and regression of well-established, castration-resistant prostate tumors. *Clin Cancer Res* 15(1), 39-47.

Spry, N.A., Galvão, D.A., Davies, R., La Bianca, S., Joseph, D., Davidson, A. & Prince, R. Long-term effects of intermittent androgen suppression on testosterone recovery and bone mineral density: results of a 33-month observational study. *BJU Int* 104(6), 806-812.

Strum, S.B., Scholz, M.C. & McDermed, J.E. (2000) Intermittent androgen deprivation in prostate cancer patients: Factors predictive of prolonged time off therapy. *Oncologist* 5, 45-52.

Taylor, L.G., Canfield, S.E. & Du, X.L. (2009) Review of major adverse effects of androgen-deprivation therapy in men with prostate cancer. *Cancer* 115, 2388-2399.

Theyer, G., Holub, S., Dürer, A., Andert, S., Haberl, I., Theyer, U. & Hamilton, G. (1997) Measurements of tissue polypeptide-specific antigen in prostate cancer patients under intermittent androgen suppression therapy. *Br J Cancer* 75, 1515-1518.

Theyer, G. & Hamilton G. (1998) Current status of intermittent androgen suppression in the treatment of prostate cancer. *Urology* 53, 353-359.

Theyer, G., Dürer, A., Theyer, U., Haberl, I., Ulsperger, E., Baumgartner, G. & Hamilton, G. (1999) Measurements of free and total PSA, tissue polypeptide-specific antigen (TPS), and CYFRA 21-1 in prostate cancer patients under intermittent androgen suppression therapy. *Prostate* 41: 71-77.

Theyer, G., Ulsperger, E., Baumgartner, G., Raderer, M. & Hamilton, G. (2000) Prolonged response to a single androgen suppression phase in a subpopulation of prostate cancer patients. *Ann Oncol* 11, 877-881.

Theyer, G., Holub, S., Olszewski, U. & Hamilton, G. (2010) Measurement of bone turnover in prostate cancer patients receiving intermittent androgen suppression therapy. *OA J Urology* 2, 155-159.

Tzou, K., Tan, W.W. & Buskirk, S. (2011) Treatment of men with rising prostate-specific antigen levels following radical prostatectomy. *Expert Rev Anticancer Ther* 11(1), 125-136.

Yu, E.Y., Gulati, R., Telesca, D., Jiang, P., Tam, S., Russell, K.J, Nelson, P.S., Etzioni, R.D. & Higano, C.S. (2010) Duration of first off-treatment interval is prognostic for time to castration resistance and death in men with biochemical relapse of prostate cancer treated on a prospective trial of intermittent androgen deprivation. *J Clin Oncol* 28(16), 2668-2673.